OPHTHALMIC PATHOLOGY WITH CLINICAL CORRELATIONS

Editor

Joseph W. Sassani, M.D.

Departments of Ophthalmology and Pathology
Penn State University
Milton S. Hershey Medical Center
Hershey, Pennsylvania

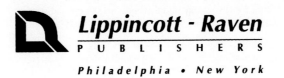

Lippincott - Raven
PUBLISHERS

Philadelphia • New York

Developmental Editor: Karen Frame
Manufacturing Manager: Dennis Teston
Production Manager: Maxine Langweil
Cover Designer: Joseph DePinho
Indexer: Alexandra Nickerson
Compositor: Tapsco
Printer: Phoenix Offset

Printed in Hong Kong

9 8 7 6 5 4 3 2 1

Library of Congress Cataloging-in-Publication Data
ISBN: 0-397-51469-7

Care has been taken to confirm the accuracy of the information presented and to describe
generally accepted practices. However, the authors, editors, and publisher are not responsible for
errors or omissions or for any consequences from application of the information in this book and
make no warranty, express or implied, with respect to the contents of the publication.

The authors, editors, and publisher have exerted every effort to ensure that drug selection and
dosage set forth in this text are in accordance with current recommendations and practice at the
time of publication. However, in view of ongoing research, changes in government regulations,
and the constant flow of information relating to drug therapy and drug reactions, the reader is
urged to check the package insert for each drug for any change in indications and dosage and for
added warnings and precautions. This is particularly important when the recommended agent is a
new or infrequently employed drug.

Some drugs and medical devices presented in this publication have Food and Drug
Administration (FDA) clearance for limited use in restricted research settings. It is the
responsibility of the health care provider to ascertain the FDA status of each drug or device
planned for use in their clinical practice. □

To my wife, Gloria, and my children, Lauren and Bill,
The center of my universe

Contents

Contributors

Harry H. Brown, O.D., M.D., *Associate Professor of Pathology and Ophthalmology, Harvey and Bernice Jones Eye Institute, University of Arkansas for Medical Sciences, 4301 West Markham, Little Rock, Arkansas 72205*

J. Douglas Cameron, M.D., *Associate Professor of Ophthalmology, Laboratory Medicine, and Pathology, University of Minnesota, 701 Park Avenue, Minneapolis, Minnesota 55415*

Martha J. Farber, M.D., *Department of Pathology, Veterans Administration Medical Center, 113 Holland Avenue, Albany, New York 12208*

Patrick M. Gardner, M.D., *Resident in Pathology, Department of Pathology, Medical College of Wisconsin, 8700 Wisconsin Ave, Box 26509, Milwaukee, Wisconsin 53226*

Ben J. Glasgow, M.D., *Associate Professor of Ophthalmology and Pathology, University of California, Los Angeles School of Medicine, 100 Stein Plaza, Los Angeles, California 90095*

W. Richard Green, M.D., *International Order of Oddfellows Professor of Ophthalmology, Professor of Pathology, The Johns Hopkins University, School of Medicine, 600 North Wolfe Street, Baltimore, Maryland 21287-9248*

LCDR Kerry E. Hunt, M.D., *Departments of Ophthalmology and Anatomic Pathology, National Naval Medical Center, Bethesda, Maryland 20889-5000*

Marilyn C. Kincaid, M.D., *Clinical Professor of Ophthalmology and Pathology, St. Louis University, 1755 South Grand Boulevard, St. Louis, Missouri 63104*

Theresa R. Kramer, M.D., *Departments of Ophthalmology and Pathology, University of Arizona, Tucson, Arizona 85719*

Scott Limstrom, M.D., *Ophthalmic Associates, 542 West 2nd Avenue, Anchorage, Alaska 99501*

William C. Lloyd III, M.D., F.A.C.S., *Clinical Professor of Ophthalmology, University of Texas Health Science Center at San Antonio, 3726 Hundred Oaks, San Antonio, Texas 78217-3410*

Curtis E. Margo, M.D., *Professor of Ophthalmology and Pathology, University of South Florida, College of Medicine, MDC Box 21, 12901 Bruce D. Downs Boulevard, Tampa, Florida 33612*

Steven A. McCormick, M.D., F.A.C.P., *Associate Professor of Pathology, Ophthalmology, and Otolaryngology/Head & Neck Surgery, New York Medical College, New York Ear and Eye Infirmary, 310 East 14 Street, New York, New York 10003*

Lois M. McNally, M.D., *Director, Medical Student Education, The New York Eye and Ear Infirmary, New York, New York 10003; Clinical Associate Professor of Ophthalmology, State University of New York Health Science Center, Brooklyn, New York 11203*

Alan D. Proia, M.D., Ph.D., *Associate Professor and Vice-Chairman, Department of Pathology, Duke University Medical Center, DUMN 3712, Durham, North Carolina 27710*

Joseph W. Sassani, M.D., *Departments of Ophthalmology and Pathology, Penn State University, Milton S. Hershey Medical Center, 500 University Drive, Hershey, Pennsylvania 17033*

Kenneth B. Simons, M.D., *Senior Associate Dean for Academic Affairs, Associate Professor of Ophthalmology and Pathology, Medical College of Wisconsin, 8701 Watertown Plank Road, Milwaukee, Wisconsin 53226-0509*

David J. Wilson, M.D., *Associate Professor of Ophthalmology, Director Christensen Eye Pathology Laboratory, Oregon Health Science University, Casey Eye Institute, 3375 SW Terwiliger Boulevard, Portland, Oregon 97201*

Preface

Whether you are a resident who is just beginning to study the visual system or a practitioner seeking to distill the clinical implications from a pathologist's report, *Ophthalmic Pathology with Clinical Correlations* is intended for you. Although there are many comprehensive textbooks on ophthalmic pathology, their very completeness makes them an unsuitable introduction. As Huck Finn said, "If words were water I'd have drowned for sure." *Ophthalmic Pathology with Clinical Correlations* is intended as a lifeboat to safely carry the nonpathologist through the "cataractous" waters of pathologic terminology. We believe, however, that after you have been introduced to ophthalmic pathology, the book will provide a valuable framework to support your knowledge of ophthalmic pathology. Each of the chapter authors has been selected for her/his demonstrated teaching ability to assist you in attaining these goals.

The challenge to these contributing authors was to provide the information that would be contained in an introductory series of lectures on ophthalmic pathology. Topics were to include those entities that were most commonly encountered and/or were the most serious. Other subjects were to be addressed in tables, etc. We have made the chapters as concise as possible. Nevertheless, those chapters dealing with Eyelid and Conjunctiva, and Immunity and Inflammation are longer than the others, reflecting the difficult terminology and overall unfamiliar nature of the material covered. Fortunately, our publisher, Lippincott-Raven Publishers, has agreed to publish over 500 color figures to help us in correlating these clinical entities with their pathologic counterparts.

Ocular diseases lend themselves well to an anatomic classification scheme with a superimposed breakdown into the traditional pathophysiologic categories of congenital, degenerative, neoplastic, traumatic, and inflammatory disorders. *Ophthalmic Pathology with Clinical Correlations* generally follows this outline; however, diabetes mellitus, pediatric disorders, and traumatic entities have been given separate chapters. Although 18 authors have contributed to this book, we have tried to speak with a consistent voice.

My fellow authors and I believe that *Ophthalmic Pathology with Clinical Correlations* will foster your appreciation for the utility and beauty of ophthalmic pathology. If our efforts help you to better care for your patients, our goals will have been accomplished.

Acknowledgments

I am most fortunate in collaborating with a gifted group of medical educators who have made my work as editor rewarding and educational. I would like to thank them for their dedication and perseverance. Lippincott–Raven Publishers has been extremely helpful to us and indulgent of the usual delays in the publishing of this text.

I believe that all of the contributing authors would like to acknowledge those who stimulated their interest in ophthalmic pathology. Fortunately, as editor, I am permitted to recognize my own mentors, Ralph Eagle, William Frayer, and Myron Yanoff, who have provided for me a gold standard of excellence as clinicians, teachers, and pathologists. I also would like to thank my fellow members of the Departments of Ophthalmology and Pathology at Penn State University for their support, fellowship, and academic stimulation. Marcia Krick and Judy Bowman have been particularly tolerant of last minute requests to send overnight mail or to pull ''just a few more articles.''

Finally, I have dedicated this book to my wife, Gloria, and my children, Bill and Lauren, who have provided meaning to my life and a continuing education in all that is important. My parents, Mary and Joseph Sassani, have given me the foundation upon whose principles I have built my personal and professional life.

Ophthalmic Pathology with Clinical Correlations,
edited by Joseph W. Sassani, M.D.
Lippincott-Raven Publishers, Philadelphia © 1997.

CHAPTER 1

The Clinician and Pathologist

Kenneth B. Simons and Patrick M. Gardner

THE PATHOLOGIST AS CONSULTANT

Many clinicians and ancillary health care providers are not familiar with the pathologist's role in managing patient care. They typically rely on the laboratory to provide test results, but often have little insight about their derivation and limitations. This lack of familiarity can lead to frustration with pathologists and the laboratory over aberrant test results, specimen inadequacy, and turnaround time for individual procedures. Pathologists may need to make their services known to the clinician. This chapter is intended to demystify the anatomic and clinical pathology disciplines for the reader and to enhance use of the laboratory.

The average practicing pathologist is trained in anatomic and clinical pathology and can be a valuable resource and consultant for laboratory use and specimen handling. Most of the clinician's interaction with pathologists usually concerns biopsy or surgical pathology results and, to some extent, microbiologic studies. Coagulation and transfusion medicine are two areas in which the pathologist may direct the evaluation of unexpected preoperative test findings and the use of blood products with greater efficiency than the clinician, who may be less experienced in these areas. With the ever-growing concerns about cost containment, many unnecessary and potentially misleading test results may be avoided by a simple phone call to the lab. The pathologist is a readily available consultant to clinicians willing to use them as a resource. As for any clinical consultation, the clinician should ask well-defined questions and understand the capabilities and limitations of the pathology staff.

K. B. Simons: Departments of Ophthalmology and Pathology, Medical College of Wisconsin, Milwaukee, Wisconsin 53226.

P. Gardner: Department of Pathology, Medical College of Wisconsin, Milwaukee, Wisconsin 53226.

SURGICAL PATHOLOGY

Surgical pathology is the branch of pathology dedicated to the gross and microscopic evaluation of tissue for evidence of disease. This includes the examination of tissue biopsies and organs removed in the operative setting for diagnostic examination and for pathologic staging of malignancies. Surgical pathology comprises much of the average pathologist's daily workload. The practice of tissue diagnosis is a dynamic interface between the clinical history and histologic data, and should closely involve the clinical staff physicians. The indications for tissue biopsy, the procedures involved in tissue interpretation, and the pathologist's role in the diagnosis of disease and patient treatment are outlined below.

Pathologic lesions of the eye and orbit can be diagnosed in the clinical setting using history and physical examination, diagnostic imaging studies, and physician experience. For lesions that are not clinically obvious, a tissue biopsy of the lesion or resection is performed to obtain diagnostic material and to guide further therapy. Indications for biopsy include, but are not limited to, the following:

1. To identify specific disease entities
2. To differentiate malignant from nonmalignant lesions
3. To differentiate primary from secondary malignancies
4. To identify inflammatory processes, with attempts to recognize specific etiologic agents
5. To clinically evaluate metastatic lesions with an attempt to identify the primary site

Biopsy of skin lesions surrounding the orbit can be obtained using the same techniques used to obtain any other skin biopsy. Biopsy of the iris or ciliary body can be performed readily, and in many instances, the entire lesion removed for pathologic study. Neoplasms of the eye also may present with vitreitis, and a diagnostic vitrectomy yields greater results in most instances than aspiration biopsy.[1] Formal tissue biopsy of the retina and choroid may be performed with the intent of excisional biopsy, or in most instances, incomplete excision for diagnosis.

Specimen Processing

Tissue specimens represent an irreplaceable source of diagnostic information. The questions that any tissue specimen will be used to answer greatly influence how it will be handled by the laboratory. Ideally, for cases other than a routine biopsy, or for specimens with which the clinician is not familiar, the pathologist should be consulted for proper specimen handling. This consultation maximizes the yield of clinically relevant information. Different hospitals also may have widely varying policies regarding tissue handling, and all clinicians who send tissue samples to the laboratory should be familiar with these policies. Some specific handling procedures that are routine at many institutions are addressed here.

Frozen section diagnoses are performed by the pathologist for cases in which immediate results will alter the course of clinical therapy. This usually entails operative cases in which the extent of the procedure depends on the tissue diagnosis. Frequently, resections for malignancy involve the use of frozen sections to evaluate the adequacy of resection margins or the confirmation of the presence of diagnostic tissue. Specimens for frozen section must be sent to the laboratory in the fresh state; saline is an appropriate transport medium. Ideally, the surgeon transports the specimen to the pathologist and can orient the tissue and discuss the clinical aspects of the case as the tissue is processed. The pathologist should be informed when any tissue requiring frozen section diagnosis is en route to the lab. Once received, the tissue is oriented, and depending on its size, the entire specimen or a representative section is submitted for analysis. The tissue is embedded in a semisolid medium and frozen at −25°C. Sections are cut on a cryostat microtome and stained with hematoxylin and eosin.

Some histologic studies also require frozen tissue. For example, lipids are removed from tissue sections during routine processing, but can be identified using special stains on frozen tissue sections. Immunofluorescence studies also require frozen tissue. Immunofluorescent studies may be useful to the clinician in diagnosing systemic lupus erythematosus or related collagen vascular diseases and pemphigoid skin lesions about the orbit. Although this method yields diagnostic tissue sections, it is not without drawbacks. Water in the tissue freezes and crystallizes, potentially distorting the histologic features. Thus, although frozen section provides information useful for immediate operative patient treatment, the clinician must weigh this benefit against the potential for compromised histology and the procedure's significant cost. The routine use of frozen sections is inappropriate for tissue diagnosis when patient treatment would not potentially be altered by the results.

In addition to frozen section specimens, hematologic and lymphoid tissues also require specific handling measures. Advances in molecular diagnostics for hematologic and lymphoid disorders have outpaced those in solid-tissue diagnostics, largely due to the greater ease of manipulating the former types of cells, which are inherently discohesive in nature. Immunophenotyping, gene rearrangement studies, and immunoperoxidase staining require special procedures. The diagnosis of suspected orbital lymphoma would be one scenario requiring special handling of lymphoid tissue. Tissue handling is of paramount importance because certain fixatives may destroy the antigenic sites, rendering these ancillary tests useless. Lymphoid neoplasms may be sent in a cell support medium to maintain cell viability and to provide tissue for multiple diagnostic modalities. Once received, the tissue can be divided into snap frozen tissue for molecular studies, tissue fixed for routine histology, and tissue for immunophenotypic analysis. Again, communication with the laboratory is imperative because high-grade lymphomas may not remain viable for extended periods even in a supportive medium. The pathologist can outline the steps necessary to ensure a maximum diagnostic yield from tissue specimens.

Macrophotography

Whole-eye specimens are extremely valuable to the clinician and pathologist regardless of the material's source. As such, careful macroexamination and documentation of the gross findings via schematic diagrams and macrophotography are essential. An excellent system for macroexamination has been detailed by Roth and Foos.[2] Their system is easily modified to accommodate recent technological advances, particularly illumination.

Macrophotography is a simple and inexpensive method for documenting the gross examination observations.[3] It also helps to meet medicolegal and academic needs. Photographic documentation of specimens is extremely important and should be routinely used by the pathologist.

Histologic Processing

Routine specimens are usually submitted to the laboratory in a fixative, such as 10% buffered formalin (formalin is a solution of 40% formaldehyde in water). Formalin crosslinks proteins and prevents autolysis (the enzymatic degradation of tissue). It is important that the tissue submitted contains an adequate volume of fixative (an approximately 20:1 fixative-to-tissue ratio). It is not unusual for the laboratory to receive large specimens stuffed into a small container with a scant amount of fixative. Specimens sitting for prolonged periods without adequate fixative begin to autolyze, compromising the histology. The examination of globes requires approximately 48 hours

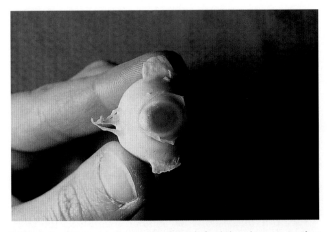

FIG. 1-1. Gross photograph of the left globe demonstrating tendinous insertions of the four recti muscles. The medial rectus insertion is on the right and is the start of the Spiral of Tillaux.

of fixation. The formalin penetrates the tissue rather quickly, and it is not necessary to section tissue or to open globes to enhance fixation. Opening the globe before fixation may destroy diagnostic tissue, rendering it useless for further interpretation.[4] Globes with suspected intraocular tumors, however, may be sectioned after only several hours of fixation to allow sufficient hardening of the tissue.

Prior to dissection, the globe is examined externally, and the gross features are detailed and documented as described earlier. Routine measurements are taken, and any external abnormalities described. The globe can be oriented using a few standard landmarks. The insertions of the tendinous portion of the superior oblique muscle and the muscular insertion of the inferior oblique muscle near the horizontal midpoint close to the optic nerve assist in the orientation of the globe (Fig. 1-1). Another helpful feature is the prominence of the long posterior ciliary arteries and nerves along the horizontal meridian on either side of the optic nerve. The relative positions of the rectus muscles' insertions as they spiral progressively more posteriorly allow further orientation, with the medial rectus attaching at approximately 5.5 mm from the limbus, the inferior rectus at approximately 6.5 mm, the lateral rectus attaching at a 7-mm distance, and the superior rectus at approximately 7.7 mm (Spiral of Tillaux).

The globe can be transilluminated to reveal the location of an intraocular lesion before sectioning.[2,5] Each pathologist may have a preferred method of opening the globe, depending on the location of the lesion within the globe. A routine technique for gross sectioning of the globe is illustrated in Fig. 1-2. Most eyes are sectioned to maintain the pupil, macula, and optic nerve in the same anterior-to-posterior section. The plane of the cut, therefore, is preferably horizontal; however, its location may be varied and determined by the location of the pathology so that the pupil–optic nerve section includes areas of interest.

For example, most limbal surgical wounds are in the superior quadrant. Therefore, eyes that have had cataract surgery are usually opened in the vertical plane so the plane of section is perpendicular to the surgical wound. This approach may be varied for certain malignancies, in which the sectioning of the globe is oriented to give the pathologist the same spatial orientation as the clinician. For tumors of the posterior segment, the anterior portion of the globe can be removed. For tumors of the anterior segment, the globe can be opened in a plane opposite the apex of the tumor. The sections of tissue containing the areas of interest and any margins of the specimen important for clinical staging should be submitted for histologic examination.[2,5] Smaller biopsy specimens are oriented and entirely submitted for tissue processing.

Tissue processing dehydrates the tissue sections and replaces the water with paraffin. Paraffin embedding stabilizes the tissue, preparing it to be cut in the desired plane of section. During the embedding process, organic solvents which dissolve most lipids are used. Following embedding, the tissue is cut in sections 4 to 6 μm thick. These sections are then adhered to a glass slide. At this stage, the tissue is colorless, and various dyes are applied to the glass slide to identify the tissue. Most sections are stained with hematoxylin and eosin dyes. Additional stains with varying affinities for tissues, organisms, and minerals can be applied to further differentiate the tissue sections. These chemical and immunochemical stains are now widely used not only in the diagnostic examination of tissue, but as research tools as well.

The process, from sectioning to cutting and staining of a routine ophthalmic specimens (other than whole globes), is usually performed overnight. Therefore, expecting results from a biopsy the same day it is taken is unreasonable. Rapid processing alternatives and frozen sections are available for cases in which the information may vastly alter the clinical management; however, these

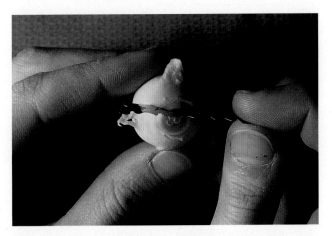

FIG. 1-2. Gross photograph showing single-edge razor blade cutting the globe into a smaller (superior) calotte and larger (inferior) calotte.

cases require direct communication with the pathology staff. A basic understanding of how specimens are handled in the laboratory enriches the yield of tissue specimens and avoids frustration over laboratory results.

In addition to the routine hematoxylin-and-eosin staining described, many other stains are available to the pathologist to highlight certain tissues and structural components. These stains may use basic chemical affinities of dyes or immunologic techniques. Some of these stains are outlined in Table 1. Immunoperoxidase studies use monoclonal or polyclonal antibodies directed at specific cellular antigens. These antibodies are physically conjugated to an enzyme commonly using glutaraldehyde or periodate. In the presence of chromogenic substrates, the enzymatic action produces a color highlighting the cells containing the antigen bound to the labeled antibody. Many variations of this technique exist; one popular method conjugates the antibodies to a horseradish peroxidase enzyme. Alternatively, the primary antibody may be unconjugated, with a second anti-idiotypic antibody labeled with enzyme (sandwich technique). A background stain is used simply to identify the tissue not recognized by the antibody. These techniques also produce their own set of artifacts. Positive and negative controls must be performed to ensure that the stains are indeed labeling the desired cells and staining the correct cellular compartment. These stains also may require more stringent control of pH, specific antibody dilutions, and special mounting media. The antigenic sites may be destroyed by certain fixatives.[6] The pathologist is responsible for the quality control of these procedures.

TABLE 1. *Commonly employed histologic stains*

Stain	Purpose of stain
Hematoxylin–eosin	Routine
Masson's trichrome	Collagen
Periodic acid–Schiff	Glycogen, fungi, neutral mucopolysaccharides
Alcian blue	Acid mucopolysaccharides
Ziehl-Neelsen, Fite, Auramine	Acid-fast bacilli
Methenamine silver	Fungi, Donovan bodies
Perls' Prussian blue	Iron
Movat's pentachrome	Elastin, collagen, muscle
IMMUNOPEROXIDASE STAINS	
Cytokeratin	Epithelial intermediate filaments
Vimentin	Mesenchymal cells
Epithelial membrane antigen	Adenocarcinoma
Carinoembryonic antigen	Adenocarcinoma
S100 protein, Chromogranin	Neural, neural-crest—derived cells
HMB-45	Melanoma cells, some nevus cells
Factor VIII	Endothelial cells
Leukocyte common antigen	Leukocytes
Desmin	Skeletal and smooth muscle

The utility of special stains is to help confirm a suspected diagnosis or to rule out other conditions in the differential diagnosis. These techniques are more costly than routine stains, requiring additional time, labor, and reagents. They should not be used as a primary diagnostic modality or as a ''fishing trip'' with no well-defined endpoint because the results may be misleading. The results must be questioned if they are not congruous with the original histology or clinical scenario. Many of the monoclonal antibodies initially were believed to be very specific for given tissues. As they have been tested on additional tissues, however, many have proved to be less specific than originally thought.

Electron microscopy is another diagnostic modality used by most university pathology departments and by some smaller community hospitals. Tissue sections are fixed in glutaraldehyde and stained with osmium tetroxide. With this technique, significant ultrastructural details can be identified in the tissue sections. This modality requires fresh or specially fixed tissue, and the pathologist can determine which cases can benefit from clinically relevant diagnostic information provided by electron microscopy. Again, communicating with the pathologist before obtaining tissue can be vital in the diagnostic evaluation of tissue specimens.

Histologic interpretation of the stained tissue sections requires the integration of all available information. Histologic patterns and cytologic features of the tissue alone may be diagnostic; however, the interpretive process is not an exact science. The clinician must be aware of the capabilities and limitations inherent in tissue examination. Pathologists are human, and histologic diagnosis is subject to the pathologist's experience, expectations, the quality of preparation, and the availability of clinically relevant information. Some clinicians withhold patient history, believing that pathologists interpret tissue preparations in a vacuum and that clinical information may bias this interpretation. This misconception may be rooted in 19th century pathology, when observations and teachings were based solely on the examination of tissue. There is no place for such practices in the current treatment of disease. Quite the contrary, histologic features may be very similar in many diseases, and the clinical pattern of disease may be the diagnostic feature. Accurate diagnosis requires that the histologic features be congruous with the given clinical history and patient profile. Just as a surgical consultant would not operate without examining the patient, the pathologist should not render a tissue diagnosis without relevant clinical data.

The pathologist's role is to ensure that any of the potentially correctable factors that may limit the usefulness of tissue examination are minimized. These include a lack of clinical history, inadequate sampling of tissue, technical errors compromising the tissue quality, inexperience, and the communication barrier.[7] Communication with the pathologist and a discussion of the patient history may prevent the inadequate sampling of lesions or, as discussed, tissue destruction by improper fixation. Pathologists are available for intraoperative consultations in cases of unusual gross pathology or in which the anatomic relation of the lesion is important.

Sampling error also may occur in the laboratory. Once received by the laboratory, tissue specimens must be adequately sampled by the pathologist. Most laboratories cut multiple sections of biopsy specimens. For larger lesions, the pathologist determines how much of the tissue will be sampled, with at least three sections of grossly identified tumor submitted. The pathologist is, therefore, examining only a fraction of the tissue present in many cases, and each section is only a few micrometers thick. To suggest that this method is completely sensitive in detecting malignant cells is ludicrous. The pathologist is responsibile for ensuring that tissue blocks have been adequately sampled. If a suspected lesion is not found in the initial sections of tissue examined, deeper sections are cut and sometimes the tissue block exhausted in an attempt to identify a diagnostic tissue. For larger lesions, additional tissue sections may be submitted. It serves no purpose for diagnostic cells to remain in an archived paraffin block with a questionable or clinically incongruous diagnosis.

Inexperience is a fact of life for pathologists. Rare lesions may never be seen throughout a pathologist's entire career, and it is imperative that pathologists recognize their own limitations. Confusing cases should be shared with colleagues and a community opinion sought. Each pathologist differs in experience, and one colleague may recollect a lesion not previously encountered by another.

Radiographic and imaging characteristics of the lesion should be sought in addition to the clinical characteristics. Some lesions may have clinical or radiographic behavior patterns that are more diagnostic than the histologic pattern seen in tissue sections. After a thorough study of the case, pathologic entities in which the diagnosis is uncertain should be submitted to a recognized authority for formal consultation. Some cases may simply be very unusual variants of disease, and the host response can reveal the true malignant potential of a tumor. Under no circumstances should a pathologist be forced to commit to a specific diagnosis in cases in which uncertainty exists. Such forced diagnoses afford the patient no benefit, and unnecessary procedures may result from an incorrect diagnosis. Tissue diagnosis must not be performed in a cavalier fashion. Labeling a patient with a specific disease may also create a burden of worry and potential insurance limitations. It is imperative that the clinician understand the limitations inherent in histologic examination of tissue and have reasonable expectations for specimen interpretation.

The pathologist is also responsible for reporting clinically pertinent information in a language familiar to the clinician. The final report should include the recognized characteristics for staging malignancies in every case. Many lesions have a variety of synonyms, and the accepted diagnosis may be followed by a list of alternatives to assist the clinician. The myth of objectivity has thrown disfavor on the use of differential or descriptive diagnosis. In some cases, however, the pathologist's ability to rule out specific diseases may be equally or more important than naming the lesion. A well-constructed differential diagnosis can at least provide the clinician with the means to further evaluate the patient. Cases that have posed a diagnostic dilemma should be followed by an explanatory comment. The pathologist should not assume that the clinician will extract the thought processes involved in the case from the microscopic description. In the litigious milieu of medicine, it also may benefit the pathologist to have a tangible record of his thought process, not merely an unsubstantiated diagnosis.

CYTOLOGY

Cytology is the branch of anatomic pathology concerned with the diagnosis of infectious, inflammatory, and neoplastic processes by examining cellular aspirates, smears, and body fluids. Gynecologic cytology, also known as the Pap smear, is the most familiar example of this principle. The use of fine-needle aspiration biopsy is well established in the diagnosis of many lesions and has clinical utility for lesions of the eye and orbit. The technique involves inserting a needle and aspirating fluid or tissue fragments. Tissue smears are prepared and fixed in alcohol or air dried. Various stains are used, and the slides are examined much like their histologic counterparts. Fluid aspirations are usually centrifuged or filtered onto a nylon membrane, which is then fixed to a glass slide. Cytology takes advantage of inherent unique nuclear and cytoplasmic details of specific cells and patterns of tissue composition. Not surprisingly, this technique has limitations, particularly the need for skilled personnel to obtain the specimens and for pathologists familiar with the diagnostic cytology.

Tumors of the eye and orbit may be clinically obvious, but require tissue for definitive identification. Fine-needle aspiration biopsy may be a useful alternative to conventional biopsy in sites deep in the orbit and cystic lesions. The aspiration itself can be done using visual, ultrasonographic, or computed tomographic guidance. Interventional radiologists are often adept at obtaining needle aspirates. The material obtained is smeared on a slide, and air-dried smears can be stained immediately to verify the presence of adequate diagnostic material.[8,9] Reported complications of this technique include minor subconjunctival hemorrhage, motility disturbances, and proptosis. A maximum needle length of 3.75 cm can prevent it from passing through the eye and entering the cavernous sinus.[10] Seeding the needle tract has been reported, but is of questionable clinical significance.[11] Clinicians may wish to discuss ocular fine-needle aspiration with cytologists to assess their level of familiarity and comfort with lesions of the eye.

Tumors of the eye are usually metastatic lesions. The most frequently encountered primary ocular malignancies are retinoblastomas and melanocytic lesions, which are the most common primary lesions in children and adults, respectively. In some cases, the clinical diagnostic imaging modalities can accurately diagnose ocular neoplasms. In the cases requiring tissue identification, aspiration biopsy may be an attractive alternative to biopsy in the surgically complex posterior aspect of the eye. The aspiration is time consuming and requires a skilled ophthalmic surgeon and cytologist familiar with ocular lesions.

FORENSIC PATHOLOGY

Forensic pathology is the subspecialty dedicated to investigating the manner and cause of death. It is used in potential criminal cases, as well as investigations of unexpected deaths of patients with no documented medical history to explain their death. The clinician may need to deal with medical examiners in cases of death associated with ocular neoplasms or traumatic death with identifiable ocular pathology. Some cases of child abuse can be diagnosed by retinal hemorrhages induced by violent shaking.

Autopsy

The public and many health professionals are most familiar with the pathologist's role as autopsy prosector or medical examiner. The autopsy has seen a great decline in popularity as a teaching tool and complement to clinical care during the past two decades. Much of this change is attributed to the marked strides in diagnostic imaging studies available to the clinician. These diagnostic modalities may be used antemortem to answer many questions pertaining to the extent of disease and the ultimate cause of death which were previously answered by postmortem examination. This does not mean the autopsy serves no valuable role in patient care or as a teaching tool. Indications for a postmortem examination include, but are not limited to the following:

1. To explain sudden or unexpected death in a patient with known illness or in a previously healthy patient
2. To confirm clinically suspected disease
3. To evaluate response to therapy in patients undergoing treatment for various disorders
4. To document the extent of disease in malignant and infectious processes
5. To document genetic or congenital abnormalities

6. To procure tissue for research purposes
7. To determine cause of death in forensic cases

The autopsy is also a valuable teaching tool, particularly in the academic setting. Medical students, interns, residents, and staff physicians can benefit from the information gained by postmortem examination, especially in cases that pose antemortem clinical diagnostic dilemmas.[12] Clinicopathologic conferences help to bridge the gap between clinicians and the pathology department and provide an opportunity for pathologists to make their role in patient treatment more visible. Tissue obtained at autopsy can be archived and may be an invaluable source of information for future basic science and clinical research projects. In cases of congenital abnormality or diseases with a genetic basis, the autopsy may be of great value to the family and can give the surviving family members peace of mind about what actually happened to loved ones. As new genes linked to disease entities are identified, the presence or absence of disease in family members assumes greater significance. Despite the growth and availability of diagnostic imaging, many clinically unsuspected lesions are identified during autopsy. Without postmortem examinations, the prevalence of a disease in the population and the true clinical significance of that disease may remain unknown.

Additional Studies

Flow cytometry uses a laser light source and photodetectors to measure cell parameters as they pass by the laser beam in fluid phase in a single file. **Forward light scatter** is a measure of size, and **side scatter** is a measure of cytoplasmic density. The cells can be sorted into subpopulations qualitatively and quantitatively. Antibodies directed at cell-surface antigens are coupled to a fluorescent dye, and the cells are sorted to distinguish one cell line from another. In this manner, subpopulations of cells are identified, and clonality can be established using the ratio of kappa to lambda immunoglobulin light chain.[13] Flow cytometry also can be used to study DNA ploidy, by exposing cells to dyes that bind DNA stoichiometrically. Cells have varying DNA content, such as 2N (diploid) and 4N (tetraploid), depending on the cell cycle. Malignant cells are often, but not always aneuploid. Studies of DNA ploidy may be helpful in differentiating benign from malignant lesions or may have prognostic significance in certain malignancies. The pathologist should be familiar with cases in which ploidy analysis adds clinically relevant data.

Lymphoid neoplasms also can be differentiated using DNA probes for known gene rearrangements, and their mutant protein products. Many of the leukemias and lymphomas are associated with specific chromosomal translocations. Demonstration of immunoglobulin and T-cell receptor gene rearrangements is used to demonstrate clonality and to subsequently monitor disease. A known genetic mutation identified in a particular malignant lesion can be assayed following therapy to assess the status of residual disease, remission, or recurrence.[14]

The polymerase chain reaction has made it possible to study very minute quantities of tissue. Through the use of oligonucleotide primers for known genomic sequences, specific regions of DNA can be amplified on an exponential scale. The native DNA is denatured using heat, and the oligonucleotide primers bind to the genomic sequence on each of the separated strands. The addition of excess oligonucleotides allows for the elongation of the primers, with a resultant copy of each of the original strands of DNA. Thus, each cycle of amplification doubles the amount of genetic material. The discovery of thermostable DNA polymerases have made this process possible. The genomic material produced by this process can then be studied using methods that separate and label the DNA. The DNA is physically separated by charge electrophoretically and can be stained (ethidium bromide) or identified by fluorescent or radioactively labeled probes. Originally a research tool, this application has quickly been applied in the clinical laboratory.

Like other technologies, molecular-based diagnostics also have limitations. These techniques require special handling of tissue in some cases, and stringent laboratory procedures must be followed to prevent contamination. Although these techniques may offer greater sensitivity and specificity, the ability to detect minute quantities of aberrant DNA may not have defined clinical significance. Identifying one cell with a given genomic alteration has questionable significance if these cells are also present in normal individuals and dealt with by the body's normal surveillance mechanisms. The pathologist can be a good resource regarding which assays have reliable results in normalizing controls and in providing information above and beyond the cheaper, traditional laboratory methods. It is this latter issue that demands attention. Laboratory testing should not only be directed at answering a specific diagnostic question; it should be performed with an understanding of the limitations, benefits, and cost of the tests performed. To justify the use of expensive molecular-based tests, additional information with clinical utility must be provided by the proposed test. With time, these techniques undoubtedly will play a greater role in the laboratory, but their addition to the diagnostic armamentarium needs to be based on practical utility.

CLINICAL LABORATORY MEDICINE

Clinicians may forget or be unaware that the pathologist oversees much of the clinical laboratory and is a reference for using it in the most efficient manner. Although most of the workload is performed by medical technologists, the pathologist often serves as director of the laboratory and as a contact for clinicians. Questions about the most appropriate test in a diagnostic workup or regarding laboratory values incongruent with clinical data can be reconciled through the pathologist.

The laboratory is sometimes viewed as an unquestioned source of patient information. Patient specimens go into the laboratory and somehow resultant data from those specimens always come out, with the process in between generally overlooked until test results are delayed, confusing data is produced, or results are incongruous with the clinical history. This is why a basic understanding of the inner workings of the laboratory is of paramount importance. One can hardly expect to interpret patient data with no knowledge of how it was derived. Just as the clinician attempting to interpret an unusual electrocardiogram may enlist the aid of a cardiologist, aberrant laboratory results should prompt a consultation of the pathologist. The pathologist is familiar with the potential pitfalls and limitations of laboratory procedures and the quality control measures instituted to ensure that valid patient data are produced. The pathologist should be consulted whenever questions arise regarding the type of specimen required for testing, the most appropriate test to order in a diagnostic workup, or the interpretation of test results.

Some tests are not performed often enough to justify the cost of an in-house assay or can not be done with the laboratory's available technology, and these specimens may be sent to an outside facility. These tests, in particular, demand attention to specimen requirements and transportation specifications. The laboratory and the pathologist can help direct the clinician in obtaining these specimens and serve as a resource for the availability of unusual tests.

The clinical laboratory is divided into hematology, chemistry, coagulation, blood bank, and microbiology sections. Larger laboratories may further subdivide these disciplines. A basic understanding of laboratory medicine is required for the clinician to submit proper specimens and to accurately interpret the patient data produced. Each test performed may have varying sensitivity and specificity, which are subject to the laboratory methodology used and the prevalence of the particular disease in the population studied. The pathologist can help the clinician to interpret the significance of test results and to select alternative methods. The following brief description of the clinical pathology disciplines and the pathologist's role in these areas is intended to familiarize the clinician with the laboratory's basic goals and the pathologist's role in it.

Hematology is concerned with evaluating the peripheral blood and bone marrow. Much of the analysis is performed on automated instruments; however, a manual examination of the peripheral blood smear remains the judging standard. Whole blood anticoagulated with EDTA is evaluated for qualitative and quantitative abnormalities of erythrocytes, leukocytes, and platelets. Automated analyzers sort the whole-blood constituents into subpopulations by using the physical and chemical properties of the cells. These sorting procedures may identify cells based on differences in size and cytoplasmic density. A specific aberrant cell population may be identified, or the analyzer may simply recognize an unspecified deviation from normal controls. Abnormalities identified through automated analyzers are explored further by manually examining the peripheral blood smear. This examination is performed by medical technologists trained in hematology. The pathologist serves as the director of the hematology service and reviews cases in which the peripheral blood diagnosis remains in question after examination by qualified technologists. Morphologic cellular changes in the peripheral smear may be diagnostic or may prompt an examination of the bone marrow to further investigate hematopoietic diseases. The examination of the peripheral blood can yield much more than a quantitative analysis of the cellular subpopulations. Unsuspected qualitative abnormalities of the cells, infectious processes, and circulating malignant cells are just a few of the anomalies that may be expressed in the peripheral blood. The pathologist should be consulted about all cases with unusual or unexpected findings.

Clinical chemistry is perhaps the most automated section of the clinical laboratory. Automated analyzers have the capacity to perform dozens of assays using variations on several methodologies and often require only microliters of patient specimen. The pathologist's role in this highly automated section is largely devoted to quality assurance, quality control, and laboratory management. The daily workload is performed by medical technologists, and deviant results, or ''panic values,'' are directly reported to clinicians. Occasionally, test results may be inconsistent with the clinical scenario. In these cases, the pathologist can help the clinician in evaluating the source of aberration. Abnormal results may be a consequence of mechanical malfunction, reagent imperfections, or improper specimen collection. Alternatively, aberrant results may be correct and may identify an occult clinical disease. Pathologists use their knowledge of clinical medicine and laboratory methodology to investigate confusing cases. The maximum benefit is achieved when open lines of communication exist between the clinical and the pathology staff.

The **transfusion medicine section,** commonly referred to as the blood bank, is dedicated to providing blood-component replacement products. Whole blood, packed red cells, platelets, frozen plasma, cryoprecipitate, and a host of specialized products are available for correcting defects in hemostasis and coagulation. The clinician should have a basic concept of how the blood bank screens and prepares blood products for patient therapy. The pathologist is a largely underutilized source of information on the optimal use of these replacement products. Many modifications of blood products such as washing,

leukocyte reduction, and irradiation may be appropriate in certain clinical settings. Too often, the pathologist is consulted when an order for blood components is questioned by the blood bank rather than ahead of time to assist in the initial choice of replacement products. Although most clinicians are comfortable with blood typing and antibody screens or crossmatch procedures, many are unfamiliar with the evaluation of alloimmune problems or autoantibodies identified by these procedures. The pathologist can aid in identifying antibodies with clinical relevance to the patient and can recommend further testing or modifications in therapy.

The direct antiglobulin test identifies antibodies attached to antigens on the red-cell surface. The indirect antiglobulin test identifies circulating antibodies. A positive result with either of these tests demands further investigation and characterization of the antibody. Cold-reacting antibodies react only at cold temperatures and may have no clinical implications for the patient. Nonetheless, they demand a thorough investigation, which takes time and may delay the availability of blood products.

The pathologist is also responsible for investigating any reported reactions or complications associated with transfusion of blood products. Investigation results must be documented in the patient's permanent record and future transfusion practices modified if necessary. The laboratory should be notified immediately when a potential transfusion reaction is encountered. An understanding of the role of the laboratory and the pathologist in providing blood replacement products can help to avoid frustration and to improve patient care.

The pathologist also is trained in the clinical diagnosis and laboratory management of **coagulation and thrombosis disorders.** These disorders may be confusing to the clinician who sees only a rare or occasional case or who receives aberrant test results from a routine preoperative screening procedure. The most important diagnostic step is an adequate patient and family history. The laboratory then can assist in further characterizing coagulation disorders. The terminology of coagulation medicine may be confusing, and in smaller hospitals only the most routine testing may be performed in-house. A good example is the lupus anticoagulant, which is seen in clinical situations other than lupus, and contrary to its name, may result in thrombosis rather than hemorrhage. This disorder is associated with antiphospholipid antibodies, which may prolong phospholipid-dependent assays such as the partial thromboplastin time. Although the antibody requires identification, it rarely causes complications in the immediate operative setting. The pathologist can assist in managing coagulation disorders and provide information for evaluating unusual cases.

The **microbiology laboratory** is concerned with identifying infectious pathogens and their susceptibility to known antimicrobial agents. These organisms include bacteria, fungi, parasites, and viruses. Similar to surgical tissue specimens, the proper handling of specimens for microbiologic analysis primarily depends on the clinical questions to be answered. The laboratory obviously does not attempt to culture every potential pathogen on every specimen submitted. Rather, it is the clinician who determines which organisms may be responsible for a patient's symptoms and who orders the appropriate tests. Many hospitals have an infectious disease service to aid in diagnosing microbial-induced illness. The pathologist can also be a resource for diagnosing infectious diseases. The laboratory should be consulted for the proper collection and transportation requirements for different microbial cultures. Ideally, specimens that require both histologic and microbiologic analysis should be divided at the time of tissue collection and submitted separately. The pathologist may divide tissue samples submitted in the fresh state, but sterility of the specimen may be compromised, and the addition of any fixative may kill organisms present in the tissue. The pathologist, once again, can assist in providing the most direct methods for achieving a clinical diagnosis and in correlating microbiologic data with that seen in histologic sections.

SUMMARY

Clearly, the basis for the relationship between the clinician and the pathologist can be summarized in a single word, **communication.**

The pathologist serves as a diagnostician and consultant in both surgical and clinical pathology. A frequent obstacle to using the pathologist as a reference source is the clinician's failure to recognize that source and the pathologist's failure to make these service visibile to the clinician. An understanding of the inner workings of the pathology laboratory can help the clinician in most effectively using the diagnostic modalities available. Frustration caused by submitting unacceptable specimens, delays in obtaining test results, or receiving aberrant results often are due to an incomplete understanding of the laboratory's and the pathologist's capabilities and limitations. A close working relationship between the clinician and pathologist can greatly enhance patient care and should be the goal of every physician.

REFERENCES

1. Foulds W. The uses and limitations of intraocular Biopsy. *Eye* 1992; 6:11–27.
2. Roth A, Foos R. A system for macroexamination of eyes in the laboratory. *Am J Clin Pathol* 1973;59:674–683.
3. Foos R. A simple macrophotographic method in the eye laboratory. *Arch Ophthalmol* 1969;81:63–69.
4. Menocal N, Ventura D, Yanoff M. *Theory and practice of histotechnology.* St. Louis: Mosby, 1980;285–291.
5. Albert D, Jakobiec F. *Principles and practice of ophthalmology: clinical practice.* Philadelphia: WB Saunders, 1994;2123–2155.
6. Nadji M, Morales A. *Immunoperoxidase techniques: a practical approach to tumor diagnosis.* Chicago: ASCP Press, 1986;1–9.
7. Koss L. *Aspiration biopsy: cytologic interpretation and histologic bases.* New York: Igaku-Shoin, 1992;659–675.
8. Rambo O. The limitations of histologic diagnosis. In: Buschke F (ed.). *Progress in radiation therapy,* Vol. 2. New York: Grune & Stratton, 1962;215–224.
9. Miden E, et al. Fine needle aspiration biopsy in ophthalmology. *Surv Ophthalmol* 1985;29:410–422.
10. Liu D. Complications of fine needle aspiration biopsy of the orbit. *Ophthalmology* 1985;92:1768–1771.
11. Karcioglu Z, et al. Tumor seeding in ocular fine needle aspiration biopsy. *Ophthalmology* 1985;92:1763–1767.
12. Hutchins G. *Autopsy performance and reporting.* Northfield, IL: College of American Pathologists, 1990;3–22.
13. Keren D. *Flow cytometry in clinical diagnosis.* Chicago: ASCP Press, 1989;12–34.
14. Knowles D. *Neoplastic hematopathology.* Baltimore: Williams & Wilkins, 1992;269–298.

Ophthalmic Pathology with Clinical Correlations,
edited by Joseph W. Sassani, M.D.
Lippincott-Raven Publishers, Philadelphia © 1997.

CHAPTER 2

Eyelid and Conjunctiva

William C. Lloyd III

GENERAL APPROACH TO SKIN AND CONJUNCTIVAL TISSUES

The diagnosis and management of lesions affecting periorbital skin, eyelid skin, and conjunctiva are an important part of vision care. Most disorders can be diagnosed promptly and treated with a few office visits. There is often a high correlation between the clinical impression and the pathologist's report. Nevertheless, successful case management hinges on diagnostic accuracy and a logical treatment plan. Both of these elements rely on a basic understanding of tissue histopathology. This chapter reviews the more common diseases affecting the eyelids, periorbital skin, and conjunctiva. Emphasis is placed on the pertinent histopathology as it relates to the clinical appearance of the lesion.

Clinical evaluation of eyelid and conjunctival diseases benefits from special advantages denied choroidal or orbital problems. Unlike other ophthalmic conditions, external lesions can easily be visually inspected with the naked eye or with a handy +20 diopter indirect ophthalmoscopy lens. Also, lid and conjunctival growths can be palpated to assess pliability and mobility.

A thoughtful history is a powerful tool that can resolve many diagnostic dilemmas. Using a nonpigmented epidermal eyelid mass as an example, rapidity of growth over a matter of weeks strongly supports a clinical diagnosis of keratoacanthoma over squamous carcinoma. These guidelines are tempered by the realization that nothing in medicine is absolute; the patient history may be noncontributory or, worse, misleading. Not infrequently the patient is unaware of or unconcerned about an abnormality, seeking care only at the urging of family members or another provider. Conversely, patients may disregard relatively inconspicuous lesions until rapid growth or discoloration is observed.

W. C. Lloyd III: Department of Ophthalmology and Ophthalmic Pathology Laboratory, University of Texas Health Science Center at San Antonio, San Antonio, Texas 78284-6230.

It is prudent, not parochial, for any patient with lesions affecting the eyelid, periorbital skin, or conjunctiva to be managed by an ophthalmologist. Several important considerations form the basis for this recommendation. The ophthalmologist has anatomic expertise and is familiar with optimal biopsy and treatment methods. He or she is most qualified to prevent, recognize, and treat any secondary ocular complications and can recognize specific conditions relevant or unique to the practice of ophthalmology (e.g., conjunctival primary acquired melanosis, oculodermal melanocytosis).

Anatomic and Histologic Similarities Between Skin and Conjunctiva

This chapter is anatomically divided into separate sections devoted to skin and conjunctiva; however, there are far more histologic and functional similarities between these two periocular structures than there are differences. Embryologically, eyelid skin and conjunctiva are derived from the same surface ectoderm that migrates over the neural crest nasal and maxillary processes. The primitive lids fuse during the eighth week of development and divide skin from conjunctiva. Differentiation of these covering layers continues until the eyelids reopen during the sixth intrauterine month as cilia emerge, surface epithelium matures, and adnexal glands begin to elaborate their products along the eyelid margin. Histologically, both structures contain squamous epithelium, dendritic melanocytes, blood and lymphatic vessels, and nerves.

Anatomic and Histologic Differences Between Skin and Conjunctiva

Significant differences between eyelid skin and conjunctiva deserve mention. The thin eyelid epidermis is covered by keratinizing squamous epithelium, which is thought to provide a protective barrier against radiation and other toxins, foreign matter, and mechanical injury.

Normal conjunctival epithelium is nonkeratinizing, but it reserves the ability to produce keratin under certain pathologic states (eg, lid dysfunction, exposure, chronic inflammation, dysplasia). Conjunctival epithelium contains a variable population of mucin-producing goblet cells that stabilize the tear film. In tissue sections, goblet cells stain vividly with the periodic acid–Schiff (PAS) method. Eyelid skin bears the normal cohort of skin appendages (cilia, sweat glands, sebaceous glands). The conjunctival subepithelial space contains lymphatic channels and a sparse population of chronic inflammatory cells that many authors believe perform a sentinel function to protect the globe from pathogenic stimuli.

Specimen Handling and Submission

Reiterating the important principles discussed in Chapter 1, all ophthalmic surgical specimens should be treated delicately. This delicacy applies equally to the techniques used to acquire the specimen, its delivery from the operative field, its transfer to the specimen container, and its transport to the pathology laboratory. Forceps crush injury and exuberant tissue cauterization obliterate any recognizable histology. Immediately after excision, fresh tissue begins to disintegrate at the cellular level. Tissue specimens not promptly preserved through freezing or chemical fixation are rendered uninterpretable. This tissue damage is especially worrisome in cases involving small suspected malignancies and questionable tumor recurrences. In summary: don't crush, don't incinerate, don't dessicate.

EYELID AND PERIORBITAL SKIN

Disease states that involve eyelid or periorbital skin pose multiple challenges to clinicians. These include patient discomfort and anxiety, clinical diagnostic accuracy, effects of previous treatment, selection of correct therapy, and avoidance of potential complications to neighboring ocular structures. A valid clinical impression and a workable differential diagnosis rely on a clear understanding of the pertinent anatomy, an accurate clinical history, and an appreciation of the clinical features that typify the condition. For example, few clinicians would clinically diagnose a teenager's pigmented eyelid skin lesion as malignant melanoma because we know that primary malignant melanoma of the eyelid is relatively rare, and it is even rarer for adolescents to be affected.

The specific diagnostic or therapeutic procedure performed is an outgrowth of the surgeon's clinical impression; for example, if one suspects sebaceous carcinoma, a full-thickness lid biopsy should be performed. Sometimes the clinician is unsure of the diagnosis and, therefore, must select a procedure that will provide adequate tissue for the pathologist to diagnose with confidence,

thus facilitating definitive treatment. Diagnostic accuracy is key, and it ultimately rests on histopathologic confirmation of representative tissue sections obtained from the surgical specimen.

Brief Overview of Gross and Microscopic Anatomy

Epidermis

The epidermis is the keratinized outer skin layer. It is thinner in the eyelid region than anywhere else on the body. Eyelid skin exhibits several distinctive characteristics (Fig. 2-1).[1] The uniform depth of epidermis across the eyelid surface highlights the absence of the familiar rete ridges at the epidermal–dermal junction. Near the eyelid margin the rete ridges reappear, and this fact may aid in tissue orientation at the microscope. Epithelial cells are the predominant cell population, and they occupy four overlapping layers within the epidermis. Beginning at the bottom, the basal **stratum germinativum** sits atop the basement membrane, and postmitotic epithelial cells migrate vertically toward the external surface and inevitable shedding. The journey normally takes 5 to 7 days, but this cycle can be significantly hastened or prolonged in response to various influences. Approaching the midlevel, the maturing polygon-shaped epithelia acquire intercellular junctions to become the spinous layer or *stratum spinosum*. These intercellular junctions can be a helpful (not absolute) finding in distinguishing epithelial cells from other cell populations when studying unknown tumors. The most superficial layer of nucleated, vital epithelium is the granular layer, the *stratum granulosum*. Under the microscope, the granular layer cells appear to have made a 90° rotation from vertical to horizontal. These cells are flattened and harbor basophilic keratohyaline granules that represent ongoing keratinization. If skin disease leads to increased cell proliferation and rapid turnover, the granular layer is bypassed. Finally, the cornified top layer of flattened anucleate epithelial cells, the **stratum corneum,** is proportionately thin and delicate in healthy eyelid and periorbital skin. A thicker horny layer is a common finding in many inflammatory and neoplastic conditions.

Other cells besides epithelial cells are present in the epidermis. Melanocytes are cuboidal neural crest cells that produce melanin. Melanin plays a vital role in protecting the skin from the harmful effects of ultraviolet irradiation. Stimulated dendritic melanocytes inoculate neighboring epithelial cells, resulting in an increased number of pigment-bearing cells but not an increase in the number of melanocytes. Normal melanocytes permanently reside within the basal epidermal layer and situate themselves as single cells evenly spaced between every seven to ten epithelial cells. Pathology is suspected whenever melanocytes appear more frequently than this inter-

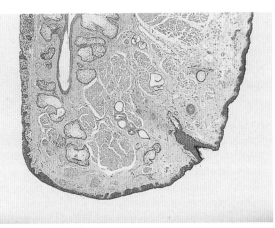
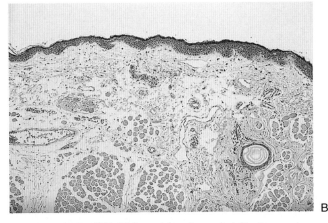

A   B

FIG. 2-1. Normal eyelid skin [eyelid margin (**A**), preorbital skin (**B**)]. Thin epidermis and delicate dermis overlie striated orbicularis muscle fibers.

val or begin to percolate superficially. Melanocytes can be difficult to identify on routine hematoxylin and eosin (H&E) sections of skin. If one searches carefully, melanocytes reveal themselves with their perinuclear halo, which forms due to cytoplasmic retraction.

In recent years, immunopathologists have greatly increased our understanding of the nature of Langerhans cells, the last major cellular constituent to the epidermis. It is believed that Langerhans cells derive from monocyte precursors in the bone marrow and perform as activated histiocytes (macrophages). These cells may be present within any layer of epithelial cells, and they may require special techniques (gold chloride or monoclonal antibodies OKT6) to confirm their presence. Langerhans cells play a pivotal role in host immune response. These dendritic cells express immune-related antigens and help host T lymphocytes to recognize soluble protein and haptenized antigens through their antigen-presenting function. When examined under transmission electron microscopy, Langerhans cells bear a familiar cytoplasmic organelle called the Bierbeck granule. It varies in size between 100 and 1000 nm; depending on its imaging perspective, it has been described as a flat disk, a bowl, a cylinder, or a tennis racket.

Dermis

Beneath the epidermis there is a delicate and slender dermis. The dermis separates the epidermis from the orbicularis muscle. It is widely taught that the eyelid is the body site where striated muscle fibers most closely approach the skin surface. In contrast to skin elsewhere on the body, the poorly defined eyelid dermis is so scant that there is no perceptible anatomic division between the superficial papillary dermis and the deeper reticular dermis. The typical upward papillary dermal projections that distort the epidermis to create rete ridges do not appear in eyelid skin. This loose connective tissue layer

is composed of elastin and collagen fibers bound within ground substance. Lymphatics, blood vessels, and peripheral nerve endings also reside within the dermis. The loose tissue organization in this region creates a potential space that is exploited during the administration of local anesthesia. Pessimistically, the dermis is a ready reservoir for edema fluid, blood, and pus. Fine vellus hairs and sweat glands also occupy the dermis (see below).

Epidermal Appendages

Skin is an organ with many important functions: mechanical protection, microbe barrier, body temperature regulation, fluid retention, and sense of touch. Assisting the skin are adnexal structures that share a common embryologic derivation with the epidermal stratum germinativum. If one closely examines microscopic sections of fully developed skin, the differentiated epidermal appendages feature a similar-appearing basal layer. This information solves an important riddle later in this chapter.

Hair growth is controlled by the dermal hair papilla at the bulbous base of the cylindrical hair follicle. During the active growth phase, melanocytes combine with hair matrix cells to produce the hair follicle. These histologic features are common to the cilia (eyelashes), the fine vellus hairs, and the eyebrow terminal hairs.

Sebaceous glands can be readily identified near the hair shafts (pilosebaceous apparatus). At the eyelid margin, the unilobar sebaceous glands that serve the cilia are known as the glands of Zeis. Sebaceous glands have a familiar histologic appearance. Under the microscope, a peripheral rim of nonlipidized basal cells surrounds lobules of sebaceous epithelium featuring a frothy, vacuolated cytoplasm. Routine specimen processing exposes the submitted tissue to alcohol, xylene, and other solvents that remove lipid while preserving the normal cytoarchitecture (Fig. 2-2).

The sebaceous glands produce an oily secretion. This

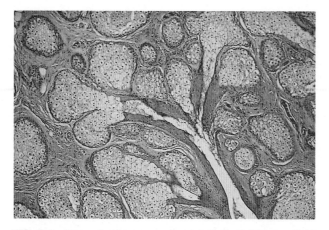

FIG. 2-2. Normal sebaceous gland. Lobules of foamy, lipid-rich sebaceous epithelium.

lipid-rich sebum is a holocrine secretion, achieved through individual cell destruction. The oily products are expressed through the excretory duct of the sebaceous lobules into the midportion of the hair follicle. Deep within the tarsus is a second network of sebaceous glands, the meibomian glands. Instead of nurturing the lashes, the ducts of the meibomian glands open directly at the skin surface so that the oily secretions can lubricate the lids and coat the tear film and retard its evaporation.

Whoever coined the phrase "working by the sweat of the brow" could just as easily have meant the eyelids, because the eyelid skin is heavily populated by sweat glands. There are two distinct types. At the eyelid margin, the glands of Moll elaborate their cytoplasmic products through apocrine secretion. Apical cytoplasmic processes undergo a decapitation phenomenon. The remaining epithelium is undisturbed. Histologically, apocrine sweat glands feature a bilayer of columnar to cuboidal cells with bright eosinophilic, PAS-positive cytoplasm. The apocrine gland synthesizes a scent, not perspiration *per se.* The gland lumens are relatively large. The sweat glands of Moll release their product into the lash follicles above the sebaceous duct. Beyond the eyelid margin, the rest of the eyelid skin relies on the eccrine sweat glands, situated in the slender dermis. These sweat glands participate in body temperature regulation and create perspiration. Eccrine glandular secretion permits the transudation of cell products through an intact membrane without decapitation "snouting." The lumens of the eccrine glands are about one-tenth the size of their apocrine counterparts. The clear perspiration can exit via the hair follicles or through its own specialized transepidermal duct, the acrosyringium.

The eyelid tarsus and the palpebral conjunctiva make up the posterior lamella of the eyelid. A complex network of highly organized collagen fibers encases the meibomian glands. Elastic fibers also are present within the tarsus. The rest of the deep eyelid tissues include smooth and striated muscle, blood vessels, lymphatics, and peripheral nerves. At the lid margin, approaching the medial canthus, the puncta is seen. The paired canaliculi are the outflow ducts for the tears. They are lined by conjunctival squamous epithelium and empty into the lacrimal sac.

Descriptive Terminology

The microscopic descriptions of most clinical alterations affecting epidermal structures rely on a common glossary of histopathologic features. The terms most frequently used are itemized below. Readers should become familiar with their correct usage. These terms are general and nonspecific; for example, the finding of acantholysis is suggestive for inverted follicular keratosis, but it also is encountered in pemphigus and herpetic skin infections. Although descriptive terms can be helpful in delineating disease processes, no single term imparts benignity or malignancy with certainty. The composite interpretation of gross and microscopic findings, viewed in the context of the clinical history, permits the pathologic diagnosis to be established.

- **Acanthosis**—thickening of the epidermis due to hyperplasia or hypertrophy of the stratum spinosum (Fig. 2-3). Acanthosis is frequently a reactive phenomenon to underlying inflammatory, infectious, or neoplastic processes.
- **Acantholysis**—loss of cohesion between epidermal and adnexal epithelial cells caused by deficient or absent intercellular bridges. Gaps form between affected cells, and coalescence leads to blister formation (Fig. 2-4).
- **Atrophy**—decreased thickness to the epidermis or dermis. This change can be ascribed to deficient proliferation of the normal cells or to premature loss of existing cells.
- **Atypia**—abnormal (atypical) appearance of the nuclei of individual cells in a disease process. Characteristic

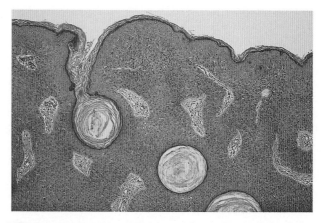

FIG. 2-3. Acanthosis. Thickening of prickle layer in seborrheic keratosis.

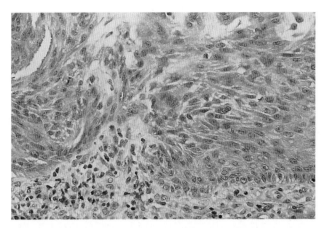

FIG. 2-4. Acantholysis. Poor intercellular cohesion.

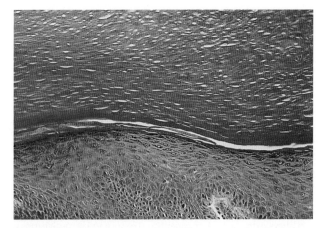

FIG. 2-6. Hyperkeratosis. Thickened horny layer (stratum corneum).

features include nuclear enlargement and hyperchromasia, irregularity of the nuclear outline, prominent nucleoli, coarse granularity of the intranuclear chromatin, and an enlarged nuclear-to-cytoplasmic ratio. Increased mitotic activity is usually observed. All these features need not be present for a cell to be considered atypical. Atypia usually connotes neoplasia; however, a long list of reactive/pseudoneoplastic conditions can create similar abnormalities. Specimens must be analyzed at both low- and high-power magnification.

- **Dyskeratosis**—abnormal (premature) keratinization of epithelial cells. Normal keratin is elaborated at the epidermal surface by mature epithelial cells. Active disease may lead to accelerated keratinocyte proliferation (Fig. 2-5).
- **Dysplasia**—disordered arrangement of epithelium. The term is applied to a population of cells and should not be used in reference to a single cell. Dysplastic epithelium is characterized by a disturbance of the normal keratinocytic maturation sequence. The conventional polarity of the different epithelial strata is also perverted. Dysplasia is a common finding in actinic

keratosis. The individual cells within a dysplastic population are not necessarily atypical.

- **Hyperkeratosis**—increased thickening of the anucleate stratum corneum (Fig. 2-6).
- **Hyperplasia**—an increase in the number of cells in any given tissue.
- **Hypertrophy**—an increase in cell size in any given tissue.
- **Papilloma**—any nipple-shaped growth caused by an upward proliferation of subepidermal papillae. Typical sections taken from papillomatous tissues reveal a central fibrovascular core enshrouded by acanthotic epithelium. Seborrheic keratosis and verruca vulgaris are two examples of clinical papillomas.
- **Parakeratosis**—increased thickening of the stratum corneum with incomplete keratinization (Fig. 2-7). Parakeratosis is histologic evidence of rapid cell turnover. As a consequence, epithelial cells retain their nuclei (in contrast to hyperkeratosis). Parakeratosis is associated with underdevelopment or absence of the granular layer.

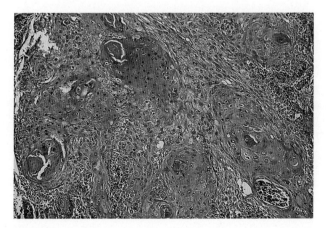

FIG. 2-5. Dyskeratosis. Abnormal intraepithelial keratinization.

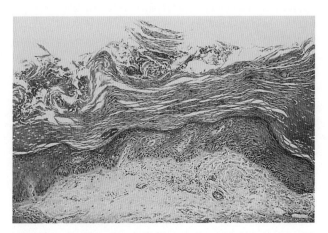

FIG. 2-7. Parakeratosis. Thickened stratum corneum with retained keratinocyte nuclei.

- **Pseudoepitheliomatous hyperplasia** (PEH)—irregular downward extension of acanthotic epidermis that mimics carcinoma. PEH represents a relatively recent concept in dermal pathology, and its introduction has led to a progressive reduction in the number of eyelid squamous carcinoma diagnoses.

Congenital Disorders

Two congenital abnormalities that affect the eyelids are eyelid coloboma and cryptophthalmia. **Eyelid colobomas** are focal disruptions in the normal development of the peripheral eyelid and eyelid margin tissues. The severity of the lid defect can range from a small notch to near-total absence of the eyelid. Eyelid colobomas can be singular or involve all four eyelids. Maldevelopment may be related to amniotic band impingement or faulty lid fusion.[2] Band-like adhesions may join the coloboma to the epibulbar conjunctiva. Eyelid colobomas are reported findings in Goldenhar syndrome and inherited cases of mandibulofacial dysostosis. A continuous fold of skin and conjunctiva bridges the unaffected leaves of eyelid. The abrupt loss of cilia, tarsus, and adnexal structures readily demarcates the edges of the coloboma.

In **cryptophthalmia,** a far rarer condition, a continuous sheet of epidermis extends between forehead and cheek, totally obscuring a malformed globe. It may be unilateral or bilateral. Anomalous failure of lid fold development results in a lack of the tarsus, eyelid adnexa, and cilia. The conjunctiva is comparably affected. Cryptophthalmia is most often present in the setting of multiple structural anomalies involving the skull and midface, the extremities, and the urogenital system. Contrast this disorder to ankyloblepharon, in which there is incomplete separation of normally developed eyelids.

Phakomatous choristoma (Zimmerman tumor) represents an accessory rest of surface ectoderm that did not accompany the normal migration of lens vesicle into the developing optic cup. This congenital abnormality occurs within the nasal lower eyelid as an enlarging rubbery nodule. The external appearance and location of this subcutaneous mass may falsely suggest a process arising from the lacrimal sac region. Excised specimens have been studied extensively. Conventional histology demonstrates cuboidal lens-like epithelium surrounded by a prominent basement membrane. The lens epithelium proliferates within a collagenous stroma and exhibits maturation changes encountered in the crystalline lens, including bladder cell and morgagnian globule formation. Ultrastructural and immunohistochemical studies confirm its true identity as lenticular anlage.[3]

Inflammatory Conditions

Inflammatory eyelid disorders represent a large element of clinical practice, but effective medical therapies limit the number of operative specimens.

The common external **hordeolum** (stye) is an acute and painful purulent infection formed in association with an obstructed sebaceous or sweat gland orifice near the cilia. Normal bacterial skin flora becomes trapped, leading to a superficial, localized abscess. The internal hordeolum arises in the meibomian gland and erupts on the palpebral conjunctival surface. Blepharitis is a frequent coexistent finding; however, many children without blepharitis experience hordeola. Surgical drainage yields copious pus laden with polymorphonuclear leukocytes and necrotic tissue.

The chronic, noninfectious counterpart to the stye is the **chalazion.** Obstruction of the sebaceous apparatus also is central to the pathophysiology of this lesion and most frequently is secondary to a mechanical blockage due to crusted debris from blepharitis. Other less common mechanical, infectious, and neoplastic causes for chalazia have been reported. Deep within the tarsus, the sebaceous glandular epithelia continue to produce their oily products for extrusion into the outflow path via holocrine secretion. These overloaded ductules rupture and the lipoidal cellular products are expressed into the surrounding tarsal soft tissues. Here the body recognizes sebum as foreign material and mounts a host foreign body granulomatous response, leading to lipogranuloma formation (Fig. 2-8). Within a dense chronic inflammatory infiltrate harboring mature lymphocytes and plasma cells, there appear discrete aggregates of large epithelioid histiocytes that appear to engulf the offending lipid material. Many of the histiocytes fuse to form multinucleated foreign body giant cells. Conventional tissue processing dissolves lipid. Clear vacuoles within the macrophages and in the extracellular space designate sites of previous lipid accumulation. Chalazia and recurrent chalazia are included in the misdiagnoses that make up the masquerade syndrome of sebaceous gland carcinoma (see below).

The conjunctiva can be affected in **sarcoidosis,** a presumed noninfectious granulomatous infiltrative process characterized by the presence of noncaseating granulomas (Fig. 2-9). Helper T-lymphocyte activation has been reported within affected tissues. Localized or diffuse, nearly any body organ can be involved. Sarcoid is discussed in greater detail in Chapter 3. The conjunctiva is often biopsied as a means of obtaining a confirmatory tissue diagnosis without the potential risks associated with other invasive procedures such as transbronchial biopsy. Authors disagree as to the value of performing so-called blind conjunctival biopsies. In general, if there appear to be no ocular or periocular clinical findings consistent with the diagnosis of sarcoid, then the yield from blind conjunctival biopsy will be low. Sarcoidosis is a diagnosis of exclu-

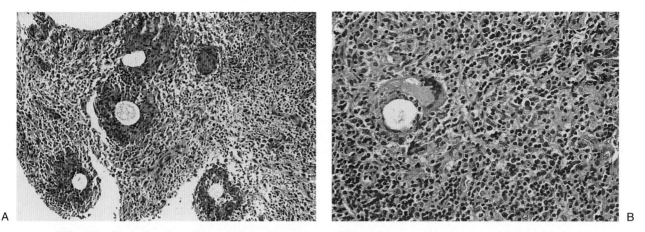

FIG. 2-8. Chalazion [low (**A**) and high power images (**B**)]. Lipid vacuoles are surrounded by foreign-body type chronic granulomatous inflammation.

sion that is made only after all other possible causes of granulomatous inflammation (eg, infectious, foreign body, vasculitis, other histiocytic proliferations) have been eliminated.

Various other granulomatous disorders involve the eyelid. **Juvenile xanthogranuloma** is a benign, reactive, nodular, inflammatory process of unknown origin. Xanthomatous lesions may appear both in the eye and the skin, frequently causing spontaneous hyphema if the iris is involved. Over 20% of cases are diagnosed in adults. The characteristic histopathology reveals an inflammatory infiltrate containing abundant epithelioid histiocytes. Xanthogranulomas are diagnosed by the presence of Touton giant cells, in which a near-complete wreath of fused histiocyte nuclei surrounds eosinophilic cytoplasm and is rimmed peripherally by pale vacuolated cytoplasm (Fig. 2-10).

The finding of Touton giant cells, in and of themselves, is nondiagnostic. **Necrobiotic xanthogranuloma** is another nodular skin proliferation that contains Touton giant cells. Not infrequently, these firm, elevated, yellowish,

and inflamed lesions are clinically mistaken for eyelid xanthelasma, which is another good reason to submit all surgical specimens for the pathologist's review. Microscopic sections of necrobiotic xanthogranuloma exhibit islands of hyaline necrobiosis amidst a granulomatous infiltrate that includes both Touton and foreign body giant cells. Necrobiotic xanthogranuloma is frequently a cutaneous marker for monoclonal gammopathy, plasma cell dyscrasias, and multiple myeloma.[4] Accordingly, patients diagnosed with necrobiotic xanthogranuloma are committed to undergo a systemic hematologic evaluation.

Some common and less common infectious causes of eyelid granulomas include mycobacteria, fungi (*Cryptococcus,* blastomycosis, coccidioidomycosis), rickettsiae (cat-scratch agent, *Bartonella henselae*), parasites (trichinosis, filariasis, cysticercosis), and protozoa (leishmaniasis).

Cutaneous viral infections are frequently encountered in clinical practice. **Herpesvirus infections** (*H. simplex, H. varicella-zoster*) of the eyelid skin characteristically

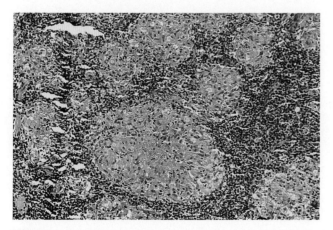

FIG. 2-9. Sarcoid granuloma. Aggregates of epithelioid histiocytes form noncaseating granulomas.

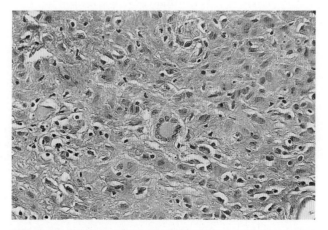

FIG. 2-10. Touton giant cell (JXG). Near-complete annulus of nuclei surround eosinophilic cytoplasm in center. Foamy wreath surrounds the periphery.

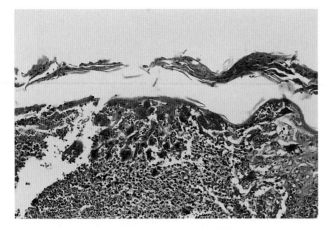

FIG. 2-11. Cowdry A-type inclusions (HSV). Densely eosinophilic intraepithelial inclusions.

produce vesiculobullous eruptions. A smear can be collected from the blister fluid to demonstrate eosinophilic Cowdry A-type intranuclear inclusions within the desquamated epithelium (Fig. 2-11). The histopathology of active herpes simplex and active herpes zoster skin lesions is indistinguishable.

Molluscum contagiosum is a familiar, waxy, domed or crater-shaped epidermal lesion that frequently arises in the eyelids and periorbital skin. Conjunctival involvement also has been reported. Shedding of virus-contaminated epithelial debris into the conjunctival cul-de-sac can lead to a unilateral follicular conjunctivitis with ipsilateral preauricular lymphadenopathy. An increased frequency of molluscum contagiosum is encountered in patients with AIDS. The virus responsible for molluscum contagiosum belongs to the poxvirus group. The histopathology of molluscum lesions is very specific. Clusters of infected epithelial cells undergo pronounced downward acanthosis, producing its familiar flask-shaped configuration when examined with the microscope at low power (Fig. 2-12).

Examination of individual epithelial cells reveals an amphophilic homogenous intracytoplasmic inclusion called the molluscum body (Henderson-Patterson corpuscle). The virus-laden, enlarging molluscum body flattens and eventually displaces the nucleus. The molluscum body becomes enmeshed in a thick, horny keratin layer as it approaches the surface.

The eyelids and periorbital skin may be sites for the common wart, **verruca vulgaris.** These nontender, elevated, firm, papillomatous papules may occur singly or in groups. Human papillomavirus (HPV) of the papova group is the causative agent. Many HPV serotypes have been identified in verrucae. Characteristic histopathologic features include elongated acanthotic papillae that resemble the spires atop a church steeple, a thick parakeratotic crust, and centrally pointing rete ridges (Fig. 2-13). Under higher power, vacuolated koilocytes reside within the superficial epidermis of the papillae, and basophilic keratohyaline granules are situated below in the hyperkeratotic valleys.

Two important parasitic processes involving the eyelids

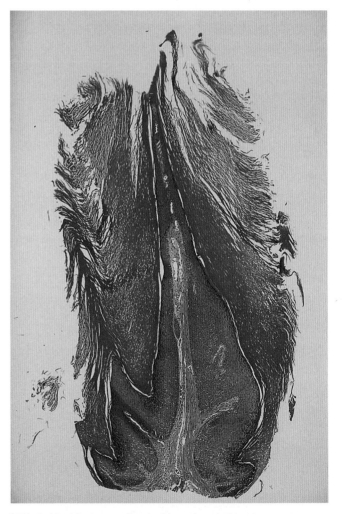

FIG. 2-13. Verruca vulgaris. Hyperkeratotic squamous papilloma featuring "church spire" configuration.

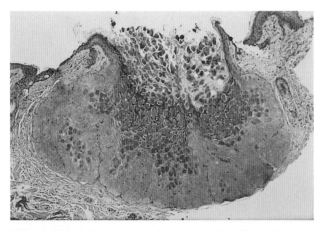

FIG. 2-12. Molluscum contagiosum. Umbilicated lesion plugged with virus-laden epithelium (Henderson-Patterson corpuscles).

are demodicosis and phthiriasis palpebrarum. The former is a ubiquitous organism incidentally encountered in eyelid skin specimens; the latter is a clinically relevant symptom-producing infestation. **Demodicosis** is caused by mites that have a preference for the pilosebaceous apparatus. *Demodex folliculorum* attach to the small hairs and lash follicles. *Demodex brevis* thrive within the sebaceous gland. Both species participate in a nocturnal migration toward the skin surface. While demodex mites wander along the lid margins, bacterial skin flora attach themselves and are transported back down into the hair follicle. Skin infections and hordeola may result.

Phthiriasis palpebrarum is the term used to describe crab lice infestation. The pubic louse (*Phthirius pubis*) commonly inhabits the groin and inguinal region: the closer arrangement of hairs in this region facilitates louse mobility. A similar pattern is present in the eyelashes, and this fact is used to explain why crab lice infest the lashes. This phenomenon is not observed with body lice and rarely with head lice. Crab lice are transmitted in the setting of poor personal hygiene, overcrowded or unsanitary living conditions, and sexual contact. At slit-lamp examination, *Phthirius pubis* can be directly visualized, along with their egg casings (nits). Blepharitis and conjunctivitis represent a host response to lice fecal debris. Secondary bacterial infection also may occur.

Acquired and Degenerative Conditions

Xanthelasma is the most common form of cutaneous xanthoma. This benign lesion is composed of perivascular aggregates of foamy dermal histiocytes that engulf extravasated plasma lipid (Fig. 2-14). Ordinarily, these pale-yellow noninflamed plaques originate in the medial eyelid skin and spread laterally in a symmetric fashion. Most often, xanthelasma are flat or nodular and exhibit minimal elevation. Any deviation from the above clinical description should arouse diagnostic skepticism. Xanthelasma

may arise *de novo* or, less frequently, in association with an underlying hereditary or dietary lipid abnormality (eg, diabetes mellitus or essential hyperlipidemia, notably types II and III). Most patients under age 40 with xanthelasma warrant screening laboratory studies to exclude lipid abnormalities and diabetes.

When considering the intensity of sun exposure and cumulative dosage of ultraviolet radiation, the facial skin arguably withstands the greatest abuse. The public is slowly adopting recommended preventive measures to protect themselves from the documented harmful effects of sunlight. Unfortunately, many adults did not benefit from the habitual use of physical and chemical sunblocks earlier in life, and so various sun-induced skin changes will be found in our patients for decades to come.

The most frequent skin alteration is **solar elastosis.** Elastic tissue in the papillary dermis of sun-exposed skin undergoes hyperplasia, leading to an increase in the number and size of curled, intertwined elastic fibers. This change is most pronounced in fair-skinned Caucasians and is universally present in Caucasians over age 40. Solar elastosis is diagnosed microscopically as a relatively acellular zone of basophilic (elastotic) degeneration in the upper dermis (Fig. 2-15). In severe cases, this degeneration can extend much deeper. Ultrastructural features confirmatory for genuine elastic tissue are absent in the area of basophilic degeneration, which is replaced by a granular extracellular matrix harboring acid mucopolysaccharides and electron-dense inclusions. Special stains for elastic tissue (Verhoeff-van Gieson) elicit a positive tissue reaction in affected dermis; however, because elastotic degeneration does not truly involve elastic fibers, the staining persists after tissue sections are exposed to the enzyme elastase.

Amyloid (''starch-like'') is a peculiar substance better described than understood. Sources of amyloid synthesis include immunoglobulin light chains, keratinocyte tonofilaments, and serum proteins. All share a similar ultra-

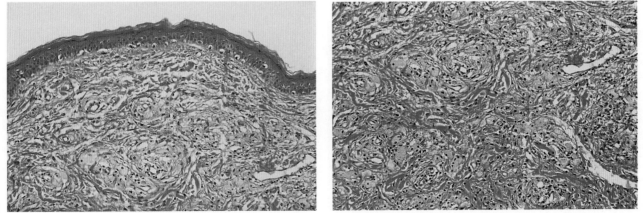

A   B

FIG. 2-14. Xanthelasma [low (**A**) and high power images (**B**)]. Lipid-rich macrophages are trapped within eyelid dermis.

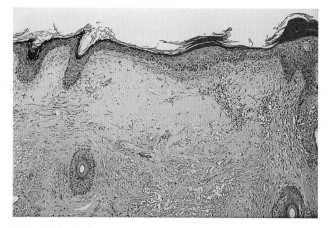

FIG. 2-15. Solar elastosis. Pale gray-blue focus of elastoid degeneration.

structural morphology: nonbranching fibrils of indefinite length with a fiber diameter varying from 7.5 to 10 nm. Periorbital cutaneous amyloid deposition most frequently occurs in two clinical settings: nonfamilial primary amyloidosis and secondary to a systemic plasma cell dyscrasia (multiple myeloma). Other amyloid disorders rarely or never involve the eyelid skin (familial primary amyloidosis, lichen amyloid, amyloidosis secondary to infection or inflammation). This pattern differs from that observed with conjunctival amyloidosis. Accumulations of amyloid within the eyelid or periorbital skin are reliable markers for multisystem involvement.[5] Jakobiec and Jones described a strictly localized form of amyloidosis that limits amyloid deposition to the ocular adnexae.[6] A helpful diagnostic clue appears during the clinical examination. Perivascular accumulations of amyloid protein lead to increased capillary fragility. When these pale cutaneous plaques are manipulated, they bruise easily, and visible evidence of earlier bleeding may be present (Fig. 2-16). Four well-known features characterize the histopathology of amyloid:

- Congophilia—orange coloration to amyloid depositions in paraffin-embedded tissue sections with the Congo red special stain
- Birefringence—light transmission due to regularity of Congo red dye molecules bound to parallel amyloid fibrils
- Dichroism—switch from green to dull red during rotation of the polarizing lens. Birefringence and dichroism are jointly appreciated when congophilic deposits are examined under a polarizing lens.
- Autofluorescence—demonstrated in tissue sections stained with thioflavine T and excited under the fluorescent microscope.

Cysts, Tumors, and Neoplasms

Benign Epidermal Lesions

Cysts frequently occur in eyelid and periorbital skin. True cysts have the following common features: a circumscribed cavity lined by some type of epithelium, and a cyst lumen that collects desquamated cells, cellular debris, and cellular products (eg, sebum, keratin, hair). An **epidermal inclusion cyst** (epidermoid cyst, infundibular cyst) is the most common cystic eyelid lesion. This true cyst represents a sequestrum of epidermis trapped beneath the epidermal layer, whether due to occlusion of the infundibulum adjacent to the eyelash or accidental epidermal implantation resulting from accidental or surgical trauma. Viable surface epithelium continues to shed keratin flakes and desquamated cells into the expanding unilocular cyst lumen (Fig. 2-17). The chronic mechanical effect of the cyst enlargement flattens the epithelial lining and promotes pseudocapsule formation. If the cyst ruptures, it usually incites a host foreign body giant cell inflammatory reaction directed against the heterotopic cyst contents. **Milia** are small epidermal inclusion cysts (usually less

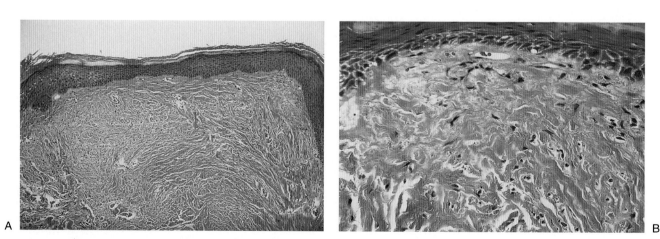

FIG. 2-16. Amyloid deposition [low (**A**) and high power (**B**) images]. Hypocellular accumulation of faintly eosinophilic material.

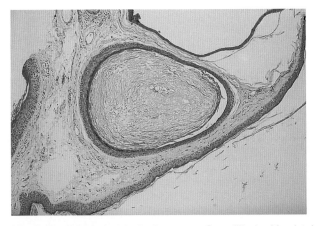

FIG. 2-17. Epidermal inclusion cyst. Cyst filled with shed keratin and desquamated epithelium. Cyst lined by surface epithelium.

than 2 mm in diameter) that are numerous on the facial and periorbital skin. They arise at the base of the infundibulum of vellus hairs at the level of the sebaceous duct. Milia are histologically indistinguishable from small epidermal inclusion cysts.

Dermoid cysts differ from epidermal inclusion cysts by virtue of their pathogenesis and histopathology. They most frequently arise in the superior temporal quadrant of the orbit, although any quadrant may be affected. Orbital dermoids may be superficial or deep, and they are always benign. Most are believed to be a congenital anomaly in which surface ectoderm is trapped within the apposing sutures of the orbital bones. This heterotopic cyst is lined by epidermis and skin appendages. The maturing cyst develops an expanding cyst cavity filled with skin cells, keratin, sweat and sebaceous secretions, and hairs (Fig. 2-18). The diagnosis can usually be established at the time of gross examination when the cyst is opened. Ruptured dermoid cysts (including incomplete surgical excisions) permit the liberation of the previously sequestered debris

and contamination of the orbit. This material elicits an intense granulomatous foreign body tissue reaction.

Other common cystic alterations involving the eyelids are **sudoriferous cysts,** or **hidrocystomas.** These are benign cystic dilatations of sweat gland origin. Because the lining epithelium yields clear fluid (perspiration), these cysts easily transilluminate. Discoloration of the cyst fluid may occur with hemorrhage. There are two types of sudoriferous cysts (Fig. 2-19).[7] The **apocrine hidrocystoma** is actually an adenoma that arises from the sweat glands of Moll near the lid margin. Clinically, these lesions appear as single or multiple elevated translucent nodules. Apocrine hidrocystomas frequently harbor a complex, arborizing lumen lined by a monolayer or bilayer of cuboidal epithelium. Under higher magnification, PAS-positive intracytoplasmic granules are a helpful feature. Epithelium lining the apocrine hidrocystoma demonstrates the decapitation or ''snouting'' phenomenon that typifies apocrine secretion. The **eccrine hidrocystoma** most likely represents a true retention cyst of the sweat gland duct. It features a solitary dilated cyst lumen, and its lining epithelium is smooth and regular. Increased fluid pressure within the eccrine hidrocystoma may flatten the lining epithelium.

Squamous papilloma (skin tag, acrochordon, fibroepithelial polyp) is an imprecise clinical term used to describe a sessile or pedunculated proliferation of benign epidermis. It is reported to be the most common benign eyelid skin lesion. Single or multiple papillomas may be present on the periorbital skin and lid margins. Microscopically, there appear elongated tongues of vascularized loose connective tissue covered by acanthotic squamous epithelium.

One familiar variant of squamous papilloma is the **seborrheic keratosis.** Most frequently discovered in older adults, seborrheic keratoses feature a palpably greasy, ''stuck-on'' appearance. It is an elevated, well-circumscribed mass of acanthotic basal epidermal cells with a verruciform surface. In Caucasians, its color is

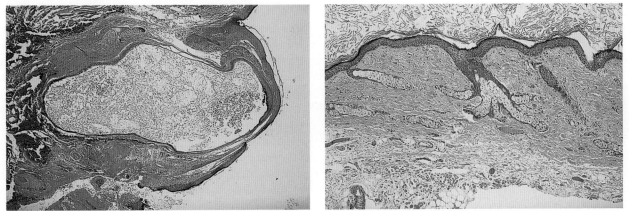

FIG. 2-18. Dermoid cyst [low (**A**) and high (**B**) power images]. Cyst lining includes surface epithelium and epidermal appendages.

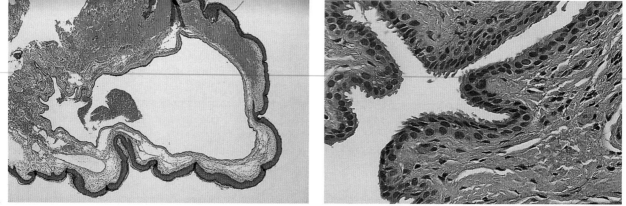

FIG. 2-19. Sudoriferous cysts [low (**A**) and high (**B**) power images]. Arborizing cyst lined by cuboidal epithelial bilayer. Apocrine variant exhibits decapitation phenomenon.

often darker than the surrounding normal skin. Three histologic subtypes have been described (hyperkeratotic, acanthotic, and adenoid), although most borrow some features from all three (Fig. 2-20). Key to the histopathology are basaloid acanthosis, papillomatosis, intraepithelial horn cyst inclusions, and variable hyperkeratosis. A histologically similar but smaller papilloma that commonly appears on the facial skin of adult blacks is called **dermatosis papulosa nigra.**

Disagreement persists regarding the nature of **keratoacanthoma.** As a distinct disease entity, it has been recognized only since 1950. Before then, lesions resembling keratoacanthomas were diagnosed as squamous cell carcinomas. This fact accounts for the continued decline in the reported incidence of squamous cell carcinoma as a primary eyelid malignancy. Is it a reactive or noncancerous neoplastic proliferation of epidermis?

Keratoacanthoma is a subset diagnosis of the larger descriptive clinical category **pseudoepitheliomatous hyperplasia.** As its name implies, pseudoepitheliomatous hyperplasia behaves and looks like an invasive malignancy but is not. Keratoacanthoma is an important diagnosis to pathologists because it illustrates the importance of correlating the clinical history with tissue histopathology. Keratoacanthomas arise along any hairy skin surface, including the periorbital skin.[8] An increased incidence of keratoacanthomas is reported in AIDS patients. At first glance, its clinical and microscopic appearances are worrisome. A firm, dome-shaped nodule surrounds a keratin-filled excavation. Characteristically, they undergo a period of rapid growth that lends to the clinician's diagnostic confidence. Keratoacanthoma growth usually peaks by 8 weeks, and it slowly involutes over a period of up to 12 months. Many patients will not tolerate the wait and justifiably seek its removal.

Complete excision is advocated for several reasons. First and foremost is diagnostic accuracy. Similarities between squamous cell carcinoma and keratoacanthoma extend to shared histopathology. Under low-power magnification, one can readily appreciate a sharply circumscribed, cup-shaped tumor architecture (Fig. 2-21). The crater may be filled with densely packed keratin overlying plump, acanthotic, epithelial cells. These abnormal epidermal cells have a pale, glassy cytoplasm. The presence of intraepidermal neutrophilic abscesses is helpful in distinguishing keratoacanthoma from squamous carcinoma. It is not alarming to discover, as in any rapidly proliferating keratinizing mass, striking invasive acanthosis with abundant mitoses, focal atypia, and dyskeratosis. Such features predominate toward the periphery of the lesion. To reiterate an earlier point, a minuscule incisional biopsy taken from this area of the lesion could mislead the pathologist into a malignant interpretation. Perineural invasion is another apparently paradoxic finding for this benign process. Marked inflammation may be situated at the base of the lesion. A final helpful feature is the observation that keratoacanthomas often sit atop the undisturbed dermal sweat glands.

The pathologist is not always successful in distinguish-

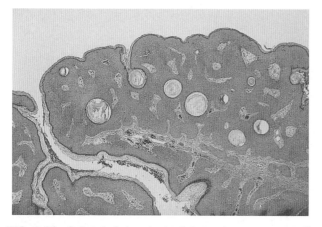

FIG. 2-20. Seborrheic keratosis. A form of squamous papilloma with basilar acanthosis and intraepithelial horn cysts.

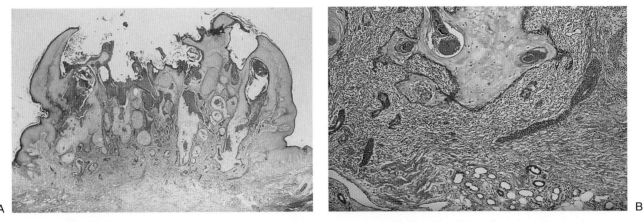

FIG. 2-21. Keratoacanthoma [low (**A**) and high (**B**) power images]. Cup-shaped epidermal proliferation filled with keratin. Affected epithelial cells feature pale, glassy cytoplasm.

ing keratoacanthoma from squamous carcinoma. Some pathologists rely on necessarily vague phraseology or descriptive terminology to render a complete report. Accurate, clear communication between pathologist and clinician is the most valuable outcome in this situation; the clinician must demand it. Once again, an excisional biopsy with adequate tumor-free margins would be likely to resolve the dilemma.

A second, less common eyelid mass included as an example of pseudoepitheliomatous hyperplasia is the **inverted follicular keratosis** (irritated seborrheic keratosis, basosquamous cell acanthoma). The eyelid margin is the most frequently involved body site. Its actual relation to the hair follicle has been disputed. Like keratoacanthoma, the inverted follicular keratosis erupts over a period of weeks to months. Moreover, the clinical presentation centers around a circumscribed, firm, exophytic papule that is often more deeply pigmented than the surrounding uninvolved skin. The typical histopathology includes a cup-shaped, markedly hyperkeratotic mass composed of proliferating basaloid cells situated adjacent to concentric whorls of squamous epithelium (squamous eddies) (Fig. 2-22).[8] Contributing to the diagnosis of inverted follicular keratosis is the finding of variable intracellular and intercellular edema, appreciated visibly as acantholysis.

Premalignant Conditions

The most common premalignant skin disorder is **actinic keratosis** (solar or senile keratosis). These oval to round scaly patches develop on sun-exposed skin surfaces and are usually less than 1 cm in diameter. The facial skin is particularly vulnerable, and multiple lesions are commonly found. Actinic keratoses arise in clinically apparent areas of chronic sun damage. Pigmentation is variable. Although actinic keratosis was once a diagnosis associated with advancing age, today these precancerous skin lesions are routinely encountered in younger adults.

Reports cite that untreated actinic keratoses lead to the development of squamous cell carcinoma in more than 20% of cases. A simple shave biopsy is usually adequate for diagnosis. The characteristic histopathology of actinic keratosis includes alternating epidermal atrophy and hyperplasia, hyperkeratosis, parakeratosis, and keratinocytic dysplasia. Epidermal hyperplasia leads to a downward proliferation of epidermal buds into the papillary dermis (Fig. 2-23). The neighboring appendageal epithelium (pilosebaceous apparatus) is spared. Features to be noted in evaluating keratinocytic dysplasia are nuclear pleomorphism (enlarged, hyperchromatic, and irregularly shaped cell nuclei), loss of cellular polarity, and loss of the normal maturation pattern. Dysplasia begins at the basal layer and may fully replace the normal overlying epidermis. The epidermal basement membrane is preserved, and a focally intense chronic inflammatory infiltrate often resides beneath an actinic keratosis. Dermatopathologists subclassify actinic keratosis by virtue of differing histologic patterns (hypertrophic, atrophic, acantholytic, li-

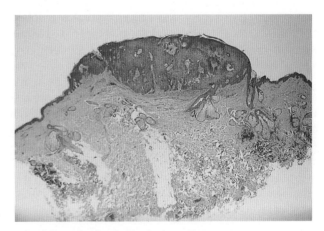

FIG. 2-22. Inverted follicular keratosis. Also known as irritated seborrheic keratosis. Noninvasive, exophytic, hyperkeratotic papule.

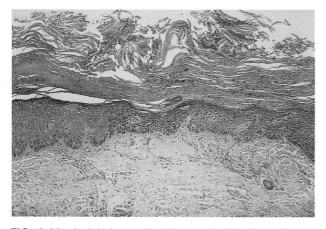

FIG. 2-23. Actinic keratosis characterized by hyperkeratosis, parakeratosis, epidermal hyperplasia involving sun-exposed skin.

chenoid, bowenoid); however, their clinical management is the same.

Bowen disease (intraepidermal squamous cell carcinoma) is another premalignant skin disorder that primarily affects the skin of Caucasians. In simplest terms, Bowen disease represents full-thickness keratinocytic dysplasia, or carcinoma in situ.[9] It usually presents as a solitary oval erythematous and scaly patch on sun-exposed skin. The patch is typically larger (1 to 2 cm) than a solitary actinic keratosis. Bowen disease arising on unexposed skin is historically associated with arsenic ingestion and carries an increased risk for coexistent internal malignancy (Rulon-Helwig syndrome). Bowen disease may arise in the company of other actinic keratoses. It is important to biopsy all clinically suspicious actinic keratoses adequately before treatment because about 5% to 10% of Bowen disease lesions harbor microinvasive squamous cell carcinoma. Wide excision with tumor-free margins is recommended. Simple freezing with liquid nitrogen in these cases is ineffective and only delays definitive treatment. There is a known historical association between Bowen disease and the development of internal malignancy. Fortunately, this cancer syndrome involves only those cases of Bowen disease arising in skin not exposed to the sun; current investigators discount any similar association with sun-exposed cases.

One question frequently raised is whether Bowen disease is merely a severe form of actinic keratosis. Although the microscopic appearance of Bowen disease can mimic actinic keratosis, most dermatopathologists prefer to separate the two conditions because they can arise independently and each has a different recommended treatment and prognosis. Three reproducible features can help discriminate between Bowen disease and actinic keratosis:

- Within the acanthotic epidermis in Bowen disease, the markedly disorganized pattern of dysplastic epithelial cells creates what has been described as a "windblown" appearance (Fig. 2-24).

- Bowen disease should exhibit individual cell dyskeratinization.
- Unlike actinic keratosis, the pathologic process in Bowen disease involves the follicular epithelium.

Basal Cell Carcinoma

Of all malignant neoplasms, **basal cell carcinoma** (basal cell epithelioma, BCC) is the most common. In retrospective series, its estimated incidence is 25% of all eyelid lesions and 90% of all lid cancers. The vast majority of BCCs arise in patients over age 40; however, the eyelid is a preferred site for BCCs in younger adults. A second unsuspected BCC is present elsewhere on the body in 60% of cases. These demographics are among the most compelling data presented in this book. Clinicians need a complete understanding of the pathophysiology and myriad appearances of BCC.[10]

BCC is a slowly progressive neoplasm that deforms and destroys normal tissues, and its surgical management often creates additional disfigurement. Although BCC rarely metastasizes (less than 0.1%), it can still be lethal. Most BCC-related mortality involves intracranial extension of lid or medial canthal tumors. Rare intraocular invasion by BCC is encountered in cases with advanced orbital involvement.

Most patients with BCC have been aware of their lesion for months or years. BCC has no precursor lesion. BCC can mimic nearly any cutaneous eruption: a papule, a crusted plaque, a cyst, an elevated nodule with or without central excavation (rodent ulcer), and even a scar. Simply stated, BCC is a necessary element in the differential diagnosis for nearly any adult acquired lid growth.

BCC tumor cells are unlike normal epidermal epithelial cells: they have deficient desmosomes, tonofilaments, and surface antigens. Current theory suggests that BCC represents a proliferation of an underdeveloped primitive stem

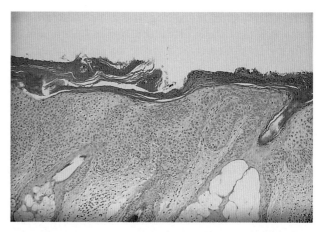

FIG. 2-24. Bowen disease demonstrating full-thickness epithelial dysplasia involving both surface epidermis and infundibulum and exhibiting "windblown epithelial disarray".

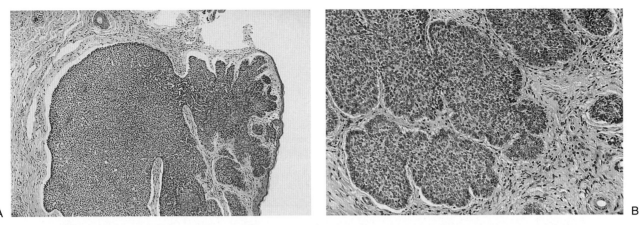

FIG. 2-25. Basal cell carcinoma [low (**A**) and high (**B**) power images]. Nests and lobules of bland, basaloid epithelium demonstrating peripheral pallisading and retraction artifact. Interlobular desmoplasia.

cell. This theory is bolstered by our knowledge that BCCs can differentiate to form squamous cells as well as pilar, sebaceous, and apocrine elements.

Low-magnification microscopy of BCC demonstrates a mass composed of relatively uniform-appearing basophilic tumor (basaloid) cells (Fig. 2-25). These tumor cells may extend from the epidermis, sweat ducts, or hair follicles. Peripheral palisading of tumor cell nuclei is an expected finding. A cleft often exists between the tumor and its adjoining stroma. This separation (retraction artifact) may be due to faulty tumor cell adhesion. Strands and lobules of BCC reside within a desmoplastic or mucinous stroma. Necrosis may appear toward the center of the tumor lobule. Under higher magnification, the basaloid tumor cells feature oval hyperchromatic nuclei with scant cytoplasm. There is minimal mitotic activity. BCC shares features with trichoepithelioma, which has hair structures within individual tumor lobules (see Fig. 2-43).

BCC has been neatly organized into five morphologic categories: nodular, nodular ulcerative, superficial multicentric, cystic, and morpheaform (Fig. 2-26). Neverthe-

less, few specimens demonstrate a pure tumor composition. What really matters is whether the tumor is circumscribed or infiltrative, and if tumor is present at the surgical margin of excision. Pigmentation of BCC does not alter management or prognosis.

Morpheaform (sclerosing) BCC deserves special mention. Instead of a circumscribed tumor nidus, the periorbital dermis is infiltrated by thin strands and fingers of BCC that may only be a few cells thick (Fig. 2-27). This variant is the most difficult to manage.[11] Clinical diagnosis in asymptomatic patients may be delayed. Conservative treatments deemed effective for other BCC subgroups (cryotherapy, topical 5-fluorouracil, dessication and curettage) invariably leave residual, recurrent neoplasm. Even a timely biopsy could be problematic because it may be easy to overlook advancing morpheaform BCC hiding amidst the cellular desmoplastic stroma.

In evaluating these lesions, one should always examine the epidermis for coexistent sun-induced changes (solar elastosis, actinic keratosis, and solar lentigo).

Children and adolescents who develop BCC should be

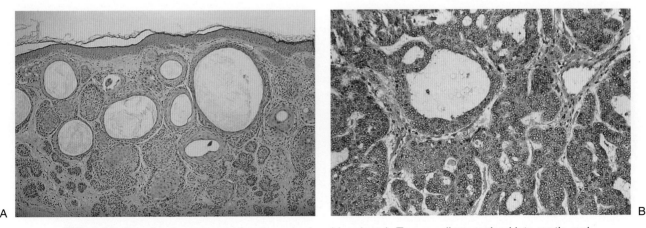

FIG. 2-26. Basal cell carcinoma (cystic and adenoid variants). Tumor cells organized into cystic and glandular patterns.

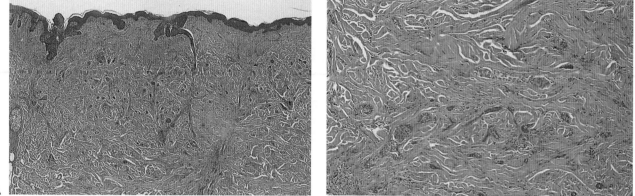

FIG. 2-27. Morpheaform BCC [low (**A**) and high (**B**) power images]. Instead of bulky tumor nodules there appear slender strands and tendrils of basal cell carcinoma. Morpheaform variant can invade deeply predating clinical detection.

suspected as having a potentially fatal heritable syndrome. Young adults with the **basal cell nevus syndrome** (Gorlin-Goltz) have inherited an autosomal dominant condition that includes multiple BCCs in association with jaw cysts, skeletal abnormalities, and a wide variety of ocular and central nervous system disorders. Ultraviolet light exposure also can lead to multiple different skin cancers in patients with defective DNA repair, as occurs in **xeroderma pigmentosum.** Finally, persons with cutaneous or oculocutaneous **albinism** are at increased risk for early skin cancers.

Squamous Cell Carcinoma

Squamous cell carcinoma (SCC) involves eyelid skin far less frequently than BCC. SCC also is a slowly enlarging skin tumor that predominantly affects older adults.[12] Chronic sun exposure is responsible for the pathophysiology of SCC. Most eyelid SCCs began as a neglected or unsuccessfully treated actinic keratosis or Bowen disease.

The lower eyelid margin is most frequently involved; however, SCC can arise anywhere in the periorbital area. In selected series, SCC is the most common upper lid malignancy, but this fact is more likely a reflection of the overall rarity of upper eyelid primary cancers. Unlike SCCs arising in extracutaneous sites (eg, pharynx, bronchus, uterine cervix), the occurrence of distant metastasis from periorbital SCC is less than 1%.

SCC appears as an elevated keratotic plaque that may be associated with extensive sun damage on the adjoining skin surface. As SCC enlarges, it acquires a shallow, encrusted ulcer with an indurated border. There may be a significant inflammatory reaction.

Sections obtained from SCC biopsy specimens disclose an invasive neoplasm composed of atypical epithelial cells. The epidermal basement membrane is violated and tongues of tumor extend into the dermis (Fig. 2-28). The abundant eosinophilic cytoplasm and pathologic keratinization impart a distinctive pink hue in conventional H& E sections. Variable degrees of differentiation may be

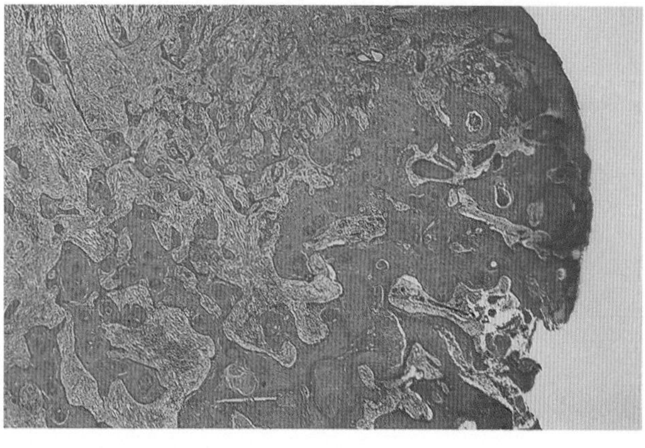

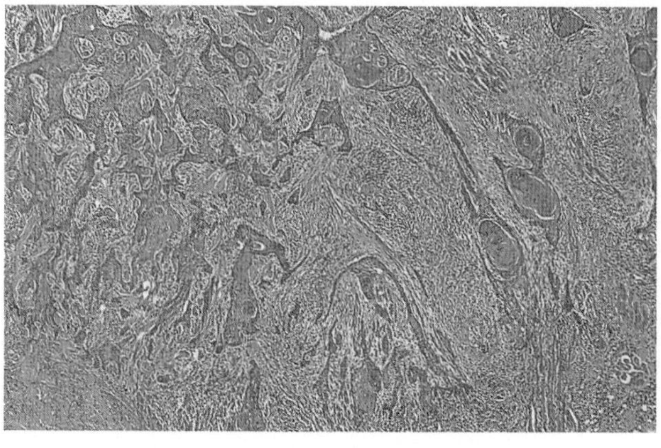

FIG. 2-28. Squamous cell carcinoma. Invasive malignant neoplasm composed of large, atypical epidermal epithelial cells. Hyperkeratosis, dyskeratosis, loss of polarity, squamous pearl formation.

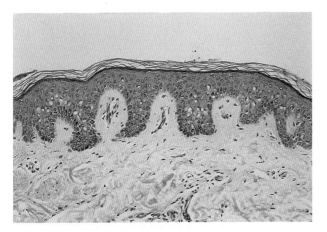

FIG. 2-29. Solar lentigo. Bulbous rete pegs with basilar pigmentation.

encountered within the same tumor. Squamous eddies encircling extracellular keratin pearls are a helpful feature. The tumor base confronts an intense chronic inflammatory infiltrate. Features of cytologic atypia include the presence of nuclear pleomorphism, hyperchromatism, dyskeratosis, and numerous abnormal mitotic figures. Complete excision usually is curative.

Melanocytic Lesions

The most common benign pigmented alteration to periorbital skin is the **ephelis** (freckle). In H&E-stained sections of small biopsy specimens, and without appropriate clinical information, it may be impossible to distinguish between ephelides and racial pigmentation. In each condition, a monolayer of benign pigmented cells occupies the basal epidermal layer. These cells include dendritic melanocytes and neighboring basal epithelial cells. Cellular atypia is not observed. Melanin granules (melanosomes) are produced by resident dendritic melanocytes and are inoculated into neighboring epithelial cells for storage and future degradation. This is the fundamental mechanism involving suntanning.

Lentigines also are pigmented patches that are derived from epidermal melanocytes (Fig. 2-29). They are flat or minimally elevated. **Lentigo simplex** is darker and larger than the ordinary freckle but is equally benign. In lentigo simplex, there are more melanocytes and a corresponding increase in melanin production. Representative tissue sections demonstrate elongation of the slender rete ridges, with melanin-bearing macrophages (melanophages) present within the papillary dermis. The **solar lentigo** is widely encountered in elderly patients. It clinically resembles lentigo simplex, but in solar lentigo the elongated rete ridges do not taper to a narrow terminus; rather, they end as a bulbous, foot-shaped process. Earlier pathologists described this finding as "dirty little feet." The final

lentiginous entity, **lentigo maligna,** is discussed below with other premalignant melanocytic disorders.

A clear understanding of the life cycle of melanocytic nevus cells simplifies the review of cutaneous nevi. First, the word *nevus* applies to any congenital abnormality of the skin. For purposes of this discussion, use of the word *nevus* will be limited to the melanocytic (nevocellular) nevus.

Cutaneous melanin pigmentation is caused by contributions from epidermal melanocytes, dermal melanocytes, and nevus cells situated in either level.[13] Although no absolute consensus exists, most embryologists believe all of these cells are of neural crest origin. During normal development, waves of neural crest cells migrate in a craniocaudal direction. Primitive melanocytes emanate from peripheral nerve tracts toward the skin surface. Nevus cells are specialized melanocytes. Viewed individually, nevus cells are indistinguishable from the normal dendritic epidermal melanocytes described earlier. Nevus cells tend to form nests and clusters.

At the earliest clinical stage, melanocytic nevus cells reside within the epidermis and are situated at the basal layer. These nevus cells may proliferate within the epidermis to form a **junctional nevus** (so named because they appear at the epidermal–dermal junction). Junctional nevi are darkly pigmented macules. The phrase "junctional activity" simply refers to the observation of nevus cells present within the epidermis (Fig. 2-30). Maturing nests of nevus cells descend into the dermis, a process characterized in the older literature as *abtropfung*. When nevus cells appear within both the epidermis and the dermis, the lesion is classified as a **compound nevus** (Fig. 2-31). Most congenital nevi are compound nevi. The compound nevus is lighter in color and slightly elevated. As the dermal migration continues, nevus cells tend to relax their nesting tendency (Fig. 2-32). Deep in the dermis, they appear as sheets of bland small blue cells, not unlike mature lymphocytes. The individual cells become more

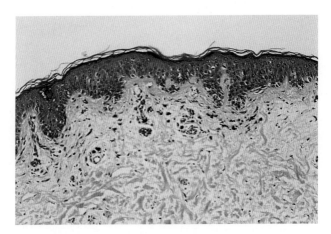

FIG. 2-30. Junctional nevus. Intraepidermal nests of benign nevus cells. Also note intradermal melanophages ingesting disgorged melanin.

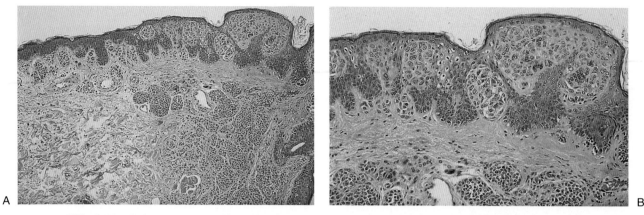

A

B

FIG. 2-31. Compound nevus [low (**A**) and high (**B**) power images]. Nests of melanocytic nevus cells reside both within the epidermis and the dermis.

compact, with a reduction of cytoplasm and melanin synthesis.

When the melanocytic nevus is totally confined to the dermis, it is an **intradermal nevus.** A thin band of collagen at the superficial nevus border often separates the intradermal nevus from the uninvolved epidermis. As expected, the intradermal nevus is pale tan and more elevated than its predecessors. An intradermal nevus may present clinically as a nodule or as a sessile papule with a verruciform surface. In fact, many intradermal nevi are misinterpreted clinically as squamous papillomas or warts.

In general, melanocytic nevi appear in infancy through early adulthood. Many completely regress, as evidenced by the infrequent discovery of nevi in elderly patients. Newly acquired pigmented skin lesions in older adults usually are not nevi.

There are several other pigmented nevi of practical significance to the clinician.[14] Their origins and histologic patterns differ from the common acquired nevi.

A **Spitz nevus** (spindle and epithelioid cell nevus, be-

nign juvenile melanoma) is another nevus variant that commonly appears on the facial and periorbital skin (Fig. 2-33). Originally thought to predominate in children, it has been recognized in all age groups. Its clinical appearance is that of a solitary pink or red-orange domed nodule. Rapid growth is characteristic. The histopathology can appear alarming to the uninitiated: it resembles a pleomorphic nevus composed of spindled and plumper epithelioid cells. Many Spitz nevi have been incorrectly diagnosed as melanomas; however, examination of the deeper dermis reveals the usual features of nevus maturation. The presence of dermal edema and telangiectasias strongly supports the diagnosis of Spitz nevus.

Not all melanocytic nevi originate in the epidermis. Some nevus cells never complete the embryonic journey to the epidermis; instead, they remain trapped within the dermis. **Blue nevi** are good examples. The bluish color imparted by these benign papules represents differential absorption and reflection of visible light (Tyndall phenomenon). Also called the dermal melanocytoma, the common blue nevus is composed of slender, wavy, dendritic melanocytes (Fig. 2-34). The diameter rarely exceeds 1 cm. Ample melanin is produced by these nevus cells, and extracellular pigment is ingested by dermal melanophages. An increased number of neighboring fibroblasts leads to focal dermal fibrosis. The cellular blue nevus generally is larger than the common blue nevus, averaging 1 to 3 cm in diameter. Nests of common blue nevus cells are separated by bundles of plump spindled cells harboring pale cytoplasm and variable melanin content. Investigators have proven that this second "neuroid" cell population also represents dendritic melanocytes. All levels of the dermis may be affected. When any common acquired nevus overlies a blue nevus, the resultant pigmented lesion is identified as a **combined nevus.**

One intriguing pigment alteration that involves the eyelids and the globe is the **nevus of Ota** (oculodermal melanocytosis). A blue-brown cutaneous discoloration is ob-

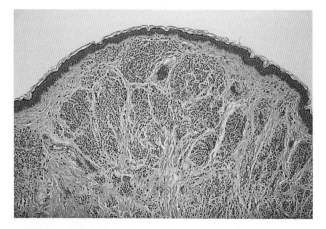

FIG. 2-32. Intradermal nevus. Nevus cells confined to the dermis. Maturing nevus cells shrink, are less cohesive, exhaust their pigment, and may resemble lymphocytes.

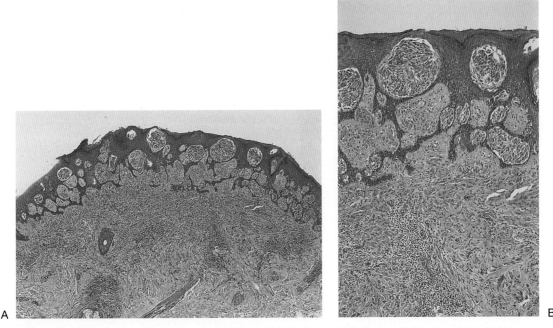

FIG. 2-33. Spitz nevus [low (**A**) and high (**B**) power images]. Spindled and plumper epithelioid nevus cells.

served most frequently along the distribution of the ophthalmic and maxillary branches of the trigeminal nerve, including the eyelid skin, periorbital skin, and ipsilateral conjunctiva and episclera. It is almost always unilateral. Blacks and Asians are more commonly affected. Isolated case reports have observed involvement of the inner ear and oral mucosa. The skin histopathology resembles the common blue nevus, in which an increased number of melanocytes populate the superficial dermis. The same process involves the entire uveal tract, resulting in heterochromia iridis and deeper choroidal pigmentation. Light reflecting off the dark-brown episcleral melanin deposition is filtered by overlying conjunctiva and

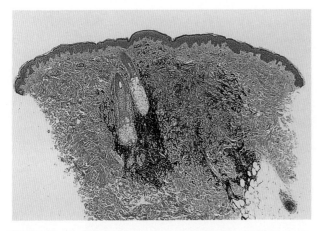

FIG. 2-34. Common blue nevus. Unlike the common melanocytic nevi, these pigmented nevus cells were trapped within the dermis and never occupied the epidermis.

Tenon's capsule to create the clinical appearance of a slate gray-blue globe discoloration. Some investigators identify nevus of Ota as a risk factor for the development of uveal malignant melanoma and primary orbital melanoma.

Two potentially worrisome lesions that appear on the eyelids and periorbital skin of adults are the dysplastic nevus and lentigo maligna.

The **dysplastic nevus** is a compound nevus with architectural disorder and melanocytic atypia. It appears as a solitary lesion in 5% of all Caucasians in the United States. The appearance of multiple dysplastic nevi in association with malignant melanoma makes up the **familial dysplastic nevus syndrome** (B-K mole syndrome). Recent reports suggest a linkage between dysplastic nevus syndrome and ocular melanoma. Dysplastic nevi can clinically resemble common nevi, with the additional findings of irregular or ill-defined borders, irregular pigmentation, accentuated skin markings, and diameter exceeding 5 mm. Under low-magnification microscopy, there is asymmetry of the lesion in which the atypical cells extend beyond the lateral border of the dermal component (Fig. 2-35). Elongated rete ridges joined by horizontally aligned n2-ests of nevus cells that overlay an acellular band of eosinophilic collagenous fibrosis are characteristic features. Dysplastic nevi can transform into malignant melanoma, but the actual incidence of this phenomenon is unproven.

Lentigo maligna (melanotic freckle of Hutchinson) appears most commonly on the face and extremities. Elderly patients are most frequently affected. This is the familiar pale-brown macule with irregular borders that grows

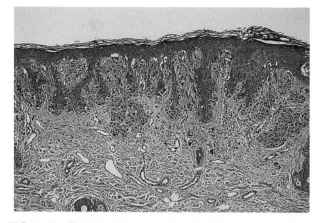

FIG. 2-35. Dysplastic nevus. Compound nevus with architectural disorder and melanocytic atypia.

slowly. Some spontaneously regress; others either exhaust their melanin or acquire additional darkened areas within the lesion. In the United States, about 5% of cases progress to the invasive **lentigo maligna melanoma.** Most of these are usually longstanding cases present for more than 10 years, as well as in larger patches (exceeding 4 cm). Tissue sections from lentigo maligna demonstrate changes in the epidermis and do not violate the basement membrane (Fig. 2-36). The basal melanocytes are increased in size and number. Proliferating melanocytes rise toward the surface. Cellular atypia is evident.

Not every patient conforms to the typical clinical characteristics of a given skin diagnosis. In dealing with any pigmented skin condition, one must not hesitate to perform (or repeat) a biopsy on any lesion that enlarges, exhibits an irregular border, becomes elevated or indurated, or exhibits variegated pigmentation.

In contrast to other body sites, invasive **malignant melanoma** arising in eyelid skin is rare: it accounts for less than 1% of primary eyelid malignancies. In the absence of nodal or distant tumor spread, the depth of invasion by melanoma is the key determinant of prognosis.

Adnexal Lesions (Including Relevant Cancer Syndromes)

There are proportionately more sebaceous glands, hair follicles, and sweat glands in the eyelid and periorbital skin than in other body surfaces. It is important to recognize the ocular and systemic conditions and syndromes that become manifest with tumors originating from adnexal epithelium.

Tumors arising from periorbital and eyelid epidermal appendages represent proliferations of pluripotential adnexal epithelium that differentiate toward the sebaceous glands, sweat glands, or hair. **Basal cell carcinoma,** on the other hand, arises from primary epithelial germ cells with little or no differentiation. Histogenesis aside, this

group of tumors has many similarities. Most are solitary in number and consist of nests and lobules of basaloid epithelium whose outer cell layer is oriented perpendicular to its contour, creating the familiar peripheral palisading, a contributory but nonspecific finding. Tumor lobules usually reside within a collagenous, hypercellular stroma. Each distinct epidermal appendage tumor develops specific morphologic features, discussed below.

Sebaceous

Three types of sebaceous glands reside in the periorbital region. The ordinary sebaceous glands appear within the pilosebaceous units of the facial and eyelid skin, as well as the caruncle. They are functionally and histologically similar to sebaceous glands found elsewhere in hair-bearing skin. The meibomian glands, situated deep within the tarsus, produce the oily component to the tear film. The glands of Zeis support the eyelash hair follicles. Each of the conditions described in this section can involve any of these sebaceous elements.

Sebaceous hyperplasia (senile sebaceous nevus) refers to a localized nonneoplastic proliferation of sebaceous glandular epithelium that usually affects older persons. If it involves the skin, sebaceous hyperplasia may appear as tan-yellow nodular plaques. Sebaceous hyperplasia arising within the tarsus creates thickening of the affected eyelid, with possible malposition (ectropion). The histologic appearance of sebaceous hyperplasia reveals enlargement in the size of the normal sebaceous lobule (Fig. 2-37). A dilated gland duct leads to a plugged follicular ostium.

Another well-circumscribed eyelid tumor arising from the sebaceous apparatus is **sebaceous adenoma.** This benign neoplasm is composed of multiple, irregular glandular lobules that host a biphasic cell population. Within each tumor lobule, mature sebaceous epithelium predominates, occupying half of the tumor mass (Fig.2-38). Also

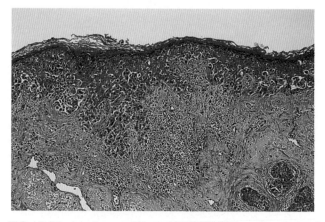

FIG. 2-36. Lentigo maligna. Noninvasive proliferation of atypical melanocytes within the epidermis.

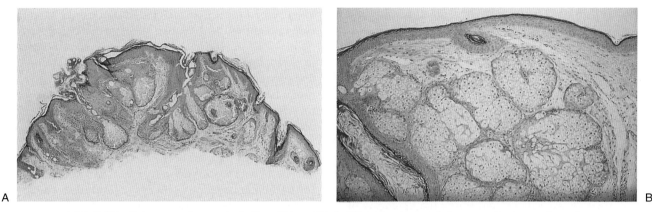

FIG. 2-37. Sebaceous hyperplasia [low (**A**) and high (**B**) power images]. Increase in size and number of normal-appearing sebaceous lobules.

present to a lesser extent are basaloid-appearing germinative cells. These can be misinterpreted as a variant of basal cell epithelioma.

The histopathology of sebaceous hyperplasia demonstrates enlarged but normal-appearing sebaceous lobules; sebaceous adenoma is characterized by multiple, irregular neoplastic lobules featuring a mix of mature and primitive adnexal epithelium.

Over the past decade, **sebaceous gland carcinoma** (masquerade syndrome) has received tremendous emphasis in the ophthalmic literature and in the training of clinicians.[15] Once considered an oddity, sebaceous gland carcinoma is now a target diagnosis that requires exclusion with every eyelid biopsy. Overlooked diagnoses of sebaceous gland carcinoma have tarnished reputations, have resulted in costly litigation, and most importantly have cost lives. It appears that the lesson has not been lost on the current generation of clinicians, as more and more biopsy specimens are received by laboratories specifically requesting ''rule out sebaceous carcinoma.'' Masquerade syndrome aptly describes the confounding clinical and histopathologic

appearances of this tumor. To both the clinician and pathologist, it may resemble other conditions (inflammatory and neoplastic); for this reason, sebaceous gland carcinoma should be considered in the differential diagnosis of most eyelid masses.

The challenges presented by sebaceous gland carcinoma may not be apparent. Nevertheless, it is a study of contradictions and lost opportunities. This malignant neoplasm primarily affects older adults, and most cases arise in the meibomian glands within the upper tarsal plate. Younger adults also may be affected, and sebaceous carcinoma also can originate in the glands of Zeis, or in the lower lid, the caruncle, or even the eyebrow. Unfortunately, the classic case of sebaceous carcinoma too frequently is the one diagnosed too late.

Pathologically, normal lobules of sebaceous gland are replaced by an anaplastic proliferation of carcinoma cells. This may clinically resemble the painless eyelid nodule encountered in chalazion. Some cases are, in fact, erroneously managed as a chalazion or recurrent chalazion without submission of the curettage specimen. Destruction of the normal piloseba-

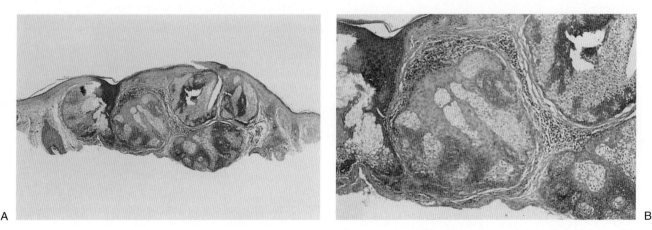

FIG. 2-38. Sebaceous adenoma [low (**A**) and high (**B**) power images]. Biphasic tumor population of mature and germinative epithelium.

ceous apparatus results in lash misdirection and madarosis (loss of cilia). Carcinoma cells migrate superficially and populate the epithelial surfaces of the eyelid margin and palpebral conjunctiva (pagetoid spread). Eventually, tumor cells may totally replace the normal squamous epithelium. Discohesive tumor cells and necrotic debris accumulate along the eyelid margin and are shed into the conjunctival cul-de-sac. The toxic contents of the lysed carcinoma cells contaminate the tear film and irritate the globe. Before long, the patient appears to have developed a unilateral blepharoconjunctivitis.

The greatest obstacle to confirming the diagnosis of sebaceous gland carcinoma is developing the necessary clinical suspicion. Most ophthalmic pathologists have little difficulty in recognizing this malignancy under the microscope with routine H&E-stained sections (Fig. 2-39). On the other hand, most surgical pathologists have limited experience with this disease because the sum of eyelid sebaceous carcinoma cases greatly exceeds those found in all other body sites combined. Once again, clear communication and timely consultation facilitate diagnostic accuracy.

No discussion of sebaceous carcinoma is complete without describing the technique for performing frozen sections of representative biopsy tissue with the oil red-O stain. This special stain imparts a vivid or-

ange color to lipid, and some laboratories rely on this step to confirm the diagnosis of sebaceous gland carcinoma. The oil red-O method works only if lipid is present; consequently, conventional paraffin-embedded permanent sections are ineligible for this technique because many of the chemicals used to process the tissue dissolve lipids. Frozen sections performed on fresh tissue are ideal. Sometimes the diagnosis of sebaceous gland carcinoma is not considered until the day after the biopsy is performed. If some of the original tissue was preserved in formalin and not submitted for permanent sections (always a good idea whenever practical), it can be retrieved, rinsed, and used for frozen sections, as lipids do not dissolve in formalin. Formalinized frozen sections adhere better to albumin-coated glass microscope slides. Oil red-O staining then can be performed.

There is great interest in the association between sebaceous gland tumors and the development of coexistent distant primary malignancies.[16] Multiple sebaceous adenomas are the clinical hallmark of **Muir-Torre syndrome.** Colon carcinoma is the most frequent accompanying neoplasm, although many other solid and hematopoietic cancers have been implicated. Much new information has been reported since Muir introduced this condition in 1967. Keratoacanthomas, BCCs with sebaceous differentiation, sebaceous hyperplasia, and seba-

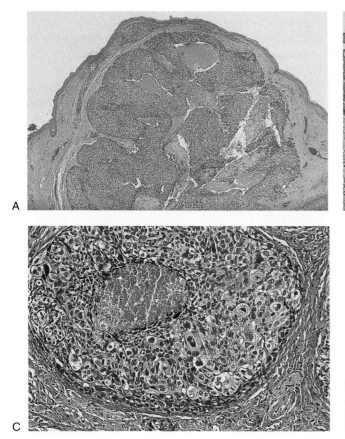
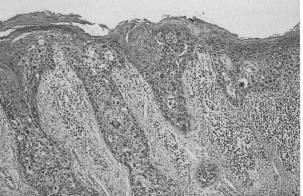

A

B

C

FIG. 2-39. Sebaceous carcinoma (three composite images). Normal sebaceous apparatus replaced by malignant cellular proliferation. Note tumor comedones and intraepithelial spread of carcinoma (pagetoid spread).

ceous carcinoma have been included as markers for the syndrome. In most cases, the cutaneous mass precedes discovery of the internal malignancy.

Sweat Gland

Syringomas, benign neoplasms arising from the eccrine sweat ducts, are the most common adnexal eyelid tumor. They usually appear as multiple small soft papules and predominantly involve the lower eyelid skin. Syringomas more often occur in adolescent and adult females. Patients report unsuccessful attempts at evacuating these small nodules with a needle-tip or tweezers, as they would a comedone. Histologically, syringomas are situated within the dermis, are composed of dilated sweat ducts, and are embedded in a dense fibrous stroma (Fig. 2-40). The ductal elements appear round, oval, or teardrop-shaped in cross-section. The ducts are lined by an attenuated bilayer of cuboidal epithelium. The duct lumen harbors amorphous proteinaceous material. In more superficial syringomas, keratin may be present within the lumen. Unattached strands and clusters of basophilic epithelium also are observed.

The lacrimal gland is a modified sweat gland. Conversely, tumors that occur in the lacrimal gland also have a propensity for the periorbital skin sweat apparatus. **Pleomorphic adenoma** (benign mixed tumor, chondroid syringoma) is more familiar to clinicians as the most common benign neoplasm originating in the lacrimal gland. Interestingly, this same lesion occurs in the head and neck skin. It presents as a small firm nonmobile dermal nodule that may measure 3 cm or larger. The histologic appearance of pleomorphic adenoma is identical to its orbital counterpart. It contains an epithelial component set amidst a mesenchymal response (Fig. 2-41). Cords and nests of basaloid epithelium reside within a mucoid stroma. The epithelial bilayer surrounds tubular lumens, many of which are cystically dilated. The inner epithelial layer is cuboidal and secretes mucopolysaccharides. The spindled

outer myoepithelial layer is believed to be responsible for producing variable stromal elements: cartilage, hyaline deposition, and dense fibrosis. A pleomorphic adenoma involving the eyelid can arise from three possible sources: eyelid skin, the supratarsal conjunctival accessory glands of Wolfring, and the palpebral lobe of the lacrimal gland. The tumor origin should be accurately identified.

Three additional benign sweat gland tumors are syringocystadenoma papilliferum, eccrine spiradenoma, and clear-cell hidradenoma (eccrine acrospiroma). These have all been reported to involve eyelid and periorbital skin but appear far less frequently. Readers with an interest in these uncommon entities can obtain additional information in the references provided.

Pilar

This review of eyelid adnexal tumors concludes with a discussion of the hair-forming elements. The periorbital skin and eyelids generate a variety of hairs: fine, nearly imperceptible vellus hairs distributed uniformly across the skin surface; eyebrow hairs, similar to the coarse terminal hairs found on the scalp and axillae; and cilia, the eyelashes. The cilia deserve special mention as they perform a supplemental sensory function. Abundant nerve endings are situated at the base of the cilia follicles. Eyelashes do not have smooth muscle attachments to the follicle wall (arrector pili), an additional anatomic exception. Ostensibly, foreign matter striking the lashes triggers immediate lid closure to protect the globe. Eyebrow hairs adopt coloration similar to scalp hair (including gray); normally, lashes remain darkly pigmented throughout life. Clinically relevant skin tumors arising from the hair follicle include trichoepithelioma, trichilemmoma, trichofolliculoma, and the pilomatricoma. Their clinical and histopathologic differentiation can be as tricky as their names.[17,18]

Trichoepithelioma (epithelioma adenoides cysticum of Brooke) is one of the most common benign hair follicle

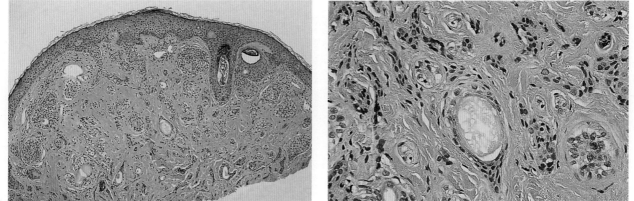

FIG. 2-40. Syringoma [low (**A**) and high (**B**) power images]. Benign sweat ductal proliferation within dermis.

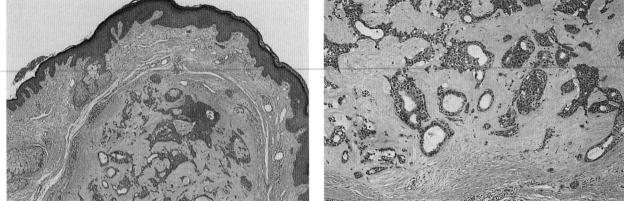

FIG. 2-41. Pleomorphic adenoma [low (**A**) and high (**B**) power images]. Similar to lacrimal gland counterpart, epithelial tumor includes glandular inner layer and outer myoepithelial stroma.

neoplasms involving the eyelid and periorbital skin. Singular or multiple in number, the clinical appearance of these fleshy nodules resembles BCC. They develop primarily in children and young adults. Multiple trichoepitheliomas can appear in the head and neck as well as the trunk. The inherited form of multiple trichoepitheliomas is transmitted in an autosomal dominant fashion. As suggested earlier, a cursory glance at histologic sections of trichoepithelioma may lead to misinterpretation (Fig. 2-42). Well-circumscribed lobules of basaloid cells exhibit peripheral palisading and surround a central keratin-filled core. The eosinophilic material within these horn cysts represents abortive hair follicle formation; it may stimulate a foreign body giant cell inflammatory reaction. Some basal cell epitheliomas differentiate so as to produce primitive hairs. Elsewhere, confluent nests of basaloid cells may exhibit a lace-like or cloverleaf pattern. Unlike basal cell epithelioma, the clefting artifact in trichoepithelioma is present within the planes of the hypercellular stroma and does not involve the basaloid cells. Nevertheless, the overlapping histopathologic features

may necessitate clinical correlation to enable the pathologist to reach a definitive diagnosis.

Trichilemmoma appears as another nodular or wart-like fleshy growth derived from the outer hair sheath of the hair follicle. The Greek noun *lemma* means rind, so whenever the suffix ''-lemmoma'' is used, the tumor should be associated with some type of covering or sheath (eg, neurilemmoma, trichilemmoma). Fortunately, the microscopic appearance of a trichilemmoma is more specific than its clinical presentation. Plate-like sheets of vacuolated, glycogen-rich epithelium stain poorly with H&E. Tumor lobules remain attached to either a hair follicle or its overlying epidermis. A delicate pink cuticle (compressed basement membrane) often outlines the peripherally palisading tumor cells (Fig. 2-43). The presence of multiple facial trichilemmomas may represent an inherited (autosomal dominant) multiple hamartoma syndrome known as Cowden disease, a cutaneous marker for an occult nonocular neoplasm. Breast cancer in women is the most frequently associated malignancy discovered in this syndrome.

Trichofolliculoma is uncommon in the periorbital

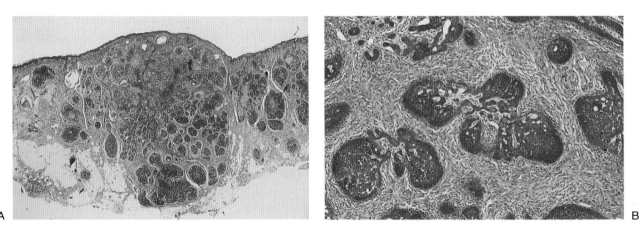

FIG. 2-42. Trichoepithelioma [low (**A**) and high (**B**) power images]. Lobules of basaloid epithelium with a keratin core.

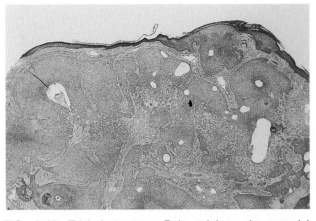

FIG. 2-43. Tricholemmoma. Pale-staining, glycogen-rich epithelium. Tumor lobules remain attached to hair follicle or overlying epidermis.

skin, but its highly characteristic clinical appearance deserves mention. Visual inspection of this solitary, firm, flesh-colored nodule will often identify a central pore from which tufts of filamentous white hairs emerge. Low-power microscopy of trichofolliculoma demonstrates a cystic process lined by keratinizing squamous epithelium. The cyst is filled with birefringent fragmented hair shafts and keratinaceous debris. Oriented toward the base of this cyst are multiple, smaller, interconnecting secondary follicles. Peripheral palisading of the basaloid epithelium is again demonstrated, as is focal vacuolization due to intracytoplasmic glycogen accumulation (Fig. 2-44).

The final hair-related tumor to be discussed is another benign histopathologic curiosity that is more frequently discussed than it is observed clinically. **Pilomatricoma** (benign calcifying epithelioma of Malherbe) is uncommon. Most pilomatricomas arise in childhood, although all ages can be affected. Facial pilomatricomas appear along the eyebrows and eyelid skin, and solitary lesions are the rule. This mobile nodule is usually very firm and

blue-red; it varies in size from 0.5 to 5 cm. Under the microscope, one finds a well-circumscribed dermal mass bordered by a connective tissue pseudocapsule. This mass is composed of a neoplastic proliferation of differentiating hair cortex cells (Fig. 2-45). Basophilic epithelial cells predominate at the periphery. A transition zone often is identified in which the basophilic cells mature into pale, anucleate, keratinized shadow cells. Extracellular aggregates of keratin are present within the tumor stroma. The ratio of basophilic cells to shadow cells generally declines with the age of the lesion. Some longstanding pilomatricomas have only shadow cells. Previous authors have noted that 75% of pilomatricomas feature dense focal calcium deposits and ossification zones interposed between the epithelial islands.

In addition to the squamous epithelium, melanocytes, adnexal elements, and various dermal elements also contribute to the pathology of the periorbital and eyelid skin. Disorders in this final subgroup are far less common in clinical practice and are even less frequently suspected as the preoperative diagnosis. Primary intradermal tumors may arise from fibrous connective tissue, nerves, blood vessels, or lymphoid elements.

Fibrous

The benign **dermatofibroma** (fibrous histiocytoma, sclerosing hemangioma) is a solitary nodule more common in the orbit than in the eyelids. These reddish, firm nodules more characteristically arise in adults, and they can appear either singly or in multiples. Dermatofibroma is composed of a vascularized admixture of spindled cells and histiocytic cells (Fig. 2-46). The multiplicity of names applied to this condition reflects variations in its histologic makeup. Dermatofibromas themselves are predominantly composed of comma-shaped tumor cells that resemble fibroblasts. Bundles of collagen become trapped between these proliferating spindled cells. Fibrous histiocytoma

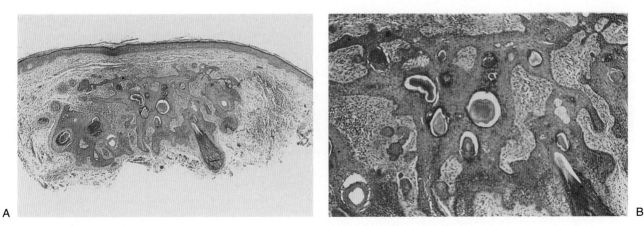

A   B

FIG. 2-44. Trichofolliculoma [low (**A**) and high (**B**) power images]. Basaloid epithelium forms cysts filled with primitive hair.

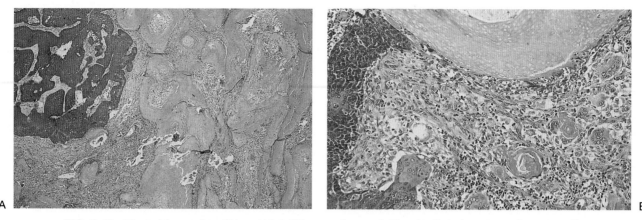

FIG. 2-45. Pilomatricoma [low (**A**) and high (**B**) power images]. Neoplastic hair cortex cells, extracellular keratin, shadow cells, calcific foci, and foreign body reaction.

connotes a preponderance of foamy, vacuolated histiocytes, and if an abundant vasculature is appreciated, the appellation "sclerosing hemangioma" is used. Regardless of the basic tumor morphology, overlying epidermal hyperplasia is a unifying histopathologic feature of most dermatofibromas.

Juvenile fibromatosis should be included in the list of "juvenile" conditions that can become manifest in adults. A rare condition, this is a benign, slow-growing, nontender nodule. Measuring less than 2 cm, this firm mass is not mobile because it usually adheres to the periosteum of the orbital bone. This clinical presentation evokes a worrisome differential diagnosis that includes malignant fibrous histiocytoma and sarcoma. Microscopic interpretation of the excised specimen can be just as challenging, and additional investigative studies (eg, electron microscopy, immunohistochemistry) may be required to establish the diagnosis. One encounters a poorly circumscribed proliferation of elongated fibroblasts featuring plump, spindle-shaped nuclei and indistinct cell borders. Wavy collagen bundles are interspersed between the intersecting fascicles of tumor cells; a storiform ("woven mat") appearance also has been described. Mitoses are rare, and tumor giant cells should not be present. These last two characteristics help distinguish it from more aggressive conditions. Incomplete excision leads to recurrence of juvenile fibromatosis, whereupon wide excision becomes necessary to achieve a cure.

Angiofibromas are the reddish papules known to most clinicians as the misnamed "adenoma sebaceum." They are one element of tuberous sclerosis (Bourneville disease), which also includes mental retardation and seizures, ostensibly due to cerebral glial hamartomas. Clusters of facial angiofibromas are situated along the nasolabial folds and mouth. Periorbital involvement is not uncommon in severe cases. The major histopathologic findings are dermal fibrosis and capillary dilatation. Elastic tissue is absent in angiofibromas. As the lesions mature, the accumulation of sclerotic collagen leads to compression of the neighboring pilosebaceous apparatus.

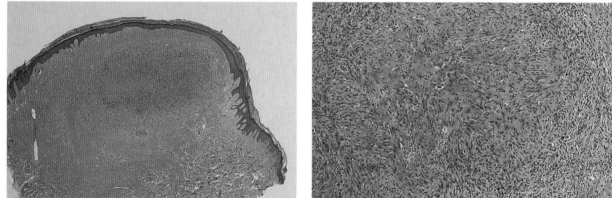

FIG. 2-46. Dermatofibroma [low (**A**) and high (**B**) power images]. Bland spindled cells amidst collagen. Note overlying epidermal hyperplasia.

Neural

Peripheral nerves are complex, highly organized structures. One axon coated by a multilaminar myelin sheath makes up the elementary nerve fiber. Nerve fibers themselves are embedded within a rich network of endoneural fibrils. Bundles of nerve fibers then are surrounded by a dense perineural sheath to form a nerve fascicle. Epineural connective tissue binds multiple fascicles to complete the organization of the composite peripheral nerve.

Peripheral nerve tumors infrequently arise in the skin. The orbit is more commonly affected, so lid abnormalities may be the earliest clinical suggestion of a deeper orbital process. One must always determine whether a neural mass is confined to the skin. The actual nerve contribution to many ''neural'' neoplasms (the axons and nerve fibers) is highly variable and frequently nil. Instead, fibroblasts, perineural cells, and Schwann cells generate the bulk of these growths. It is the particular mixture of these supporting elements that contributes to a specific tumor's identity. Beyond histopathology, the greater significance of cutaneous neural tumors lies with their affiliation with neurocutaneous syndromes (phakomatoses). This section will deal with the three most common periorbital cutaneous neural tumors: neurofibroma, neurilemmoma, and traumatic neuroma. These and other related conditions are discussed in greater detail in Chapter 12.

The cutaneous **neurofibroma** is a soft, firm, nonencapsulated dermal mass that can arise singly or in multiples.[19] It is frequently tender. Most initially appear in childhood, and they slowly enlarge throughout life. These tumors show great variability in size: small pedunculated neurofibromas that appear at the lid margin are *molluscum fibromas;* huge pendulous masses coursing the length of affected peripheral nerve segments characterize *elephantiasis neuromatosa.* Histologically, the neurofibroma is essentially a neoplasm of nerve sheath tissue.

Neurofibromas are subdivided into several descriptive categories, but they represent expressions of the same fundamental process. The **isolated neurofibroma** is a haphazard accumulation of bland, elongated spindled cells with oval, wavy nuclei. Mast cells are easily identified within this circumscribed tumor (Fig. 2-47). As mentioned earlier, few myelinated nerve fibers are demonstrated. Isolated neurofibromas are not always solitary. The *diffuse neurofibroma* is an infiltrative process that often extends deep into the orbital soft tissues. Individual neurofibromas may appear as solid proliferations of nerve sheath elements or less cellular proliferations set within a myxoid stroma.

None of these cutaneous neurofibromas automatically invites or excludes a systemic disorder; however, **plexiform neurofibromas** have great clinical relevance. The plexiform neurofibroma is a destructive infiltrative process composed of hyperplastic peripheral nerve terminal branches. They traditionally arise in deeper, larger nerves. In addition to marked enlargement of the involved peripheral nerve axons, there is corresponding proliferation of the surrounding perineurium, enveloping Schwann cells, and endoneural fibroblasts (Fig. 2-48). The actual number of nerve fibers within a plexiform neurofibroma is not increased. The diagnosis of plexiform neurofibroma, with rare exception, is tantamount to a diagnosis of von Recklinghausen peripheral neurofibromatosis.

The correct designation for Schwann cells is neurilemma. These cells ensheath or surround the individual axons and provide myelin to the peripheral nerves. **Neurilemmoma,** therefore, describes a neoplasm composed of proliferating Schwann cells (**schwannoma**). Neurilemmomas are usually single and small, rarely exceeding 5 cm in diameter. They remain attached to a peripheral nerve, and any mechanical impingement on the host nerve may evoke symptoms. At the time of surgical excision, the tumor can be observed arising from the nerve sheath and independent of the nerve itself. Neurilemmomas have been described in patients with neurofibromatosis; conversely, neurofibromas have schwannian elements. The histopathology of the neurilemmoma reveals a well-

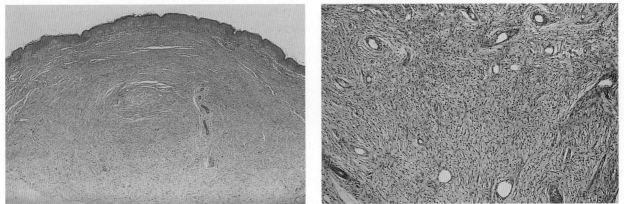

FIG. 2-47. Neurofibroma [low (**A**) and high (**B**) power images]. Elongated endoneural fibroblasts.

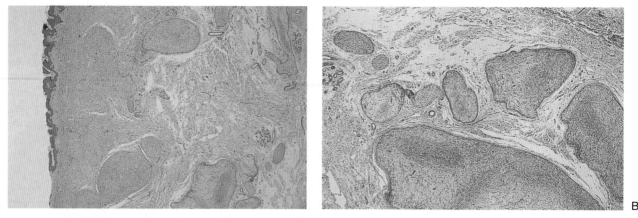

FIG. 2-48. Plexiform neurofibroma [low (**A**) and high (**B**) power images]. Sharply demarcated nests of proliferating endoneural fibroblasts and Schwann cells, myxoid background.

encapsulated mass that features a biphasic tumor population—the so-called Antoni A and Antoni B patterns.[19] Antoni A is the densely cellular region of compact spindled tumor cells. Individual tumor cells have a slender, wavy nucleus (Fig. 2-49). Regimented bundles of palisading Schwann cells create a familiar tissue pattern. Two parallel rows of tumor cells are configured with their nuclei at opposite poles. Centrally, the indistinct cell borders create a homogenous, eosinophilic core called a *Verocay body*. This finding is supportive but not pathognomonic of the diagnosis of neurilemmoma. Antoni B portions of the neurilemmoma are more edematous and disorganized. There appear fewer tumor cells, and they appear scattered amidst a mucinous stroma. Neurilemmomas rarely undergo malignant change.

The final cutaneous nerve tumor discussed here is the traumatic neuroma (amputation neuroma). Described as an exuberant response to tissue injury, the traumatic neuroma is a sharply demarcated but nonencapsulated proliferation of perineural cells and collagen separating widely scattered axons. Clinically, these dermal nodules are exquisitely sensitive to touch. Most patients relate a history of previous surgery or trauma to the region.

Vascular

Cutaneous vascular abnormalities involving the eyelids can be congenital or acquired. The risk of amblyopia adds an important dimension to the clinical management of these conditions in infants and preschool children.

The most common vascular lesion affecting the eyelids is the **capillary hemangioma** (strawberry hemangioma). It is a true hamartoma because it is a proliferation of normal tissue at a normal anatomic location. Most are observed at birth or within the first weeks of life, and over 90% are noted by age 6 months. Red or purplish, they are pliable and have a pebbly surface. Subcutaneous or orbital hemangiomas have a dusky color and may cause exophthalmos. The size of a capillary hemangioma can vary markedly, ranging from a few millimeters to a large elevated hemifacial mass. The natural course of capillary hemangioma exhibits a period of progressive growth of the lesion (age 0 to 2 years), followed by slow regression and shrinkage of the mass (age 2 to 6 years). Large eyelid capillary hemangiomas may lead to occlusion and astigmatism and consequent amblyopia. Therapeutic intervention with the use of intralesional corticosteroid injections, cryotherapy, and laser ablation may help reduce the tumor bulk. By age 6 years, the process normally stabilizes. Previously taut overlying eyelid skin becomes overstretched and flaccid, imparting a crêpe paper appearance. Histopathologically, one finds a nonencapsulated proliferation of capillaries and pericytes (Fig. 2-50). Larger collecting vessels are usually present; however, confluent lobules of capillaries predominate, best appreciated under higher magnification. Brisk mitotic activity may be present. Treated and regressing lesions may demonstrate larger vessels with an accompanying fibrotic stroma.

Unlike capillary hemangioma, the **cavernous heman-**

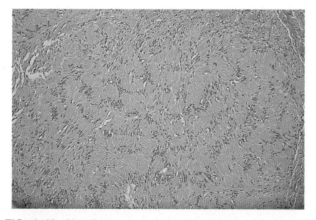

FIG. 2-49. Neurilemmoma. Antoni A pattern with densely packed spindled cells organized into fascicles. Parallel rows of polarized nuclei form Verocay bodies.

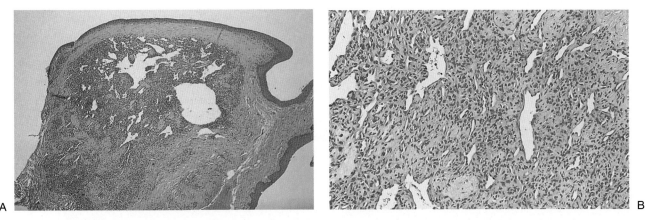

FIG. 2-50. Capillary hemangioma [low (**A**) and high (**B**) power images]. Nonencapsulated proliferation of capillaries and larger collecting vessels.

gioma is a vascular malformation most often diagnosed in adults. It is a slowly enlarging, indolent mass that does not spontaneously regress. It may enlarge after the Valsalva maneuver. Rarely a *de novo* eyelid mass, its appearance usually connotes a larger orbital process. Chronic progressive expansion leads to the formation of a dense pseudocapsule. The cavernous hemangioma is composed of large, dilated, endothelium-lined vascular spaces filled with blood (Fig. 2-51). The spaces are separated by delicate septa that contain smooth muscle cells. Venous blood perfuses sluggishly through this lesion (as demonstrated by radiologic and echographic imaging studies), and thrombosis is common. The absence of any significant stromal inflammatory infiltrate or lymphoid follicles favors the diagnosis of cavernous hemangioma over lymphangioma.

Nevus flammeus (port-wine nevus) refers to the congenital cutaneous hemangioma seen in association with Sturge-Weber syndrome (encephalotrigeminal angiomatosis). It is always present at birth. It may appear flat or minimally elevated. Histologically, the nevus flammeus is an intradermal cavernous hemangioma (Fig. 2-52). It does not blanch to digital pressure, and its color tends to be a darker purple than the infantile capillary hemangioma. Most of these lesions are ipsilateral and respect the sagittal midline; however, bilateral cases do occur. Upper eyelid involvement is highly predictive for the development of an ipsilateral open angle glaucoma.

Another hamartoma that affects the eyelid is the **lymphangioma.** Its pathogenesis remains obscure. It has endothelium-lined vascular spaces without pericytes. The endothelial cells do not demonstrate immunoreactivity to factor VIII-related antigen (as seen in capillary and cavernous hemangiomas), but all three lesions react to *Ulex europaeus* agglutinin I.

Three types of **cutaneous lymphangiomas** have been described: lymphangioma circumscriptum (dermal), cavernous lymphangioma (deep tissues), and cystic hygroma (more common in the neck). Lymphangioma circumscriptum is a localized, noninflamed cluster of vesicular nodules that may resemble other papillomatous skin conditions. Patients often report a longstanding history of the growth. Wide surgical excision is usually curative. Most cavernous lymphangiomas are diagnosed in infancy or

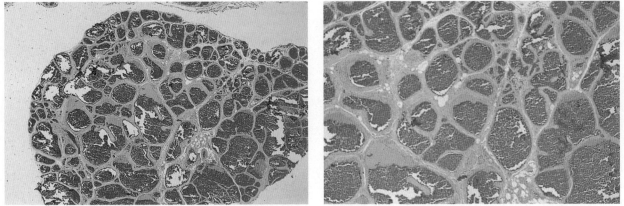

FIG. 2-51. Cavernous hemangioma [low (**A**) and high (**B**) power images]. Pseudoencapsulated vascular lesion features large blood-filled spaces separated by delicate fibrous septa.

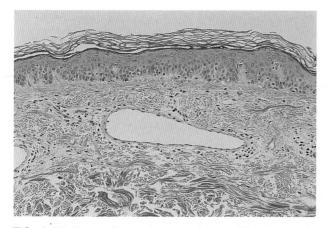

FIG. 2-52. Nevus flammeus. Intradermal dilated vascular spaces.

early childhood, and they progressively enlarge over time. This is the most common form of lymphangioma to affect the ocular adnexa and orbit. Lesions can vary from small, isolated, compressible cystic nodules to very large and complex multilobed masses that communicate across several facial regions.

Experienced surgeons approach periorbital lymphangiomas with enormous trepidation. Most surgical attempts to debulk the mass are merely palliative. This is a highly infiltrative process that extends into the surrounding muscle, adipose, and fibrous connective tissues. Visual loss is a risk due to amblyopia, tumor mass effect, and potential surgical complications. The histopathologic appearance of the lymphangioma characteristically features variably sized and irregularly shaped vascular spaces set within a fibrous stroma. Blood or serous fluid may be present within the vascular spaces. If intralesional hemorrhage has occurred, erythrocytes and blood breakdown products can be demonstrated.

Because vascular spaces and hemorrhage are common to both hemangiomas and lymphangiomas, can they be differentiated histopathologically? One helpful diagnostic feature seen in lymphangiomas is the presence of stromal lymphoid follicles, many surrounding germinal centers (Fig. 2-53).

An important cutaneous manifestation of AIDS is **Kaposi sarcoma** (KS). Currently, researchers attribute HIV suppression of vascular endothelial contact inhibition as the most likely causative factor for this lethal neoplasm. KS is a vascular malignancy composed of proliferating capillaries, slit-like vascular spaces, and a spindled stroma (Fig. 2-54). Extravasated erythrocytes are an expected finding. At an initial glance, it may resemble a capillary hemangioma or a pyogenic granuloma. Histopathologically, the differential diagnosis includes spindle cell (squamous) carcinoma, hemangioendothelioma, bacillary angiomatosis (cat-scratch agent *B. henselae*), and angiosarcoma. Before the AIDS epidemic, KS predominantly affected older men of Ashkenazic Jewish and Mediterra-

nean descent. It classically began in the extremities and rarely involved the facial region. Today, eyelid or conjunctival involvement with KS may be the earliest physical manifestation of AIDS.[20] KS develops in 30% of all AIDS patients in the United States. Lesions appear in the eyelid and conjunctiva in 20% of AIDS-associated KS. It presents initially as a minimally elevated red-violet patch that may resemble a simple bruise. Currently, the clinical diagnosis of periocular KS is indicative of full-blown AIDS. KS follows a far more aggressive clinical course in HIV-infected patients than in other patient subgroups. In addition to treating local and presumed systemic KS, a comprehensive evaluation is performed to assess the patient's immune status and to identify other treatable AIDS-related disorders.

Lymphoid

Various lymphoproliferative disorders can arise in the eyelid. These diseases may involve or ignore the epidermis. This section highlights the primary lymphoid conditions that originate in the eyelid, as opposed to direct extension of an orbital or sinus condition, or secondary involvement from distant spread.

There are no lymph nodes in the eyelid, and this fact may explain why primary lymphoid neoplasms are relatively rare in this anatomic region. Conversely, the duplicate blood supply and ample lymphatics within the eyelids lend themselves to secondary involvement by a neighboring or distant process.

The clinician cannot be expected to interpret any lymphoid process with accuracy as malignant or benign. Instead, he or she is best served by becoming familiar with the steps that should be taken in the planning and execution of tissue biopsy for any suspected ocular adnexal lymphoproliferative process.

Before contemplating any biopsy, a thorough medical

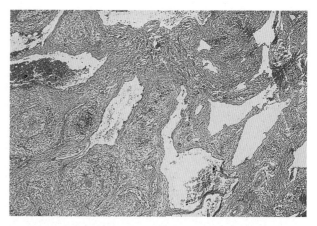

FIG. 2-53. Lymphangioma. Germinal centers reside within the fibrous septa that divide the endothelial-lined fluid spaces.

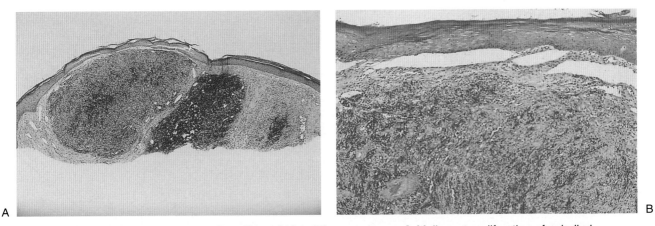

A   B

FIG. 2-54. Kaposi sarcoma [low (**A**) and high (**B**) power images]. Malignant proliferation of spindled cells with slit spaces and extravasated blood.

history, a complete physical examination, and appropriate imaging studies should be performed to confirm that the mass is indeed confined to the eyelid. These steps help exclude the possibility of widespread lymphoma or, just as likely, primary orbital or sinus-related lymphoma manifesting clinically as a more limited entity. Knowles and coworkers have reported that patients with primary eyelid lymphoid tumors, benign or malignant, always complained of a palpably enlarged mass and ptosis but did not typically experience proptosis or diplopia.[21]

In general, there are few small lymphomas; in other words, the tissue changes that induce the patient's initial presentation are not subtle. There should be adequate tissue for biopsy. Sampling of any mass should harvest sufficient tissue for the performance of conventional histopathology and special studies. Scrape and touch cytologic preparations performed on fresh tissue can usually provide immediate preliminary information regarding the presence of malignancy. Laboratory protocols vary by institution; however, one popular approach divides the fresh specimen into several fragments. Separate portions are placed in 10% buffered formalin and B5 fixative (formaldehyde with mercuric chloride) for routine permanent sections. Another portion should be placed in RPMI-1640* solution or another suitable culture media for flow cytometry. The remainder is snap-frozen with cyclohexane immersion for molecular hybridization analysis. If the specimen is so small that it cannot be divided, it is prudent to perform a touch prep and submit the entire specimen in formalin for permanent sections. The simplest way to coordinate these steps is to seek preoperative consultation with a pathologist who regularly deals with lymphoid tumors involving other body sites.

There is a collection of benign dermatoses that resemble malignant lymphoma and are called **pseudolymphoma** (lymphocytoma cutis). Pseudolymphoma presents clinically as a reddish nodule or plaque. It may be single or multiple, and the facial skin is most often affected. Clinical differentiation from non-Hodgkin's lymphoma is impossible because both conditions may begin in this fashion. The histopathology gives no significant assistance in qualifying the lesion as benign or malignant. Under the microscope, pseudolymphoma appears as a nodular infiltrate within the reticular dermis (Fig. 2-55). This infiltrate is separated from the overlying epidermis by the narrow collagenous Grenz zone in the superficial dermis. These nodules contain aggregates of lymphoid cells that include small and large lymphocytes and histiocytes. Germinal centers also are encountered. The discovery of plasma cells and eosinophils within the infiltrate favors a benign process. On the other hand, local areas of cytologic atypia with brisk mitotic activity may be indistinguishable from malignant lymphoma. This is one of those perplexing disorders whose final diagnosis is based on its clinical behavior. Pseudolymphoma lesions eventually regress, sometimes years later, and usually do not progress to disseminated nodal disease.

Because this is an ophthalmic pathology text, representative cases are presented to illustrate the clinical spectrum of ocular adnexal lymphoid disease. Low-power examination of the overall specimen provides an enormous amount of useful information and should not be overlooked in the rush to examine the specimen under higher magnification.

Lymphoid hyperplasia accounts for half of all adnexal lymphoid proliferations; the rest are diagnosed as malignant lymphoma. **Benign reactive lymphoid hyperplasia** (BRLH) can appear as a unilateral or bilateral mass. Vigorous debate surrounds the issue as to whether BRLH can progress to malignant lymphoma. Consensus is not crucial because patients with primary eyelid BRLH and

*RPMI-1640 is a widely available transport media solution named for Roswell Park Memorial Institute. It is refrigerated until needed, then warmed to room temperature before fresh tissue is introduced. At least 2 mL of fresh tissue is needed to perform flow cytometry. The fresh tissue should be cut into small cubes to optimize cell viability.

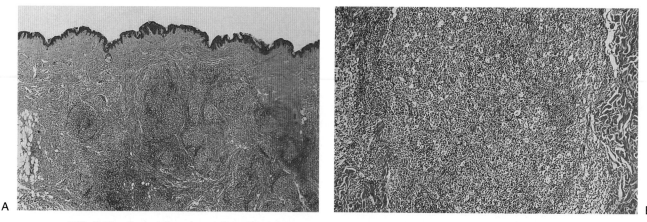

FIG. 2-55. Pseudolymphoma [low (**A**) and high (**B**) power images]. Collagenous Grenz zone separates nodular lymphoid infiltrate from overlying epidermis.

primary eyelid malignant lymphoma have the same risk (67%) of subsequently developing extraocular lymphoma. Considering all ophthalmic and orbital structures, a lymphoid proliferation arising in the eyelid has the greatest likelihood of progressing to disseminated lymphoma.[21]

Histologically, BRLH exhibits a follicular architecture (Fig. 2-56). Within a polymorphous proliferation of mature (small, round, and blue) lymphocytes, plasma cells, rare eosinophils, and histiocytes appear paler-staining germinal centers that harbor tingible body macrophages. These macrophages impart the ''starry sky'' appearance to the germinal center. Endothelial cell proliferation also is an expected finding. Because BRLH shares features similar to low-grade non-Hodgkin's lymphoma, immunohistochemical staining and flow cytometry are used to determine whether the lymphoid proliferation is polyclonal (benign) or monoclonal (malignant). A definitive diagnosis should not be based on a single laboratory finding, particularly if it conflicts with other available data. For example, if all histopathologic indices point to a benign process, one should not label a lymphoid mass malignant simply because focal monoclonality is observed with immunostaining.

Bridging the unequivocally benign from unmistakably malignant is **atypical lymphoid hyperplasia.** Poorly defined lymphoid follicles, if any, are observed amidst a monotonous proliferation of mature lymphocytes. In atypical lymphoid hyperplasia, the small lymphocytes exhibit cytologic irregularities (Fig. 2-57). These cells exhibit a more open chromatin pattern, irregular nuclear shapes, inconspicuous nucleoli, and more numerous mitoses. Multinucleated histiocytes are an additional finding not encountered in BRLH.

Primary **malignant lymphoma** arising in the eyelid is nearly always a non-Hodgkin's lymphoma. Patients are usually in their sixth decade or older. Primary malignant lymphoma may arise in the ocular adnexa *de novo* or in association with various autoimmune disorders, including AIDS. Font and coworkers reported two cases of primary adnexal B-cell lymphoma in patients with preexisting benign lymphoepithelial lesions of the parotid glands.[22] As elsewhere in the orbit, most of these tumors feature a

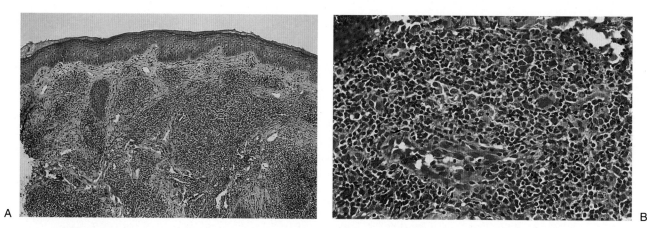

FIG. 2-56. Benign reactive lymphoid hyperplasia [low (**A**) and high (**B**) power images]. Polymorphous proliferation of mature lymphocytes, plasma cells, and histiocytes.

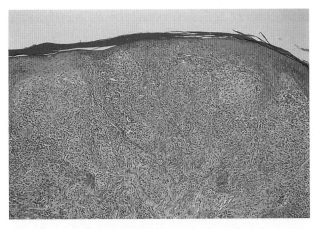

FIG. 2-57. Atypical lymphoid hyperplasia. Monotonous proliferation of lymphocytes. Many have cytologic irregularities.

diffuse monoclonal B-cell proliferation (Fig. 2-58). Non-Hodgkin's lymphomas have been categorized under the Working Formulation for Clinical Use. A detailed review of the myriad criteria used to diagnose the many lymphoma subtypes is unwarranted here. The diagnosis of non-Hodgkin's lymphoma arising in an extranodal site relies on the pathologist's appreciation of complex histopathologic features combined with results of immunohistochemical analysis and gene rearrangement studies. Treatment, clinical course, and prognosis for extraocular dissemination hinge on the tumor histology, the clinical stage, and the anatomic site of primary disease. Interested readers should consult the references for more detailed discussions.

Mycosis fungoides is a cutaneous T-cell lymphoma with a progressive, indolent clinical course. The periorbital skin is commonly involved, and the eyelid is the most frequently involved ophthalmic structure in this condition. Three clinical stages are described: an early pruritic eczematous stage, a plaque stage, and the ulcerated tumor stage. Patients exhibit universal erythroderma. Sys-

temic involvement usually accompanies the plaque stage but occasionally occurs earlier. Globe involvement (keratitis, uveitis, retinal infiltrates) correlates with an advanced disease state. Sézary syndrome refers to leukemic progression of the cutaneous mycosis fungoides. The histopathology of eyelid skin with mycosis fungoides features changes in both the epidermis and dermis (Fig. 2-59). Psoriasiform epidermal hyperplasia may include irregular acanthosis. Atypical T lymphocytes may reside within the epidermis (epidermotropism). In mycosis fungoides, these large anaplastic tumor cells (Sézary cells) harbor a convoluted nucleus with many deep indentations of its nuclear membrane. Aggregates of these atypical cells surrounded by a halo make up **Pautrier microabscess,** a supportive finding for this diagnosis. Pautrier microabscesses also are seen in other inflammatory dermatoses. A band-like or perivascular infiltrate of atypical lymphocytes, plasma cells, and eosinophils within the edematous dermis is characteristic.

The American form of **Burkitt lymphoma** usually presents in children as an abdominal mass; however, periocular involvement has been reported infrequently. Periocular Burkitt lymphoma also has been diagnosed in immunosuppressed patients with clinical and laboratory evidence of AIDS. The Epstein-Barr virus has been identified within the tumor cell genome of this B-cell malignancy. Chromosomal translocation t(8;14) is a consistent finding in this tumor.

Hematopoietic

Malignant proliferations within the lymphopoietic or myelopoietic arms of erythropoiesis make up the family of diseases called **leukemia.** Leukemia is subcategorized based on the responsible cell line and whether the clinical course is acute or chronic. It is a malignancy that begins in the bone marrow, disseminates via the circulation, and can reach nearly every anatomic site in the body. In al-

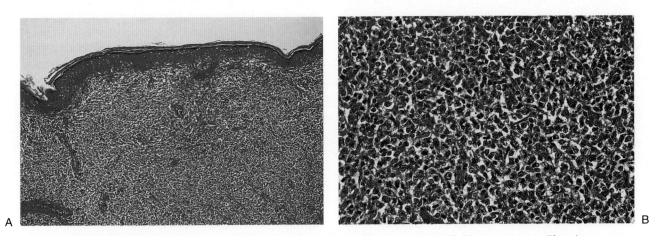

FIG. 2-58. Non-Hodgkin's lymphoma [low (**A**) and high (**B**) power images]. Monotonous proliferation of neoplastic lymphocytes.

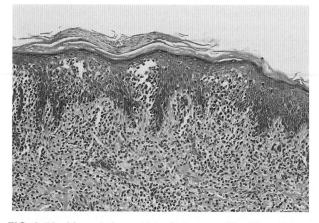

FIG. 2-59. Mycosis fungoides. Cutaneous T-cell lymphoma. Intraepithelial Pautrier's microabscesses. Band-like dermal infiltrate.

most every instance, patients presenting to the clinician with leukemia have already been diagnosed. Many have already been treated and have been in remission. Ocular symptomatology may indicate progression or recurrence of disease. Consistent with the earlier discussion of lymphoproliferative disease, we will not attempt here to unravel the bewildering and continuously changing clinical and diagnostic criteria for the leukemias. What space is budgeted for this important topic is reserved for reinforcing concepts important to the clinician.

Ocular and orbital morbidity may develop either from direct tumor infiltration or consequent to anticancer therapies. The acute leukemias are more likely than the chronic leukemias to involve the eye and orbit. Lid involvement by leukemia is usually an extension of orbital disease, and it is most commonly accompanied by painful exophthalmos. Eyelid swelling and erythema have been observed, but it is rare for an isolated palpable mass to form. Reddish-brown macular eruptions appearing on the eyelid skin that mimic the rash seen in secondary syphilis are called **lymphoma cutis.** Countless chemotherapeutic regimens have been established for treating leukemia, and 5-fluorouracil is often used. Toxic effects from systemic 5-fluorouracil include cicatricial ectropion, ankyloblepharon, lid necrosis, and punctal occlusion.

Multiple myeloma is a widely disseminated plasma cell malignancy that originates in the bone marrow. Systemic disease is manifested as tumor infiltration and the accumulation of abnormal immunoglobulins synthesized by the neoplastic plasma cells. Nearly all patients with multiple myeloma demonstrate abnormal electrophoretic patterns of serum immunoglobulins and Bence-Jones proteinuria. Most patients are elderly and initially present with symptoms of disseminated disease. Myeloma involvement of the eyelid and periorbital skin spares the epidermis (Fig. 2-60). Sheets of atypical plasma cells with abundant Russell bodies pervade the dermis. Immaturity of the malignant cells may disguise their identity. Cuta-

neous amyloid deposition should always alert the clinician to the diagnostic possibility of multiple myeloma. As with other diseases discussed in this section, skin findings often accompany more clinically significant orbital involvement.

Miscellaneous

The eyelids are an uncommon site for **metastatic cancer,** accounting for less than 1% of all eyelid tumors. Intraocular metastasis is much more common. There are no genuine surprises when the primary sites of cancer are tabulated: breast, lung, distant melanoma, gastrointestinal, and renal. The remaining malignancies are even less common. Usually, the patient's primary cancer diagnosis has already been established, perhaps years earlier. Cutaneous metastases may appear as a solid nodule, diffuse skin induration, or a nonhealing ulcer.[23]

A particularly curious malignant neoplasm arising in the eyelid or periorbital skin is the **Merkel cell tumor** (primary neuroendocrine carcinoma of skin, trabecular carcinoma). Normal Merkel cells reside in the epidermis near hairs, and they may be involved in our sense of touch. The exact role for these cells remains uncertain. Like epithelium elsewhere, intracytoplasmic keratin filaments have been demonstrated. Older patients are most often affected. Merkel cell tumors can appear as a single lesion or in multiples (up to 100) widely distributed over the body surface. The upper eyelid is more often affected by this firm, nontender, rapidly expanding mass. It has a deep cranberry-red color. Some authorities argue that neoplastic Merkel cells differentiate as both neuroendocrine and epithelial cells, a concept bolstered by immunohistochemical confirmation of both cytokeratin and neurofilament proteins. Ultrastructural analysis of Merkel cells reveals intracytoplasmic dense core granules measuring 100 to 200 nm in diameter, a reliable feature in the histopathologic interpretation of this tumor. The granules identify Merkel cells as belonging to the APUD (amine precursor uptake and decarboxylation) family. Merkel cell tumors demonstrate positive immunoreactivity to neuron-specific enolase. Conventional histopathology usually suffices for establishing the diagnosis due to its distinctive morphologic appearance (Fig. 2-61). This poorly circumscribed tumor is composed of nests and anastomosing cords of uniform, plump basophilic cells that feature scant cytoplasm and indistinct cell borders.[24] Nuclear atypia and brisk mitotic activity are usually observed. The tumor margins do not contact the epidermis.

Pyogenic granuloma is a double misnomer: not only is it neither pyogenic nor a granuloma, its name is reversed to designate a somewhat different cutaneous disorder known to dermatologists. The ophthalmic pyogenic granuloma is an exuberant proliferation of granulation tissue that most frequently develops after accidental or

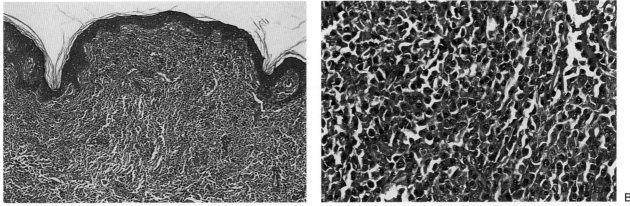

FIG. 2-60. Cutaneous involvement by multiple myeloma [low (**A**) and high (**B**) power images]. Infiltrative sheets of neoplastic plasma cells.

surgical trauma. It is an exaggerated tissue healing response. Rapid growth is typical for this smooth, red-purple lobulated mass. It is composed of radiating capillaries and fibroblasts with a mixed inflammatory infiltrate that includes mature lymphocytes and polymorphonuclear leukocytes (Fig. 2-62). Its rich vascularity leads to easy bleeding with minimal manipulation. Clinical correlation is very useful with a presumptive pyogenic granuloma because its microscopic appearance may simulate that of KS, hemangiopericytoma, and capillary hemangioma. Pyogenic granulomas also appear on the conjunctival surface.

CONJUNCTIVA

The critical role of conjunctiva in maintaining ocular health is widely underestimated and underappreciated—until the ophthalmologist has the opportunity to manage a complex case involving widespread conjunctival disease such as an alkali burn or severe xerophthalmia. Key functions of healthy conjunctiva include:

- Maintaining adequate wetting of the globe
- Tear film synthesis and distribution
- Providing a smooth interface between eyelids and the globe surface
- Providing limited mechanical protection for the globe and orbit
- Participating in lymphatic drainage of the eyelids
- Most importantly, maintaining continuous immune surveillance and immunoreactivity to a wide variety of antigenic stimuli.

Conjunctival secretions include the aqueous component (accessory lacrimal glands) and mucous component (goblet cells) of the tear film. Also, the resident population of plasma cells elaborates abundant immunoglobulins that can rapidly bind to foreign proteins and trigger the inflammatory cascade. The globe rarely survives very long after the demise of its conjunctiva.

This section presents the histopathology of the more common conjunctival disorders. Parallel entities presented earlier in the eyelid section are cross-referenced.

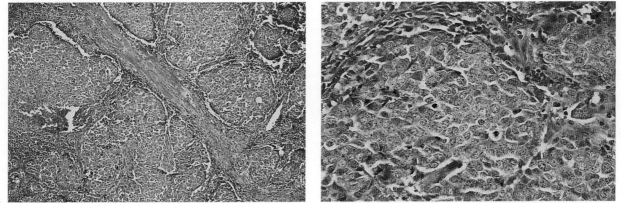

FIG. 2-61. Merkel cell tumor [low (**A**) and high (**B**) power images]. Nests of basophilic tumor cells with scant cytoplasm. Brisk mitotic activity.

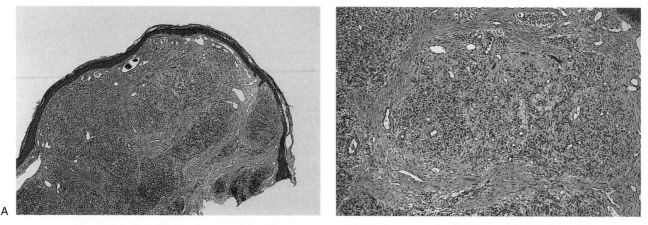

FIG. 2-62. Pyogenic granuloma [low (**A**) and high (**B**) power]. Exuberant granulation tissue composed of fibroblasts, capillaries, and a mixed inflammatory infiltrate.

Brief Overview of Gross Anatomy

The conjunctiva extends from the eyelid margin to the corneoscleral limbus. The histologic appearance of normal conjunctiva varies with its anatomic region (Fig. 2-63). The thin palpebral conjunctiva lines the inner tarsal surface and adheres directly to the tarsus. This thin mucosal layer is predominantly low cuboidal epithelium without a substantia propria. Abundant goblet cells reside within the palpebral conjunctiva.

The fornical conjunctiva is the cul-de-sac region where the conjunctiva is reflected from the eyelid onto the globe surface. Here the tissue is loose and redundant. Its only true attachment is at the orbital septum. Such laxity permits free movement of the globe in relation to the eyelids. The surface epithelium acquires a more cuboidal appearance, and the population density of the goblet cells increases. Beneath the epithelium is the vascularized connective tissue layer called the substantia propria. Within the substantia propria is a rich complement of immunocompetent cells (mature lymphocytes, mast cells, plasma cells) and extracellular immunoglobulins (IgG, IgA, and IgM) that protect the globe from infection. Collagenous and elastic tissues, peripheral nerves, vessels, and accessory lacrimal glands of Krause reside deep in the fornical substantia propria. Vital anatomic landmarks within the conjunctival fornix include the ducts of the lacrimal gland (superior temporal fornix) and the ducts that subserve the accessory lacrimal glands of Krause and of Wolfring (superior and inferior fornices). Any tissue injury to the fornical conjunctiva (eg, traumatic, cicatricial, toxic, inflammatory) that interferes with the normal expression of the maintenance tears may result in dry eye, exposure keratopathy, dellen formation, tissue melting, and even corneal perforation.

The outermost protective coat of the globe is the bulbar conjunctiva. At the medial and lateral canthi, the bulbar conjunctiva remains loosely adherent to facilitate globe excursions. One of these folds, the medial plica semilunaris, is a crescent-shaped fold of bulbar conjunctiva that disappears during abduction. It has been likened to the nictitating membrane found in lower vertebrates. Microanatomists claim that the greatest concentration of goblet cells appears within the plica. Any type of manipulation of the plica should be avoided because scarring in the area may lead to gaze restriction. Toward the corneoscleral limbus, the epithelial layer thickens and the dendritic Langerhans cells appear. Goblet cells disappear, and none are usually found at the limbus. The rest of the conjunctiva thins as it conforms to the shape of the globe, making the limbal conjunctiva nearly transparent. The limbal conjunctiva is densely adherent to the globe.

The familiar pink, fleshy **caruncle** is believed to be an undescended lower eyelid remnant (Fig. 2-64). This theory helps explain the complex anatomy of this medial canthal structure. Beneath nonkeratinizing squamous epithelium appear epidermal appendages (hair follicles, sebaceous and sweat glands) within a collagenous stroma. Smooth muscle and adipose are usually found in its deeper layers. The caruncle should not be excised unless there are compelling indications. Functional and cosmetic problems await the hasty surgeon. The caruncle helps direct tear outflow, and epiphora is a common postsurgical complaint. Moreover, the caruncle softens the appearance of the medial canthal angle. After excision of the caruncle, the external appearance may resemble that of a toy doll or lend the false impression of an artificial eye.

The conjunctiva is perfused by different divisions of the ophthalmic artery. Contributing from the eyelid are palpebral branches of the nasal and lacrimal arteries. On the surface of the globe, the anterior ciliary artery gives off branches to the conjunctiva where the anterior ciliary artery crosses the tendinous insertions of the rectus muscles. Conjunctival veins are more numerous than arteries. Conjunctival veins drain aqueous fluid from the anterior chamber. These can be studied at slit-lamp examination.

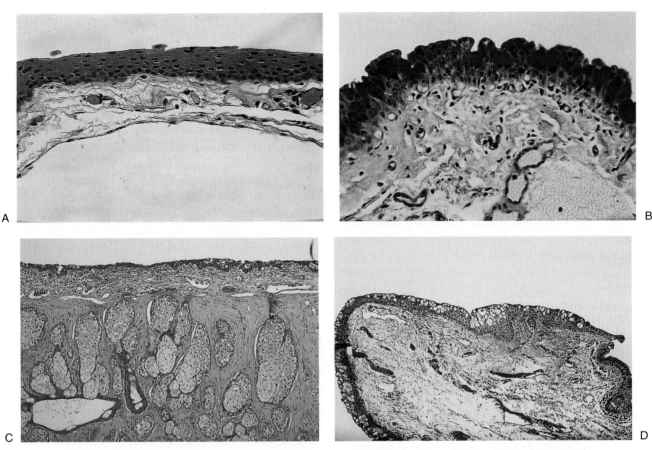

FIG. 2-63. Normal conjunctiva (four image composite). (**A**) *Limbal,* nonkeratinizing stratified squamous epithelium without goblet cells; (**B**) *fornical,* PAS stain demonstrates increased number of goblet cells. Normal sentinel inflammatory cells within substantia propia; (**C**) *palpebral,* slender mucosa covers posterior tarsal surface; (**D**) *plica semilunaris,* greatest density of goblet cells.

Both laminar flow and a dilutional effect can be observed where the emissarial veins of Ascher empty into the episcleral veins. Most of the conjunctiva *per se* drains into the palpebral veins and, ultimately, into the superior and inferior ophthalmic veins. Superficial and deep conjunctival lymphatics reside in the substantia propria. The eye-

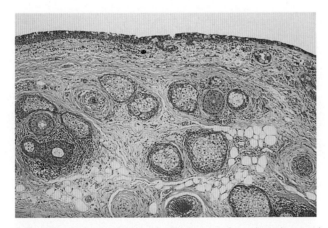

FIG. 2-64. Normal caruncle. Features of conjunctiva and skin are present. Nonkeratinizing squamous epithelium overlying dermal appendages.

lids and conjunctiva share a lymphatic drainage pattern. The anatomic region representing the medial half of each orbit drains to the submandibular and superior cervical lymph nodes, whereas the lateral half drains to the preauricular nodes.

Caution should be used in performing periorbital skin incisions, particularly with respect to the horizontal raphe emanating from the lateral canthus. Vertical incisions crossing this landmark sever the underlying lymphatic channels and result in pronounced eyelid lymphedema.

Microscopic Anatomy

The conjunctival surface is covered by nonkeratinizing squamous epithelium. The depth of this epithelial layer varies topographically, as described above. Basal columnar or cuboidal epithelium migrates superficially and flattens as it matures. In the presence of a noxious stimulus, the conjunctival epithelium may elaborate keratin as a mechanical barrier. **Leukoplakia** is the clinical term used to describe the resultant whitish plaque. Leukoplakia is not a histopathologic diagnosis, nor does it connote a precancerous or malignant process. Goblet cells were previously discussed. The mucus they produce stabilizes the tear film and imparts a smooth optical surface to the cornea. Microvilli on the conjunctival epithelial cell membrane help mucus cling to the ocular surface. Crypts are present between adjoining superficial tarsal epithelia. Whether shallow or deep, the walls of these crypts are lined by microvilli. Researchers believe these crypts play an active role in trapping and neutralizing pathogenic microorganisms, including viral particles.

Dendritic melanocytes are scattered among the basal epithelium of normal limbal and bulbar conjunctiva. In a fashion reminiscent of epidermal melanocytes, stimulated dendritic cells synthesize melanin and then inoculate adjoining conjunctival epithelial cells. Normal melanocytes remain as single cells within the basal layer. Any aggregation or superficial migration signifies active melanocyte proliferation.

Situated within the substantia propria of the conjunctiva are the accessory lacrimal glands of Krause and Wolfring. The glands of Krause are found in the cul-de-sac. There are far more of these structures in the upper fornix than in the inferior cul-de-sac. The glands of Wolfring reside in the portion of the palpebral conjunctiva between the tarsal border and the cul-de-sac. It is merely conjunctival epithelium that overlies the inner tarsal surface. The watery secretion from the accessory lacrimal glands drains through ducts that have their orifices at the conjunctival fornix. This is how the aqueous component of the tear film is replenished.

The remaining structures within the subepithelial space include blood vessels, lymphatics, and peripheral nerves, in a meshwork of collagen and elastic fibers.

Congenital Disorders

Congenital anomalies of the conjunctiva may present as isolated innocuous growths or they may be elements of complex ocular or multisystem developmental anomalies.

Cryptophthalmia is a serious malformation in which a continuous sheet of epidermis extends between the forehead and cheek, totally obscuring a malformed globe. It was previously discussed under congenital eyelid abnormalities.

Choristomas are nonneoplastic proliferations of normal tissue in an abnormal location. Choristomas are present at birth. One of the most common choristomas is the **limbal dermoid.** Usually, it is a single, solid, immobile epibulbar mass at the inferotemporal limbus, with encroachment onto the peripheral cornea. Exceptions abound regarding the number and location of these lesions. Round to oval, they measure up to 15 mm in diameter. The limbal dermoid is an ectopic rest of surface ectodermal tissue that includes epidermis and epidermal appendages (pilosebaceous apparatus, sweat

glands) set within a dense collagenous stroma (Fig. 2-65).[3,25] Interestingly, lid colobomas may coexist in the same area. Some authors speculate that the limbal dermoid may be the lid margin's "missing piece." The limbal dermoid is integrated superficially into the outer half of the sclera and cornea. Efforts at surgical treatment are usually restricted to debulking the growth and restoring normal globe contour. Complex choristomas resemble limbal dermoids. They harbor additional heterotopic tissues such as cartilage, smooth muscle, adipose, and lacrimal gland tissue.

Limbal dermoids may present as the ocular manifestation of Goldenhar syndrome (oculoauriculovertebral dysplasia). In addition to bilateral limbal dermoids, patients exhibit preauricular skin tags or pits, misshapen ears, and cervical vertebral malformations. Since its description in 1952, additional observed findings have included dermolipomas, lid colobomas, cleft lip and palate, and cardiac and renal anomalies.

A **dermolipoma** (lipodermoid) is an epibulbar choristoma that involves conjunctival and orbital structures. The superotemporal quadrant is its most common locale; it is usually unilateral. Unlike the solid limbal dermoid, the yellowish dermolipoma is a soft, compressible, protuberant tumor.[3,25] Its name identifies its contents, skin and adipose tissue. Smooth, attenuated squamous epithelium overlies skin adnexa, smooth muscle, and mature adipose tissue (Fig. 2-66).

An epibulbar **osseous choristoma** is more accurately categorized as an anomaly of scleral tissue. These lesions appear at birth as small, mobile, epibulbar nodules that favor the superior temporal quadrant. Most embryologists equate this choristoma with a variant of the solid dermoid—a benign growth of mature compact bone. The presence of other heterotopic tissues is rarer still. Osseous choristoma is not associated with other ocular or orbital developmental anomalies.

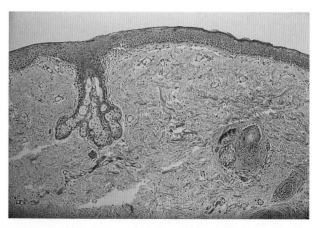

FIG. 2-65. Solid limbal dermoid. Epibulbar conjunctiva covers ectopic dermis and dermal appendages.

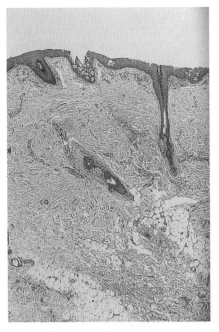

FIG. 2-66. Dermolipoma. Mature adipose incorporated into heterotopic mass of skin appendages.

Inflammatory Conditions

Conjunctivitis is a host-mediated immune response to a noxious stimulus. Conjunctival hyperemia, edema, and exudation are its clinical hallmarks. Common agents that provoke conjunctival inflammation include microorganisms (bacteria, viruses, chlamydia, fungi, mycobacteria, spirochetes, protozoa, and parasites), allergens, foreign particles, and toxic substances, including topical medications. Additional antigenic stimuli include host proteins that are no longer tolerated by persons with autoimmune disorders. Various schemes have been used to categorize conjunctival inflammation clinically, and these have attempted to correlate the tissue response to the cause and duration of the mucosal irritation. Unfortunately, these artificial paradigms cannot rigidly impose order and logic to human disease. There is tremendous imprecision, overlap, and redundancy in any overview of conjunctival pathology: acute versus chronic, infectious versus noninfectious, toxic versus autoimmune, and so forth.

Management of most inflammatory ocular surface disorders is guided by clinical impression based on physical examination and the results of any culture samples. Cytologic smear preparations have enormous diagnostic utility. In general practice, conjunctival biopsy is reserved for unresponsive or atypical cases. Tissue changes observed at this point in the clinical course may be nonspecific or noncontributory. Special stains for pathogens may corroborate culture results if infection has persisted.

Acute conjunctivitis, as its name implies, develops within hours and exhibits the familiar vascular, humoral, and cellular responses traditionally associated with acute inflammation. Vascular dilatation and increased permeability lead to edema and the emigration of neutrophils. Mononuclear phagocytes help digest antigenic material. These activities are modulated by the elaboration of chemical mediators. Acute conjunctivitis is identified histopathologically by the nature of the inflammatory cell infiltrate (predominantly polymorphonuclear leukocytes) and by the presence of a flimsy proteinaceous pseudomembrane (Fig. 2-67). In more severe forms of acute conjunctivitis (e.g., *Staphylococcus aureus, Corynebacterium diphtheriae, Streptococcus pneumoniae*), an adherent true membrane may form that incorporates devitalized surface epithelium. A purulent discharge is a common presenting symptom in acute conjunctivitis. The term **hyperacute conjunctivitis** is reserved for a rapid exacerbation featuring copious suppuration, lid swelling, ocular pain, and preauricular lymphadenopathy due to infection by organisms such as *Neisseria.*

Allergic hypersensitivity can induce an acute conjunctivitis within minutes. In addition to pronounced bilateral hyperemia and chemosis, there is an acute inflammatory infiltrate that features abundant mast cells (tissue basophils) and eosinophils. Previously sensitized B lymphocytes elaborate IgE antibodies that bind to the mast cells. Antigen/IgE cross-linking leads to mast cell degranulation and the elaboration of preformed histamine and serotonin, as well as secondary mediators such as leukotrienes.

Although acute conjunctivitis can complete its clinical course in days, **chronic conjunctivitis** evolves over days to weeks and may persist indefinitely. Most cases of chronic conjunctivitis started as an acute conjunctivitis; however, the acute response was insufficient to neutralize the immune threat. The vascular and cellular changes that characterize chronic conjunctivitis require time to develop. Instead of the immediate mobilization of circulating neutrophils seen in acute conjunctivitis, the inflammatory infiltrate contains proliferating lymphocytes, plasma cells, and activated histiocytes. Fibroblasts and capillaries also proliferate. Chronic conjunctivitis pro-

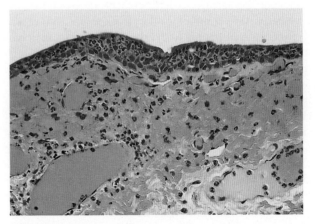

FIG. 2-67. Acute conjunctivitis. Acute inflammatory infiltrate. Dilated vessels within substantia propria.

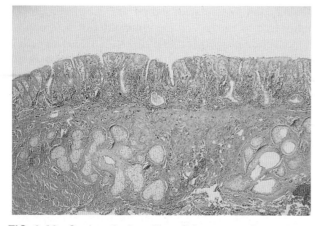

FIG. 2-68. Conjunctival papillae. Edematous, elevated conjunctiva with prominent central vessels.

motes goblet cell hyperplasia and increased mucous production. Accordingly, chronic conjunctivitis leads to recognizable alterations in the conjunctival epithelium and stroma.

The palpebral conjunctival epithelium is tethered to the tarsus by a lacework of fibrous attachments. Flat-topped conjunctival papillae form on the palpebral conjunctiva in response to perivascular transudation and the pronounced inflammatory infiltrate that elevates the unbound epithelium. The infiltrate contains eosinophils, mast cells, and mononuclear cells (Fig. 2-68). Conjunctival papillae are encountered in **vernal keratoconjunctivitis** (VKC). Chronic irritation from hard contact lenses or ocular prostheses leads to the formation of giant papillae, an exaggerated tissue response.

What are the differences between seasonal, vernal, and giant papillary conjunctivitis? Acute seasonal allergic conjunctivitis represents an antibody-mediated type I hypersensitivity reaction that may be triggered by airborne pollen, animal dander, molds, and similar agents. Conjunctival papillae do not appear during the acute phase, and spontaneous recovery is expected. The same allergens may coat the surface of hard contact lenses and ocular prostheses, thus combining allergen exposure with repetitive mechanical trauma to the palpebral conjunctival epithelium. This mechanism underlies the pathophysiology of giant papillary conjunctivitis. Treatment requires removal of the offending device. VKC is a chronic, cell-mediated response that exhibits features of both type I (IgE, eosinophils) and type IV (T lymphocytes) hypersensitivity. Patients with active VKC have conjunctival papillae on the lid. Limbal papillae can also appear and are characterized by the presence of mounds of eosinophils atop the limbal papillae (Horner-Trantas dots). Progressive VKC can lead to corneal involvement (shield ulcer) with scarring and possible perforation.

Another visible marker for chronic conjunctivitis is the presence of conjunctival follicles. Although the conjunc-

tiva has no lymph nodes, its superficial substantia propria is populated by immunocompetent cells and extracellular immunoglobulins that protect the globe from infection. After antigenic stimulation, aggregation of these lymphocytes and plasma cells forms discrete subepithelial nodules, the substrate of conjunctival follicles. Some follicles feature germinal centers that include debris-laden tingible body macrophages (Fig. 2-69).

Bacterial infections usually are associated with bilateral acute suppurative conjunctivitis. Other infectious causes of conjunctivitis manifest themselves as a unilateral or asymmetric chronic follicular conjunctivitis. Pathogens in this category include viruses and chlamydia. Ipsilateral preauricular lymphadenopathy is an expected finding. Allergy to topical ocular medications (medicamentous) is an important noninfectious cause of chronic follicular conjunctivitis.

Not all inflammatory conjunctival nodules are follicles, and not all represent a reactive lymphoid process. **Conjunctival granulomas** also can appear as multiple nodular elevations of the fornical conjunctiva in the clinical setting of a red eye. A granuloma is a collection of activated macrophages (epithelioid histiocytes) that attempt to phagocytose and degrade a target antigen. These can be infectious or noninfectious. Microorganisms known to incite a granulomatous chronic conjunctivitis include mycobacteria, fungi, rickettsiae, syphilis, *Leptothrix, Pasteurella tularensis, Haemophilus ducreyi,* and cat-scratch agent *Bartonella henselae.* Any of these pathogens can lead to **Parinaud oculoglandular syndrome,** unilateral chronic granulomatous conjunctivitis with ipsilateral preauricular lymphadenopathy. Noninfectious granulomas may be due to sarcoidosis, xanthogranulomatous infiltrates, and retained foreign bodies. These were discussed in the eyelid section.

A necrotizing vasculitis with granulomatous inflammation in the epibulbar or scleral tissues should alert the clinician to the possibility of a potentially lethal systemic autoimmune disorder such as **Wegener granulomatosis.**

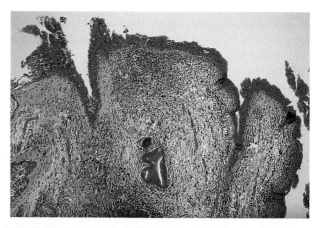

FIG. 2-69. Conjunctival follicles. Focal benign lymphoid hyperplasia within substantia propia.

Orbital and adnexal involvement may precede the discovery of cavitary pulmonary and renal lesions. These patients demonstrate elevated serum levels of antineutrophil cytoplasmic antibody, a highly sensitive marker for this disease.

Acquired and Degenerative Conditions

Dry eye irritation is a presenting ocular complaint familiar to clinicians. Patients develop symptomatic dry eyes when there is undersecretion of tears, aberrant tear film composition, or excessive tear film evaporation. **Xerosis** is the global (and nonspecific) medical term applied to dry eye conditions due to underlying conjunctival and lacrimal gland abnormalities. In these conditions, the conjunctival accessory lacrimal glands of Krause and Wolfring, together with the main lacrimal gland, secrete an inadequate aqueous component to the maintenance tear film. Xerosis can result from involutional lacrimal gland atrophy or from active ocular or systemic disease.

The term **keratoconjunctivitis sicca** was coined by Sjögren over 60 years ago to describe patients with xerosis, xerostomia, and arthritis. Subsequent investigators periodically tampered with the original nosology. Currently, keratoconjunctivitis sicca and extraocular xerostomia affecting oral, anal, and vaginal surfaces without an underlying systemic autoimmune rheumatic disease make up primary Sjögren syndrome. Secondary Sjögren syndrome adds the concomitant systemic autoimmune rheumatic disease. Rheumatoid arthritis and scleroderma are the two most frequently implicated autoimmune connective tissue diseases. Biopsy of minor labial salivary glands is routinely performed to establish the diagnosis. Positive specimens harbor a benign lymphocytic infiltrate surrounding myoepithelial islands. The infiltrate replaces normal salivary gland tissue. Similar changes occur in the main and accessory lacrimal glands. Consistent histopathologic changes to the affected conjunctiva have been described by several investigators. The conjunctival epithelium demonstrates internalization and disappearance of goblet cells, along with flattening and keratinization of the surface cells. A nongranulomatous chronic inflammatory infiltrate composed of mature lymphocytes and plasma cells is present in the substantia propria. When secondary Sjögren syndrome is due to scleroderma, perivascular fibrosis within the substantia propria is present.

Xerophthalmia differs from xerosis. Deficient mucous production from the conjunctival goblet cells leads to squamous metaplasia and keratinization of the mucosal epithelium. Xerophthalmia is due to vitamin A deficiency (hypovitaminosis A), a condition not limited to Third World populations. Although endemic dietary deficiencies of vitamin A account for the enormous numbers of childhood cases of xerophthalmia in underdeveloped countries, impaired absorption of ingested fat-soluble vitamin A appears in a significant number of adults in Western cultures with liver dysfunction secondary to chronic alcohol consumption. This condition is often manifested as Bitot spots and corneal melting. Dramatic clinical improvement results when topical and parenteral vitamin A is administered.

Superior limbic keratoconjunctivitis is a mysterious inflammatory disorder affecting the palpebral and bulbar conjunctiva. Most cases appear bilaterally and predominate in adult females. Its clinical course can be highly variable. Xerosis and filamentary keratitis can complicate management. Topical medications, cryotherapy, and excision of involved conjunctiva have yielded mixed outcomes. Biopsy specimens from active cases reveal acanthotic squamous epithelium featuring dyskeratosis and infiltration by neutrophils (Fig. 2-70). Newly diagnosed patients should be evaluated for associated thyroid dysfunction.

Some inflammatory disorders that afflict the conjunctiva represent derangements in recognition or tolerance of native proteins. **Ocular cicatricial pemphigoid** (benign mucosal pemphigoid, bullous pemphigoid) is an example. This systemic disorder can affect periorbital skin, conjunctiva, and corneal epithelium.[26,27] The fundamental problem is the presence of predominantly fixed antibodies (particularly IgG and IgA) and complement (C_3) directed against epithelial basement membrane. Idiopathic and drug-related forms have been described. Friable subepithelial bullae eventually rupture (Fig. 2-71). In the conjunctiva, this can lead to scarring and symblepharon formation. Fresh-frozen conjunctival biopsies exposed to direct and indirect immunofluorescence testing and immunoperoxidase amplification techniques are confirmatory. **Pemphigus vulgaris** is a related autoimmune dermatologic disorder in which host antibodies lyse the epidermal intercellular bonds and create intraepithelial blisters. The eyelid skin may become involved, although conjunctiva and other mucosal sites are usually spared.

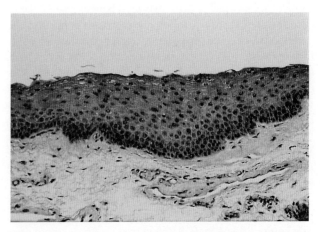

FIG. 2-70. Superior limbic keratoconjunctivitis. Polymorphonuclear leukocytes within hyperplastic surface epithelium.

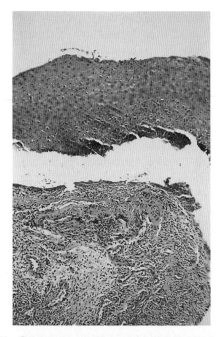

FIG. 2-71. Ocular cicatricial pemphigoid. Early changes include epithelial hyperplasia, loss of goblet cells, epithelial blister formation, chronic inflammatory infiltrate, and granulation tissue formation beneath the epithelium. (Courtesy of HE Grossniklaus, MD, Atlanta, GA)

The conjunctiva is often compromised as a result of medical or surgical treatment for some unrelated ocular or orbital disorder. Excessive surgical manipulation of the conjunctiva and the prolonged use of lid specula can traumatize the accessory lacrimal glands and lead to postoperative xerosis. Cataract surgery patients routinely encounter this problem. Supervoltage orbital radiation therapy, proton beam radiation therapy, and plaque brachyradiotherapy have had widespread popularity among ocular oncologists. Patients enrolled in any radiation therapy protocol must be carefully counseled regarding possible ocular complications resulting from treatment. Acute and latent tissue changes have been described. In the days following radiation exposure, the conjunctiva becomes hyperemic and edematous. The surface epithelium also becomes edematous, and many cells are sloughed. Over a period of weeks to months, depending on the cumulative dose of radiation, the typical features of xerosis can appear, squamous metaplasia with keratinization. Severe cases acquire epidermalization of the conjunctiva. Spontaneous fibrosis may develop in the subepithelial tissues. Late obliterative changes to the conjunctival and epibulbar vessels may result in ischemic necrosis of the conjunctiva and cornea.

Another important exogenous threat to healthy conjunctiva is the use of topical and parenteral medications. The key problems include direct toxicity from active drug ingredients, drug metabolites, preservatives, and drug vehicles as well as depositions of drugs and their metabo-

lites. Chronic noninfectious conjunctivitis has been traced to habitual use of pilocarpine, eserine, and idoxuridine. These same agents have caused ocular cicatricial pemphigoid. Conjunctival shrinkage is another unwanted side effect of this same trio of drugs and is seen also in patients using timolol and dipivefrin. Topical anesthetics, aminoglycoside antibiotics, and antimetabolites (5-fluorouracil and mitomycin C) poison healthy surface epithelium and may destabilize connective tissues long after exposure.[28] The contact lens solution preservative thimerosal may be responsible for immediate and delayed hypersensitivity reactions involving the ocular surface. Many of the most frequently prescribed systemic cancer chemotherapeutic agents are toxic to the conjunctiva. Imperia and coworkers have tabulated an impressive list of ocular complications related to chemotherapy.[28] Cited ocular surface disorders include keratoconjunctivitis sicca, blepharoconjunctivitis, and chronic conjunctivitis. Compounds known to accumulate within the conjunctiva include silver (epithelial basement membrane), gold (all levels), mercury, amiodarone (epithelium), tetracycline and minocycline (within cystic inclusions, both autofluoresce), epinephrine (pigmented adrenochrome within cystic inclusions), quinacrine, and chlorpromazine (Fig. 2-72).

In addition to drug compounds, other physiologic and pathologic substances may accumulate within the conjunctiva. Elevated serum bilirubin (kernicterus, jaundice) results in a bilateral yellow discoloration of the conjunctival and episcleral soft tissues. Conjunctival biopsy may help establish the diagnosis of several inborn errors of metabolism and lysosomal storage diseases. The deposition material may not be clinically apparent in the conjunctiva, as it often is on the cornea; however, appropriate microscopic and ultrastructural preparations of conjunctiva can be expected to correlate well with the clinical corneal observations. Systemic conditions known to deposit altered metabolic products in the conjunctiva include alkaptonuria (phenylalanine), cystinosis (cysteine),

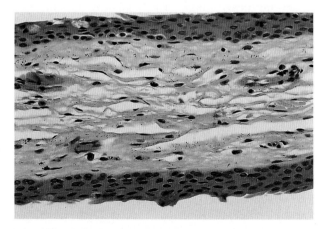

FIG. 2-72. Argyrosis. Miniscule polychromatic granules are seen at the level of epithelial basement membrane and within substantia propia.

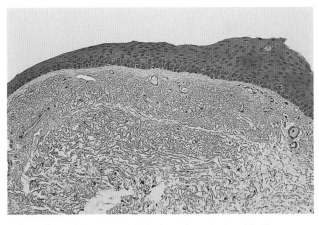

FIG. 2-73. Pterygium. Limbal conjunctival epithelium overlying nodule of degenerated collagen (solar elastosis).

gout (urate crystals), mucopolysaccharidosis (especially I-H, I-S, and VI), mucolipidosis (especially types II, III, IV), sphingolipodosis (Fabry, Niemann-Pick), and Addison disease (basal melanin). In suspected cystinosis, the biopsy specimen must be preserved in absolute alcohol to prevent the loss of the water-soluble cysteine crystals. Finally, patients with multiple myeloma or other dysproteinemias may demonstrate crystallized immunoglobulin within the conjunctiva and cornea.

Subepithelial **conjunctival amyloidosis** is most often an isolated finding that represents a localized primary deposition. Secondary amyloid deposition may occur after chronic inflammation or as an ocular manifestation of multiple myeloma or lymphoma.[5] The amyloid material demonstrates the characteristic histochemical features outlined above. Nodular or plaque-like accumulations may involve one or both eyes. These nontender, pale masses bleed with gentle manipulation due to small-vessel rigidity.

The conjunctiva is susceptible to the damaging effects of ultraviolet radiation acquired during sun exposure. The vulnerable bulbar conjunctiva in the region of the open interpalpebral fissure is the typical site for **pterygium** (Fig. 2-73). This thickened mass of vascularized conjunctival and peripheral corneal tissue usually arises along the nasal limbus in adults. The pterygium is not a cellular proliferation; rather, it is an accumulation of actinically damaged subepithelial connective tissue.[29] **Solar elastosis** (elastotic degeneration), described earlier, is the operative tissue alteration. Acellular and faintly basophilic material reacts positively to special stains for elastic tissue (Verhoeff-von Gieson method); however, it resists digestion by the enzyme elastase. Curled, fragmented collagen bundles, acid mucopolysaccharide deposition, and dystrophic calcification may be present. Pterygia recur, and so timing of their excision must balance the concerns of recurrence against preservation of the visual axis. **Pingueculae** (from the Greek word meaning fat) are similar growths that are yellower and spare the cornea. All ex-

cised pterygia and pingueculae should be submitted for pathologic examination. The overlying surface epithelium also has sustained chronic sun exposure, and pathologic examination of these specimens is required to identify epithelial changes that range from atrophy to invasive squamous carcinoma.

Tumors and Neoplasms

Epithelial

Cystic

Simple **epithelial inclusion cysts** of the conjunctiva may be congenital or acquired. Acquired cysts usually arise in areas of previous surgical or accidental trauma. The superomedial quadrant is the most common location for these benign lesions. A solitary unilocular cyst is lined by nonkeratinizing cuboidal epithelium (Fig. 2-74). Goblet cells are often included, leading to mucous accumulation within the cyst lumen. Cyst drainage is a temporizing measure; complete excision usually is recommended.

Conjunctival dermoid cysts (cystic dermoids) are uncommon cystic orbital lesions. They are believed to be developmental in nature; however, they usually do not become clinically apparent until adulthood. They may cause significant exophthalmos and diplopia. The cyst lining of conjunctival dermoids is nonkeratinizing squamous epithelium (in contrast to orbital cystic dermoids), and the cyst wall contains heterotopic epidermal appendages such as hair shafts, pilosebaceous apparatus, and sweat glands (Fig. 2-75).[25] A modest chronic inflammatory infiltrate resides within the surrounding connective tissue.

Tarsal **conjunctival concretions** are visible at slit-lamp examination. These small yellowish nodules are more common in older patients and rarely warrant excision. They represent inspissated collections of degenerated cel-

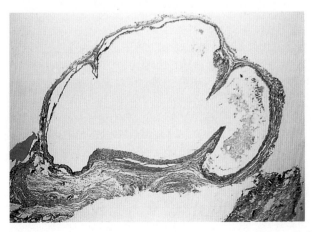

FIG. 2-74. Conjunctival epithelial inclusion cyst. Distended cyst lumen lined by nonkeratinizing squamous epithelium.

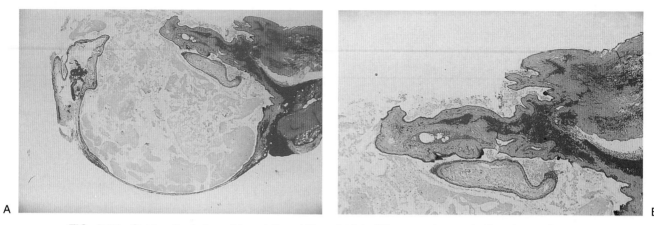

A   B

FIG. 2-75. Conjunctival dermoid cyst [low (**A**) and high (**B**) power images]. Cyst lumen includes caseous debris and desquamated epithelium. Adnexal appendages are observed within cyst wall.

lular debris within the deep intercellular crypts on the outer mucosal surface. Calcification may occur in these concretions.

Noncystic

Several conjunctival lesions are clinically described as papillomas. Many benign and malignant disorders can assume a papillomatous configuration, misleading the clinician. Diagnostic accuracy and the development of an optimal treatment plan hinge on the histopathologic interpretation of a representative biopsy specimen.

Squamous papillomas are benign proliferations of surface epithelium. All ages can be affected, as can any region of the conjunctiva. Most are believed to be virally induced; HPV is most frequently implicated. This virus is responsible for similar growths at other mucosal sites, such as the uterine cervix, oral mucosa, and penis. Conjunctival and extraocular papillomas share gross and microscopic features. These lesions may be pedunculated or sessile. Multiple branching fronds of acanthotic epithelium enshroud an inflamed fibrovascular core (Fig. 2-76).

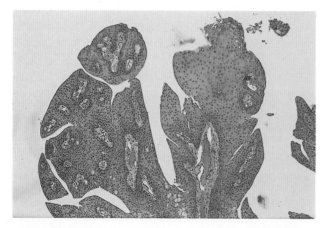

FIG. 2-76. Squamous papilloma. Fingerlike projections of acanthotic squamous epithelium enshroud central blood vessel.

Intraepithelial cytoplasmic vacuoles surround the small hyperchromatic nuclei, a feature described as koilocytic atypia. Although gynecologic pathologists and dermatopathologists have long studied the pathophysiology of HPV infections involving the skin and genitalia, ophthalmic pathologists have only recently begun to investigate viral papillomas of the conjunctiva. Numerous serotypes of HPV have been identified, some of which are specifically associated with malignant transformation of the papilloma into invasive squamous carcinoma. HPV-16 is one example, and more are expected to be proven to be oncogenic. Conjunctival papillomas tend to recur. Repeat excision and local cryotherapy has been recommended.

Leukoplakia is another overused descriptive clinical term. To the ophthalmic pathologist, leukoplakia carries no diagnostic significance: it simply means the lesion clinically appeared as a whitish plaque on the conjunctiva. The native nonkeratinizing squamous epithelium is rapidly proliferating and producing abundant keratin. This process is observed in benign, premalignant, and malignant conditions.

One cause of leukoplakia that appears more frequently in certifying examinations than in the waiting room is **hereditary benign intraepithelial dyskeratosis.** Bilateral epibulbar leukoplakic patches overlie markedly dilated vessels, imparting a pinkish discoloration. The temporal globe is more commonly affected, and corneal encroachment is not uncommon. The buccal mucosa is similarly afflicted. An autosomal dominant inheritance pattern was documented in the mixed-race Haliwa Indians (a geographic acronym for *Hali*fax and *Wa*shington counties in northeastern North Carolina). Microscopic examination of biopsy specimens reveals a markedly thickened squamous epithelium with prominent extracellular and intracellular keratinization (Fig. 2-77). Cellular atypia is not observed, and the basement membrane is not violated.

One example of disease progression that leads to cancer is **conjunctival intraepithelial neoplasia** (CIN). Long-term exposure of the bulbar conjunctiva within the inter-

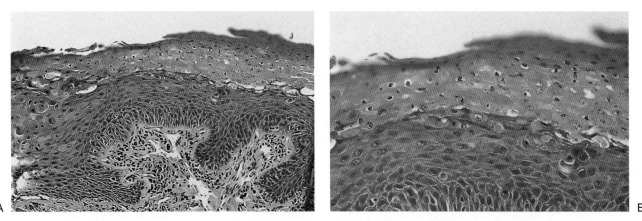

A   B

FIG. 2-77. Hereditary benign intaepithelial dyskeratosis [low (**A**) and high (**B**) power images]. Noninvasive proliferation of abnormal conjunctival epithelium. Hyperkeratosis, parakeratosis, and dyskeratosis without dysplasia.

palpebral fissure to ultraviolet radiation results in epithelial dysplasia (*dysplasia* means "poorly formed"). The normal tissue architecture, cell polarity, and maturation pattern are replaced (partially or totally) by cells having abnormal sizes and shapes, haphazard distribution, and disordered maturation. Although the dysplastic epithelial changes noted in HPV infection begin at the outer surface, sun-induced CIN begins at the basal layer and extends upward. These cases of clinical leukoplakia often present in older adults as gray-white, gelatinous or velvety patches, typically originating near the limbus. Disease progression may completely encircle the cornea and advance onto the corneal surface. Under the microscope, there appears an abrupt transition between relatively normal unaffected conjunctiva and a markedly acanthotic diseased epithelium (Fig. 2-78).[29] Dysplasia is categorized based on the proportion of epithelial involvement: mild dysplasia (less than 15% of total thickness), moderate dysplasia (up to 50% involvement); and severe (greater than 50% involvement). The epithelial basement membrane remains intact. A focally intense chronic inflammatory infiltrate hugs the base of the lesion.

When the conjunctival epithelium is completely replaced by dysplastic CIN, the condition is described as **carcinoma in situ** (Fig. 2-79). All that separates carcinoma in situ from invasive squamous carcinoma is the integrity of the basement membrane. Once the dysplastic conjunctival epithelium violates the basement membrane, the condition becomes **conjunctival squamous carcinoma.** Neoplastic proliferation leads to vertical growth of the mass, creating an elevated, exophytic tumor and concurrent epibulbar extension. The clinical appearance of early invasive squamous conjunctiva may not differ significantly from any of the previously discussed epibulbar masses. The same architectural and cytologic features present in CIN with severe dysplasia are preserved throughout squamous cell carcinoma (Fig. 2-80). These lesions are usually well-differentiated carcinomas. Intercellular bridges and individual cell keratinization are evi-

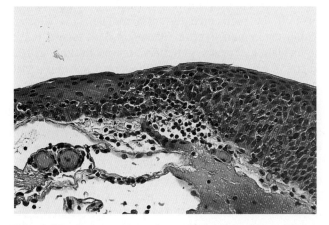

FIG. 2-78. Conjunctival intraepithelial neoplasia. Abrupt transition between normal and dysplastic surface epithelium.

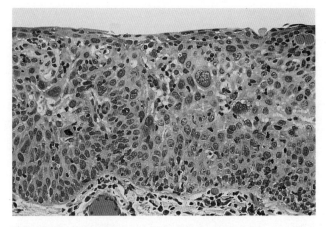

FIG. 2-79. CIN with severe dysplasia (carcinoma in situ). Full-thickness dysplasia with loss of polarity and disordered maturation, noninvasive.

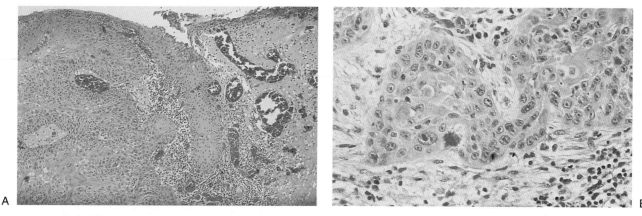

FIG. 2-80. Conjunctival squamous cell carcinoma [low (**A**) and high (**B**) power images]. Invasive mass composed of malignant epithelial cells. Individual tumor cells feature abundant eosinophilic cytoplasm and nuclear atypia.

dent. Intraocular invasion and metastatic lymphatic spread by conjunctival squamous carcinoma are rare. Two rarer and more aggressive variants are spindle cell carcinoma and mucoepidermoid carcinoma.

Conjunctival involvement by **sebaceous carcinoma** is a critical element of the **masquerade syndrome.** As mentioned earlier, sebaceous gland carcinoma is prone to diagnostic delays by both clinician and pathologist. Carcinoma cells exploit this delay by advancing beyond the pilosebaceous apparatus and joining the surface epithelium of both the conjunctiva and eyelid skin (Fig. 2-81). These discohesive cancer cells shed easily and disgorge their irritating cytoplasm into the tear film. Patients present with unilateral blepharoconjunctivitis, the hallmark of pagetoid spread of sebaceous carcinoma.[15] The greasy lid debris seen at slit-lamp examination represents exfoliated tumor. Full-thickness eyelid biopsy is recommended to confirm the diagnosis. Frozen sections stained with oil red-O demonstrate intracellular lipid, although at this stage of disease conventional H&E staining usually suffices. Margo and coworkers have suggested that it is pos-

sible for sebaceous gland carcinoma to arise primarily from the conjunctival epithelium, based on their experience with a case of documented conjunctival intraepithelial sebaceous carcinoma without an underlying eyelid tumor.[30]

Melanocytic

Pigmented lesions of the conjunctiva frequently evoke the concern of both patient and clinician. In this section, the benign, premalignant, and malignant melanocytic conjunctival processes are discussed, with emphasis on primary acquired melanosis. Only a few epithelial and subepithelial pigmented alterations have malignant potential; the challenge is to identify the troublemakers. The clinical history and physical examination greatly aid the clinician in distinguishing patients needing surgery from those deserving reassurance and a more conservative approach.

The first question raised in the evaluation of epibulbar pigmentation is one of anatomy: where, specifically, is the lesion located? Gentle manipulation of the conjunctiva with a cotton-tipped applicator usually provides the answer. If the pigmented lesion is mobile, it is situated within the conjunctival or subconjunctival layers. If the pigmentation remains stationary, one is dealing with a scleral or episcleral process. Oculodermal melanosis (nevus of Ota) was discussed earlier.

The quantity and intensity of melanin pigment does not correlate with the histopathologic grade. For example, an amelanotic conjunctival malignant melanoma may clinically resemble any of a variety of benign lesions. On the other hand, the banal compound nevus cells may disgorge abundant pigment that is phagocytosed by macrophages within the substantia propria (melanophages). This phenomenon creates an enlarging pigmented patch on the conjunctiva that may exceed the actual dimensions of the benign nevus.

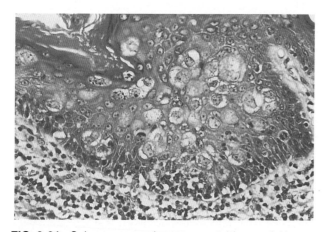

FIG. 2-81. Sebaceous carcinoma, pagetoid spread. Vacuolated malignant tumor cells reside within surface epithelium.

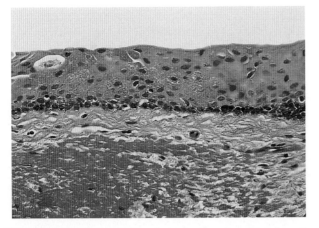

FIG. 2-82. Benign racial melanosis. Increased basilar pigmentation, bilateral.

Another valuable determination is the exact nature of the pigmentation. Not all discoloration is due to melanin. Brown or black conjunctival/episcleral pigmentation may be due to topical medications (argyrosis, adrenochrome deposition), parenteral drugs (tetracycline, amiodarone, phenothiazines), foreign bodies, inborn errors of metabolism (cystinosis, ochronosis, jaundice), or chronic hemorrhage (hemosiderin). Finally, abnormal discoloration of the globe may actually be visible uvea, as occurs in scleral thinning conditions (staphyloma, osteogenesis imperfecta, scleromalacia perforans), focal senile translucency, Axenfeld nerve loops, or epibulbar extension of primary uveal malignant melanoma. This section addresses only the conjunctival alterations directly caused by melanin-bearing cells.

None of the following pigment alterations is a precursor lesion for malignant melanoma.[31] **Benign racial melanosis** is a bilateral nonproliferative conjunctival pigmentation that affects nearly all blacks and is found less commonly in other darkly complected persons. The conjunctiva at the corneoscleral limbus is most intensely pigmented in an annular distribution. There is a moderate increase in the number of basal dendritic melanocytes, and these cells discharge melanin granules (melanosomes) that are taken up by the neighboring epithelial cells (Fig. 2-82). Pigment may trespass onto the corneal surface. Inflammation and ultraviolet irradiation may intensify the pigmentation. In the absence of a complete clinical history, it is impossible to distinguish between a small biopsy specimen from benign racial melanosis and the conjunctival ephelis (freckle). **Secondary acquired melanosis** of the conjunctiva results from excess melanin production from reactive, hyperplastic dendritic melanocytes. Stimuli responsible for this condition include drugs (chlorpromazine), sun exposure, elevated hormone levels, and chronic conjunctival inflammations (trachoma, VKC, foreign bodies), or it may occur in association with other nonmelanocytic lesions such as cysts, papillomas, or CIN.

The histogenesis of conjunctival nevi parallels that previously described in the skin, although the terminology is slightly different. Plump, polygonal melanocytic nevus cells typically reside at the epithelial basal layer. Nevus cells proliferate into nests and clusters. They may remain stationary within the epithelium, but more commonly they mature and descend into the substantia propria and subconjunctival layers. As melanocytic nevus cells descend, they tend to "kidnap" adjoining epithelial cells and goblet cells. As this process continues, the nevoid melanocyte cytoplasm shrinks; the cells resemble lymphocytes. The nesting pattern deteriorates. Older cells tend to release their pigment and halt new melanin synthesis. As a consequence, the mature nevus extends deep beneath the epithelium, appears as a bland sheet of small blue cells, and bears little pigment. Observing this maturation sequence in stages permits one to learn the characteristic features of the common conjunctival nevi.[32]

Common Nevi

Junctional nevi are the darkest and most superficial melanocytic nevi of the conjunctiva. Such a nevus is nearly always present at birth or early infancy. It is a dark-brown, sometimes black, macule. The junctional nevus is completely intraepithelial (Fig. 2-83). It is situated predominantly at the basal epithelial layer (the junction of the epithelial and subepithelial layers), although clusters of nevus cells extend vertically toward the surface. As previously explained, junctional nevus cells are the most immature and pose the greatest risk (albeit a low risk) for malignant transformation. This fact, combined with concern for the child's appearance, appropriately results in early excision. With all other common conjunctival nevi, the risk of developing malignant melanoma is extraordinarily low. The diagnosis of a newly acquired junctional nevus in an adult should be approached with skep-

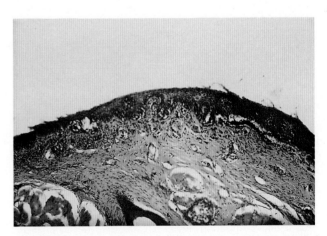

FIG. 2-83. Junctional nevus. Small nests of intraepithelial nevus cells. Biopsy taken from darkly pigmented conjunctival macule that was present in infancy.

ticism, as primary acquired melanosis has similar microscopic features and is far more likely in this age group. In general, the body's tendency to form new melanocytic nevi decreases steadily with age. Moreover, most existing benign nevi tend to fade over time. Variations to these time-tested precepts always deserve careful scrutiny.

The most frequently diagnosed common conjunctival nevus is the **compound nevus.** Most congenital nevi are compound nevi. This benign growth represents the next stage of maturation, with nevus cells present both within the epithelium and beneath in the subepithelial space (Fig. 2-84). The compound nevus may darken and enlarge with the onset of puberty. A reassuring clinical finding that supports the diagnosis of compound nevus is the presence of numerous cysts within the pigmented patch. Histologically, nests of nevus cells straddle the epithelial basement membrane. Subepithelial cysts are lined by nonkeratinizing squamous epithelium and often include goblet cells. Compared with the junctional nevus, the compound nevus appears less dark and is minimally elevated.

The conjunctival counterpart to the cutaneous intradermal nevus is the **subepithelial nevus.** Nevus cells have finished maturing and have completely abandoned the conjunctival epithelium (Fig. 2-85). The subepithelial space is distended by pale, shrunken nevus cells mimicking a neuroidal or lymphocytoid proliferation. Epithelium-lined cysts may persist.

Any of the common conjunctival nevi may be accompanied by a focally intense chronic nongranulomatous inflammatory infiltrate.

Two helpful guidelines aid in clinical decision-making regarding the management of suspicious conjunctival pigmentations. First, nevi tend to arise early in life and fade with time; most nevi disappear by the sixth decade. In older adults, any newly emergent pigmented patches on the conjunctiva should be approached with caution. Second, there are few, if any, benign newly acquired pig-

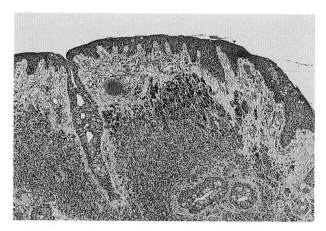

FIG. 2-85. Subepithelial nevus. Benign nevus cells situated in subepithelial layer.

mented growths involving the palpebral or fornical conjunctiva in patients over age 40. All such lesions warrant biopsy. If a benign diagnosis is returned, the clinician should reevaluate the accuracy of the patient's history or ask for the biopsy to be reviewed, or both. The clinician should visit the pathologist to examine the biopsy slides.

The current generation of practitioners has witnessed a rapid evolution of our understanding of **primary acquired melanosis** (PAM). Increased attention has been paid to the conjunctival pigment alteration given this name by Jakobiec and coworkers.[32] Earlier names included *precancerous melanosis* and *benign acquired melanosis.* Attention to PAM is well deserved, as it is the most common precursor lesion for conjunctival malignant melanoma.

As part of any clinical assessment for conjunctival pigmentation, the clinician must carefully determine if the process is unilateral or bilateral. One simple rule minimizes diagnostic confusion over PAM and other pigmented lesions: PAM is nearly always unilateral. Variability is the watchword regarding the clinical appearance of PAM, as it will change color, size, and affected regions (but will not involve the fellow eye). PAM arises from dendritic melanocytes, not from nevoid melanocytes. It may begin as a noncircumscribed dusky discoloration and develop into darker flat patches. Over a period of months, PAM tends to wax and wane. Single or multiple patches may fade only to reappear in a different quadrant.

The onset of PAM is in the fourth or fifth decade. The clinical course lasts years, even decades. Such a slow and indolent disease process can lead to a delay in diagnosis. No racial groups are exempt, but PAM in blacks rarely progresses to malignant melanoma. Not all cases of PAM become malignant melanoma; however, there are no clinical features that can identify the high-risk cases. Conjunctival biopsy is the only accurate method to diagnose PAM.

Histopathologically, PAM is divided into two groups: low-risk PAM without atypia, and high-risk PAM with atypia. The former accounts for about one third of all

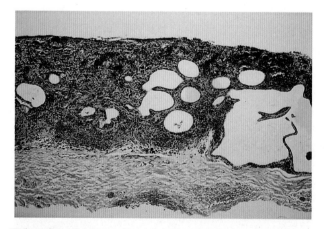

FIG. 2-84. Compound nevus. Descending nevus cells recruit neighboring surface epithelial cells with consequent subepithelial cyst formation. Visualization of cysts is a clinical indicator of benignity.

biopsied PAM cases. Here one finds a proliferation of generally uniform dendritic melanocytes confined to the basal epithelial layer (Fig. 2-86). These benign-appearing pigmented cells remain confined to the base, although adjacent pigment-bearing epithelial cells migrate toward the surface. It is often difficult to distinguish between melanocytes and pigment-bearing epithelial cells in routine H&E-stained sections. Perinuclear cytoplasmic retraction, if observed, is suggestive of melanocytes. Once again, clinical data are valuable in establishing the correct diagnosis. PAM without atypia does not progress to malignant melanoma.

Nearly two thirds of PAM biopsy cases belong to the high-risk category, PAM with atypia (malignant melanosis, melanoma in situ). Architectural and cytologic abnormalities are encountered. The proliferating atypical melanocytes assume a variety of cellular forms: polyhedral cells, spindle cells, large dendritic melanocytes, and even epithelioid cells. In addition to the abnormal morphology, these cells percolate toward the conjunctival surface (Fig. 2-87). The normal ratio of epithelial cells to melanocytes is inverted. In advanced states, malignant cells replace almost the entire conjunctival epithelium. The epithelial basement membrane remains intact. Involved conjunctiva should be excised or treated with cryotherapy. Additional clinical studies can identify the presence of epithelioid cells, a growth pattern exceeding basilar hyperplasia, and distant intraepithelial (pagetoid) extension by PAM with atypia as poor prognostic factors for the eventual development of invasive malignant melanoma.

Caution is advised in managing patients who have PAM without atypia. Biopsy confirmation is favorable information, but it applies only to the tissue biopsied; it does not preclude the development of separate or subsequent areas of PAM with atypia. Periodic surveillance conjunctival biopsies have been advocated as a preventive measure.

Conjunctival **malignant melanoma** can arise from preexisting PAM, from preexisting conjunctival nevi, or de

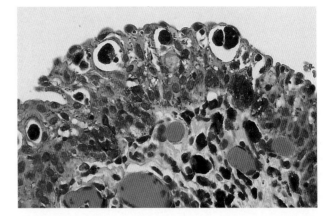

FIG. 2-87. Primary acquired melanosis with atypia. Melanocytic proliferation involves full thickness of surface epithelium, unilateral. High risk for developing melanoma in untreated cases.

novo without any apparent preexisting lesion. The neoplastic melanocytes can be of the nevocytic or dendritic type. Malignant tumor cells violate the epithelial basement membrane and extend into the subepithelial layers, thus creating an enlarging painless nodule (Fig. 2-88). Conjunctival malignant melanoma does not typically invade the globe. Tumor may seed the orbit directly, or more commonly it reaches the systemic circulation via the lymphatic drainage. Cell types encountered in melanomas from other ocular and extraocular sites have been identified in the conjunctival species: spindle, polyhedral, epithelioid, and balloon cells. It is inaccurate to apply the modified Callender classification developed for posterior uveal melanomas to the conjunctiva. Mortality due to metastatic spread of conjunctival malignant melanoma exceeds 25%. Factors that correlate with a poorer prognosis include a palpebral or fornical location, preexistent PAM with atypia featuring pagetoid extension, predomi-

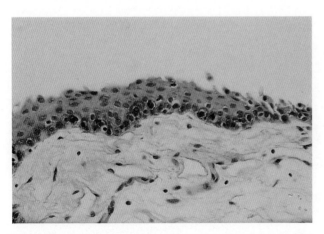

FIG. 2-86. Primary acquired melanosis without atypia. Melanocytic proliferation confined to basilar layer, unilateral. Low risk for melanoma.

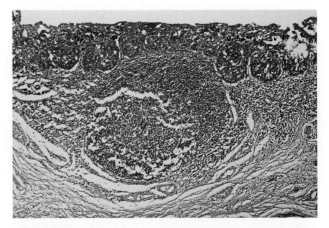

FIG. 2-88. Conjunctival malignant melanoma. Invasive palpebral mass composed of atypical melanocytes. Precursor lesion was junctional nevus for which treatment was refused.

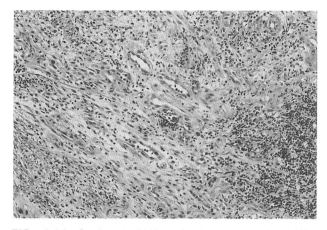

FIG. 2-89. Conjunctival Kaposi sarcoma. Hypercellular spindle-cell neoplasm with slit vascular spaces and extravasated erythrocytes.

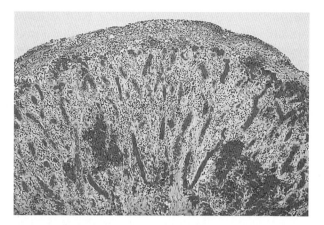

FIG. 2-90. Pyogenic granuloma. Several weeks following chalazion curettage; rapidly growing vascular mass composed of fibroblasts, capillaries, and a mixed inflammatory infiltrate.

nance of epithelioid cells, and tumor invasion deeper than 0.8 mm.[33]

Conjunctival malignant melanoma is far rarer than uveal melanoma. Any evaluation of suspected epibulbar conjunctival melanoma must exclude the possibility of extraocular extension from a primary uveal melanoma.

A large collection of noncancerous pigmentations may clinically resemble a conjunctival malignant melanoma. Patients with these **pseudomelanomas** frequently report a history of a longstanding "mole" that abruptly changed in size or color. Clinical conditions that may play a role in pseudomelanoma include chronic hemorrhage, retained foreign bodies, and nevi responding to hormonal changes or inflammation.

Lymphoid

The conjunctiva is an infrequent site of origin for both benign and malignant lymphoid proliferations. Patients are usually older adults and free of ocular symptomatology. Elevated pink-tan fleshy nodules may appear in any conjunctival region but predominate in the fornix.[34] Bilaterality carries no diagnostic or prognostic significance; in fact, the clinical examination yields limited information and cannot reliably differentiate between reactive lymphoid hyperplasia and malignant non-Hodgkin's lymphoma. Tissue biopsy is necessary to characterize the mass as benign or malignant.

Important recommendations involving the diagnostic workup for suspicious lymphoid proliferations involving the ocular adnexa were presented earlier. There is considerable overlap between eyelid and conjunctival lymphoid disease that will not be repeated here.

It is important to discern if the "salmon patch" lesion in the cul-de-sac is actually a primary conjunctival lymphoproliferation. Orbital, eyelid, and sinus masses, as well as distant malignancies, can manifest in this same fashion. Knowles and coworkers reported that patients with pri-

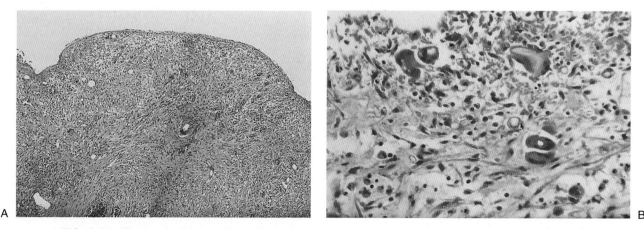

FIG. 2-91. Foreign body granuloma [low (**A**) and high (**B**) power images]. Trapped synthetic fibers incite focally intense host foreign-body hypersensitivity reaction. Multinucleated giant cells surround birefringent fibers.

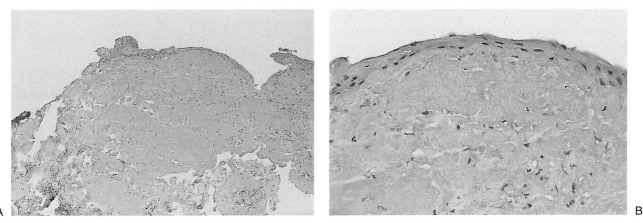

FIG. 2-92. Ligneous conjunctivitis [low (**A**) and high (**B**) power images]. Aberrant host response to chronic inflammation. Accumulation of hyalinized collagen.

mary conjunctival lymphoid tumors (benign or malignant) usually present with a visible mass but almost never complain of diplopia, ptosis, or exophthalmos.[21]

Unlike the eyelid, conjunctival non-Hodgkin's lymphoma has a relatively good prognosis, with extraocular lymphoma developing in only about 20% of cases.

Vascular

The conjunctiva can give rise to many of the vascular disorders discussed earlier in the chapter. Capillary hemangiomas and lymphangiomas usually appear in conjunction with coexistent lid and orbital masses, but isolated forms of both exist. Their histopathology was previously discussed. Conjunctival and epibulbar involvement in Sturge-Weber syndrome (encephalotrigeminal angiomatosis) is predictive for a secondary open angle glaucoma. Arteriovenous malformations within the hemangiomas elevate normal episcleral or conjunctival venous pressure and retard aqueous outflow.

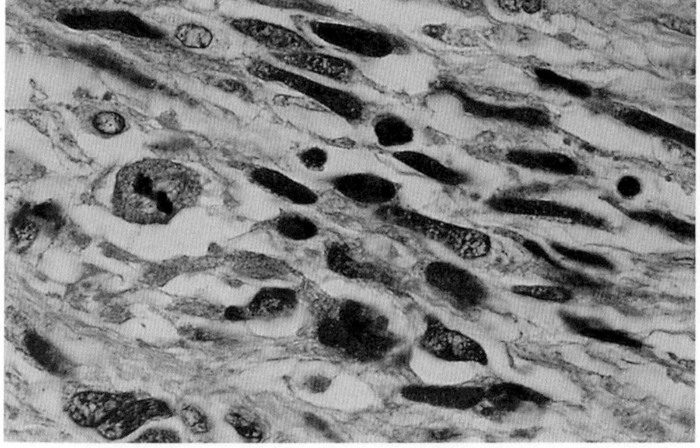

KS was mentioned in the eyelid portion of this chapter, but several points deserve repeat emphasis. The AIDS epidemic has reintroduced KS into the mainstream practice of clinical medicine. Most cases of conjunctival KS arise in homosexual and bisexual males infected with HIV. It may be the earliest clinical sign of active AIDS.[20] Organ transplant recipients also have developed conjunctival KS that may spontaneously regress after cessation of systemic immunosuppresive therapy. KS may clinically simulate a subconjunctival hemorrhage, except that it tends to enlarge rather than resorb. KS is a malignant vascular neoplasm consisting of a neoplastic proliferation of endothelial cells. KS forms a solid mass consisting of capillaries and slit-like vascular spaces within a spindled stroma (Fig. 2-89).

Miscellaneous

After accidental or surgical trauma to the conjunctiva, patients occasionally develop a rapidly enlarging mass that bears the confusing misnomer **pyogenic granuloma.** These have occurred after chalazion curettage, pterygium excision (recurrent pterygium), and strabismus surgery. Described in the earlier literature as "proud flesh," microscopic examination of excisional biopsy specimens reveals a benign and exuberant proliferation of granulation tissue (Fig. 2-90). It is characterized by the presence of abundant capillaries, fibroblasts, and inflammatory cells amidst an edematous stroma. Pyogenic granulomas also have been diagnosed in the setting of conjunctival foreign body granulomas, specifically those caused by the introduction of synthetic filamentous materials used in the manufacture of blankets and stuffed toys. We have seen several pediatric and adult cases like this presenting as suspicious, enlarging fornical conjunctival masses. Sections from biopsy demonstrate a large pyogenic granu-

FIG. 2-93. Conjunctival rhabdomyosarcoma. Embryonal variant most common. Poorly differentiated mesenchymal neoplasm. Malignant rhabdomyoblasts exhibit many bizarre forms.

loma resting atop a foreign body giant cell reaction to birefringent polarizable filamentous foreign material (Fig. 2-91).

Ligneous conjunctivitis is a rare and puzzling aberrant host response to chronic inflammation. Ligneous conjunctivitis typically appears bilaterally in young females. The clinical course is unpredictable. A patient may experience a single episode or endure decades of ocular discomfort due to the accumulation of hyalinized collagen within the palpebral conjunctiva. Granulation tissue is a component of this recurrent mass (Fig. 2-92). The cause remains obscure, as does any universally successful therapy. Most cases eventually spontaneously regress, and this fact prompts many clinicians to favor conservative management.

It is a mistake to believe that **rhabdomyosarcoma** can arise only within the orbit. Documented extraorbital sites of origin include intraocular tissues, eyelids, and conjunctiva. The superior and superonasal fornix are most frequent sites. The embryonal histologic pattern is most commonly encountered (Fig. 2-93).

REFERENCES

1. Griffith DG, Salasche SJ, Clemons DE. *Cutaneous abnormalities of the eyelid and face.* New York: McGraw-Hill, 1987.
2. Johnson CC. Developmental abnormalities of the eyelids. *Ophthalmol Plast Reconstr Surg* 1986;2:219.
3. Mansour AM, Barber JC, Reinecke RD, Wang FM. Ocular choristomas. *Surv Ophthalmol* 1989;33:339.
4. Alper MG, Zimmerman LE, LaPiana FG. Orbital manifestations of Erdheim-Chester disease. *Trans Am Ophthalmol Soc* 1983;81:64.
5. Sandgren O. Ocular amyloidosis, with special reference to the hereditary forms with vitreous involvement. *Surv Ophthalmol* 1995; 40:173.
6. Jakobiec FA, Jones IS. Introduction to ultrastructure, inflammation, and neoplasia. In: Jones IS, Jakobiec FA, eds. *Diseases of the orbit.* Hagerstown, MD: Harper & Row, 1979.
7. Saornil MA, Kurban RS, Westfall CT, Mihn MC Jr. Pathology of the lids. In: Albert DM, Jakobiec FA, eds. *Principles and practice of ophthalmology.* Philadelphia: WB Saunders, 1994.
8. Murphy GF, Elder DE. *Non-melanocytic tumors of the skin.* Washington, DC: Armed Forces Institute of Pathology, 3rd series, 1991.
9. Lever WF, Schaumberg-Lever G. *Histopathology of the skin,* 7th ed. Philadelphia: JB Lippincott, 1990.
10. Margo CE, Waltz K. Basal cell carcinoma of the eyelid and periocular skin. *Surv Ophthalmol* 1993;38:169.
11. Glover AT, Grove AS. Orbital invasion by malignant eyelid tumors. *Ophthalmol Plast Reconstr Surg* 1989;5:1.
12. Reifler DM, Hornblass A. Squamous cell carcinoma of the eyelid. *Surv Ophthalmol* 1986;30:349.
13. Bernardino VB Jr, Lloyd WC III, Naidoff MA. Melanocytic lesions of the eyelids. In: Fraunfelder FT, Roy FH, eds. *Current ocular therapy,* 4th ed. Philadelphia: WB Saunders, 1995.
14. Elder DE, Murphy GF. *Melanocytic tumors of the skin.* Washington, DC: Armed Forces Institute of Pathology, 3rd series, 1991.
15. Kass LG, Hornblass A. Sebaceous carcinoma of the ocular adnexa. *Surv Ophthalmol* 1989;33:477.
16. Jakobiec FA, Zimmerman LE, LaPiana F, Hornblass A, Breffeilh RA, Lackey JK. Unusual eyelid tumors with sebaceous differentiation in the Muir-Torre syndrome. *Ophthalmology* 1988;95:1543.
17. Simpson W, Garner A, Collin JR. Benign tumors in the differential diagnosis of basal cell carcinoma of the eyelids: a clinicopathological comparison. *Br J Ophthalmol* 1989; 73:347.
18. Sassani JW, Hidayat AA, Jakobiec FA. Unusual eyelid tumors. In: Albert DM, Jakobiec FA, eds. *Principles and practice of ophthalmology.* Philadelphia: WB Saunders, 1994.
19. Jakobiec FA, Font RL. Orbit. In: Spencer WH, ed. *Ophthalmic pathology,* 3rd ed. Philadelphia: WB Saunders, 1986.
20. Shuler JD, Holland GN, Miles SA, Miller BJ, Grossman I. Kaposi sarcoma of the conjunctiva and eyelids associated with the acquired immunodeficiency syndrome. *Arch Ophthalmol* 1989;107:858.
21. Knowles DM, Jakobiec FA, McNally L, Burke JS. Lymphoid hyperplasia and malignant lymphoma occurring in the ocular adnexa (orbit, conjunctiva, and eyelids). *Hum Pathol* 1990;21:959.
22. Font RL, Laucirica R, Rosenbaum PS, Patrinely JR, Boniuk M. Malignant lymphoma of the ocular adnexa associated with the benign lymphoepithelial lesion of the parotid glands. *Ophthalmology* 1992;99:1582.
23. Mansour AM, Hidyat AA. Metastatic eyelid disease. *Ophthalmology* 1987;94:667.
24. Mamalis N, Redlock RD, Holds JB, Anderson RL, Crandall AS. Merkel cell tumor of the eyelid: a review and report of an unusual case. *Ophthalmol Surg* 1989;20:410.
25. Jakobiec FA, Bonnano PA, Sigelman J. Conjunctival adnexal cysts and dermoids. *Arch Ophthalmol* 1978;96:1404.
26. Mondino BJ. Cicatricial pemphigoid and erythema multiforme. *Ophthalmology* 1990;97:939.
27. Foster CS. Cicatricial pemphigoid. *Trans Am Ophthalmol Soc* 1986; 84:527.
28. Imperia PS, Lazarus HM, Lass JH. Ocular complications of systemic cancer chemotherapy. *Surv Ophthalmol* 1989;34:209.
29. Grossniklaus HE, Green WR, Luckenbach M, et al. Conjunctival lesions in adults: a clinical and histopathologic review. *Cornea* 1987;6:78.
30. Margo CE, Stern AL, Stern GA. Intraepithelial sebaceous carcinoma of the conjunctiva and skin of the eyelid. *Ophthalmology* 1992;99: 227.
31. Folberg R, Jakobiec FA, Bernardino VB, Iwamoto T. Benign conjunctival melanocytic lesions: clinicopathologic features. *Ophthalmology* 1989;96:436.
32. Liesegang TJ. Pigmented conjunctival and scleral lesions. *Mayo Clin Proc* 1994;69:151.
33. Jakobiec FA, Folberg R, Iwamoto T. Clinicopathologic characteristics of premalignant and malignant melanocytic lesions of the conjunctiva. *Ophthalmology* 1989;96:147.
34. Campbell RJ. Tumors of the eyelids, conjunctiva, and cornea. In: Garner A, Klintworth GK, eds. *Pathobiology of ocular disease.* New York: Marcel Dekker, 1994.

Ophthalmic Pathology with Clinical Correlations,
edited by Joseph W. Sassani, M.D.
Lippincott-Raven Publishers, Philadelphia © 1997.

CHAPTER 3

Immunology and Intraocular Inflammation: Granulomatous and Nongranulomatous

Theresa R. Kramer and Scott Limstrom

PRINCIPLES OF GENERAL IMMUNOLOGY

Immunity is the capacity to distinguish foreign material from self and to neutralize, eliminate, or metabolize that which is foreign. An appropriately functioning immune system makes the body unsusceptible to the invasive or pathogenic effects of foreign microorganisms and to the toxic effect of antigenic substances. The defense against infection is an incredibly complex process. Throughout the ages, the human body has been exposed to countless challenges from infectious organisms such as bacteria, fungi, viruses, and parasites. To survive these challenges, various defense mechanisms have evolved. Such mechanisms can be broadly classified into two groups—an innate immune system and an acquired immune system.

Innate Immunity

The innate immune system includes the mechanisms for evading infection, which are nonspecific, lack memory, and do not discriminate self from nonself.[1] The first barrier an infecting organism encounters is the skin and mucosal membranes. These barriers prevent infection through local production of antimicrobials, competition from commensal organisms, and the mere presence of a physical barrier. The body also produces a variety of secretions that contain antimicrobial factors. Probably the most well known of these substances is **lysozyme,** present in tears, saliva, and nasal secretions. Lysozyme is a low molecular weight cationic protein. It acts locally by degrading the mucopolysaccharide cell wall of gram-

positive bacteria. Other secretory factors include lactoperoxidase, lipase, gastric acidity, and spermine.[2]

Once an organism overcomes the external barriers to infection, it encounters an innate cellular defense mechanism. These cells include the mononuclear phagocyte system, granulocytes, and natural killer (NK) cells.

The cells of the **mononuclear phagocyte system** develop from progenitors in the bone marrow and enter the circulation as monocytes, which eventually develop into macrophages. Monocytes are large cells with an oval nucleus and abundant cytoplasm filled with azurophilic granules. Monocytes have a serum half-life of 1 to 3 days before they migrate into various tissues and differentiate into macrophages. Fixed macrophages, or cells of the reticuloendothelial system, also are important in innate immunity. Macrophages actively phagocytize and destroy foreign material and present antigen to cells of the acquired immune system.[3]

The **polymorphonuclear neutrophil** (PMN) accounts for 60% to 65% of white cells in circulation. The cell gets its name from its characteristic multilobed nucleus. Its progenitors also form in the bone marrow. The PMN contains many granules, which function in the phagocytosis and destruction of invaders. Primary granules contain various hydrolytic enzymes. Secondary granules contain many of the same enzymes but lack myeloperoxidase.[4]

The third component of the innate cellular defense is the **NK cell.** The precursor of this cell is not known; however, it is believed to be a lymphocyte. The NK cell appears as a large granular lymphocyte with a round or indented nucleus and abundant cytoplasm. The cytoplasm is filled with azurophilic granules containing hydrolases. The NK cell acts in the destruction of certain tumor and viral-infected cells.[5]

Immunocytology is a special type of histology that has produced monoclonal antibodies to immune-cell antigens, which can delineate B cells from T cells and help to

T. R. Kramer: Departments of Ophthalmology and Pathology, University of Arizona, Tucson, Arizona 85719.

S. Limstrom: Department of Ophthalmology, University of Arizona, Tucson, Arizona 85719.

identify cells in different stages of lymphoid differentiation. These antigens are distinguished by the prefix CD (cluster designation) and are summarized in Table 1. Immunocytochemical characterization of many forms of intraocular inflammation also has been completed[6-12] as has immunocytochemical staining of vitreous cells for diagnostic purposes.[13]

Acquired Immunity

As the invading organism encounters the cells of the innate immune system, another parallel defense system, the acquired immunity, begins to function. In contrast to innate immunity, acquired immunity is specific for the

TABLE 1. *Some immune cell antigens detected by monoclonal antibodies*

Antigen designation*	Comments
Primary T cell-associated	
CD2	Receptor for sheep erythrocytes; present on all T cells (peripheral and intrathymic) and NK cells
CD3	Present all peripheral T cells; associated with the T-cell antigen receptor
CD4	Present on 60% of peripheral cells and some monocytes; a marker for T helper-inducer cells
CD5	Present on all T lymphocytes, peripheral and intrathymic
CD7	Present on all T lymphocytes
CD8	Present on 30% of peripheral T cells; marker for cytotoxic cells
CD25	Receptor for interleukin 2; present on activated T cells and monocytes
Primary B cell-associated	
CD19	Present on B cells, from pre-B stage to mature B cells; absent from plasma cells
CD20	Appears on pre-B cells after CD19; otherwise similar to CD19 in distribution
CD10	Common acute lymphoblastic leukemia antigen (CALLA); present on pre-B cells
Primary monocyte- or macrophage-associated	
CD13	Present on blood monocytes and granulocytes
CD33	Present on myeloid stem cells and mature monocytes
CD11b	Present on monocytes, granulocytes, and some NK cells; receptor for complement (C3b)
Primarily NK cell-associated	
CD16	Present on all NK cells and granulocytes; low-affinity receptor for Fc portion of 1gG
Present on all leukocytes	
CD45	
CD11a	

* The antigens are designated by the prefix *CD* (cluster designation) based on Third International Workshop on Human Leukocyte Differentiation Antigens as reported by Shaw S. *Immunol Today* 1987;8:1.

(From Cotran RS, Kumar V, Robbins SL. *Robbins pathologic basis of disease.* Philadelphia: WB Saunders, 1989)

antigen encountered. The acquired system also possesses memory (upon subsequent exposure, the response is amplified) and discriminates self from nonself.[1] The ability to form a specific immunologic response, which discriminates self and contains memory, develops from a complex interplay of DNA rearrangements and cellular interactions.

Molecular Biology of Acquired Immunity

The initial event in forming the immune response involves processing the antigen. An **antigen** is defined as any substance capable of invoking an immune response. It is important to differentiate the antigenicity of an antigen from its immunogenicity. **Antigenicity** refers solely to the ability of an antigen to bind to an antibody. In contrast, **immunogenicity** refers to its ability to stimulate an immune response. Three qualities of an antigen confer immunogenicity. These include foreignness, high molecular weight, and chemical complexity.[14]

The acquired response begins when antigen-presenting cells ingest and break down a foreign substance. The antigenic material is processed and presented externally as an epitope in conjunction with **major histocompatibility complex (MHC)** class II proteins.[15] An **epitope** is the area of the antigen involved in antibody binding. It is a very small region consisting of 4 to 5 amino acids or a monosaccharide.[16] Once the epitope is expressed externally, it is bound by T and B lymphocytes. T-helper cells are restricted to binding the epitope in the presence of MHC class II. T-suppressor and B cells are not MHC restricted. MHC is a group of genes that code for cell surface proteins, which act as identifiers in allorecognition and antigen presentation. T-helper cells have an MHC receptor consisting of a glycoprotein. It is this receptor, termed **CD4,** which is restricted to binding the epitope in conjunction with MHC class II.[17]

With the MHC providing the ability to discriminate self, how does this response develop specificity and memory? The answer again lies in the interaction of the lymphocytes with the epitope. For many years, two theories—the template theory and the clonal selection theory—existed to explain how lymphocytes formed antibody specific to the antigen. The template theory suggested that antibodies were formed through differential folding of protein chains to correspond to the specific antigen.[18] This theory could not explain the development of memory or the large rise in antibody production that occurs early in the immune response. The clonal selection theory maintains that a pool of lymphocytes is formed and that each lymphocyte is capable of producing only one antibody specific to one antigen. This pool of lymphocytes is capable of interacting with a specific antigen, can develop a large initial production of antibody, and is capable of an enhanced secondary response through the formation of memory cells. This theory had difficulty explaining how cells of identical genetic make-up could differentiate into cells specific for a wide array of antigens. The latter question remained unanswered until Tonegawa and Hozumi reported the first direct evidence that variable and constant regions of the antibody light chains are coded separately and subsequently are joined.[19] In other words, during cell development, the genes undergo rearrangement resulting in a pool of lymphocytes, each coding for a different antibody.[20] The clonal selection theory is now generally accepted as the explanation for how antibody is produced.

As previously mentioned, the CD4 cell binds epitope in conjunction with MHC class II. A B cell specific to the antigen also binds the epitope, via antibody expressed on its cell surface. A complex interaction then takes place whereby the T cell secretes various substances resulting in B-cell activation, growth, and differentiation into a high-rate antibody-secreting cell.[21]

Antibody Structure

Antibodies are protein molecules capable of binding antigen. The basic structure of the antibody molecule consists of a tetramer consisting of two identical heavy chains and two identical light chains bound through disulfide bonds (Fig. 3-1). Light chains have a molecular weight of about 23,000 and are designated kappa or lambda. Heavy chains are about twice the size of light chains. There are five isotopes of heavy chains designated gamma, mu, delta, alpha, and epsilon. A hinge region exists where the heavy chains are bound together. Both the heavy and the light chains display variable regions at the N-terminus of the monomer. Hypervariable regions within the variable regions are important in antigen binding.[21,22]

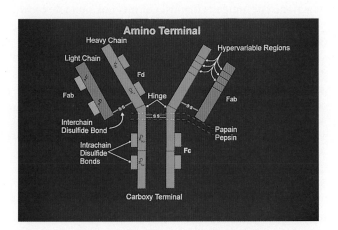

FIG. 3-1. Graphic representation of an antibody molecule including the heavy chain, the light chain, as well as highlights of the important regions of the molecule.

The differentiation of the heavy chain into five types allows immunoglobulins to be divided into five classes. All of the antibody classes exist as monomers except immunoglobulin M (IgM), which forms a pentamer, and secretory immunoglobulin A (IgA), which forms a dimer.

IgG is the prototypical antibody. It accounts for 75% of total serum immunoglobulin and is the only immunoglobulin capable of crossing the placenta, thereby providing neonatal immunity. The two main functions of IgG are to opsonize foreign material and to fix complement.[16]

IgA exists both in the serum, and in various secretions (eg, tears, saliva, colostrum). Serum IgA accounts for about 20% of serum antibody. It is important in complement fixation via the alternate pathway. Secretory IgA exists as two IgA molecules joined by a secretory component and a J chain. As the IgA monomers pass through the mucosa in various secretions, they are joined by the secretory component produced by the epithelium.[23] Secretory IgA prevents infection by interfering with pathogen adherence and colonization.

IgM is a serum immunoglobulin. It accounts for about 10% of serum antibody. Five IgM molecules are joined by disulfide bonds and a J chain. IgM is the initial antibody formed in an immune response. It functions in opsonization and complement fixation. Because of its pentameric configuration, IgM is very efficient at forming bridges between antigenic determinants resulting in agglutination.[2]

IgD accounts for only 1% of the serum antibody; however, it does occur in large quantities on the surface of B lymphocytes. This observation indicates IgD may play a role in antigen recognition and B-cell activation.[24]

IgE or **reaginic antibody** is present in serum only in trace amounts. IgE possesses a high affinity for both mast cells and basophils. When antigen binds the IgE attached to these cells, they release several factors important in hypersensitivity and allergy. IgE does not function in complement fixation.[25]

When antigen is encountered, B lymphocytes are activated into synthetically active immunoblasts, which eventually develop into antibody-secreting plasma cells. The initial antibody formed is IgM. Shortly thereafter, the plasma cells secrete IgG. As IgG production increases, a parallel decline in IgM production occurs (Figs. 3-2 and 3-3). Upon reexposure to the antigen, IgG is formed from the onset, permitting a more rapid response which is thought to be secondary to memory cells formed during the initial exposure.[26]

Complement

The term **complement** describes a group of plasma and cell membrane proteins, which play a variety of roles in defense. The activation of the complement system progresses in a cascade fashion, similar to the coagulation

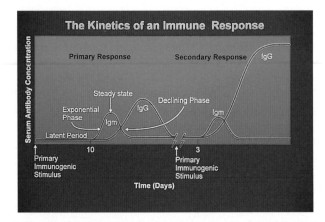

FIG. 3-2. Graphic representation of the kinetics of the primary and secondary immune response including early increase of IgM titer and later rise of IgG after a primary immunogenic stimulus.

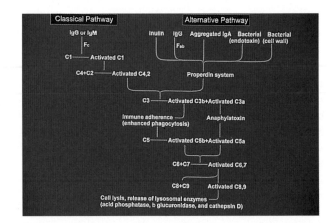

FIG. 3-4. Graphic representation of the classical pathway and the alternative pathway of the complement cascade with cell lysis and release of lysosomal enzymes as the final common pathway.

cascade and fibrinolysis. Complement can be activated via antigen/antibody complexes, termed the **classical pathway.** Endotoxin, bacterial cell wall, polysaccharide, and IgA can activate complement via the **alternate pathway** (Fig. 3-4). This mechanism is not specific for the antigen and, therefore, falls under the realm of innate immunity.[27]

Complement proteins are designated C and are numbered 1 through 9 in the order in which they are activated. During complement activation, numerous substances that play an integral role in the immune response are produced. Probably the most important of the activated components are C3a and C5a, known as the **anaphylotoxins.** These proteins get their name by their ability to induce mast-cell and basophil degranulation during anaphylaxis. C3a also functions in immune regulation. C5a has several functions, which include chemotaxis, neutrophil adherence and activation, and stimulation of leukotriene production.[28]

Complement also can cause cell lysis. A complex is

formed at the point of C5 activation consisting of C5b6789. The complex induces formation of hollow cylinders in the cell membrane leading to osmotic cell lysis.[16] Several of the other components of complement play small but important roles in the immune response.

Hypersensitivity Reactions

The same immunologic mechanisms that provide protection against invading pathogens also may produce deleterious effects termed **hypersensitivity reactions.** They are divided into four different classes based on the cellular and molecular mechanisms unique to each class.

Type I Hypersensitivity

Type I or immediate hypersensitivity is mediated through the effects of IgE. When antigen binds cell-bound IgE, various substances are released initiating the type I reaction. The antigens that trigger this reaction are known as **allergens.** A variety of substances, such as pollens, foods, drugs, and chemicals can act as allergens.[29]

During initial exposure to the allergen, IgE specific to the antigen is produced. This antibody ultimately becomes bound to mast cells and basophils. On subsequent exposure, antigen binds to the cells, bridging two IgE molecules, resulting in degranulation and release of chemical mediators. The release of mediators is coupled to adenosine $3':5'$-cyclic phosphate (cyclic AMP), which results in the aggregation of microtubules in the cell membrane through which mediators are released.[30]

The type I reaction can vary from minor itching and rash to systemic anaphylaxis. The mediators of immediate hypersensitivity include histamine, bradykinin, serotonin, eosinophil chemotactic factor, platelet aggregation factor, and prostaglandins.[31]

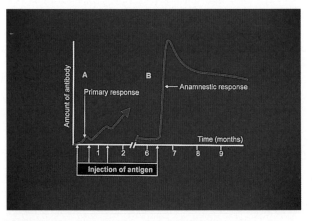

FIG. 3-3. Graphic representation of the primary and anamnestic responses after injection of antigen.

Atopy is an immediate hypersensitivity reaction characterized by the propensity to respond to many allergens. Atopy can manifest as allergic rhinitis, asthma, hives, angioedema, and eczema.[2] The development of atopy is thought to be genetically linked. Low levels of serum IgA during infancy have been linked to later development of atopy.[32]

Type II Hypersensitivity

Cytotoxic reactions initiated through the binding of IgG or IgM are classified as type II hypersensitivity. This type of hypersensitivity results when antibody binds the surface antigens of normal cells resulting in phagocytosis or in complement activation and cell lysis.[33] Many diseases fall under the heading of type II hypersensitivity. The most common are transfusion reactions, Rh incompatibility, systemic lupus erythematosus, and idiopathic thrombocytopenic purpura.[1]

Drug reactions may occur by this mechanism. An immune reaction is initiated when a drug binds to the cell surface in the form of a hapten. A **hapten** is a low molecular weight substance that becomes immunogenic when bound to a high molecular weight carrier.[2] Drugs associated with type II hypersensitivity include chloramphenicol, phenacetin, chlorpromazine, and quinidine.[31]

Type III Hypersensitivity

Type III or immune complex reactions were discovered in 1903 by Maurice Arthus. He immunized rabbits with repeated intradermal injections of horse serum. Initially, a mild erythema and edema developed. As time progressed, repeat injections resulted in hemorrhagic necrosis.[31] It is now known that this reaction is secondary to the formation of immune complexes.

The pathogenesis of immune complex disease begins with the formation of soluble antigen–antibody complexes. This process generally occurs in the presence of antigen excess. The immune complexes must be small enough to avoid phagocytosis and large enough to initiate the complement cascade.[33] Once formed, the immune complexes deposit in various tissues resulting in an inflammatory response.

The deposition of immune complexes can be localized, as in hypersensitivity pneumonitis, or diffuse, as in serum sickness. Serum sickness is characterized by fever, rash, splenomegaly, lymphadenopathy, arthritis, and glomerulonephritis. Intravenous infusion of immune complexes in rabbits has been shown to increase ocular vascular permeability in the region of the ciliary body.[34] This finding may explain the development of nongranulomatous iritis seen in serum sickness.[33]

Type IV Hypersensitivity

In contrast to the other classes of hypersensitivity, type IV is carried out predominately by T cells. Because the response occurs days after antigen exposure, type IV also is termed delayed type hypersensitivity. The pathogenesis of the type IV response begins with exposure to the antigen. The response is specific to the antigen, which must be presented in the context of MHC class II proteins.[35] The T cell that is specific for the antigen is activated and differentiates into memory cells that distribute throughout the body. The T cells that initiate the response display the CD4 marker. Cytotoxic and suppressor cells, which display the CD8 marker, are important in subsequent responses. During secondary exposure to the antigen, memory cells are activated, divide, and release lymphokines. **Lymphokines** are a large group of inflammatory mediators that have a variety of effects on inflammatory cells. Their individual names describe their actions. For example, macrophage chemotactic factor stimulates migration of macrophages to the site of inflammation. Other lymphokines include macrophage activating factor, migration inhibition factor, interleuken-2 (stimulates T-cell division), and gamma interferon (activates macrophages).[36]

Delayed type hypersensitivity plays an important role in the defense against fungi, viruses, protozoans, and certain bacteria. Contact sensitivity and allograft rejection represent pathologic delayed type hypersensitivity reactions.

In contact sensitivity, lipid soluble environmental agents penetrate the skin and form bonds with skin proteins. The agent, in effect, becomes a hapten conjugated to a carrier protein. It is thus capable of stimulating an immune response. Contact sensitivity presents clinically as flare, papular, or vesicular reactions at the site of exposure.[37]

The antigen that initiates allograft rejection is thought to be the class II human leukocyte antigen present on the cells of donor tissue.[38] Graft rejection occurs in three types: hyperacute, acute, and chronic. In **hyperacute rejection,** the host has preformed antibodies to the donor tissue due to ABO blood antigen mismatch. This results in immediate rejection characterized by vascular spasm and occlusion. Acute rejection occurs 10 to 30 days after transplantation. The pathogenesis of **acute rejection** involves a delayed type hypersensitivity response initiated against the HLA antigen of the donor tissue. This process presents as a lymphocytic and mononuclear infiltration of the donor perivascular tissue. **Chronic rejection** occurs over a period of months to years with a gradual loss of tissue function.[36]

Corneal graft rejection is an example of delayed type hypersensitivity and is the most common cause of corneal allograft failure in the late postoperative period. Graft rejection may present with epithelial or endothelial manifestations. Epithelial rejection presents clinically as an elevated line that moves across the cornea. Round subepithelial deposits also may be seen. Endothelial rejection presents clinically with corneal edema due to endothelial cell dysfunction. Fine keratic precipitates and anterior chamber reaction also are seen. Keratic precipitates may aggregate into a distinct line known as the **Khodadoust line.** The etiology of graft rejection is thought to be a combination of antibody and cell-mediated hypersensitivity reactions.[39]

Histopathologically, epithelial rejection consists of a line of polymorphonuclear leukocytes followed by a line of lymphocytes. The epithelial cells are disorganized and irregular with loss of superficial layers. The endothelial rejection line is infiltrated with lymphocytes. The endothelial cells are rounded and globular. Lymphocytes, monocytes, and fibrin may precipitate on the endothelial surface.[31]

If treated early, rejection usually responds well to immunosuppressive therapy. A combination of topical, subconjunctival, and systemic corticosteroids often can reverse even advanced rejection.

GENERAL PRINCIPLES OF INTRAOCULAR INFLAMMATION

Inflammation is defined as a localized protective response elicited by injury to or destruction of tissues. The process serves to destroy, dilute, and sequester the injurious agent and to partly isolate the injured tissue. It involves a complex series of events, including dilatation of arterioles, capillaries, and venules resulting in increased blood flow and vascular permeability, exudation of fluid and plasma proteins, and migration of leukocytes into the inflammatory region. Inflammation is a dynamic process resulting from a complex interplay of vascular, humoral, and cellular factors. It can be elicited by many physical, chemical, and biologic stimuli.

The nature and extent of the inflammatory process are defined by the interplay of the direct cellular damage causing the inflammatory response, indirect cellular destruction produced by the mechanisms that enhance the inflammatory process, and the host's capacity to mount an immunologic response. Thus, in the normal situation, the inflammatory response, although destructive, should neutralize an inciting agent.

It is well known that, under certain conditions, the immune response itself can be harmful as in autoimmune diseases. In addition, when the host immune mechanism is inhibited or modulated, as in the acquired immunodeficiency syndrome and other immunocompromised situations, the process can be deficient and damaging.

Terminology and Definitions

The suffix *-itis* generally is used to designate an inflammatory process. If several tissues are simultaneously involved, the one that is the most prominently or initially affected is designated first in the terminology. It is important to separate "true" intraocular inflammatory processes from pseudoinflammatory processes such as pseudouveitis, in which the inciting agent is ischemia or neoplasia. Examples of pseudoinflammatory processes include the pseudohypopyon produced by a leukemia, retinoblastoma, or metastatic neuroblastoma[40] or pseudouveitis produced by the anterior segment ischemic syndrome.[41,42] Table 2 delineates the terms used to denote inflammation involving specific ocular structures.

Histopathologic Characteristics of Tissue Changes

For the purposes of classification, the histopathologic changes seen in inflammation have been characterized as **granulomatous** and **nongranulomatous.** Clinically, small keratic precipitates characterize nongranulomatous inflammation, and larger, clumped, greasy-appearing aggregates are typical of granulomatous inflammation. These terms, however, are misleading because they imply a pathologic entity that can only be recognized by biopsy of the involved tissue.

Granulomatous Inflammations

A **granuloma** is a mass or nodule that usually is less than 2 mm in diameter, is composed of macrophages or modified macrophages known as **epithelioid cells,** and may contain **multinucleated giant cells** (Fig. 3-5). Histopathologically, the lesion usually is surrounded by a rim of mononuclear cells, mainly lymphocytes. Actively growing fibroblasts and capillary buds also may be identified within a granuloma. The term **granulomatous inflammation** refers to inflammation in which granulomas are present and usually occurs in response to certain defined infectious agents. The differential diagnosis of granulomatous intraocular inflammations includes bacteria (tuberculosis, syphilis, and leprosy), mycoses (candidiasis, histoplasmosis, coccidioidomycosis, cryptococcosis, and toxoplasmosis), and parasites (toxocariasis, onchocerciasis, and cysticercosis).[43] Granulomatous inflammations also can be induced by a reaction to autologous intraocular tissue such as in phacoanaphylactic endophthalmitis, resorbing vitreous hemorrhage, cholesterol granuloma, sympathetic ophthalmia, and chalazion. Immunologic processes of unclear etiology include sarcoidosis, Vogt-Koyanagi-Harada (VKH) syndrome, Still's disease, scleritis/uveitis in rheumatoid arthritis,[44] Chédiak-Higashi syndrome, and juvenile xanthogranuloma.[43] These entities also have been associated with granulomatous inflammation. Intraocular foreign bodies can incite a granulomatous inflammatory response.[43,45,46]

Three histologic patterns have been associated with granulomatous inflammation including the nodular pat-

TABLE 2. *Terminology of intraocular inflammations*

Inflammation	Definition	Examples and remarks
Endophthalmitis	Involvement of all intraocular tissues except the cornea and sclera	Posttraumatic; phacoanaphylactic endophthalmitis; metastatic, endogenous, and organism-induced endophthalmitis
Panophthalmitis	Involvement of all intraocular tissues including the cornea and sclera; often accompanied by involvement of the orbit with proptosis	Posttraumatic, perforating corneal ulcers; involvement of the globe secondarily in inflammatory orbital processes, eg, Wegener's granulomatosis and mucormycosis
Uveitis	General term for all inflammations of the uveal tract	—
Panuveitis	Inflammation involving the entire uveal tract	—
Anterior uveitis	Inflammation of the iris and ciliary body; iridocyclitis	—
Iritis	Inflammation of the iris	Exudative process primarily in the anterior chamber; minimal involvement of the anterior vitreous
Cyclitis	Infiltration of the ciliary body	Exudates also located within the anterior vitreous
Pars planitis	Massive infiltration of peripheral retina and vitreous; often with connective tissue scarring between the pars plana and equator of the lens	Associated with retinal perivasculitis
Choroiditis	Inflammatory process begins in the choroid; in later stages, there may be involvement of the retina (chorioretinitis)	Presumed ocular histoplasmosis syndrome; granulomatous choroiditis in tuberculosis; sympathetic ophthalmia
Chorioretinitis	Primarily a choroidal inflammatory process; secondary involvement of the retinal pigment epithelium and sensory retina; commonly chorioretinal scarring and reactive proliferation of the retinal pigment epithelium	Granulomatous inflammation caused by syphilis, sarcoidosis, and endogenous mycoses
Retinitis	Inflammation largely confined to the sensory retina and pigment epithelium	Measles retinitis; cytomegalic inclusion disease retinitis; herpes simplex retinitis; rubella retinitis
Retinochoroiditis	Primary inflammation involvement in the sensory retina; choroid secondarily involved	Acquired toxoplasmosis
Retinal vasculitis and perivasculitis	Inflammation of the retinal vessels	Sarcoidosis; Behçet's disease
Papillitis	Inflammation of the optic nerve; isolated inflammation of the nerve head alone is unusual; commonly involves the deeper nerve substance and the peripapillary retina (neuroretinitis) common	Optic neuritis and multiple sclerosis

(Modified from Naumann GOH, Naumann LR. Intraoccular inflammations. In: Naumann GOH, Apple DJ, eds. *Pathology of the eye*. New York: Springer-Verlag, 1986)

tern, which is usually seen in tuberculosis infections, the zonal pattern, typified by phacoanaphylactic uveitis, and the diffuse pattern, which is classically seen in sympathetic ophthalmia.

Epithelioid cells are modified macrophages which have abundant eosinophilic cytoplasm that make them resemble epithelium. Like macrophages, they are derived from blood monocytes. Many times during the inflammatory process, the epithelioid cells aggregate forming giant cells including the Langhans' giant cell, the foreign-body giant cell, or the Touton giant cell. In the **Langhans' giant cell,** the nuclei are arranged around the periphery (Fig. 3-6). In the **foreign-body giant cell,** nuclei are randomly arranged throughout the syncytium and may contain foreign material (Fig. 3-7), and in the **Touton giant cell,** there is a rim of cytoplasm that contains lipid peripheral to the ring of nuclei (Fig. 3-8).

Nongranulomatous Inflammations

The most common type of intraocular inflammation seen in iridocyclitis/uveitis or other ocular inflammatory processes is nongranulomatous. On histopathologic examination, the inflammatory reaction consists primarily of a lymphocyte and plasma cell infiltration (Fig. 3-8). The plasma cells in the reactive tissue are responsible for immunoglobulin production and secretion. Within tissue, these cells can be recognized in various stages of evolution toward this process. When large quantities of immu-

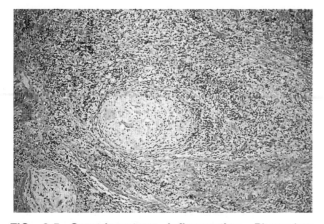

FIG. 3-5. Granulomatous inflammation. Photomicrograph of a granuloma with a central area composed of epithelioid cells and multinucleated giant cells. A surrounding rim of mononuclear cells, chiefly lymphocytes, is identified in the periphery. Fibroblasts and capillaries also are identified within the granuloma.

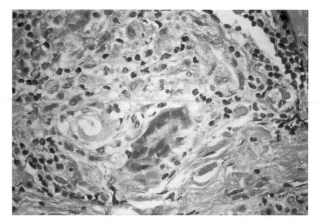

FIG. 3-7. Foreign body giant cell. Photomicrograph demonstrating the nuclei in a foreign-body giant cell, which are randomly arranged throughout the cytoplasmic syncytium. The surrounding cells are epithelioid histiocyte and lymphocytes.

noglobulin accumulate intracellularly, causing the cytoplasm to become eosinophilic, a plasmacytoid cell results. As the intracellular protein production continues, the nucleus often is extruded by the cell, forming an eosinophilic structure termed a **Russell body.** The Russell body generally is considered a histopathologic hallmark of longstanding disease. Mast cells also may play an important role in the nongranulomatous inflammatory process and can be identified in the inflamed tissue.

Severity and Course of Inflammatory Disease

The severity and course of intraocular inflammation can be subclassified into three defined periods: (1) acute intraocular inflammation, (2) subacute intraocular inflammation, and (3) chronic intraocular inflammation. **Acute inflammation** generally is thought to begin within

minutes of the injury and lasts for several days or weeks before resolving. There are five cardinal signs of acute phase of inflammation: (1) **rubor** or redness, (2) **calor** or heat due to an increased rate and volume of blood flow, (3) **tumor,** swelling or edema due to the exudation of the fluid and the cellular components of the blood into the extravascular space, (4) **dolor,** which is pain, and (5) **functio laesa,** loss of function.[42,47]

The principal feature of acute inflammatory responses are vasodilation, increased blood flow, increased vascular permeability, and the exudation of blood proteins and leukocytes. The emigration of leukocytes into the inflammatory focus has been divided into three stages: (1) margination, during which leukocytes pass from the center of the vessel to contact the endothelial lining; (2) adherence of white blood cells to the microvasculature; and (3) diapedesis, or migration of the leukocytes through

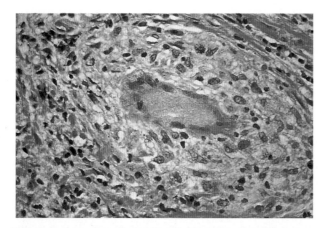

FIG. 3-6. Langhans' giant cell. Photomicrograph demonstrating the nuclei in a Langhans' giant cell arranged around the periphery of the cytoplasmic syncytium.

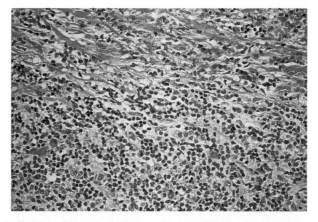

FIG. 3-8. Chronic inflammatory infiltrate. The collagen lamellae are infiltrated with a chronic inflammatory infiltrate. The infiltrate is composed of small round lymphocytes, plasma cells, and occasional epithelioid histiocytes.

the interendothelial junctions into the extravascular space. Initially, neutrophils are the predominant inflammatory cell; however, after 24 hours, they are replaced by monocytes and monocyte derivatives. The neutrophils and monocytes in particular are drawn to the region of injured tissue by specific chemical mediators or chemotactic agents within the tissue.

Chemotaxis is followed by the process of **phagocytosis,** which also is divided into three phases: (1) attachment of the phagocytes to the foreign or antigenic particles, (2) ingestion and intracellular degradation of the particle, and (3) extracellular release of the leukocyte breakdown products.[48]

Various chemical mediators of inflammation are released during the process of extracellular exudation. All of these chemical mediators have specific actions that enhance the acute inflammatory response.[48] These substances include plasma proteases involved in the kinin system, the complement system, and the clotting system; preformed cell mediators, including histamine, serotonin, and lysosomal components; and newly synthesized cell mediators, including prostaglandins, leukotrienes, platelet-stimulating factor, and cytokines.[48] The balance of synthesis and degradation of these mediators of inflammation helps to determine the nature, time course, and severity of the inflammatory response. Thus, acute inflammation may subside with complete resolution, in which case, the area of inflammation is healed by scarring or abscess formation, or the inflammation may persist and the character of the inflammation may change and progress to subacute or chronic inflammation.

Subacute inflammations are those in which the destructive force or inciting agent continues to elicit a modified inflammatory response over a period of weeks or months.

Chronic or recurrent intraocular inflammation usually follows an acute or subacute phase; however, some inflammatory processes may present a more chronic appearance throughout their entire course. The characteristic histologic appearance of chronic inflammation consists of the presence of lymphocytes, macrophages, and plasma cells, often associated with a proliferation of fibroblasts and small capillaries. Other types of cells that may be found in chronic inflammation include plasma cells, eosinophils, and mast cells.[48–50]

Phases of the Inflammatory Process

Three phases are common to all inflammatory processes and include: (1) an **exudative phase** in which cells and serum proteins migrate from the intravascular space to the extravascular space,[34,51] (2) an acute **adaptive phase,** in which cytotoxicity and tissue necrosis ensue, and which may vary in its severity, duration and ultimately progresses to subacute or chronic inflammation, and (3) a *reactive phase* of homeostasis restoration that involves reactive proliferation and restoration of tissue substance with newly formed parenchymal tissue, scarring, fibrosis, or granulation tissue.[47,52]

Exudation

In anterior uveitis, there is exudation of either lymphocytes, plasma cells, or polymorphonuclear leukocytes into the aqueous humor of the anterior chamber. The cells are typically deposited inferiorly in the anterior chamber by gravitational effects and may form a hypopyon. One must always be careful to differentiate an inflammatory hypopyon from a pseudohypopyon, which by definition is not composed of inflammatory cells. Large cells, such as macrophages, or particles with a diameter of more than about 20 μm may clog the intertrabecular spaces of the trabecular meshwork and can produce an acute secondary open-angle glaucoma[43]; however, secondary open-angle glaucoma in anterior uveitis occurs in only about 20% of cases.

Exudation within the stroma of the anterior uvea, including the iris and the ciliary body, also can occur. An inflammatory exudate in the stroma of the iris inhibits free movement of the iris and causes the typical miosis of iritis. Posterior synechiae can result from adherence of the posterior iris to the lens capsule and can cause pupillary block and angle-closure glaucoma. Inflammation of the ciliary body leads to decreased production of aqueous humor and ciliary muscle spasm. Infiltrates within the pars plicata of the ciliary body may cause a decrease in aqueous formation, which explains the fact that normal intraocular pressure, or **hypotony,** are commonly seen in anterior uveitis.[43] Choroidal detachment often occurs as a result of hypotony and can lead to relaxation of the zonules and displacement of the lens.

Intermediate, also known as **posterior, uveitis** results from exudation into the vitreous. Depending on the origin of the inflammation, the anterior or posterior hyaloid face may confine the exudates to the preretinal or retrolenticular space. Longstanding vitreous infiltrations often settle inferiorly. In general, bacterial infections tend to cause a diffuse infiltration of the vitreous resulting in extensive liquefaction necrosis. On the other hand, mycotic infections can cause multifocal microabscesses, a feature that can help in distinguishing bacterial from mycotic infections. Inflammatory conditions result in posterior vitreous detachment and inflammatory infiltrates may become loculated inferiorly behind the posterior vitreous face.[43]

Exudation beneath the retinal or choroid may result in **retinal** or **choroidal detachments.** Alternatively, the exudative process may cause separation of the basal lamina of the retinal pigment epithelium and the remainder of Bruch's membrane, leading to a retinal pigment epithelial detachment. When Bruch's membrane and the intracellular tight junctions of the retinal pigment epithelium are unable to confine the inflammatory exudate that is pouring out of the choriocapillaris, a serous detachment of the sensory retina may occur.[43] Serous retinal detachment causes a reduction of oxygen and nutritional supply to the retina from the choriocapillaris and may result in degeneration of the photoreceptors and outer retinal layers.

Edema also may be present within the retina. Outer retinal edema often is more severe than that involving the inner retina in choroidal inflammatory processes because the external limiting membrane of the retina often limits the spread of the exudate to the inner layers of the retina. The morphology of the intracellular and intercellular edema of the retina is determined by the various horizontal limiting membranes and the vertical boundary structures including the Müller cells' processes within the retina. These boundary structures often succeed in preserving the general retinal architecture.[43] **Cystoid macular edema** results when fluid accumulates in the outer plexiform layer or Henle's fiber layer and creates the typical honeycomb appearance seen on fluorescein angiography.[53] The end result of this process may be retinoschisis.[54] Retinal vasculitis and perivasculitis are very common features associated with intraocular inflammatory processes.

Optic nerve edema or inflammatory swelling of the optic disk may be due to two mechanisms. Mild inflammatory infiltrates of the retrobulbar optic nerve may occur; however, anterior extension often is limited by the blood–retinal barrier. Disk swelling also can occur as a passive phenomenon and often can accompany hypotony resulting from the inflammation of the anterior uvea.[43]

Experimental studies on the mechanisms of the exudative process in the eye have been reported by many authors.[55–57]

Cytotoxicity and Tissue Necrosis

Cytotoxic immunologic mechanisms, though intended to destroy noxious agents, often result in some destruction of the normal host tissue.[58] Inflammatory exudates in the anterior chamber often become adherent to the corneal endothelium and can cause focal destruction of the corneal endothelium. This results in decompensation and swelling of the corneal stroma. The stroma and pigment epithelium of the iris and ciliary body often remain relatively intact in the nongranulomatous inflammatory processes[59]; however, in granulomatous inflammation or viral-induced inflammation, sectoral or diffuse iris necrosis can occur.[60] Chronic recurrent inflammations of any type can lead to focal or diffuse atrophy of the iris and ciliary body. When inflammatory exudates occur in the vitreous, the result is a structural change known as lacunar degeneration of the vitreous. Subsequently, posterior vitreous detachment and epiretinal membrane formation can result. The choroidal changes from inflammation in bacte-

rial endophthalmitis can be severe. In contrast, with most viral retinopathies, the choroid is surprisingly spared. Toxoplasmic retinochoroiditis causes marked focal destruction about the retina and the choroid. Choroidoretinal scars, with hypopigmentation and hyperpigmentation of the retinal pigment epithelium are due to pigment proliferation and clumping and often result from both chorioretinitis and retinochoroiditis.[43]

In primary choroidal inflammatory diseases, the pigment epithelium and outer layers of the retina are damaged secondarily. The bipolar layer, the ganglion cell layer, and the nerve fiber layer often remain intact owing to the presence of the external limiting membrane. In contrast, primary inflammations affecting the retina (retinitis) are characterized by various types of cellular infiltrates throughout the entire retinal structure. Viral-induced retinitis, including herpes simplex and herpes zoster retinitis, as well as toxoplasma-induced retinitis are typically characterized by necrosis of all retinal layers.[43,61]

Reactive Proliferation and Chronic Inflammatory Changes

The third phase of inflammation generally is **reparative** in nature and involves reactive proliferation of parenchymal tissue and replacement with fibrous tissue. The reparative process may result in restoration of normal function, but more often results in destructive sequelae.[43,62]

Reactive proliferation of the pigment epithelium can result in the formation of chorioretinal scars, cyclitic membranes, and Dalen-Fuchs nodules. In this process, proliferating pigment epithelial cells undergo metaplasia, lose their melanin granules, and assume a spindle shape. There is extensive deposition of collagen fibers presumably due to fibrous metaplasia of the pigment epithelium. Basement membrane material often is found within the fibrous bundles because the pigment epithelium has the capability to produce basement membrane material. **Osseous metaplasia** of the retinal pigment epithelium also may occur especially in phthisical eyes.[43,62] Proliferation of the iris pigment epithelium can cause posterior synechiae formation between the iris pigment epithelium and the anterior capsule of the lens. Secondary proliferation and fibrous metaplasia of the lens epithelium can produce an **anterior capsular cataract. Cyclitic membranes** are formed by the proliferation of the nonpigmented ciliary epithelium and may extend across the entire width of the eye. Proliferation of the pars plana epithelium anterior to the ora serrata often is associated with longstanding retinal detachment, and the mound of proliferated retinal pigment epithelium beneath the detached retina is known as a **ringschwiele**.[43] **Perivascular pseudoretinitis pigmentosa** occurs secondary to several types of disease entities including various inflammatory process. Proliferating retinal pigment epithelial cells migrate into the retina in a perivascular fashion creating the typical bone spicule pattern seen clinically.

Dalen-Fuchs nodules are focal cellular accumulations that often can take the form of a pile of cannon balls that accumulate between Bruch's membrane and an elevated retinal pigment epithelium.[43] These lesions typically are seen in **sympathetic ophthalmia.** The origin of the Dalen-Fuchs nodule is not completely understood, but it is thought to be an accumulation of histiocytes or a proliferation of a retinal pigment epithelium[64,65] (Fig. 3-9).

Reactive proliferation of vascular connective tissue also occurs. Potential sites of **neovascularization** and the **proliferation of fibrovascular tissue** include the following: (1) the anterior surface of iris stroma producing rubeosis iridis, (2) the inner surface of the ciliary body producing **cyclitic membranes,** (3) the surface of the peripheral retina as in pars planitis, (4) the surface of the posterior retina and optic nerve head producing **vasoproliferative retinopathy,**[43,66] and (5) the choriocapillaris producing a **subretinal neovascular membrane.**

Rubeosis iridis consists of neovascular budding from the anterior surface of the iris stroma, and most often appears at the pupillary margin or on the surface of the far peripheral iris.[67] This fibrovascular membrane on the anterior iris surface may undergo contraction that results in tugging of the posterior iris pigment epithelium from the posterior surface of the iris around the pupillary margin onto the anterior surface resulting in **ectropion uvea.**[67] Chronic inflammatory processes of the pars plana typically cause proliferation of the ciliary epithelium and fibrovascular tissue.[70] These epithelial and fibrovascular elements migrate along the anterior hyaloid face toward the equator of the lens, eventually forming a complete **cyclitic membrane** in the retrolental space. Contraction of myofibroblasts within the membrane may exert traction

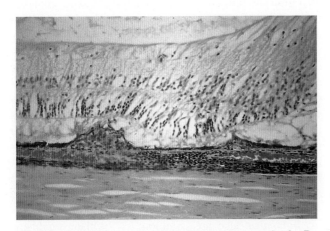

FIG. 3-9. Dalen Fuchs' nodule. Photomicrograph of a Dalen Fuchs' nodule consisting of a clump of epithelioid histiocytes beneath the retinal pigment epithelium. (From Margo CD, Grossniklaus HE. Ocular histopathology: a guide to differential diagnosis. Philadelphia: WB Saunders, 1991)

on the ciliary body and produce a ciliochoroidal detachment with subsequent severe hypotony.[43]

There are numerous causes of **proliferative vitreoretinopathy,** a condition characterized by proliferation of fibrovascular tissue and neovascularization. The two basic forms of proliferative vitreoretinopathy are due to: (1) organization of intraocular hemorrhages, exudates, inflammatory infiltrates, and other noxious substances with associated formation of granulation tissue and (2) retinal neovascularization that occurs as a consequence of intraocular hypoxia or ischemia.[43]

Neovascularization generally occurs as a response to a relative lack of oxygen. The combined presence of both viable tissue in the affected region and partial hypoxia induces the formation of an **angiogenic factor** that initiates the neovascularization process. Clinically and histopathologically, proliferative vitreoretinopathy has two distinct characteristics: (1) an abnormal location, in which the new vessels are present where vessels normally do not exist, and (2) increased vascular permeability. In contrast, normal retinal vessels have an intact lining with tight junctions formed by zonula occludens, which prevent leakage of fluid into the surrounding retina. These tight junctions are absent in neovascular vessels and extravasation of fluid and lipid occurs.[43] The vascular channels break through the internal limiting membrane of the retina and grow along the surface of the retina. In addition to this flat growth, the buds often proliferate anteriorly onto the vitreous scaffolding forming the arborizing fibrovascular fronds, which are typical of proliferative retinopathy.[43] The preretinal membranes are composed of proliferating vascular elements, vitreous hyalocytes, retinal glial elements, and macrophages derived from the blood. When simultaneous retinal defects are present, metaplastic proliferating retinal pigment epithelium may grow through these holes and contribute to the fibrovascular membranes.[69]

Subretinal neovascularization is a common sequelae of inflammation of the retina and choroid. Almost all focal inflammatory processes of the choroid and retina can induce neovascularization derived from the choroid.[70] This is particularly true when basement membrane attachments of the retinal pigment epithelium are compromised or there is an interruption of Bruch's membrane. Subretinal neovascularization can lead to subretinal hemorrhages.[43]

Reactive proliferation of glial tissue, or **reactive gliosis,** most often occurs when there is damage to the pigment epithelium.[43] The cells of the retinal pigment epithelium are strongly inclined toward reactive hyperplasia. In contrast, the elements of the sensory retina possess less tendency toward reactive proliferation, but in some cases, extensive glial proliferation from the sensory retina does occur. **Massive reactive gliosis** of the retina is a relatively unusual process. It involves a massive proliferation of retinal glial tissue, often simulating a tumor. It may occur following hemorrhage or severe intraocular inflammation.[71]

TYPES OF INTRAOCULAR INFLAMMATION

Infectious Intraocular Inflammations

Endophthalmitis and panophthalmitis describe the extent of intraocular inflammation and usually refer to infectious processes. **Endophthalmitis** refers to inflammation involving an ocular cavity (anterior chamber or vitreous cavity) and one of the ocular coats (sclera or episclera). **Panophthalmitis** is a more extensive process involving the eye and extending into the orbit. Intraocular inflammation due to infectious agents also can be subclassified as exogenous or endogenous depending on the route of entry of the infectious agent into the eye.[72] **Exogenous intraocular inflammations** are due to entrance of a noxious agent into the eye from the external environment. **Exogenous** endophthalmitis and panophthalmitis generally occur when there is perforating injury, traumatic laceration, or surgical injury to the globe,[73,74] or when a corneal ulcer progresses to perforation. In **endogenous intraocular inflammation,** the noxious agent gains access to the eye primarily through blood vessels, particularly the posterior ciliary arteries, the retinal arteries, and the anterior ciliary arteries.[75] Offending agents also may gain entrance to the eye by way of the nervous system. Endogenous endophthalmitis and panophthalmitis are more common in immunosuppressed and diabetic patients.[76]

Virtually all types of organisms, including bacteria, fungi, viruses, protozoa, parasites, and even insects can cause intraocular infection and inflammation. Many times, the intraocular inflammation is presumed to be induced by an organism although no specific organisms can be identified.

Intraocular Inflammation Caused by Bacteria and Fungi

Purulent, nongranulomatous, intraocular inflammation usually is caused by infection with bacteria and fungi. Purulent bacterial endophthalmitis was a relatively common eye disease in the preantibiotic era.[77,78] Today, such endophthalmitis usually arises as a complication of immunosuppression or trauma, which are discussed later. Bacterial and fungal infections also may have a granulomatous or nongranulomatous component to the inflammation. Typically, bacterial infections progress much more rapidly than do those involving fungi.

Bacterial endophthalmitis occurs in various clinical settings. Reported series have suggested the distribution of cases to be 62% following intraocular surgery, 20% following penetrating trauma, 10% following planned or inadvertent filtering blebs, and 8% as a result of metastatic infection.[48,73,79,81,82] The incidence of endophthalmitis following cataract surgery has been reported to be between 0.06% and 0.33%. Clinical signs of endophthalmitis include conjunctival hyperemia and chemosis, cell and flare in the anterior chamber, hypopyon, fibrin deposition, vitritis, scattered retinal hemorrhages, loss of the red reflex, and rarely, corneal opacification.[83] In most instances, clinical signs occur within 24 to 48 hours; however, the clinical presentation may be markedly delayed in infection by indolent organisms such as *Propionibacterium*.

Anterior chamber or vitreous **paracentesis** often is diagnostic in bacterial endophthalmitis.[84] In eyes with a clinical diagnosis of infectious endophthalmitis, approximately 64% have a positive culture.[48,73,79,80,81] Of these, approximately 56% to 90% of the isolates are gram-positive, 7% to 29% are gram-negative, and 3% to 13% are fungal.[48,73,77,79–81] *Staphylococcus epidermidis, Staphylococcus aureus,* and streptococci are the most common gram-positive organisms in postsurgical patients. *Streptococcus* sp. are most common in cases following filtering blebs,[85] and *Bacillus* organisms have been reported to account for 26% to 46% of posttraumatic cases.[86,87] *Proteus* sp., *Pseudomonas aeruginosa,* and *Hemophilus* sp. are the most common gram-negative isolates, and *Hemophilus* is particularly common after filtration surgery.[85] *Nocardia asteroides* has an unusual clinical presentation because it causes a peculiar dissolution of the lens.[88] Histopathologically, bacterial endophthalmitis is characterized by acute purulent exudates consisting primarily of polymorphonuclear leukocyte and necrotic intraocular tissue (Fig. 3-10).

Subretinal retinitis (Roth spot) is characteristic of endogenous endophthalmitis and usually is induced by emboli of causative organisms. The bacterial or mycotic offender penetrates the capillary wall causing retinal hemorrhages as well as infiltration of the organisms into the retina and vitreous, yielding the typical white-centered hemorrhage. The organisms rapidly proliferate to form an abscess. Endogenous endophthalmitis is rare, and usually occurs in immunosuppressed or otherwise systemically compromised host, including intravenous drug abusers and diabetics. In a review of 72 cases of endogenous endophthalmitis, 18 of which were bilateral, meningitis was present in 19, endocarditis and urinary tract infections in 10 cases, and a bacteremia of unknown origin in 19 patients.[89] Metastatic *Candida* endophthalmitis is probably the most common form of endogenous intraocular infections[90,91] (Fig. 3-11). Bacteria including *Bacillus* sp., *Neisseria meningiditis, Staphylococcus* sp., *Escherichia coli, Klebsiella pneumonia, Serratia* sp., and *Haemophilus influenzae* also are common.[48,89,96] Other organisms that have been reported as causative agents include *Clostridium perfringens,* anaerobic organisms,[76] and *Petriellidium boydii*.[82]

Fungal infection of the retina, choroid, and vitreous

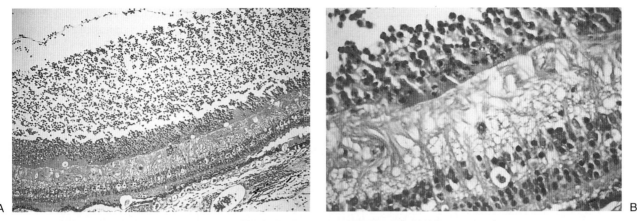

FIG. 3-10. Acute bacterial endophthalmitis with vitreous inflammation. (**A**) Photomicrograph demonstrating numerous acute inflammatory cells in the vitreous and on the surface of the retina. (**B**) Acute inflammatory cells are present on the surface of the retina. The nerve fiber layer and inner limiting membrane tend to limit the spread of the inflammation into the outer retinal layers.

occurs in several types of patients, including postoperative patients, patients with systemic mycotic infections, intravenous drug users, and patients who have endured surgical or nonsurgical ocular trauma.[24,93] Occasionally, patients without any known risk factors develop an endogenous fungal endophthalmitis. Fungal infections can present as a chronic panuveitis. There are fluffy, deep retinal or choroidal, yellow-white lesions, and the vitreous may contain fungal abscesses. Mycotic postoperative infections appear after a latency of weeks or months and are associated with microabscesses.[24]

Intraocular fungal infections account for 10% to 15% of endophthalmitis cases in most series, and *Candida* sp., *Fusarium* sp., *Aspergillus* sp., and *Paecilomyces lilacimum* are the most commonly reported organisms isolated. The relative frequency of each organism in posttraumatic and postoperative infections has not been established.[87,94] Other organisms that have been reported to cause endogenous fungal endophthalmitis include *Aspergillus* sp., *Coccidioides immitis*, *Cryptococcus neoformans*, *Histoplasma capsulatum*, *Sporotrichum schenckii*, *Blastomyces dermatitidis*, *Torulopsis* sp., and *Mucor* sp.[48,95–97]

Candida sp. endophthalmitis is the most common cause of disseminated fungal infection, and the predisposing factors for ocular involvement are identical to those causing systemic disease.[90,91,98] The diagnosis is suspected on clinical grounds and confirmed by blood culture or by vitreous biopsy. *Candida* sp. retinochoroiditis typically begins with focal yellow-white, deep, retinal or choroidal infiltrative lesions. They are usually multiple, and there often are one or more associated vitreous abscesses or vitreous "fluff balls." Retinal hemorrhages and cotton-wool exudates often are present. Subsequent complications include purulent retinal detachment, purulent endophthalmitis with hypopyon, vitreous abscess, and panophthalmitis. Histopathologic examination reveals neutrophils, macrophages, lymphocytes, and either yeast

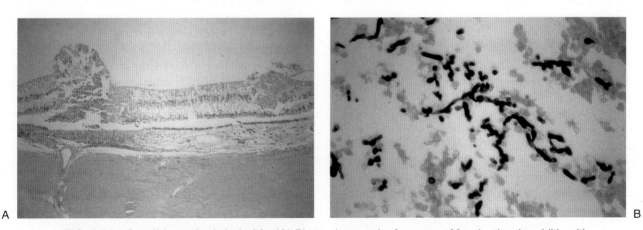

FIG. 3-11. *Candida* endophthalmitis. (**A**) Photomicrograph of an area of focal retinochoroiditis with acute necrosis of the retina and infiltration of the retina and choroid with acute inflammatory cells (left). Nearby, a focal area of retinitis also is identified. (**B**) *Candida* hyphae are readily identified with Gomori methenamine silver stain.

forms or pseudohyphae consistent with *Candida* sp. endophthalmitis (Fig. 3-11).

Nonpurulent, granulomatous, intraocular inflammation also can be caused by infection with bacteria and fungi. Bacteria represent a relatively rare cause of such endogenous uveitis.[57,72] Granulomatous endophthalmitis has been associated with tuberculosis,[99] syphilis,[100,101] and leprosy.[102] Rare other bacterial causes of such inflammation have been demonstrated including leptospirosis,[103] *Clostridium perfringens,* listeriosis,[104] and brucellosis.[105]

For many years, **tuberculosis** was a common systemic disease and a very common cause of uveitis.[102,106,107] Tuberculosis now occurs infrequently, and ocular involvement occurs only in association with active miliary tuberculosis. The choroid usually is the primary site of involvement.[102,108] A recent resurgence of tuberculous uveitis has accompanied the increased prevalence of immunosuppression and human immunodeficiency (HIV) infection. In addition, many multidrug-resistant strains have emerged. Histologically, tuberculous uveitis is characterized by granulomatous inflammation.[109] Typical **caseous lesions** may be present as isolated nodules or diffuse infiltrates, and the organisms can be demonstrated by **acid-fast stains.**

Syphilis has been reported to cause episcleritis, scleritis, interstitial keratitis, iridocyclitis, vitritis, retinitis, papillitis, panuveitis, cystoid macular edema, and retinal detachment. *Treponema pallidum* has been demonstrated in the aqueous and ocular tissues.[110–112]

Ocular involvement in **leprosy** can occur in 10% to 90% of patients.[113–116] Prendergast has reviewed the various reports in the literature dealing with all forms of ocular involvement with leprosy.[116] Patients with **lepromatous leprosy** developed eye lesions in later stages of the disease, whereas **tuberculoid** patients developed ocular involvement early. Lepromatous patients typically have iridocyclitis and superficial punctate keratitis, whereas tuberculoid patients have problems related to lagophthalmos and corneal anesthesia.[113] Uveal involvement is much more common in the lepromatous than in the tuberculoid form of leprosy and includes anterior and posterior uveal involvement. Choroidal involvement was demonstrated in the histopathologic study of 28 eyes by Prendergast,[116] in which he observed choroidal inflammatory lesions in 15 eyes, of which 9 had acid-fast bacilli present. Anterior nongranulomatous uveitis also can occur in association with Rocky Mountain spotted fever.[117]

Lyme disease is a bacterial infection caused by the spirochete *Borrelia burgdorferi.*[118–120] It is transmitted to humans by the *Ixodes dammini* tick. Clinically, the disease is divided into three phases. The **first stage** is localized. After infection, the spirochete spreads locally through the skin causing the characteristic rash known as **erythema migrans. Stage two** begins days to weeks after the primary infection and **systemic spread** to many organs can occur during this stage. Clinically, the most

common manifestations include cardiac and neurologic involvement. Patients also may experience secondary annular skin lesions. Stage three, or the persistent stage, is characterized by prolonged episodes of arthritis and chronic neurologic manifestations such as ataxia, chronic encephalomyelitis, spastic paresis, and dementia.[121,122]

Lyme disease has been associated with numerous ocular findings. During stage two, the most common ocular findings are conjunctivitis and uveitis. Other ocular findings observed during early stages include episcleritis, iridocyclitis, and retinal vasculitis.[123] Bell's palsy and optic neuritis also may occur during the neurologic stages of the disease.[124,125] Bilateral keratitis, characterized by patchy stromal infiltrates of the cornea from Bowman's layer to Descemet's membrane is a late manifestation.[126] Less common ocular findings include diffuse choroiditis, cystoid macular edema, and exudative retinal detachments.[127,128] Most patients have elevated antibody titers to *Borrelia burgdorferi* by several weeks after the infection. The diagnosis of the disease is based on both immunofluorescent assays and **enzyme-linked immunosorbent assays (ELISA).**

Systemic **fungi** including blastomycosis, cryptococcosis,[129] coccidioidomycosis, sporotrichosis, and histoplasmosis all can cause a necrotic chorioretinitis or retinochoroiditis with diffuse zonular-type granulomatous inflammation. In ocular histoplasmosis the organism has only rarely been demonstrated.[130,131] Ocular involvement by many fungi has been confirmed pathologically including *Aspergillus* sp.,[132] *Blastomyces dermatitidis,*[133,134] *Coccidioides immitis,*[135–138] *Cryptococcus neoformans,*[139,140] and *Sporotrichum schenckii.*[141–143] *Toxoplasma gondii* also has been demonstrated histopathologically in ocular tissue.[144–150]

Histoplasmosis often has ocular manifestations.[151] Reid and co-workers described the first case of ocular lesions that are now recognized as the typical presumed ocular histoplasmosis syndrome. There are four major clinical characteristics: (1) disseminated choroiditis which produces the characteristic "histo spots,"[130] (2) **maculopathy,** (3) **peripapillary pigment changes,** and (4) **clear vitreous.** Histoplasma has been identified histopathologically in the eyes of patients who have been immunosuppressed. The ocular lesion manifested was that of an endophthalmitis.[152–154] In addition, orbital involvement by histoplasmosis has been reported.

Intraocular Inflammation Caused by Viruses

Intraocular inflammation can be caused by infection with **viral organisms.** Intraocular viral inflammations may be isolated and confined to the globe and adnexa, or they may occur as a component of a generalized systemic disease. The most important histopathologic characteristic, which can assist in the diagnosis of viral diseases, is the presence of **inclusion bodies** that may be intracytoplasmic or intranuclear.[52,155] Viruses may cause a necrotizing or a granulomatous inflammatory reaction. Viruses that have been reported to cause intraocular inflammatory disease include herpes simplex, herpes zoster,[156,157] cytomegalovirus,[158–160,165] rubella,[162–167] varicella,[168] Rift Valley fever,[169,170] Cruetzfeldt-Jakob disease,[171] and measles (subacute sclerosing panencephalitis).[172–175]

Herpes simplex is probably the most common cause of viral intraocular inflammation in Europe and North America.[176,177] The most frequent ocular manifestation is keratitis or keratouveitis, and the associated inflammation is nongranulomatous with an infiltrate composed primarily of lymphocytes and plasma cells.[178] Histologic examination of the cornea in herpes keratitis can reveal an inflammatory infiltrate even in eyes that are uninflamed clinically. In addition, herpes virus particles have been demonstrated in the iris pigment epithelium and stromal cells[52] and in the aqueous humor.[179] Secondary open-angle glaucoma also can be seen. Herpetic retinitis has been described in congenital herpes infections and in adults with immune deficiency conditions.[180] Histologically, one can observe intranuclear inclusions within retinal ganglion cells and bipolar cells, particularly in the macular region.[177,181,182]

Intraocular Inflammation Caused by Parasites

Intraocular inflammation also can be caused by **parasitic infection.**[183] Parasitic diseases that are known to have ocular manifestations include *Loa loa,*[184] gnathostomiasis,[185] amebiasis, cysticercosis,[186] onchocerciasis, dirofiliarisis,[187] and toxocariasis, all of which are known to cause anterior chamber inflammation or hemorrhage. Iritis has been reported in amebiasis, angiostrongyliasis,[188] hookworm, ascariasis, schistosomiasis,[189] cysticercosis, giardiasis, gnathostomiasis, leishmaniasis, *Loa loa,* myiasis,[190,191] onchocerciasis, tapeworm trichinosis, toxocariasis,[192–195] trypanosomiasis, and Bancroft's filariasis. Vitreous hemorrhage and vitritis have been associated with infestation by ascariasis, schistosomiasis, *Loa loa,* trichinosis, cysticercosis, gnathostomiasis, onchocerciasis, and toxocariasis. Finally, choroidal and retinal degeneration, exudates, nodules, detachment, or hemorrhage are seen with angiostrongyliasis, amebiasis, babesiosis, cysticercosis, leishmaniasis, *Loa loa,*[196] myiasis,[190,197] onchocerciasis, trichinosis, toxocariasis, hookworm, ascariasis, schistosomiasis,[189,198] giardiasis, gnathostomiasis,[185,199] malaria, and trypanosomiasis.

Onchocerciasis, or **river blindness,** is a disease that affects about 20 million people worldwide, with some 10% considered visually handicapped as a direct result of the disorder. The disease is caused by the nematode *Onchocerca volvulus.* It is spread by the black flies of the *Simulium* species. Many clinical findings of ocular onchocerciasis have been reported. Microfilarial infestation in the cornea is most commonly the cause of visual loss over time. In the cornea, there is a punctate keratitis that may progress to sclerosing keratitis with more intense infestation. An iridocyclitis can be seen with secondary atrophy of the iris, glaucoma, and secondary cataract. Alterations of the posterior pole include optic neuropathy and large areas of chorioretinitis.[201–205]

Noninfectious Intraocular Inflammation

Isolated Intraocular Inflammation

The term **anterior uveitis** encompasses both iritis and iridocyclitis and is generally thought of as a nonspecific, nongranulomatous, diffuse anterior uveitis. It is the most common form of uveitis and accounts for approximately three fourths of cases. Inflammation occurs in the iris or the ciliary body with few vitreous inflammatory cells, which are usually confined to the retrolental space or anterior vitreous. A single episode of anterior uveitis is uncomfortable but produces very few sequelae. Recurrent anterior uveitis can produce cataracts or glaucoma. Clinically, keratic precipitates and anterior chamber cell and flare are common. Idiopathic anterior uveitis is associated with the HLA-B27 haplotype, and the patients are more often young males. Clinical signs of anterior uveitis are pain, redness, and photophobia. Keratotic precipitates and posterior synechia are common sequelae.[56,57,208]

Other **ocular diseases** that are associated with a diffuse anterior uveitis include Fuchs' iridocyclitis[209,210] and Posner-Schlossman syndrome.[211,212] Systemic diseases that have been reported to be associated with a diffuse anterior uveitis include ankylosing spondylitis,[213] Reiter's syndrome,[214,215] juvenile rheumatoid arthritis,[102,216–220] Crohn's disease,[221–223] ulcerative colitis,[223] and psoriasis.[46] A summary of the clinical characteristics of these diseases is included in Table 3. Posterior and peripheral uveitis is found in association with multiple sclerosis.[224–226] Whipple's disease is associated with vitritis and retinitis.[227–229]

Pathologic studies have been done on only a few eyes with anterior uveitis. The inflammation is most prominent in the iris and ciliary body. Plasma cells and lymphocytes appear to be the most common inflammatory cells. Scattered giant cells have been noted.[216,230] Pathologic examination of ocular tissue from Fuchs' iridocyclitis patients has disclosed plasma cells and lymphocytes, thus supporting a probable inflammatory etiology for this syndrome.[231] Electron microscopy of iris biopsy specimens in patients with this disease show a decrease in stromal melanocytes and a decrease in the size of individual melanosomes. Plasma cells, mast cells, and lymphocytes are present in the tissue.[232] Alterations in immunoglobulin levels in the aqueous[233] and immune complex formation have been

TABLE 3. *Clinical characteristics of diseases associated with anterior uveitis*

Disease	Age (yr)	Sex	Ocular redness	HLA-B27	Systemic findings	Steroid response
Idiopathic	Any	Either	Yes	No	None	Yes
HLA-B27, ocular only	15–40	M > F	Yes	Yes	None	Yes
Ankylosing spondylitis	15–40	M > F	Yes	Yes	Spondylitis, sacroiliitis	Yes
Reiter's syndrome	15–40	M > F	Yes	Yes	Arthritis, urethritis, mucocutaneous lesions	Yes
Juvenile rheumatoid arthritis	3–16	F > M	No	No	Pauciarticular arthritis, ANA* positive	Yes
Fuchs' iridocyclitis	Any	Either	No	No	None	Yes
Posner-Schlossman syndrome	Adult	Either	No	No	None	Yes
Schwartz syndrome	Adult	Either	No	No	None	No
Ocular ischemia	>60	Either	Yes	No	Carotid insufficiency	No
Kawasaki syndrome	1–18	Either	Yes	No	Skin rash, lymphadenopathy, fever, cardiac lesions	Yes

* ANA, antinuclear antibody.

(From Nusenblatt RB, Palestine AG. *Uveitis: fundamentals and clinical practice.* Chicago: Year Book Medical Publishers, 1989)

associated with some of the inflammatory disorders related to anterior uveitis.

Intermediate uveitis describes ocular inflammation that is primarily confined to the vitreous and peripheral retina. Other terms such as **chronic cyclitis** and **peripheral uveitis** have also been used to describe this type of ocular inflammation. A subset of intermediate uveitis in which there is a large white opacity over the pars plana and ora serrata (a snowbank) has been termed **pars planitis.**[46,57,235–238] Intermediate uveitis has been reported to account for 8% of uveitis in one referral practice.[239] It is rarely reported in families, and there is no consistent HLA haplotype. Most patients present with blurred vision or floaters without pain or photophobia. The condition is bilateral in approximately 75% of patients.[239] Signs of anterior segment inflammation are minimal or absent in adults, but may be present in children. Keratotic precipitates also occur. The most important finding in this disease is a cellular infiltrate in the vitreous and peripheral retina. Vitreous cells are, by definition, always present in active intermediate uveitis. Vitreous **snowballs** and an inferior white **snowbank** often are present in the inferior vitreous (histopathology is discussed later). Complications include glaucoma, cataracts, vitreous hemorrhage, peripheral retinal neovascularization, and rhegmatogenous and nonrhegmatogenous retinal detachment. Macular edema is the most common cause of visual loss.[66] Histologic examination of the snowbank has demonstrated that it is composed of fibroglial and vascular components and contains fibrous astrocytes that form new collagen.[238,240,241] The peripheral retinal veins show lymphocytic cuffing and infiltration. Inflammation of the choroid and ciliary body is mild. The vitreous snowballs contain epithelioid cells and multinucleated giant cells, but these cells have not been found in the uvea.[240] Immunohistologic examination of one case demonstrated glial tissue in the snowbank as

well as lymphocytes and the presence of class II antigen on the vascular endothelium.[58,239,242]

Several forms of retinitis that have no known causative organisms and that manifest with a variety of clinical presentations are known as the **white dot syndromes.** These include multiple evanescent white dot syndrome (MEWDS) reported by Jampol[243] and other authors,[244] multifocal choroiditis and panuveitis,[245] acute retinal pigment epitheliitis,[247,248] acute posterior multifocal placoid pigment epitheliopathy (APMPPE), described by Gass and other authors, the subretinal fibrosis and uveitis syndrome,[252,253] acute macular neuroretinopathy,[254,255] and diffuse unilateral subacute neuroretinitis (DUSN).[256–258]

Finally, there are **several retinochoroidal** or **choroidal inflammatory processes without known causative organisms.** These include vitiliginous (birdshot) retinochoroidopathy[259–262] and serpiginous choroidopathy.[263–265] Histologic examination of a specimen from a patient with serpiginous choroidopathy shows an extensive loss of the retinal pigment epithelium and destruction of the overlying retina. The choriocapillaris as well as part of the choroid is filled with a round cell infiltrate, suggesting an inflammatory component to this disorder. Immunologic studies have been performed.

Sympathetic ophthalmia[266] is a specific bilateral inflammation of the entire uveal tract of unknown etiology, characterized clinically by an insidious onset and a progressive course with exacerbations.[267] Pathologically, there is a nodular or diffuse infiltration of the uveal tract with lymphocytes and epithelioid histiocytes.[268] The disease almost invariably follows a perforating wound involving the uveal tissue. A nonsurgical perforating wound is the most common cause, and a surgical wound is the second most common cause in most series.[269,270] Often, there is a clinical history of vitreous and uvea extruding from the wound during the primary repair. Several authors have postulated an increased incidence of sympathetic ophthalmia after vitrectomy, especially when used during the primary repair of a ruptured globe.[49,271–273] Sympathetic ophthalmia also has been reported to occur after retinal reattachment surgery, after evisceration,[274] and following argon laser cyclophotocoagulation. Sympathetic ophthalmia sometimes is accompanied by the presence of phacoantigenic uveitis.[275,276]

Males have a higher incidence of sympathetic ophthalmia after trauma than females, but this is probably related to higher injury rates in males. For surgical cases, the rates are equal in both sexes.[269,270] Most authors have reported the greatest number of sympathetic ophthalmia cases occurring between 2 weeks and 3 months after injury[269,278,279]; however, it has been reported to occur as late as 18 years after injury.

The clinical presentation of sympathetic ophthalmia was reviewed by Marak.[278] The earliest clinical signs may be a minimal nongranulomatous uveitis, a minimal vitritis, or rarely, an optic neuritis and circumpapillary choroiditis. It usually presents as a moderate-to-severe anterior and posterior uveitis with keratic precipitates, which may be of any character but are often of the mutton fat variety.

Although the fundus often is obscured by vitreous inflammation, when observable, there are few-to-many drusen-like subretinal exudates that may extend and coalesce, producing an exudative retinal detachment. These subretinal exudates correlate histologically with Dalen-Fuchs nodules and are most often found in the midperipheral retina.[278,280]. Papillitis often is a prominent feature.[278]

The typical histopathologic findings in sympathetic ophthalmia consist of a diffuse cellular infiltrate composed predominantly of lymphocytes and scattered nests of epithelioid cells. In the infiltrate, there may be numerous eosinophils, but plasma cells and polymorphonuclear leukocytes are rarely present.[279] **Dalen-Fuchs nodules** also may be present (Fig. 3-9). The lack of either necrosis or retinal involvement and the sparing of the choriocapil-

laris are features that typically differentiate sympathetic ophthalmia from other causes of uveitis.[276,281] Several authors have described cases of sympathetic ophthalmia[269,271,282] that were somewhat atypical with features including obliteration of the choriocapillaris, involvement of the retina, and chorioretinal scarring. A summary of these findings are included in Table 4. Immunohistopathologic findings have been reported.[64]

The differential diagnosis of sympathetic ophthalmia includes VKH syndrome. The histopathologic picture of sympathetic ophthalmia and of Harada's disease is often identical, especially in the early stages.[65,283–286] In VKH disease, however, there are characteristic clinical signs associated, including alopecia, poliosis, vitiligo, dysacousia, or meningeal symptoms.[287] Bilateral lens-induced endophthalmitis also can have an identical histopathologic picture; however, there usually is evidence of rupture of the lens capsule in the allegedly sympathizing eye.[276,281,288]

Noninfectious Intraocular Inflammation and Systemic Disease

There are many **systemic inflammatory or immune-related diseases** including systemic lupus erythematosus, Sjögren's syndrome, and systemic sarcoidosis that have associated ocular inflammatory manifestations.

Systemic **sarcoidosis** often has been associated with ocular granulomatous inflammation.[289,290] The incidence of ocular involvement in sarcoidosis is variable with reports ranging from 11% to 78%. The most comprehensive reviews report ocular involvement in 27.8% and 38% of cases.[291–293] In addition, approximately 2% to 7% of patients with ocular inflammatory disease who are referred to a uveitis clinic have sarcoidosis.[72,293,295]

Almost all **ocular tissues** can be involved with sarcoidosis; however, the most frequent site of involvement is the uveal tract.[296] Table 5 shows a summary of the frequency of involvement of various ocular tissues as reported by several review series.

TABLE 4. *Findings in typical cases of sympathetic uveitis*

Finding	Croxatto[389] (100 cases)	Lubin[262] (105 cases)
Eosinophils	34%	46%
Plasma cells	60%	65–85%
Focal choriocapillaris obliteration	40%	
Chorioretinal scarring	7%	<5% (Makeley, 41%)[390]
Dalen Fuchs' nodules	26%	35%
RPE disruption/heaping	19%	84%
Retinal perivasculitis	55%	50%
Retinal inflammation	18% (Winter, 30%)[271]	42%
Optic nerve perivasculitis	25%	12%
Optic nerve pial septae inflammation	17%	21%
Meningeal inflammation	22%	18%
Lens-induced endophthalmitis	14%	46%

TABLE 5. *Ocular site/type of involvement in sarcoidosis*

Segment	Obenhauf et al.[281]	Other authors
ANTERIOR SEGMENT		
Anterior granulomatous uveitis or iridocyclitis	52%	72%[388]
Acute iridocyclitis	15%	27.6%[388]
Keratoconjunctivitis sicca	15.8%	5.7%[388]
Phlyctenular/nonspecific conjunctivitis of conjunctival lesions	6.9%	11.3%
POSTERIOR SEGMENT	25.3%	—
Chorioretinitis	10.9%	—
Periphlebitis	10.4%	—
Chorioretinal nodules	5.5%	—
Vitreous cells or opacities	3.0%	—
Vitreous hemorrhage	1.5%	—
Retinal neovascularization	1.4%	—
Optic nerve head neovascularization		27.2%[289]
CNS involvement		2%[49]
CNS involvement with retinal involvement	20%	37%[288]
Optic nerve and nerve head involvement	7.4%	5%
ORBIT	1.0%	—

The **central nervous system** is clinically affected in 5% of cases, but autopsy studies have disclosed lesions in the central nervous system in 15% of cases.[297] The spectrum of involvement includes mononeuropathies, polyneuropathies, cranial nerve palsies, pituitary-hypothalamic syndromes, seizure disorders, and the clinical manifestations of a space-occupying lesion.[298] The most frequently involved cranial nerve is the seventh nerve, and the second most commonly involved is the optic nerve.[299,300] Kaufmann noted a 37% incidence of central nervous system (CNS) sarcoidosis when the fundus is involved, compared with a 3.5% overall incidence of CNS sarcoid in unselected sarcoidosis patients.[301]

Optic nerve and **optic nerve head** involvement have been reported to occur in about 5% of patients with sarcoidosis, although one study reported an incidence of almost 40% by fluorescein angiographic studies.[302–304] The mechanisms of optic nerve involvement include: (1) optic disk edema or papillitis secondary to intraocular inflammation, (2) true papilledema caused by increased intracranial pressure, (3) retrobulbar neuritis, (4) primary infiltration of the optic nerve, and (5) optic atrophy secondary to one of the other four forms, to glaucoma, or to compression by adjacent granulomatous lesions.[305] **Conjunctival biopsy** often is positive, particularly in those who subsequently are diagnosed as having sarcoidosis.[306]

Behçet's disease was first discovered by a dermatologist who noted characteristic findings including a recurrent hypopyon iritis and oral and genital ulcerations.[307–309] The cause of the disease is not known. Environmental as well as viral causes have been implicated. The HLA-B5 phenotype and its subtype, HLA-BW51 are more common in patients with the disease. HLA-B12 is associated with neurocutaneous Behçet's, and HLA-B27 is associated with the arthritic type.[310,311] Behçet's disease presenting with ocular manifestations has been associated with HLA-B5.[312] A diagnosis of the disease is based solely on clinical findings. **Four types** of Behçet's have been identified: (1) **complete,** (2) **incomplete,** (3) **suspect,** (4) **possible.** The characterization of the disease into the four subtypes is based on major and minor criteria. These criteria include oral, dermal, ocular, genital, joint, gastrointestinal, vascular, and CNS involvement.[313,314]

The ocular manifestations of the disease may be unilateral; however, the disease invariably progresses to bilateral involvement.[315] All of the eye structures can be involved.[316] Anterior segment manifestations of the disease include an iridocyclitis with hypopyon. Clinically, the patient presents with periorbital pain, redness, photophobia, and blurred vision. On examination, the patient displays conjunctival and ciliary injection with aqueous flare and cells. Fine keratic precipitates may be present on the corneal endothelium. A hypopyon is characteristic.[317] In the posterior pole, a vitritis is present during the acute phase. A retinal vasculitis affecting both the arteries and veins also may be present. There is a patchy perivascular sheathing with inflammatory exudates surrounding retinal hemorrhages. Yellow-white, deep retinal exudates and retinal edema also may be present. The vasculitis may lead to thrombosis of vessels with secondary ischemic retinal changes. Optic nerve involvement includes papillitis.

Histopathologically, the disease is characterized as a necrotizing, obliterative vasculitis. The vessels show an inflammatory cell infiltration. Acutely, the iris has neutrophils present in the stroma and surrounding the vessels. Subsequently, a monocytic and lymphocytic infiltrate develops and later is followed by atrophy and fibrosis of the iris, which may be accompanied by anterior synechiae formation. Proliferation of collagen fibers can result in the formation of a cyclitic membrane.[318–320] The long-term consequences of Behçet's disease include cataract formation, secondary glaucoma, optic atrophy, retinal breaks, rhegmatogenous retinal detachment, and retinal neovascularization.

INFLAMMATION OF SPECIFIC OCULAR TISSUES

Conjunctival Inflammation

The **conjunctiva** is located in an external, exposed position and is prone to many primary and secondary inflammations caused by several exogenous and endogenous infectious and toxic agents. The histopathologic features are variable and depend on the duration of the inflammation and on the site of origin.[49]

Clinically, **acute conjunctivitis** is characterized by congestion, hyperemia, tearing, edema, and increased mucous secretion. If the inflammation is particularly intense, ulceration of the epithelial surface occurs. Histopathologically, one can identify dilated lymphatic channels, an edematous substantia propria, and a marked inflammatory cell infiltrate in the interstitium. In an acute bacterial conjunctivitis, a polymorphonuclear leukocyte infiltrate often is seen. Viral infections elicit a mononuclear cell response, and allergic stimuli produce an increased number of eosinophils or basophils.[49]

Chronic conjunctivitis is clinically characterized by the presence of conjunctival inflammation lasting longer than 2 months. Histopathologically, chronic inflammation is identified by an increased number of goblet cells, hyperplasia of the epithelium, and the formation of pseudoglands of Henle and retention cysts filled with inspissated and calcific concretions.

Inflammation in the stroma is often manifested by the formation of papillae and follicles. **Papillae** are produced by infiltration of the palpebral conjunctiva by inflammatory cells and transudate in a perivascular distribution, whereas **follicles** are discrete aggregates of lymphoid tissue within the superficial stroma of the conjunctiva. Clinically, a papilla has a characteristic small vessel in the center, whereas in the follicle, the conjunctival vessels can be seen to surround and encircle the mound.

Granulomatous inflammations of the conjunctiva are uncommon and are most often associated with disseminated granulomatous diseases including sarcoidosis or tuberculosis. More rarely, the conjunctiva may serve as a portal of entry for systemic granulomatous infections such as cat-scratch fever, tularemia, or coccidioidomycosis. These entities may cause enlargement of the ipsilateral preauricular lymph nodes. The combination of conjunctivitis and ipsilateral enlargement of the lymph node is known as **Parinaud's oculoglandular syndrome.** A **chalazion** usually is a lipogranulomatous inflammation originating in the tarsus; however, it also may occur in the conjunctiva. Mycotic infections of the conjunctiva and episclera are rare, and most occur in association with mycotic keratitis or blepharitis. Granulomatous inflammation of the conjunctiva can be caused by protozoa and parasites. Chlamydia can also cause granulomatous conjunctival inflammation and inclusion conjunctivitis.[49,321,322]

Chronic inflammatory changes of the conjunctiva include atrophy and epidermalization. When epidermalization occurs, there is loss of goblet cells and conversion to stratified squamous epithelium, with keratinization and the formation of rete ridges and pegs within the stroma. Reparative scarring and shrinkage of the conjunctiva results in shortening of the fornices and formation of symblepharon.

Corneal Inflammation

The clinical signs of **corneal inflammation** include epithelial edema, diffuse stromal haziness, and folds in Descemet's membrane. Perilimbal hyperemia occurs because the conjunctiva contains anastomoses between the superficial vessels of the conjunctiva and the deep vessels of the ciliary/episcleral circulation. Because of this vascular arrangement, many corneal inflammations are associated with an iritis or anterior chamber hypopyon.[39,49]

In the acute phase of corneal inflammation, the initial cellular migration consists of interlamellar polymorphonuclear leukocytes that appear within 8 to 12 hours of injury. During the later stages, or 12 to 16 hours after injury, the cells of the monocytic system, including macrophages and lymphocytes, are present. Finally, after 36 hours, the entire inflammatory reaction usually is composed of lymphocytes and plasma cells.[39,49] Neovascularization, which occurs in response to edema, cellular infiltration, and tissue necrosis, is seen at this stage and later. As healing ensues and inflammation subsides, the vascular channels regress and become less conspicuous. **Ghost vessels** may remain clinically visible for many years.

Corneal inflammations are either nonulcerative or ulcerative and are associated with a variety of infectious and noninfectious conditions. Inflammation often results in disruption of the corneal epithelium, cellular infiltration, and opacification of subepithelial tissues.

Nonulcerative inflammations of the cornea include the superficial keratopathies and interstitial keratitis. Various agents can cause these inflammatory changes of the cornea.

Clinically, **superficial keratopathy** can appear as punctate, linear, dendritic (branching), or geographic types of lesions. The number, distribution, and size of the lesions and the extent of involvement of the epithelial and subepithelial tissues are variable. Punctate epithelial keratopathy can occur in association with mild bacterial or viral infections, and more severe punctate epitheliopathy can occur in epidemic keratoconjunctivitis caused by adenoviruses (serotypes 8 and 19). Histologically, there is a loss of the superficial corneal epithelium, and there may be an associated mild anterior stromal inflammatory infiltrate. Herpes simplex and chlamydial infection can involve the full thickness of the epithelium. Dendritic lesions are usually seen in association with herpes simplex infections of the cornea but rarely can be seen in herpes zoster. Histologically, there is erosion of the epithelium along the course of the dendritic or geographic pattern down to the basal layer. Epithelial giant-cell formation often can be seen adjacent to the areas of epithelial erosion, and acidophilic intranuclear viral inclusions known as **Lipschütz bodies** are present.[49]

Inflammation is often limited to a specific zone on the cornea. In vernal conjunctivitis, subepithelial infiltrates of eosinophils known as **Tranta's dots** occur in the superior cornea. Peripheral stromal infiltrates with deposition of adjacent immune complex rings occur in patients with rheumatoid arthritis and Wegener's granulomatosis. Midperipheral ring-shaped zonal opacities known as **Wessely rings** may occur in association with hypersensitivity states. Trachoma is associated with involvement of the superior limbus with follicles, which are composed of lymphocytes, and with histiocytes. Later, during the reparative phase, vascularization of the limbus and superior cornea can occur. Finally, after regression of the follicles, the characteristic depressed round scars known as **Herbert's pits** are seen. Histopathologically, the vascularization is associated with gradual destruction of the peripheral corneal stroma and adjacent Bowman's layer and with replacement with granulation tissue.[49]

Stromal keratopathy, or **nonulcerative stromal keratitis,** results when conjunctival and superficial corneal infections extend to the stroma. The epithelium characteristically remains intact while the stroma becomes edematous, and folds in Descemet's membrane can develop. Infectious causes of nonulcerative keratitis include viruses, bacteria, fungi or parasites. Another form of nonulcerative stromal keratitis is **interstitial keratitis** in which the middle and deep corneal stroma become vascularized. Herpes zoster, herpes simplex, syphilis, tuberculosis, onchocerciasis, and leprosy are known to produce interstitial keratitis.[39,323] Syphilitic stromal keratitis or interstitial keratitis classically results from congenital luetic infection, and appears between ages 5 to 15 years. Histopathologically, the entire cornea becomes thickened and edematous with diffuse or localized lymphocytic infiltration in the middle and deep stromal layers. Later, vascularization of the stroma appears in the deeper layers (Fig. 3-12). The infiltration can cause folding of Descemet's membrane and Bowman's layer.[305] Proliferation of corneal fibroblasts, deposition of collagen, and gradual conversion to a vascularized scar occur during the healing process.[49]

Ulcerative corneal inflammation can be caused by either infectious or noninfectious causes. Histopathologically, the epithelium and stroma in the area of injury swell, become necrotic, and ulcerate. The corneal lamellac around the ulcer are infiltrated by acute inflammatory cells and are necrotic. Acute and chronic inflammatory cells are noted at the limbus, and diffusion of inflammatory cells into the anterior chamber may result in a hypopyon. As the ulceration ensues and the necrosis progresses, much of the entire thickness of the cornea may be involved. The remaining cornea, consisting of a few posterior lamellae and Descemet's membrane, may then bulge forward forming a **descemetocele.** Later, as the lesion begins to heal, new vessels enter from the limbus and fibroblasts derived from the stroma fill in the ulcer to form a connective tissue scar.[49]

Infectious corneal ulcerations can result from bacterial, viral, fungal, or parasitic invasion.[93,326,327] **Bacterial corneal ulcers** can result from infection by almost all virulent pyogenic organisms. The most frequent offenders are staphylococci, pneumococci, beta-hemolytic streptococci, pseudomonas, *Moraxella* sp., and other gram-negative organisms.[39] Herpes simplex keratitis is the only purely viral infection that produces stromal ulceration. Mycotic ulcers often present clinically as patchy white infiltrates associated with the formation of satellite lesions. Histologically, the lesions are focal zones of necrosis composed of fragments of lamellae and acute inflammatory cells. Intact organisms are rarely seen within the necrotic foci, but can be found in the surrounding stroma. Descemet's membrane can be penetrated by some types of fungi. **Protozoa,** such as ameba, can cause an ulcerative keratitis.[328-330] Ocular infections have been caused by *Acanthamoeba castellani* and *Acanthamoeba histolyticum.* Histopathologically, the diagnosis can be made from wet mounts of corneal scrapings. Amebic cysts and trophozoites can be seen at the base of the ulcerated zone.[331,332] Identification is aided by special stains including the Giemsa stain.[330,333,334]

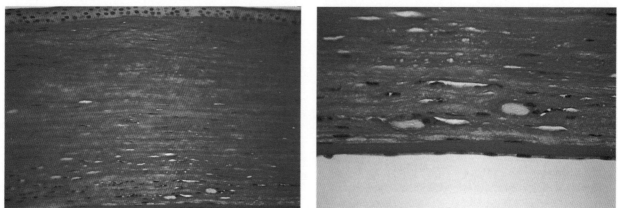

A   B

FIG. 3-12. Interstitial keratitis. (A) Photomicrograph demonstrating inflammatory cells infiltrating the deep vascularized stroma. **(B)** Higher power photomicrograph demonstrating endothelial-lined capillary channels in the posterior stroma and thickening of Descemet's membrane.

Noninfectious corneal ulcerations include the **catarrhal** or **marginal ulcer,** which is often seen in association with blepharoconjunctivitis and is thought to be caused by hypersensitivity to a staphylococcal toxin. Histopathologic examination reveals necrosis of the involved tissues and infiltration by polymorphonuclear leukocytes. Later, healing occurs by fibroblastic proliferation, collagen deposition, and secondary vascularization.[49] A **Mooren's ulcer** is a special form of peripheral corneal ulceration.[335]

The **sequelae of corneal ulceration** includes replacement of the tissue loss with fibrosis and vascularization. An **inflammatory pannus** is defined as an ingrowth of inflammatory elements between the epithelium and Bowman's layer of the cornea. It occurs as a primary ingrowth of cellular elements and is aggravated by chronic endothelial decompensation. Typically, Bowman's membrane is destroyed in the process. **Band keratopathy,** defined as a dystrophic deposition of calcium in Bowman's layer, is a secondary reaction to many types of degenerative or inflammatory processes. **Keratoectasia** is bulging of a thin scarred portion of the cornea, and a **descemetocele** is a herniation of the Descemet's membrane through the floor of a corneal ulcer. It is usually covered by a thin layer of fibrinous exudate and corneal epithelium. A leukoma is a dense corneal scar and is termed an **adherent leukoma** if intraocular tissue is adherent to its internal surface. Historical review almost always reveals a prior corneal perforation.[49]

Inflammation and the Lens

Inflammatory processes involving the anterior segment of the eye rarely elicit an intralenticular inflammatory response because the lens capsule plays an important role in protecting the lens cells from infectious processes. The lens epithelium may undergo a spectrum of changes including proliferation of differentiated cells, fibrous metaplasia, posterior migration, and focal or diffuse necrosis.[49] The term **complicated cataract** often is used to denote a lens opacity induced by associated ocular disease. Irritation produced by posterior synechiae and by traction of the iris musculature on the lens can create localized fibrous metaplasia of the anterior lens epithelium, leading to an **anterior subcapsular cataract.** Posteriorly, the mature, differentiated cortical lens cells may take on a rounded configuration often accompanied by discontinuity of their cell membrane producing what is known as a **postinflammatory cataract** or a **posterior subcapsular cataract.**[49]

Bacterial and mycotic agents rarely cause capsular rupture because the capsule is an effective barrier to invasion; however, necrotizing endogenous ocular infection is rarely associated with capsular rupture. The entry and implantation of infectious agents into the lens may induce the formation of an intralenticular abscess. Inflammation or any edematous process that causes thickening of the pars plicata and pars plana of the ciliary body, with or without hypotony, can lead to relaxation of the zonular fibers and thereby cause luxation or subluxation of the lens. Lenticular subluxation often is worsened when zonular fibers are destroyed by an inflammatory exudate.[43,49]

There are several **lens-induced intraocular inflammatory** processes which all can result in lens-induced glaucoma. The terminology for these processes varies and has included phacoanaphylactic endophthalmitis, phacotoxic reaction, phacogenic glaucoma, phacotopic glaucoma, lens-induced uveitis, and endophthalmitis phacoanaphylactica. These terms have been replaced by phacolytic glaucoma and phacoantigenic endophthalmitis. The older terms, granulomatous lens-induced endophthalmitis or phacoallergic endophthalmitis, correlate with the currently used term phacoantigenic endophthalmitis. In addition the terms nongranulomatous lens-induced endophthalmitis or **phacotoxic endophthalmitis** correlate with the terms lens-particle glaucoma and phacolytic glaucoma.[49,336]

Phacoantigenic endophthalmitis is an intractable uveitis that is due to the liberation of nondenatured lens protein after lens capsule disruption. The entity may follow a surgical or accidental capsular interruption in which the liberated lens protein acts as a primary antigen.[337,338] It develops after a latent period during which there is sensitization of the immune system. Antibodies to autologous lens protein of the IgG class can be detected.[339,340] The classic histologic pattern of this reaction is a **zonal granulomatous inflammation** centered around lens material, often adjacent to the site of capsule rupture. Polymorphonuclear leukocytes accompany the giant cells at the center of the granuloma. These cells are surrounded by a layer of lymphocytes and histiocytes, which in turn, are surrounded by reactive connective tissue[52,341] (Fig. 3-13). Mononuclear inflammatory cells may be present along the nerve fiber layer and inner surface of the retina.[375] It is most important to exclude a concurrent sympathetic ophthalmia in any case of phacoantigenic endophthalmitis, because the histopathology can be similar and the two entities can occur concurrently.

Lens particle glaucoma requires surgical or traumatic disruption of the lens capsule followed by the release of cortical material into the aqueous humor. Precipitating events include extracapsular cataract extraction, traumatic capsular rupture, and laser posterior capsulotomy. The histologic pattern consists mainly of macrophages and fragments of lens cortical material within the anterior chamber and trabecular meshwork.

Phacolytic glaucoma, or **nongranulomatous lens-induced endophthalmitis,** is a process in which a nongranulomatous inflammation occurs in the fluid surrounding the lens.[342] It is most often associated with a hypermature or Morgagnian cataract. Lens protein that

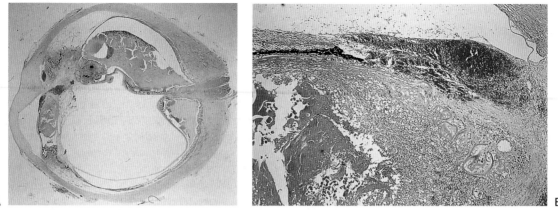

A   B

FIG. 3-13. Lens induced uveitis. (A) Whole mount demonstrating inflammatory reaction centered mainly around the area of the lens. **(B)** The classic histologic pattern of a zonal granulomatous inflammation is centered around a capsular rupture. Inflammatory cells form a zonal granuloma around the lens material with associated polymorphonuclear leukocytes, epithelial cells, giant cells, lymphocytes, and plasma cells. Granulomatous infiltration of the uveal tract also is present and raises the suspicion of a concurrent sympathetic uveitis.

has broken down and become liquified may pass through the capsule and elicit a macrophage response often resulting in secondary glaucoma (Fig. 3-14). Aspirated aqueous reveals macrophages that have engulfed lens protein.[341,343]

Inflammatory Glaucomas

Inflammation of the iris and ciliary body often is accompanied by the deposition of inflammatory cells and proteinaceous exudate in the trabecular meshwork. This material may form a partial or total mechanical barrier to the passage of aqueous through the trabecular meshwork and causes **secondary open-angle glaucoma** in about 20% of cases.[49] Conversely, hyposecretion of aqueous by

the ciliary body can be caused by persistent hypotony, which can progress to **phthisis bulbi.**

In chronic recurrent inflammatory processes, focal areas of peripheral anterior synechiae are formed and eventually may cause **secondary angle-closure glaucoma.** In addition, posterior synechiae may form with adherence of the iris to the capsule of the lens causing a condition known as **secluseo pupillae. Occluseo pupillae** occurs when the synechiae extend for the entire circumference of the pupil and the pupillary space is filled with a connective tissue membrane. The aqueous trapped in the posterior chamber causes the midperipheral iris to be pushed forward against the trabecular meshwork producing **iris bombé,** angle closure, and **pupillary block glaucoma.**[43,49]

The major inflammatory disorders associated with glaucoma include idiopathic anterior uveitis, Fuchs' heterochromic iridocyclitis, sarcoidosis, glaucomatocyclitic crisis (Posner-Schlossman syndrome), herpetic keratouveitis, idiopathic inflammatory precipitates in the anterior chamber angle, syphilitic interstitial keratitis, juvenile rheumatoid arthritis, scleritis and episcleritis.[48] Hemolytic glaucoma also can occur.[344]

Vitreous, Retinal and Choroidal Inflammation

Inflammation of the Vitreous

Inflammation of the vitreous is usually passive and is characterized by liquefaction, opacification, and shrinkage. Acute inflammatory exudates quickly become necrotic, and polymorphonuclear leukocytes often degenerate the vitreous. The inflammatory cells tend to aggregate along the course of collagenous fibrils, particularly in the

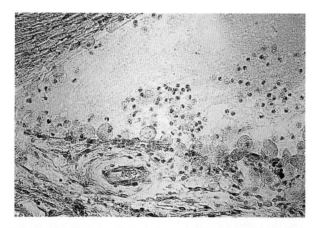

FIG. 3-14. Nongranulomatous lens induced endophthalmitis (phacolytic glaucoma). Macrophages with engulfed lens protein are present in the anterior chamber angle and amidst the beams of the trabecular meshwork.

area of the retina and ciliary body. Abscesses may be discrete and encapsulated with a connective tissue wall or may diffusely fill the entire vitreous.[43,49] Mononuclear phagocytes, lymphocytes, and plasma cells may appear later. During the reparative stage, capillary proliferation and connective tissue infiltration may extend into the vitreous. Cyclitic membranes derived from the ciliary body may form in the anterior portion of the vitreous. Contraction of myofibroblasts within connective tissue may result in detachment of the ciliary body and anterior choroid accompanied by hypotony.[49] Inflammatory cells, pigment granules, or pigment-bearing macrophages may enter the vitreous following a primary inflammation of the choroid or ciliary body. Serum proteins may enter the vitreous if the retina or ciliary body becomes inflamed.

Vitreous inflammations may be grouped into **primary vitreous inflammations** or **vitreous inflammations secondary to systemic disease.** Each of these categories is then subdivided into infectious and noninfectious categories and further classified into exogenous or endogenous.[49] Infectious causes of vitreous inflammation include bacterial, mycotic, and parasitic infections and were discussed earlier in this chapter.

Noninfectious inflammation of the vitreous results from inflammation of the adjacent retina, ciliary body, and pars plana. It is often bilateral and is characterized by minimal anterior chamber cellular reaction and nongranulomatous inflammation in the anterior and inferior vitreous, clinically known as **snowbanking.** Histopathologic examination reveals condensed vitreous containing mononuclear cells intermixed with fibroglial tissue, vessels, and nonpigmented cellular epithelium.[238,240,345]

Noninfectious granulomatous inflammation of the vitreous also can occur in patients with systemic sarcoidosis who develop retinitis. Histologically, the infiltrates in sarcoidosis are composed of histiocytes with associated fibrocollagenous connective tissue most often derived from the adjacent retina and ciliary body. Idiopathic diffuse nonnecrotizing vitritis without vitreous base exudation and organization has been reported.[346]

Inflammation of the Retina

Most **inflammations of the retina** involve a vascular response similar to that seen in other inflamed tissues. The vascular response produces vasodilation resulting in margination and migration of leukocytes. The perivascular area shows an accumulation of white cells that forms sheathlike cuffs around the vessels. This is known clinically as **perivascular sheathing.**[49] Edema soon follows, and fluid gradually diffuses into adjacent nonvascular areas and accumulates in large pools. Pressure exerted by the fluid may cause degeneration of retinal elements, producing large spaces containing cellular debris, fibrin, and inflammatory cells. Hemorrhage into the retinal layers

may occur. These may be small linear hemorrhages in the nerve fiber layers or larger, round hemorrhages in the outer retinal layers. Hemorrhage may break through the internal limiting membrane into the vitreous.[49] Persistence or recurrence of such hemorrhages leads to additional necrosis and inflammation, followed by repair, scarring, and deformity. The neurons respond to the inflammatory process mainly by degeneration of the axons and dendrites and by swelling of the cell bodies followed by disintegration of the cytoplasm and nucleus.[49] Retinal glial cells respond in a similar manner. Surrounding the affected zones is an early and rapid proliferation of the retinal astrocytes, producing the condition known as **retinal gliosis.**[347] Infarction of the axons of the nerve fiber layer may occur, leading to the production of **cotton-wool spots.** Histologically, the patches are known as **cytoid bodies.** Healing occurs by the removal of edema fluid by adjacent vessels and by the removal of degenerated cells and other debris by the macrophages. Any disease characterized by intraocular organization of fibrovascular connective tissue (eg, a cyclitic membrane or proliferative retinopathy) produces large quantities of collagen. Organization and contraction of the collagen produces distortion and folding of the retina, tractional retinoschisis, and traction retinal detachment.[49]

If the inflammation is severe, the retinal pigment epithelium is destroyed and the pigment granules are phagocytized by adjacent cells or by macrophages. Adjacent retinal pigment epithelial cells often undergo hypertrophy and hyperplasia to form clumps. Most inflammations that affect the retina involve the adjacent choroid, and the healing process eventually leads to fusion of the outer limiting membrane of the retina to the lamina vitrea of the choroid.[49] There is a loss of Bruch's membrane and of the choroidal blood vessels. These normal structures are replaced by a dense connective tissue scar. Hyaline and calcific degeneration are commonly associated.

Infections of the retina can be generally classified into **primary** and **secondary.** The primary infections are endogenous, and they lead to an acute suppurative process that either is localized or becomes diffuse. Localized white-centered retinal hemorrhages are due to septic emboli and are referred to as **Roth spots.**[43,49] **Secondary infections** most often are **exogenous** or are endogenous by extension from the anterior portion of the eye or through the optic nerve or uveal tract. Secondary inflammations also can occur from chorioretinal inflammations in which the choroid is primarily involved and the inflammation extends internally to the retina. Retinal inflammation may be secondary to disease of the anterior segment. Retinal edema most often occurs in the macular and peripapillary regions. **Cystoid retinal edema** is prominent in the macular region and is a common complication of intraocular inflammation. The cystoid changes are most evident in the outer plexiform layer, are lined by Müller cell columns, and clinically show a honeycomb or flower-petal appearance.[49] Breakdown of the bordering Müller cell processes causes the intraretinal cysts to become confluent producing secondary retinoschisis and irreversible vision loss in the affected area. Chronic cystoid macular edema can lead to macular cysts and lamellar or complete hole formation. **Postchoroiditis retinoschisis** can develop after focal choroiditis in which the involved segment of the retina becomes edematous and cystic. The area of schisis typically overlies the chorioretinal scar resulting from the primary inflammation.[43,49]

Inflammation of the Choroid

Many of the uveal inflammations were discussed in the earlier sections on intraocular inflammation. It is important to know that many of the **HLA antigens** are associated with uveitis including HLA-Bw54 and HLA-Dwa in VKH syndrome,[348,349] HLA-A29 in birdshot retinochoroidopathy,[262] HLA-A11 in sympathetic uveitis, HLA-B7, DRw2 in the ocular histoplasmosis syndrome, HLA-B5 and Bw51 in Beçhet's disease, HLA-B7 in serpiginous choroidopathy, and HLA-B27 in adult iridocyclitis, ankylosing spondylitis, and inflammatory bowel disease.[49,350] A review of the immunology of chorioretinal disorders has been reported by Corwin.[351]

Inflammation of the Optic Nerve

Infections of the optic nerve are divided into two groups: (1) those that involve the nerve by direct extension from contiguous structures (eye, orbit, and brain), and (2) those that involve the nerve by hematogenous spread (bacterial, viral, fungal, and protozoal).[49]

Bacterial infections caused by a variety of organisms have been documented. The degree of tissue damage and reactive connective tissue proliferation varies with the organism and the intensity of the inflammation. **Viruses** rarely affect the optic nerve alone.[49] The retina and optic nerve may be involved with acute viral infections, persistent viral infections, and slow virus infections. Herpes zoster, influenza, and vaccinia viruses are believed to cause optic nerve inflammations. Intranuclear and intracytoplasmic inclusion bodies have been found by light microscopy in the brain, optic nerves, retina, and choroid. Electron microscopic studies have demonstrated viral particles in the optic nerve. Immunohistochemical methods have demonstrated intranuclear and cytoplasmic viral nucleocapsids in the retina of a child who died of subacute sclerosing panencephalitis caused by paramyxovirus (measles).[172]

Individuals whose immune mechanisms have been compromised appear to be more susceptible to infections with **fungi.** Patients with diabetes are particularly susceptible to infections with *Phycomycetes* species. These organisms gain access to the optic nerve from the adjacent infected paranasal sinuses and have a propensity to invade vascular channels resulting in ischemic optic neuropathy. Other fungal agents, such as *Cryptococcus* and *Coccidioides* organisms, also have been observed to invade the optic nerve.[49] Intraocular infection with *Cryptococcus neoformans* occurs by direct extension from the central nervous system along the meningeal sheaths.

Granulomatous inflammations of the optic nerve head and optic nerve may be caused by a variety of infectious (fungi, syphilis, and tuberculosis) and noninfectious (foreign body and sarcoidosis) intraneural processes.[49] Wegener's granulomatosis and lethal midline granuloma may extend into the nerve. Involvement of the optic nerve occurs in 5% of patients with systemic sarcoidosis.[352]

Optic neuritis and optic atrophy occur in association with a number of disorders of uncertain etiology. Destruction of myelin sheaths may occur clinically as a result of nutritional deficiencies, viral infections, immunopathologic reactions, toxins, or genetically determined enzyme deficiencies. Early destruction of myelin sheaths is associated with degenerative changes in the oligodendroglia. The disintegrated myelin is phagocytized by microglial cells, which are mobilized in large numbers. Later, there is an astrocytic and fibroblastic response. Other morphologic alterations common to these diseases are a perivenous distribution of lesions and perivascular location of inflammatory cells.

The clinical features and pathologic findings of **multiple sclerosis** were first described by Charcot in 1868 and have more recently been reviewed by Spencer[49] and reported by others.[226,353] Pathologic examination reveals widely scattered irregular plaques measuring from 1 to 5 mm. Myelin stain reveals loss of myelin, and glial stains demonstrate gliosis. Perivascular inflammatory cell infiltrate also can be demonstrated.

Inflammation of the Episclera and Sclera

Inflammations of the sclera can be divided into **primary scleral inflammations** and **scleral inflammations secondary to systemic disease.** Isolated primary inflammations of the scleral collagen and of the vascular and neural structures that traverse the sclera occur infrequently. Inflammations of these areas more often are part of a systemic disease, such as rheumatoid arthritis. In addition, the sclera is frequently affected by spillover inflammation originating in adjacent structures including the cornea, conjunctiva, uveal tract, and the orbit. The intrascleral perforating vessels and nerves often serve as passageways for extraocular extension.[49,354]

The most frequently seen clinical form of **primary episcleritis** manifests as a recurrent, spontaneous, noninfectious inflammation of a sector of the anterior episclera. The process also may involve all quadrants. The frequency is equal in both sexes, with a mean age of onset in the fifth decade.[49] Clinically, **simple episcleritis** is accompanied by pain and focal dilatation of episcleral vessels, and the inflammation often subsides spontaneously. Histologically, the inflammation is nongranulomatous and is characterized by vascular dilatation, perivascular lymphocytic infiltration, and the accumulation of serous fluid in the extracellular spaces. Healing occurs without scarring.[49]

Nodular episcleritis occurs in conjunction with focal granulomatous inflammation of the underlying scleral stroma.[355] The nodules are usually single and localized to one sector of the eye.[49] Histopathologic features are similar to those seen in subcutaneous rheumatoid nodules.[356–358] Comparable inflammation may extend into the limbus or peripheral cornea.

Scleritis is a more severe disease than episcleritis, and it is more likely to lead to vision loss from associated keratitis, uveitis, cataract, or retinal detachment. The process is generally divided into anterior scleritis and posterior scleritis. It is more prevalent in women and often develops later in life.[49] Many patients have associated systemic connective tissue disease including systemic lupus erythematosus, polyarteritis nodosa, relapsing polychondritis, and Wegener's granulomatosis. Scleritis also has been observed in patients with tuberculosis, syphilis, gout, and ochronosis.[49]

Clinically, in **anterior scleritis,** there is increasing redness of a quadrant or sector of the sclera and episclera, associated with photophobia and severe pain. In a less severe and more common form of the disease, inflammation and swelling involves the bulbar conjunctiva and episclera. The more severe nodular form is definitely of scleral origin.[49] Focal or diffuse scleral thinning often occurs, but uveal prolapse (**scleromalacia perforans**) is relatively uncommon, occurring in only 15% to 20% of cases.[49]

Posterior scleritis or inflammation in the posterior portion of the sclera can produce disturbances in motility, proptosis, retrobulbar pain, and visual field loss.[359,360]

Most patients with posterior scleritis have a history of anterior scleritis. The process is usually unilateral. Edema of the optic disk, optic neuritis, nonrhegmatogenous retinal detachment, choroidal detachment, diplopia, exophthalmos, and intermittent retinal and choroidal detachments may occur. The inflamed posterior sclera may become grossly thickened. By ultrasound examination, inflammation of the posterior choroid often results in an ill-defined boundary between uvea and sclera.[49]

All forms of scleritis are histologically similar but vary in distribution, intensity, and extent.[49] In **nodular scleritis,** focal or zonal necrotizing granulomatous inflammation surrounds a discrete focus of scleral collagen of varying size.[361] These focal zones are usually surrounded, in turn, by a broad zone of fibrinoid necrosis and chronic inflammatory cell infiltration causing the tissues to thicken in a fusiform configuration (Fig. 3-15).[49] When the collagen lamellae have been destroyed by the inflammation, the swelling recedes and the uvea may herniate into the defect producing a condition known as **scleromalacia perforans.** Often, the thinned sclera surrounding the defect bulges outward, forming a **staphyloma.**[49]

Brawny scleritis has been applied to the diffuse form of the process in which large areas of scleral collagen are infiltrated by a granulomatous inflammatory process, causing the sclera to become markedly thickened.[49] It varies somewhat in configuration from the discrete nodular form, but the basic granulomatous process is the same. In late cases or after the inflammation has subsided, scleromalacia can occur, and relatively large limbal, equatorial, or posterior staphylomas may form.

Inflammation of the Orbit

Noninfectious Orbital Inflammation

The orbit frequently is the site of idiopathic inflammations, which can be primary and strictly localized or sec-

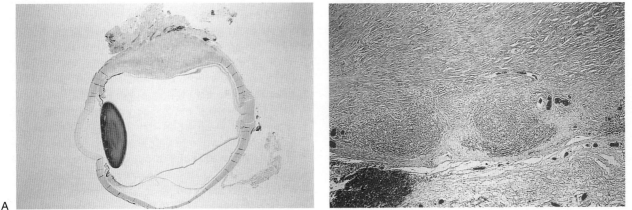

A

B

FIG. 3-15. Diffuse and nodular scleritis. (A) Whole mount showing fusiform thickening of the preequatorial sclera. **(B)** Necrotizing granulomatous inflammation amidst the scleral collagen lamellae.

ondary as a manifestation of a systemic disease.[362,363] **Idiopathic orbital inflammation or pseudotumor** is an example of a primary orbital inflammation. Graves' disease, which accounts for more than 50% of cases of proptosis, is an example of orbital inflammation associated with systemic disease.[49,365]

Graves' orbitopathy remains an enigma from the point of view of causation and immunologic parameters.[49] Men and women are equally affected. Patients have insidious development of irritation of the eyes, stare or upper lid retraction, lid lag, and proptosis. Corneal exposure and epithelial breakdown may occur. In the infiltrative form of orbitopathy, the extraocular muscles are thickened by inflammatory cells and scarring. Proptosis and extraocular motility disturbances can result.[49] A reduction of visual acuity can result from compression of the optic nerve at the orbital apex by the swollen extraocular muscles as they impinge on the optic nerve within the annulus of Zinn.[365] Fortunately, fewer than 10% of Graves' patients develop infiltrative orbitopathy. A detailed system of classifying the eye changes of Graves' disease is widely used.[366]

Studies on the pathologic features of Graves' disease[365,367–369] have revealed that the inflammation is virtually always restricted to the muscle bellies of the extraocular muscles. The inflammation consists mostly of lymphocytes and plasma cells with occasional mast cells. Secretion of mucopolysaccharide has been demonstrated; however, with progressive irritation of the fibroblasts, they modulate from mucopolysaccharide production toward collagen production. Electron microscopic studies reveal that the tendons inserting onto the globe, the optic nerve meninges, and the orbital fat are generally uninflamed.[367,370] The lacrimal gland shows moderate numbers of lymphocytes and plasma cells, with interstitial fluid collection but no fibrosis. Examination of the optic nerve in an exenteration specimen has shown axonal loss.

Pseudotumor is a term used to describe inflammatory swelling of the orbital contents that produces proptosis and the false clinical impression of a neoplasm. Some investigators have categorized lymphoid tumors as lymphoid pseudotumors.[49,371–375]

Idiopathic orbital inflammations, or **pseudotumors,** have no recognizable local causes nor any obvious underlying systemic disease. Orbital pseudotumors account for 5.2% to 6.3% of orbital tumors in several large series.[376,377] It is probably the most frequent cause of proptosis after Graves' disease. Patients with idiopathic orbital inflammation may be children or adults who present acutely, subacutely, or chronically. The disease may be unilateral, recurrent in one orbit, bilateral, or may alternate from one orbit to the other.[362,363] The disease can be further characterized according to which orbital structure is predominantly involved, such as dacryoadenitis, periscleritis, trochleitis, perineuritis.[363] Involvement of the cavernous sinus is known as **Tolosa-Hunt syndrome.**[378,379]

Lesions also may be diffuse, involving more than one site. Multifocality of orbital involvement also is typical of idiopathic orbital inflammation. Edema and a mild polymorphic inflammatory infiltrate composed of lymphocytes, plasma cells, eosinophils, and occasionally polymorphonuclear leukocytes are typical.[362,363,372]

As the disease progresses and fibrosis ensues, the inflammatory cells become more widely separated by tracts of collagen, which radiate outward from the fibrous tissue septa and blood vessels into the orbital fat.[49] The connective tissues of the muscles thicken, and there is hyperplasia of the periacinal and periductal tissue.[49]

The **immunopathologic mechanisms** responsible for idiopathic orbital inflammation are only vaguely understood.[9] Immunocytologic studies of idiopathic orbital inflammation and idiopathic dacryoadenitis revealed a predominance of B lymphocytes.[9] Patients with idiopathic orbital inflammations may be at risk for such systemic diseases as rheumatoid arthritis, regional enteritis, and lupus erythematosus although fewer than 10% have any underlying disease.[380,381]

Infectious Orbital Inflammation

In **infectious orbital inflammation** an identifiable bacterial, fungal, or parasitic cause usually can be discovered. **Viral** infections of the orbital contents are virtually unknown. **Bacterial** infection of the orbit and its surrounding compartments is clearly the most common cause. Orbital cellulitis occurs more commonly in children than adults.[49] Infections (both bacterial and fungal) generally spread to the orbit from the surrounding sinuses, lids, or conjunctiva. Spread by an exclusively hematogenous route is exceedingly rare.[362] In children, bacterial orbital cellulitis and preseptal cellulitis occur far more commonly than primary and secondary neoplasms. In adults, idiopathic inflammations, such as Graves' disease and pseudotumor, rival infectious orbital cellulitis in frequency of occurrence.[49,382]

Infectious orbital inflammation generally is divided into two categories: preseptal cellulitis and deep orbital cellulitis. In **preseptal cellulitis,** inflammatory signs are localized to the preseptal portion. In **deep orbital cellulitis,** infection spreads from the involved sinus into the orbital soft tissues posterior to the orbital septum.[362,382–384] Both forms of disease may follow upper respiratory infections with sinus involvement. In the **preseptal form,** there is erythema and swelling of the eyelids and chemosis of the conjunctiva without significant impairment of vision, proptosis, or extraocular motility disturbance. In **deep orbital cellulitis,** disturbance of ocular function is generally seen, including proptosis, massive swelling of the eyelids, palpable mass, visual decrease, extraocular motility disturbance, afferent pupillary defect, optic nerve head swelling, and papillitis.[49,381] There is associated pain and

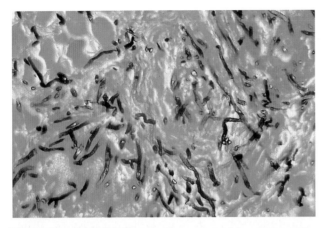

FIG. 3-16. Orbital inflammation caused by *Aspergillus* species. Fibrous connective tissue from the orbit of a patient with a subperiosteal orbital abscess. The branching and the septated characteristics of the fungus are demonstrated.

proptosis. Sinus opacification occurs and most frequently involves the ethmoid sinus and the maxillary sinus. *Haemophilus influenzae, Streptococcus* sp., *Staphylococcus aureus, Clostridia, Bacteroides, Enterobacteriaceae, Proteus,* and *Klebsiella* organisms all have been reported as causative agents. Streptococci and staphylococci are the most frequent pathogens, but consideration should be given to *H. influenzae, E. coli,* and anaerobic organisms.[49]

The histopathologic evaluation of tissues excised from the orbit in the course of surgical intervention in orbital cellulitis generally reveals abundant infiltration of polymorphonuclear leukocytes, with or without focal necrosis of the orbital fat. Necrosis is extremely prominent if the infection progresses to incipient abscess formation (Fig. 3-16).[49]

An orbital cellulitis can progress to an orbital abscess or focal loculation.[385] Orbital abscess formation and subperiosteal abscesses may result from incompletely treated orbital cellulitis or from subacute infectious sinusitis following upper respiratory infections. An abscess situated either in the orbital fat or subperiosteally usually is a surgical emergency and requires drainage along with evacuation of the contiguous inflammatory focus in the sinus.

Many **fungi** are known to cause orbital infections.[386–388] **Mucormycosis** (also known as **phycomycosis**) is a very serious fungal infection because of its associated high fatality rate. The fungi are present ubiquitously in nature, can be readily cultured from the human upper respiratory system, and normally are noninvasive. The ophthalmically important form is the rhinoorbitocerebral variety, although other systemic forms exist.[49,389,390] Almost all patients have an underlying systemic disease, especially diabetic ketoacidosis. Children may not manifest a systemic disease.[391] The mildest form is oropharyngitis, nasopharyngitis, or sinusitis.[392,393] The ethmoidal and sphenoidal sinuses are the most common sites from which such

invasion of the orbit occurs. An **orbital apex syndrome** including external and internal ophthalmoplegia, decreased vision, decreased sensation, ptosis, exophthalmos, chemosis, and facial pain may occur. The fungal hyphae have a distinct propensity to invade vascular walls, particularly those of arteries. Brain involvement can occur from extension to the cavernous sinus. The organism is a large (30 to 50 μm wide), nonseptate, branching hypha that stains vividly with routine hematoxylin and eosin (Fig. 3-17). Invasion of the orbital vessels and arteries, the optic nerve, the extraocular muscles, and even transscleral invasion to the choroid may be observed.[49] Because of the associated prominent necrosis, polymorphonuclear leukocytes rather than granulomas are prominent in the infiltrate.

Vasculitis

The most common forms of **vasculitis** include temporal arteritis, Wegener's granulomatosis,[394,396–398] and polyarteritis nodosa. Rarely, veins are primarily involved, producing thrombophlebitis.[49] **Temporal (cranial) arteritis** is the most common variety. In temporal arteritis, the short posterior ciliary arteries become involved with a granulomatous inflammation centered in the muscularis and internal elastica. The condition may lead to the development of anterior ischemic optic neuropathy.[399]

OCULAR, FUNGAL, AND PARASITIC INFECTIONS IN PATIENTS WITH HUMAN IMMUNODEFICIENCY VIRUS OR ACQUIRED IMMUNODEFICIENCY SYNDROME

The advent of the **acquired immunodeficiency syndrome (AIDS)** pandemic has resulted in the emergence

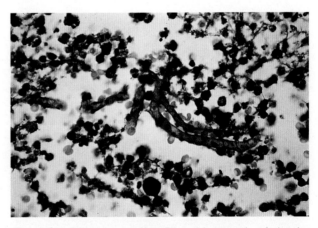

FIG. 3-17. Mucormycosis. Photomicrograph of the hyphae of mucormycosis that are characterized by their large size, lack of septation, and affinity for hematoxylin. The organism has a tendency to invade vascular structures and may cause thrombosis.

of ocular involvement by previously obscure fungal, viral, and parasitic diseases.[400–406] **Cytomegalovirus (CMV)** infection is a major cause of morbidity and mortality in AIDS. Cytomegalovirus retinitis occurs in approximately 15% to 20% of AIDS patients and, in contrast to the noninfectious lesions of AIDS, demands aggressive treatment to prevent severe vision loss.[406–409] Ocular involvement with the fungus *Cryptococcus neoformans* occurs more frequently as a late complication in AIDS patients and is often associated with CNS involvement.[410] The first report of ocular *Pneumocystis carinii* in a patient with AIDS was by Macher et al.[411] *Toxoplasma gondii* was previously thought to be a self-limited, recurrent process that arose focally from a remote chorioretinal scar, but recently has been reported as a retinal necrosis syndrome in AIDS patients.[412–416]

Ophthalmic manifestations in AIDS patients that are infection related include herpes zoster ophthalmicus,[415,416] herpes simplex keratitis,[417,418] fungal keratitis, bacterial keratitis,[419] molluscum contagiosum,[420] cytomegalovirus retinitis, toxoplasma retinochoroiditis, acute retinal necrosis, HIV retinitis, syphilitic retinitis,[421–427] *Pneumocystis carinii* choroiditis, *Mycobacterium avium intracellulare* choroiditis,[406] fungal and bacterial endophthalmitis,[428] fungal choroiditis, and neuroophthalmic disorders.[408,428–432] Coccidiodomycosis also is known to cause multifocal choroiditis (Fig. 3-18).

Anterior Segment Disease

Corneal Microsporidiosis

Microsporidia are obligate intracellular protozoa/parasites that are increasingly recognized as opportunistic pathogens in patients with AIDS. They have been associated with enteritis, hepatitis, peritonitis, and recently, keratoconjunctivitis.[433] Microsporidia produce infective spores that are known to infect both invertebrate and vertebrate species. Cases of human microsporidiosis were exceedingly rare until the advent of AIDS, with only five reported cases of isolated infectious keratitis.[354] Microsporidiosis has been reported subsequently as an opportunistic infection in the cornea, conjunctiva, and intestinal mucosa in AIDS patients. Five additional cases of corneal microsporidiosis were reported during the last several years, and three of these were associated with AIDS or seropositivity for HIV.[433,435,436]

Clinically, patients present with blurred vision, photophobia, and irritation. The most common manifestation of microsporidiosis keratitis is the presence of diffuse course epithelial opacities or punctate epitheliopathy and irregular staining with fluorescein. Occasionally, a corneal stromal infiltrate is present. There is an associated fusiform swelling and hyperemia of the inferior forniceal conjunctiva, with or without a slight follicular reaction. Fine keratic precipitates and minimal cell and flare also can be present. Conjunctival or corneal cultures are often negative or misleading. Scrapings reveal large ovoid intracellular and extracellular gram-positive bodies. Many of them contain a vacuole and a densely stained nucleus. A single small periodic acid-Schiff (PAS)-positive polar body is seen within many of the inclusions.[435] Histopathologic studies of corneal biopsy specimens reveal spores interspersed between intact stromal lamellae without an inflammatory reaction.[434] The spores are elongated and oval and measure 3.5 to 4.0 μm in length and 1.5 μm in width. Under polarized light, the spores contain polychromatic, linear birefringent particles that appear to represent the polar tubule. Spores are located both within keratocytes and extracellularly. Vacuoles containing gray granular organisms are present within the cytoplasm of superficial epithelial cells. These vacuoles and their contents replace the usual eosinophilic cytoplasm with minimal

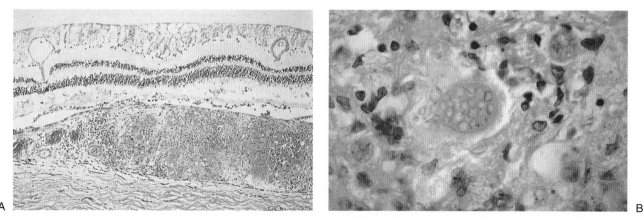

A   B

FIG. 3-18. Coccidiomycosis with multifocal choroiditis. (A) A choroidal granuloma with central necrosis composed of epithelioid histiocytes, lymphocytes, and polymorphonuclear leukocytes. **(B)** Coccidiomycosis spherules in various stages of their life cycle. Some spherules contain conspicuous endospores.

nuclear distortion. The organisms stain well with Giemsa stain and in tissue sections with Gram stain. Ultrastructural characteristics of mature spores include a thin electron-lucent endospore and a polar vacuole (with 5 to 6 coils). The coiled polar tubule is pathognomic for microsporidia infection.[434]

No definitive treatment for microsporidia keratitis is known to date. It has been reported that trimethoprim/sulfisoxazole alone can result in improvement in systemic cases,[434] but there are no reports of microsporidial keratoconjunctivitis cases that have been successfully eradicated with antiparasitic agents. Symptomatic relief can be obtained with artificial lubricants.

Posterior Segment Disease

Noninfectious AIDS Retinopathy

A retinal microangiopathy characterized by the presence of cotton-wool spots, retinal hemorrhages, microaneurysms, telangiectasias, and areas of capillary nonperfusion is often seen in AIDS patients. These manifestations may appear independently of retinal infections and are most logically classified as noninfectious AIDS retinopathy. Cotton-wool spots are the most common of these manifestations and may be found in more than 50% of the cases in clinical series and in up to 100% in autopsy series.[404]

The appearance of cotton-wool spots in AIDS patients does not differ clinically or by fluorescein angiography from the cotton-wool spots found in diabetes and hypertension. Isolated cotton-wool spot formation does not usually affect vision, although patients may occasionally notice a relative scotoma corresponding to its location in the retina. No treatment is required, although it is important to differentiate between cotton-wool spot formation and early CMV retinitis.

Cotton-wool spots are superficial, grayish-white opacities with feathery margins oriented along the direction of the nerve fiber layer. They rarely extend beyond the posterior pole. Resolution of the cotton-wool spots may leave biomicroscopic evidence of a focal depression in the inner retinal surface indicative of a nerve fiber layer infarction.

Histopathologically, cotton-wool spots are identical to the cytoid bodies found in diabetes and hypertension.[402] Cytoid bodies represent accumulations of cytoplasmic debris caused by obstructed orthograde and retrograde axoplasmic flow in ganglion cell axons. They are a nonspecific reaction to injury most commonly associated with ischemic insults, but they also may follow traumatic, thermal, or toxic episodes.

The other lesions of noninfectious AIDS retinopathy are readily visible by fluorescein angiography. Ultrastructural studies of AIDS microangiopathy have revealed small vessels with swollen endothelial cells, occluded lumens, thickened basal lamina, and degenerating pericytes.[406] Histologic examination of such Roth spots revealed acute inflammatory cells and cotton-wool spots as the cause of the white centers.[400,401]

Perivasculitis, which has often been seen in association with CMV retinitis, is also common in noninfectious AIDS retinopathy in Africa. In studies of African adults and children with AIDS and AIDS-related complex, 16% to 33% were found to have perivasculitis without evidence of CMV infection. Perivasculitis has not been reported as a manifestation of noninfectious AIDS retinopathy in the United States. To date, it is unclear why there is a variance in these findings between the AIDS population in Africa and in the United States.[404]

The presence of retinal edema, macular exudates, and cotton-wool spots has been termed ischemic maculopathy. It is noteworthy that this is the only sequela of noninfectious AIDS retinopathy that results in visual symptoms.

Cytomegalovirus Retinitis

Cytomegalovirus (CMV) retinitis is the most common cause of retinal inflammation in patients with AIDS.[158,406,408,409,437,438] CMV can cause severe vision loss, with 40% of patients losing central vision by the time of death.[439] CMV retinitis is a slow, progressive, necrotizing retinal inflammation that may affect the posterior pole, the periphery, or both and may be unilateral or bilateral. Involved areas appear as white interstitial, intraretinal, or superficial lesions with areas of infiltrate and necrosis along the vascular arcades in the posterior pole. In addition, prominent retinal hemorrhages often are seen within the necrotic areas or along their leading edges.[440] Other direct manifestations of CMV retinitis include retinal edema, attenuated vessels, perivascular sheathing, and exudative retinal detachment. Additionally, vitritis, anterior uveitis, papillitis, and optic atrophy have been reported. The optic atrophy may be seen as a late manifestation secondary to widespread retinal destruction.[441] As the retinitis progresses, an area of atrophic, avascular retina may remain, with underlying retinal pigment epithelial atrophy or hyperplasia. Peripheral CMV retinitis tends to have a less intense white appearance than its more posterior counterpart and appears as areas of granular white retinitis that may or may not demonstrate associated retinal hemorrhage. It also is common in AIDS patients who may initially complain only of floaters with or without a visual field deficit. The recent prospective studies using indirect ophthalmoscopy in such patients indicate that peripheral retinitis may be the most common form of CMV retinitis.[407] In addition to the classically described retinitis, several authors have reported disk neovascularization in patients with AIDS and CMV retinitis.[442] In approximately

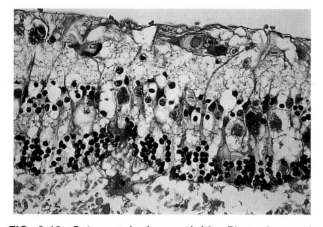

FIG. 3-19. Cytomegalovirus retinitis. Photomicrograph of retina with focal photoreceptor necrosis. Pathognomonic cytomegalic cells are identified.

15% of AIDS patients, the presence of CMV retinopathy was the initial manifestation of HIV infection.[438] CMV also can occur concurrently with other forms of chorioretinitis.[443]

Histopathologically, the CMV primarily affects the neurosensory retina, although the retinal pigment epithelium and the choroid are rarely involved. Full-thickness necrosis of the retina in AIDS-associated CMV retinitis is typical. Pathognomic cytomegalic cells, with only a few polymorphonuclear inflammatory cells, are found in the lesions (Fig. 3-19). Intracytoplasmic and intranuclear DNA-positive viral inclusions are found within cytomegalic cells.[401,407] Choroidal involvement is rare. Antigens to CMV have been demonstrated in the retina by immunofluorescence, by immunoperoxidase staining, and by DNA hybridization techniques. Diagnosis also can be made by culturing the virus from ocular tissue.[444]

Acute Retinal Necrosis and Progressive Outer Retinal Necrosis

Acute retinal necrosis (ARN) caused by herpes simplex virus and **progressive outer retinal necrosis (PORN)** caused by varicella-zoster virus are acutely developing, devastating retinal inflammations occasionally seen in the AIDS patient.[406,445–448] Examination of the fundus reveals confluent areas of necrotizing retinitis, characterized by early patchy choroidal and deep retinal lesions, and late diffuse thickening of the retina. Optic neuritis often is present. One third of cases are bilateral. Most cases of retinitis begin in the posterior pole, with little or no clinical evidence of associated vasculitis. In all patients, there is a typical cherry-red spot in the macula.[449] The disease is characterized by relentless progression to atrophy. In all reported cases of AIDS, the final picture has been an atrophic necrotic retina, pale optic nerve, and narrowed retinal vasculature. There is no associated aqueous or vitreous inflammation or retinal detachment.[407,450] ARN and PORN are very similar clinical processes; however, the cherry-red spot is more prominent in PORN, and the perivascular region is characteristically spared in PORN and involved in ARN.[450–452]

Indirect immunofluorescence with a monoclonal antibody, has been used to confirm the varicella-zoster antigen within the retinal tissue[453,454] and the vitreous.[456] Examination of the tissue by transmission electron microscopy has revealed intranuclear and intracytoplasmic viral particles measuring approximately 80 to 100 nm in diameter within the nuclear layer of the retina. Histopathology of several enucleation specimens disclosed a clinically normal anterior segment, except for a few lymphocytes. The vitreous was clear, but the retina showed variable degrees of inflammation and necrosis. Similarly, a variable inflammatory response was found in the choroid with an intense lymphocytic infiltrate in some areas of the choriocapillaris. The optic nerve showed a marked necrosis and a lymphocytic infiltrate. Later, there is atrophy (Fig. 3-20). There were no inclusion bodies observed in the choroid, retina, or optic nerve. Varicella-zoster antigens have been detected in a vitreous aspirate from one case.[450] Detection of herpes virus by the polymerase-chain reaction also has been reported.[456,457]

Cryptococcus neoformans

Cryptococcus neoformans is a yeastlike fungus that is pathogenic in humans as well as many lower animals. The fungus infects both immunosuppressed and healthy hosts, producing a clinical or subclinical pneumonitis and hematogenous dissemination that tends to involve the CNS. The CNS cryptococcal infection is the fourth most

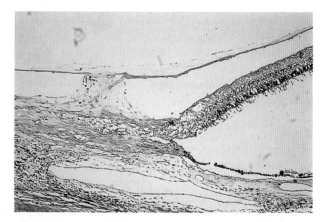

FIG. 3-20. Acute retinal necrosis. Photomicrograph of the atrophic retina in an enucleated specimen from a patient with acute retinal necrosis. The retina in the affected area is thinned, atrophic, and fibrotic. The retinal pigment epithelium is absent and replaced by a chorioretinal scar. In the adjacent area, the retina is normal and artifactually detached.

commonly recognized life-threatening infection in AIDS patients.[410] Cryptococcal meningitis is the usual clinical manifestation of CNS; however, 40% of patients have abnormal ocular findings, including photophobia, diplopia, blepharoptosis, amblyopia, nystagmus, ophthalmoplegia, anisocoria, papilledema, neuroretinitis, choroiditis, and endophthalmitis.[458] Ocular involvement is either the result of increased intracranial pressure related to meningitis from direct extension to the optic nerve via the subarachnoid space or is associated with widespread disseminated diseases and produces choroiditis, chorioretinitis, or endophthalmitis.[139,459,460]

The characteristic fundus changes in cryptococcal choroiditis have been described as deep, hypopigmented, yellow-white, slightly elevated lesions at the level of the choroid. They are approximately one fifth to one whole disk diameter in size. These lesions block choroidal fluorescence during fluorescein angiography. The choroiditis may progress to involve the retina, producing chorioretinitis, and subsequently a diffuse uveitis, vitritis, endophthalmitis, and rarely, an exudative retinal detachment.[140,459] A solitary vitreoretinal abscess has been documented as the initial manifestation of cryptococcal infection.[461] There is one unique case of intraocular cryptococcus presenting as an iris inflammatory mass in a patient with the AIDS. The diagnosis was established by anterior chamber tap and confirmed by histopathology of the enucleated eye. Optic nerve involvement is manifested clinically as optic atrophy, papilledema, or retrobulbar neuritis.[410,462–465]

Histopathologic studies of eyes with cryptococcal infections have documented choroiditis, neuroretinitis, optic nerve invasion, and diffuse intraocular invasion. The choroidal inflammatory reaction is characterized by a diffuse granulomatous process, with fungi concentrated in the choroid and subretinal space. Additionally, microabscesses in the choriocapillaris have been described. This organism ranges in size from 5 to 15 mm and has a surrounding mucinous capsule that is 3 to 5 mm in width and is identifiable by India ink, PAS, and mucicarmine staining.[140] Organisms can be round or budding.[461]

Pneumocystis carinii

Pneumocystis carinii is a unicellular organism that exhibits many morphologic features of a protozoan, but is considered by some researchers to be a fungus.[466] P. carinii infection is the most common infection in patients with AIDS and causes pneumonia in more than 80% of the cases studied.[466] Ocular involvement is rare, but is becoming more significant with the increased incidence of AIDS. Ocular involvement may be the initial presenting sign in patients with disseminated P. carinii infection. The characteristic fundus changes in P. carinii infection consist of numerous slightly elevated, plaquelike yellow-to-white choroidal lesions that vary from

1 to 3 mm in diameter and are located primarily in the posterior pole. Some of the lesions are round, whereas others are geographic and multilobulated. The lesions are often covered by relatively normal retinal pigment epithelium. Large lesions may show areas of retinal pigment epithelial mottling. Intraocular inflammation does not accompany the choroidal lesions.[466–468] Orbital involvement also has been reported.[469]

Histopathologic characteristics of P. carinii choroiditis have been described in several autopsy specimens[466] and one transscleral biopsy.[470–472] The lesions are eosinophilic, acellular, and contain vacuolated frothy material. Foci of hemorrhage and calcifications may be present in the larger lesions. The lumina of choroidal vessels may be partially or totally obliterated by the eosinophilic material (Fig. 3-21). Gomori's methenamine silver staining method demonstrates mature P. carinii cysts in the lesions, but trophozoites usually are not stained by this method.[466]

Electron microscopic examination can provide a definitive diagnosis. The choroidal lesions contain different ultrastructural stages of the organism. Most of the organisms are pleomorphic trophozoites covered with surface projections that contain empty spaces or electron-lucent areas, and have few internal structures. Precysts show a distinct wall without intrinsic bodies or trophozoites. Mature cysts with numerous intracystic trophozoites are infrequently seen.[377] Treatment consists of trimethoprim/sulfamethoxazole or pentamidine. Potential adverse effects associated with these agents include neutropenia, thrombocytopenia, skin rash, fever, and renal failure.

Toxoplasma gondii

Toxoplasma gondii is an obligate intracellular parasite that causes infections in both humans and animals. Most cases of T. gondii infection are reactivations of congenital toxoplasmosis. Congenital toxoplasmosis results from the transplacental transmission of maternal T. gondii infection that was acquired just before or during gestation. Clinical manifestations of congenital toxoplasmosis include retinochoroiditis, hydrocephalus, microcephaly, cerebral calcifications, seizures, psychomotor retardation, organomegaly, jaundice, rash, and fever. Acquired infection generally is subclinical and asymptomatic; however, in 10% to 20% of patients with acute infection, there is an acute, flulike illness that is self-limited.[345]

Ocular disease is estimated to occur in 2% to 3% of patients with systemic toxoplasmosis. Retinochoroiditis and papillitis are the most common clinical manifestations. The characteristic toxoplasmosis fundus lesion in the immunocompetent host is a focal retinitis that appears as a white, fluffy lesion with surrounding retinal edema and an overlying vitritis usually adjacent to an old, inactive scar. **Three morphologic variants** have been de-

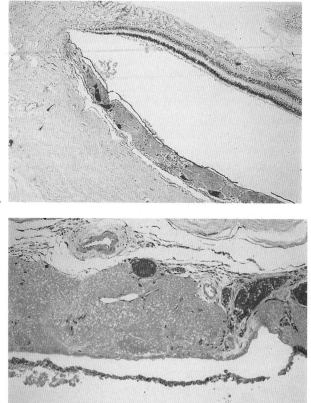

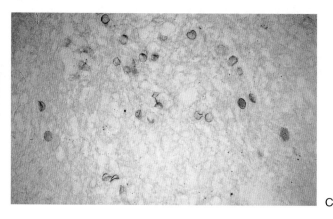

FIG. 3-21. *Pneumocystis carinii* **choroiditis.** (**A**) Typical pneumocystis choroidal lesion composed of eosinophilic acellular vacuolated frothy material that can often be identified within the lumina of choroidal vessels. (**B**) Higher power view of typical pneumocystis choroidal lesion composed of eosinophilic acellular vacuolated frothy material. (**C**) Mature pneumocystis carinii cysts.

scribed: (1) large destructive lesions greater than one disk diameter with associated vitritis, (2) punctate inner retinal lesions, and (3) punctate outer retinal lesions. Toxoplasma papillitis presents with a white inflammatory mass either within or adjacent to the optic nerve, sometimes in a sectoral distribution, and associated with disk edema and adjacent retinal edema. Dense visual-field defects may be associated with optic nerve involvement. Other neuroophthalmic manifestations also are known.[471]

Several life-threatening illnesses, including encephalitis, pneumonitis, and myocarditis, may develop in immunocompromised hosts. Ocular toxoplasmosis has been reported to accompany systemic toxoplasmosis in AIDS patients in less than 1% of cases[473]; however, toxoplasma retinitis is second only to CMV retinitis as a cause of retinitis in AIDS patients.[412,413] Ocular toxoplasmosis can accompany AIDS-related intracranial toxoplasmosis in 10% to 20% of patients.[413]

Clinically, AIDS-related ocular toxoplasmosis most often presents as an acute necrotizing retinitis. Toxoplasma retinochoroiditis in patients with AIDS may have several clinical manifestations, including discrete single lesions, multifocal discrete lesions, or diffuse areas of retinal necrosis.[413] The latter has been described as large, confluent patches of white, necrotic-appearing retina with scattered intraretinal hemorrhages. Vascular sheathing, vitritis, and anterior segment uveitis are common.[474] Unlike acquired toxoplasmosis in the immunocompetent host, the process is only rarely associated with an old scar. Secondary complications include chronic iridocyclitis, cataracts, glaucoma, band keratopathy, cystoid macular edema, retinal detachment, optic atrophy, branch retinal artery obstruction, periphlebitis, periarteritis, and choroidal neovascularization.[413]

Histopathologically, there is microscopic evidence of retinal necrosis with destruction of the normal retinal architecture. There may or may not be an associated mononuclear inflammatory cell infiltrate composed of lymphocytes, macrophages, and epithelioid cells in toxoplasma retinochoroiditis. Optic nerve involvement includes necrosis of nerve-fiber bundles, congestion of fibrovascular pial septa, and marked thickening of meningeal sheaths with infiltration by acute and chronic inflammatory cells.[412,413,473,475] Toxoplasma-related scleritis also has been reported.[476] *T. gondii* cysts and tachyzoites may be identified within the retina and optic nerve[473,475] (Fig. 3-22). Ultrastructural characteristics of *Toxoplasma tachyzoites* include a triple-walled pellicle, an intracytoplasmic conoid, amylopectin granules, dense granules, and rhoptries.[475] *T. gondii* DNA fragments have been demonstrated in infected eyes by the polymerase chain reaction technique.

Ocular Histoplasmosis

Disseminated histoplasmosis is one of the life-threatening opportunistic infections associated with AIDS. In recent years, there have been two reports of **ocular**

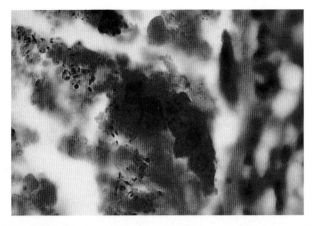

FIG. 3-22. Photomicrograph of multiple *Toxoplasma gondii* cysts overlying Bruch's membrane at the level of the retinal pigment epithelium.

histoplasmosis in AIDS patients with disseminated histoplasmosis.

Clinically, the ocular findings include creamy white intraretinal and subretinal infiltrates that measure from one sixth to one fourth disk diameter in size. The retinal infiltrates are occasionally surrounded by hemorrhage and generally have very indistinct borders.[477] As the disease progresses, the number of retinal infiltrates can increase. Evidence of disseminated histoplasmosis can be demonstrated by bone marrow biopsy, which shows histoplasmosis histopathologically. Other ways of confirming infection are by positive blood cultures or on the basis of radiographic findings. The intraocular diagnosis is established by enucleation or by biopsy only.

Typically, the retinal lesions contain histoplasma yeast in all layers; sometimes it extends to the subretinal and subhyaloid spaces. Often, the lesions are perivascular. The organisms are free or phagocytized within white cells and may be seen with or without infiltrative lymphocytes and histiocytes. Associated retinal nerve fiber layer infarcts can be found adjacent to perivascular infiltrates. Retinal lesions may show intraretinal migration of retinal pigment epithelium with disruption of Bruch's membrane. Intracytoplasmic yeasts often are present in retinal pigment epithelial cells. Focal choroiditis with histiocytes, lymphocytes, plasma cells, and rare histoplasma yeasts can be seen in areas adjacent to the retinitis.[477,478]

References

1. Barret JT, ed. *Textbook of immunology,* ed 4. St. Louis: Mosby, 1983.
2. Amos DB, Schwartz RS, Janicki BW. *Immune mechanisms and disease.* New York: Academic Press, 1979.
3. Carr I. The biology of macrophages. *Clin Invest Med* 1978;1:59.
4. Wheater PR, Burkitt HG, Daniels VG. *Functional histology,* ed 2. New York: Churchill Livingston, 1987.
5. Trinchieri G. Biology of natural killer cells. *Adv Immunol* 1989; 47:187–376.
6. Tolede de Abreu M, Belfort R, Matheus PC, et al. T-lymphocyte subsets in the aqueous humor and peripheral blood of patients with acute untreated uveitis. *Am J Ophthalmol* 1984;98:62–65.
7. Nussenblatt RB, Salinas-Carmona M, Leake W, et al. T lymphocyte subsets in uveitis. *Am J Ophthalmol* 1983;95:613.
8. Belfort R, et al. T and B lymphocytes in the aqueous humor of patients with uveitis. *Arch Ophthalmol* 1982;100:465.
9. Jakobiec FA, Leftkowitch J, Knowles DM II. B-and T-lymphocytes in ocular disease. *Ophthalmology* 1984;91:635–654.
10. Kaplan HJ, Waldrep JC, Nicholson JKA, et al. Immunologic analysis of intraocular mononuclear cell infiltrates in uveitis. *Arch Ophthalmol* 1984;102:572–575.
11. Kaplan HJ, et al. Recurrent clinical uveitis: cell surface markers on vitreous lymphocytes. *Arch Ophthalmol* 1982;100:585–587.
12. Deschenes J, Char DH, Kaleta S. Activated T lymphocytes in uveitis. *Br J Ophthalmol* 1988;72:83–87.
13. Davis JL, Solomon D, Nussenblatt RB, et al. Immunocytochemical staining of vitreous cells: indications, techniques, and results. *Ophthalmology* 1992;99:250–256.
14. Sela M. Antigenicity: some molecular aspects. *Science* 1969;166: 1365.
15. Rosenthal AS. Regulation of the immune response-role of the macrophage. *N Engl J Med* 1980;303:1153–1156.
16. Benjamini E, Leskowitz S. *Immunology: a short course.* New York: Alan R. Liss, 1988.
17. Hubbard RA, Marchalonis JJ. Molecular biology of T-cell recognition elements. *J Immunol Immunopharmacol* 1988;8:248–256.
18. Pauling L. A theory of the structure and process of formation of antibodies. *J Am Chem Soc* 1940;62:2643–2657.
19. Marx JL. Antibody research garners Nobel prize. *Science* 1987; 238:484–485.
20. Ada GL, Nossal G. The clonal selection theory. *Sci Am* 1987;257: 62.
21. Nossal G. The basic components of the immune system. *N Engl J Med* 1987;316:1320–1325.
22. Porter RR. Chemical structure of globulin and antibodies. *Br Med Bull* 1963;19:197–201.
23. South MA, et al. The IgA system. *J Exp Med* 1966;123:615–627.
24. Mosier DA, et al. Fungal endophthalmitis following intraocular lens implantation. *Am J Ophthalmol* 1977;83:1–8.
25. Dorrington KJ, Bennich HH. Structure-function relationships in human immunoglobulin E. *Immunol Rev* 1978;41:3–25.
26. Stites DP, Terr AI. *Basic and clinical immunology.* Newark, NJ: Appleton and Lange, 1991.
27. Ross GD. Clinical and laboratory features of patients with an inherited deficiency of neutrophil membrane complement receptor type 3 (CR3) and the related membrane antigens LFA-1 and p150,95. *J Clin Immunol* 1986;6:107–113.
28. Hugli TE, Müller-Eberhard HJ. Anaphylatoxins: C3a and C5a. *Adv Immunol* 1978;26:1.
29. Marsh DG, Meyers DA, Bias WB. The epidemiology and genetics of atopic allergy. *N Engl J Med* 1981;305:1551–1559.
30. Lichtenstein LM. Sequential analysis of the allergic response: cyclic AMP, calcium and histamine. *Int Arch Allergy Immunol* 1975; 49:143–154.
31. Smolin G, O'Connor GR. *Ocular immunology.* Philadelphia: Lea & Febiger, 1981.
32. Taylor B, Norman AP. Transient IgA deficiency and pathogenesis of infantile atopy. *Lancet* 1973;2111–113.
33. Dixon FJ, Jacinto J, Vazquez J, et al. Pathogenesis of serum sickness. *AMA Arch Pathol* 1958;65:18–28.
34. Howes EL, McKay DG. Circulating immune complex effects on ocular vascular permeability in the rabbit. *Arch Ophthalmol* 1975; 93:365.
35. Benacerraf B, Levine BB. Immunological specificity of delayed and immediate hypersensitivity reactions. *J Exp Med* 1962;115: 1023.
36. Guttmann RD. Immunology, ed 3. Kalamazoo: Upjohn 1987.
37. Claman HN, Miller SD, Conlon PJ, et al. Control of experimental contact sensitivity. *Adv Immunol* 1980;30:121–157.
38. Von Rood JJ, van Leeuwen A. The serology of HLA-DR[1,2]. *Clin Immunobiol* 1980;4:113–122.
39. Smolin G. The defense mechanism of the outer eye. *Trans Ophthalmol Soc UK* 1985;104:363–366.

40. Alio JL, et al. Anterior chamber metastasis from neuroblastoma. *J Pediatr Ophthalmol Strabismus* 1982;19:299–301.

41. Michelson PE, et al. Ischemic ocular inflammation: a clinicopathologic case report. *Arch Ophthalmol* 1971;86:274.

42. Knox DL. Ischemic ocular inflammation *Am J Ophthalmol* 1975; 60:995.

43. Naumann GOH, Naumann LR. Intraocular inflammations. In: Naumann GOH, Apple DJ, eds. *Pathology of the eye.* New York: Springer-Verlag, 1986:99–184.

44. Brubaker R, Font RL, Shepherd EM. Granulomatous sclerouveitis. *Arch Ophthalmol* 1971;86:517.

45. Eagle RC Jr, Yanoff M. Cholesterolosis of the anterior chamber Graefes. *Arch Klin Exp Ophthalmol* 1975;193:121–134.

46. Nussenblatt RB, Palestine AG. *Uveitis: fundamentals and clinical practice.* Chicago: Year Book Medical Publishers, 1989.

47. Robbins SL, Cotran RS, Kumar V. *Robbins' pathologic basis of disease,* ed 5. Philadelphia: WB Saunders, 1994.

48. Albert DM, Jakobiec FA. *Principles and practice of ophthalmology: basic sciences.* Philadelphia: WB Saunders, 1994.

49. Spencer WH. *Ophthalmic pathology: an atlas and textbook,* ed 3. Philadelphia: WB Saunders, 1985.

50. Rahi AHS, Morgan G, Levy I, Dinning W. Immunological investigations in post traumatic granulomatous and nongranulomatous uveitis. *Br J Ophthalmol* 1978;62:722–728.

51. Howes EL, Cruse VK. The structural basis of altered vascular permeability following intraocular inflammation. *Arch Ophthalmol* 1978;96:1668–1676.

52. Apple DJ, Rabb MF. *Ocular pathology: clinical applications and self-assessment,* ed 3. St. Louis: Mosby, 1986.

53. Fine BS, Brucker AJ. Macular edema and cystoid macular edema. *Am J Ophthalmol* 1981;92:466–481.

54. Zimmerman LE, Naumann GOH. Pathology of retinoschisis. In: McPherson A, ed. *New and controversial aspects of retinal detachment.* New York: Hoeber, 1968.

55. Green K, Kim K. Pattern of ocular response to topical and systemic prostaglandin. *Invest Ophthalmol* 1975;14:36–40.

56. Maumenee AE. Clinical entities in uveitis: an approach to the study of intraocular inflammation. XXVI Memorial Lecture. *Am J Ophthalmol* 1970;69:1–27.

57. Perkins ES. Recent advances in the study of uveitis. *Br J Ophthalmol* 1974;58:462.

58. Rahi AHS, Holborow EJ, Perkins ES, et al. Immunological investigation in uveitis. *Trans Ophthalmol Soc UK* 1976;96:113–122.

59. Hogan JJ, Kimura SJ. Cyclitis and peripheral choroiditis. *Arch Ophthalmol* 1961;66:667.

60. Norn MS. Iris pigment defects in uveitis. *Acta Ophthalmol (Copenh)* 1971;49:895–901.

61. Lee WR, Grierson I. Macrophage infiltration in the human retina. *Graefes Arch Clin Exp Ophthalmol* 1977;203:293–309.

62. Lamberts DW, Foster CS. Chronic unilateral external ocular inflammation. *Surv Ophthalmol* 1979;24:157–166.

63. Finkelstein EM, Boniuk M. Intraocular ossification and hematopoiesis. *Am J Ophthalmol* 1969;68:683–690.

64. Jakobiec FA, Marboe CC, Knowles DM II, et al. Human sympathetic ophthalmia: an analysis of the inflammatory infiltrate by hybridoma-monoclonal antibodies, immunochemistry, and correlative electron microscopy. *Ophthalmology* 1983;90:76–95.

65. Perry HD, Font RL. Clinical and histopathologic observation in severe Vogt-Koyanagi-Harada syndrome. *Am J Ophthalmol* 1977; 83:242–254.

66. Shorb SR, et al. Optic disk neovascularization associated with chronic uveitis. *Am J Ophthalmol* 1976;82:175–178.

67. Gartner S, Henkind D. Neovascularization of the iris (rubeosis iridis). *Surv Ophthalmol* 1978;22:291–312.

68. Gärtner J. The fine structure of the vitreous base of the human eye and pathogenesis of pars planitis. *Am J Ophthalmol* 1971;71: 1317.

69. Pülhorn G, Teichmann KD, Teichmann I. Intraocular fibrous proliferation as an incisional complication in pars plana vitrectomy. *Am J Ophthalmol* 1977;83:810–814.

70. Kennedy JE, Wise GN. Retinochoroidal vascular anastomosis in uveitis. *Am J Ophthalmol* 1971;71:1221–1225.

71. Yanoff M, et al. Massive gliosis of the retina, a continuous spectrum of glial proliferation. *Int Ophthalmol Clin* 1971;11:211–229.

72. Schlaegel TF Jr, Coles RS. Uveitis and miscellaneous general diseases. In: Duane TD, ed. *Clinical ophthalmology.* Hagerstown, MD: Harper & Row, 1976:6.

73. Allen HF, Mangiaracine AB. Bacterial endophthalmitis after cataract extraction. II. Incidence in 36,000 consecutive operations with special reference to preoperative topical antibiotics. *Trans Am Acad Otolaryngol* 1973;77:581–588.

74. O'Connor GR. Factors related to the initiation and recurrence of uveitis. *Am J Ophthalmol* 1983;96:577–599.

75. Remky H. Etiological diagnosis of endogenous uveitis. *Int Ophthalmol Clin* 1965;5:789.

76. Jones DB, Robinson NM. Anaerobic ocular infections. *Trans Am Acad Ophthalmol Otolaryngol* 1977;83:309–331.

77. Puliafito CA, Baker AS, Haaf J, Foster CS. Infectious endophthalmitis; review of 36 cases. *Ophthalmology* 1982;89:921–929.

78. Locatcher-Khorazo D, Seegal BC. *Microbiology of the eye.* St. Louis: Mosby, 1972.

79. Bohigian GM, Olk RJ. Factors associated with a poor visual results in endophthalmitis. *Am J Ophthalmol* 1986;101:332–341.

80. Diamond JG. Intraocular management of endophthalmitis: a systematic approach. *Arch Ophthalmol* 1981;99:96–99.

81. Rowsey JJ, Newsom DL, Sexton DJ, et al. Endophthalmitis: current approaches. *Ophthalmology* 1982;89:1055–1066.

82. Forster RK. Etiology and diagnosis of bacterial postoperative endophthalmitis. *Ophthalmology* 1978;85:320–326.

83. D'Amico DJ, Libert J, Kenyon KR, et al. Retinal toxicity of intravitreal gentamicin: an electron microscopic study. *Invest Ophthalmol Vis Sci* 1984;25:564–572.

84. Allansmith MR, Skaggs C, Kimura SJ. Anterior chamber paracentesis (diagnostic value in postoperative endophthalmitis). *Arch Ophthalmol* 1970;84:745–748.

85. Mandelbaum S, Forster RK, Gelender H, Culbertson WW. Late-onset endophthalmitis associated with filtering blebs. *Ophthalmology* 1985;92:964–972.

86. Affeldt JC, Flynn HW Jr, Forster RK, et al. Microbial endophthalmitis resulting from ocular trauma. *Ophthalmology* 1987;94:407.

87. Brinton GS, Topping TM, Hyndiuk RA, et al. Posttraumatic endophthalmitis. *Arch Ophthalmol* 1984;102:547–550.

88. Meyer SL, Font RL, Shaver RP. Intraocular nocardiosis: report of three cases. *Arch Ophthalmol* 1970;83:536–541.

89. Greenwald MJ, et al. Metastatic bacterial endophthalmitis: a contemporary reappraisal. *Surv Ophthalmol* 1986;31:81–101.

90. Edwards JE Jr, Foos RY, Montgomery JZ, Guze LB. Ocular manifestations of *Candida* septicemia: review of seventy-six cases of hematogenous *Candida* endophthalmitis. *Medicine* 1974;53:47.

91. Jones BR. Principles in the management of oculomycosis. XXXI Edward Jackson memorial lecture. *Am J Ophthalmol* 1975;79: 719–751.

92. Grossniklaus H, Bruner WE, Frank KE, Purnell EW. *Bacillus cereus* endophthalmitis appearing as acute glaucoma in a drug addict. *Am J Ophthalmol* 1975;100:334–335.

93. Naumann GOH, Green WR, Zimmerman LE. Mycotic keratitis: a histopathologic study of 73 cases. *Am J Ophthalmol* 1967;64:668.

94. Ryan SJ. *Retina.* St. Louis: CV Mosby, 1989;484.

95. Cassady JR, Forester HC. *Sporotrichum schenckii* endophthalmitis. *Arch Ophthal* 1971;85:71–74.

96. Naidoff MA, Green WR. Endogenous *Aspergillus* endophthalmitis occurring after kidney transplant. *Am J Ophthalmol* 1975;79:502.

97. Bodia RD, Kinyoun JL, Qingli L, et al. Aspergillus necrotizing retinitis: a clinico-pathologic study and review. *Retina* 1989;9: 226–231.

98. McDonald HR, et al. Vitrectomy for epiretinal membrane with *Candida* chorioretinitis. *Ophthalmology* 1990;97:466–469.

99. Woods AC. Chronic bacterial infections. I. Ocular tuberculosis. In: *Systemic ophthalmology.* London: Butterworth, 1951.

100. Moore JE. Syphilitic iritis: a study of 249 patients. *Am J Ophthalmol* 1931;14:110.

101. Turner TB. Race and sex distribution of lesions of syphilis in 10,000 cases. *Bull Johns Hopkins Hosp* 1930;46:159–184.

102. Sachsenweger R. Uveitis in infants and children. *Int Ophthalmol Clin* 1965;5:851.

103. Alexander A, Baer A, Fiar F, et al. Leptospiral uveitis. *Arch Ophthalmol* 1978;96:2081.

104. Goodner EK, Okumoto M. Intraocular listeriosis. *Am J Ophthalmol* 1967;64:682–686.

105. Solanes MP, Heatley J, Arenas F, Ibarra GG. Ocular complications in brucellosis. *Am J Ophthalmol* 1953;36:675.

106. Donahue HC. Ophthalmologic experience in a tuberculosis sanitorium. *Am J Ophthalmol* 1967;64:742–748.

107. Dvorak-Theobald G. Acute tuberculous endophthalmitis: report of a case. *Am J Ophthalmol* 1958;45:403–407.

108. Ni C, Albert DM. Uveal tuberculosis. *Int Ophthalmol Clin* 1982;22:103–123.

109. McMoli TE, Mordi VPN, Grange A, et al. Tuberculous panophthalmitis. *J Pediatr Ophthalmol Strabismus* 1978;15:383–385.

110. Blodi FC, Hervouet F. Syphilitic chorioretinitis: a histologic study. *Arch Ophthalmol* 1968;79:294–296.

111. DeLuise VP, Clark SW III, Smith JL, et al. Syphilitic retinal detachment and uveal effusion. *Am J Ophthalmol* 1982;94:757.

112. Deschenes J, Seamone CD, Baines MG. Acquired ocular syphilis: diagnosis and treatment. *Ann Ophthalmol* 1992;24:134–138.

113. Shields JA, Waring GO III, Monte L-G. Ocular findings in leprosy. *Am J Ophthalmol* 1974;77:880–890.

114. Allen JH. The pathology of ocular leprosy. II. Miliary lepromas of the iris. *Am J Ophthalmol* 1966;61:987–992.

115. Binford CH. Pathology—the doorway of the understanding of leprosy: Ward Burdick Award address. *Am J Clin Pathol* 1969;51:681–698.

116. Prendergast JJ. Ocular leprosy in the United States: a study of 350 cases. *Arch Ophthalmol* 1940;23:112–137.

117. Cherugini TD, Spaeth GL. Anterior nongranulomatous uveitis associated with Rocky Mountain spotted fever: first report of a case. *Arch Ophthalmol* 1969;81:363–365.

118. Burgdorfer W, Barbour AG, Hayes SF, et al. Lyme disease: a tickborne spirochetosis? *Science* 1982;216:1317–1319.

119. Steere AC, Grodzicki MS, Kornblatt AN, et al. The spirochetal etiology of Lyme disease. *N Engl J Med* 1983;308:733–740.

120. Steere AC. Lyme disease. *N Engl J Med* 1989;321:586–596.

121. MacDonald AB. Lyme disease: a neuro-ophthalmologic view. *J Clin Neuro-ophthalmol* 1987;7:185–190.

122. Pachner AR, Steere AC. The triad of neurologic manifestations of Lyme disease: meningitis, cranial neuritis, and radiculoneuritis. *Neurology* 1985;35:47–53.

123. Winward KE, Smith JL, Culbertson WW, et al. Ocular Lyme beryllioses. *Am J Ophthalmol* 1989;108:651–657.

124. Clark JR, Carlson RD, Saski CT, et al. Facial paralysis in Lyme disease. *Laryngoscope* 1985;95:1341–1345.

125. Bertuch AW, Rocco E, Schwartz EG. Eye findings in Lyme disease. *Conn Med* 1987;51:151–152.

126. Orlin SE, Lauffer JL. Lyme disease keratitis. *Am J Ophthalmol* 1989;107:678–680.

127. Aaberg TM. The expanding ophthalmologic spectrum of Lyme disease. *Am J Ophthalmol* 1989;107:77–80.

128. Bialasiewiez AA, Ruprecht KW, Naumann GOH, et al. Bilateral diffuse choroiditis and exudative retinal detachments with evidence of Lyme disease. *Am J Ophthalmol* 1988;105:419–420.

129. Avendano J, Tanishima T, Kuwabara T. Ocular cyptococcosis. *Am J Ophthalmol* 1978;86:110–113.

130. Klintworth G, Gollingsworth A, Lusman P, Bradford N. Granulomatous choroiditis in a case of disseminated histoplasmosis. *Arch Ophthalmol* 1973;90:45–48.

131. Meredith TA, et al. Ocular histoplasmosis: clinicopathologic correlation of 3 cases. *Surv Ophthalmol* 1977;22:189–205.

132. Zinneman HH. Sino-orbital aspergillosis: report of a case and review of the literature. *Minn Med* 1972;55:661–668.

133. Font RL, Spaulding AG, Green WR. Endogenous mycotic panophthalmitis caused by *Blastomyces dermatitidis*: report of a case and a review of the literature. *Arch Ophthalmol* 1967;77:217–222.

134. Lewis H, et al. Latent disseminated blastomycosis with choroidal involvement. *Arch Ophthalmol* 1988;106:527–530.

135. Bell R, Font RL. Granulomatous anterior uveitis caused by *Coccidioides immitis*. *Am J Ophthalmol* 1972;74:93.

136. Green WR, Bennet JE. Coccidioidomycosis: Report of a case with clinical evidence of ocular involvement. *Arch Ophthalmol* 1967;77:337.

137. Rodenbiker HT, Ganley JP. Ocular coccidioidomycosis. *Surv Ophthalmol* 1980;24:263–290.

138. Zakka KA, Foos RY, Brown WJ. Intraocular coccidioidomycosis. *Surv Ophthalmol* 1978;22:313–321.

139. Hiles DA, Font RL. Bilateral intraocular cryptococcosis with unilateral spontaneous regression: Report of a case and review of the literature. *Am J Ophthalmol* 1968;65:98.

140. Shields JA, Wright DM, Augsburger JJ, et al. Cryptococcal chorioretinitis. *Am J Ophthalmol* 1980;89:210–218.

141. Font RL, Jakobiec FA. Granulomatous necrotizing retinochoroiditis caused by *Sporotric schenckii*. *Arch Ophthalmol* 1976;94:1513–1519.

142. Levy JH. Intraocular sporotrichosis: report of a case. *Arch Ophthal* 1971;85:574–579.

143. Streeten BW, Rabuzzi DD, Jones DB. Sporotrichosis of the orbital margin. *Am J Ophthalmol* 1974;77:750–755.

144. Hogan JJ, et al. Recovery of *Toxoplasma* from a human eye. *Arch Ophthalmol* 1958;60:548.

145. Desmonts G, Couvreur J. Congenital toxoplasmosis: A prospective study of 378 pregnancies. *N Engl J Med* 1974;280:1110.

146. Dobbie J. *Toxoplasma* retinochoroiditis: Successful isolation of *Toxoplasma gondii* from subretinal fluid of the living human eye. *Ann Ophthalmol* 1970;2:509.

147. Jabs DA. Ocular toxoplasmosis. *Int Ophthalmol Clin* 1990;30:264–270.

148. Schlaegel TF Jr. Toxoplasmosis. In: Duane TD, ed. *Clinical ophthalmology*, Vol. 4. Hagerstown, MD: Harper & Row, 1976 [rev 1981].

149. Rao N, Font RL. Toxoplasmic retinochoroiditis electron microscopic and immunofluorescent studies. *Arch Ophthalmol* 1977;95:273–277.

150. Zimmerman LE. Ocular pathology of toxoplasmosis. *Surv Ophthalmol* 1961;6:832.

151. Goodwin RA Jr, et al. Disseminated histoplasmosis: clinical and pathologic correlations. *Medicine* 1980;59:1–33.

152. Ryan SJ. Histopathological correlates of presumed ocular histoplasmosis. *Int Ophthalmol Clin* 1975;15:125–137.

153. Schlaegel TF Jr. *Ocular histoplasmosis*. New York: Grune & Straton, 1977.

154. Sheffer A, Green WR, Fine SL, et al. Presumed ocular histoplasmosis syndrome. *Arch Ophthalmol* 1980;98:335–340.

155. Witmer R, Iwamoto T. Electron microscopic observation of herpes-like particles in the iris. *Arch Ophthalmol* 1968;79:331.

156. Naumann GOH, et al. Histopathology of herpes zoster ophthalmicus: A report of 21 cases and review of the literature. *Am J Ophthalmol* 1968;65:533.

157. Edgerton AE. Herpes zoster ophthalmicus: report of cases and review of literature. *Arch Ophthalmol* 1945;34:114.

158. Murray HW, et al. Cytomegalovirus retinitis in adults: a manifestation of disseminated viral infection. *Am J Med* 1977;63:574.

159. Smith ME, et al. Ocular involvement in congenital cytomegalic inclusion disease. *Arch Ophthalmol* 1966;76:696.

160. Wyhinny GJ, et al. Adult cytomegalic inclusion retinitis. *Am J Ophthalmol* 1973;76:773.

161. Boniuk I. The cytomegaloviruses and the eye. *Int Ophthalmol Clin* 1972;12(2):169.

162. Wolff SM. The ocular manifestations of congenital rubella: A prospective study of 328 cases. *Trans Am Ophthalmol Soc* 1972;70:577.

163. Yanoff M, et al. Rubella ocular syndrome: Clinical significance of viral and pathologic studies. *Trans Am Acad Ophthalmol Otolaryngol* 1968;72:896.

164. Zimmerman LE. Histopathologic basis for ocular manifestations of congenital rubella syndrome. The Eighth William Hamlin Wilder Memorial Lecture. *Am J Ophthalmol* 1968;65:837.

165. Boniuk M, Zimmerman LE. Ocular pathology in the rubella syndrome. *Arch Ophthalmol* 1967;77:455–473.

166. Boniuk V. Systemic and ocular manifestations of the rubella syndrome. *Int Ophthalmol Clin* 1972;12:67–76.

167. Boniuk V. Rubella. *Int Ophthalmol Clin* 1975;15:229–249.

168. Edwards TF. Ophthalmic complications from varicella. *J Pediatr Ophthalmol* 1965;2:3.

169. Siam AL, Meegan JM, Gharbawi KF. Rift Valley fever ocular manifestations: observations during the 1977 epidemic in Egypt. *Br J Ophthalmol* 1980;64:366–374.

170. Deutman AF, Klomp HJ. Rift Valley fever retinitis. *Am J Ophthalmol* 1981;92:38–42.

171. Fratkin J, Smith A. Slow virus infections. *Surv Ophthalmol* 1977; 21:356–365.

172. Font RL, Jenis EH, Tuck KO. Measles maculopathy associated with subacute sclerosing panencephalitis. *Arch Pathol* 1973;96· 168.

173. Green SH, Wirtschafter JD. Ophthalmoscopic findings in subacute sclerosing panencephalitis. *Br J Ophthalmol* 1973;57:780–787.

174. Nelson DA, et al. Retinal lesions in subacute sclerosing panencephalitis. *Arch Ophthalmol* 1970;84:613.

175. Landers MB III, Klintworth GK. Subacute sclerosing panencephalitis (SSPE): a clinicopathologic study of the retinal lesion. *Arch Ophthalmol* 1971;86:156.

176. Kimura SJ. Herpes simplex uveitis: A clinical and experimental study. *Trans Am Ophthalmol Soc* 1962;60:440–470.

177. Meyers RL, Chitjian PA. Immunology of herpes virus infections: immunity to herpes simplex virus in eye infections. *Surv Ophthalmol* 1976;21:194–204.

178. Tarkkanen A, Laatikainen L. Late ocular manifestations in neonatal herpes simplex infection. *Br J Ophthalmol* 1977;61:608–616.

179. Kaufman HE, Kanai A, Ellison ED. Herpetic iritis: demonstration of virus in the anterior chamber by fluorescent antibody techniques and electron microscopy. *Am J Ophthalmol* 1971;71:465–469.

180. Grutzmacher RD, et al. Herpes simplex chorioretinitis in a healthy adult. *Am J Ophthalmol* 1983;96:788–796.

181. Johnson BJ, Wisotzkey HM. Neuroretinitis associated with herpes simplex encephalitis in an adult. *Am J Ophthalmol* 1977;83:481.

182. Cogan DG, et al. Herpes simplex retinopathy in an infant. *Arch Ophthalmol* 1964;72:641.

183. Estrada WB. Uveitis in tropical diseases. *Int Ophthalmol Clin* 1965;5:863.

184. Botero D, et al. Intraocular filaria, a *Loaiana* species, from man in Columbia. *Am J Trop Med Hyg* 1984;33:578–582.

185. Tudor RC, Blair E. Gnathostoma spinigerum: an unusual cause of ocular nematodiasis in the Western Hemisphere. *Am J Ophthalmol* 1971;72:185–190.

186. Manschot WA. Intraocular cysticercus. *Arch Ophthalmol* 1968; 80:772–774.

187. Font RL, Neafie RC, Perry HD. Subcutaneous dirofilariasis of the eyelid and ocular adnexa. *Arch Ophthalmol* 1980;98:1079–1082.

188. Singalavanija A, Wangspa S, Teschareon S. Intravitreal angiostrongyliasis. *Aust N Z J Ophthalmol* 1986;14:381–384.

189. Newton JC, Kanchanaranya C, Previte LR. Intraocular *Schistosoma mannsoni*. *Am J Ophthalmol* 1968;65:774–778.

190. Gass JDM, Lewis RA. Subretinal tracks in ophthalmomyiasis. *Trans Am Acad Ophthalmol Otolaryngol* 1976;81:483–490.

191. Steahly LP, Peterson CA. Ophthalmomyiasis. *Ann Ophthalmol* 1982;14:137.

192. Ashton N. Larval granulomatosis of the retinas due to *Toxocara*. *Br J Ophthalmol* 1960;44:129.

193. Ashton N, Cook C. Allergic granulomatous nodules of the eyelid and conjunctiva. The XXXV Edward Jackson Memorial Lecture. *Am J Ophthalmol* 1978;87:1.

194. Duguid JM. Features of ocular infestation by *Toxocara*. *Br J Ophthalmol* 1961;45:789.

195. Maguire AM, et al. Recovery of intraocular *Toxocara canis* by pars plana vitrectomy. *Ophthalmology* 1990;97:675.

196. Poltera AA. The histopathology of ocular loiasis in Uganda. *Trans Roy Soc Trop Med Hyg* 1973;67:819.

197. Wood TR, Slight JR. Bilateral orbital myiasis. *Arch Ophthalmol* 1970;84:692–693.

198. Jakobiec FA, et al. Granulomatous dacryoadenitis caused by *Schistosoma haematobium*. *Arch Ophthalmol* 1977;95:278.

199. Bathrick ME, Mango CA, Mueller JF. Intraocular gnathostomiasis. *Ophthalmology* 1981;88:1293–1295.

200. Goodart RA, Riekhof FT, Beaver PC. Subretinal nematode: an unusual etiology for uveitis and retinal detachment. *Retina* 1985; 5:87.

201. Garner A, Duke BOL, Anderson J. A comparison of the lesions produced in the cornea of the rabbit eye by microfilaria of the forest and Sudan savanna strains of *Onchocerca volvulus* from Cameroon. II. The pathology. *Tropenmed Parasitol* 1973;24:385.

202. Connor DH. Onchocerciasis. *N Engl J Med* 1978;298:379–381.

203. Bird AC, et al. Morphology of posterior segment lesions of the eye in patients with onchocerciasis. *Br J Ophthalmol* 1976;60:2.

204. Anderson J, Font RL. Ocular onchocerciasis. *In* Binford CH, Connor DH, eds. *Pathology of tropical and extraordinary diseases*. Washington, D.C.: Armed Forces Institute of Pathology, 1976; 373.

205. Rodger FC. The pathogenesis and pathology of ocular onchocerciasis. *Am J Ophthalmol* 1960;49:104–35,327–37,560.

206. Kimura SJ, Hogna MJ. Uveitis in children: Analysis of 274 cases. *Trans Am Ophthalmol Soc* 1964;62:174.

207. Guyton J, Woods A. Etiology of uveitis: A clinical study of five-hundred and sixty-two cases. *Arch Ophthalmol* 1941;26:982.

208. Maumenee A, Silverstein AM. *Immunopathology of uveitis*. Baltimore: Williams & Wilkins, 1964.

209. Kimura SJ, et al. Fuchs' syndrome of heterochromic cyclitis. *Arch Ophthalmol* 1955;54:179.

210. Loewenfeld IE, Thompson HS. Fuchs' heterochromic cyclitis: A critical review of the literature. I. Clinical characteristics of the syndrome. *Surv Ophthalmol* 1973;17:394–457; II. Etiology and mechanisms. *Surv Ophthal* 1973;18:2.

211. Posner A, Schlossman A. Syndrome of unilateral recurrent attacks of glaucoma with cyclitis symptoms. *Arch Ophthalmol* 1953;39: 517.

212. Kass MA, Becker B, Kolder AE. Glaucomacyclitic crisis and primary open-angle glaucoma. *Am J Ophthalmol* 1973;75:668–673.

213. Brewerton DA, Caffrey M, Hart FD, et al. Ankylosing spondylitis and HLA-27. *Lancet* 1973;1:904–907.

214. Lee DA, Barker SM, Su WPD, et al. The clinical diagnosis of Reiter's syndrome. *Ophthalmology* 1986;93:350–356.

215. Ostler HB, et al. Reiter's syndrome. *Am J Ophthalmol* 1971;71: 986.

216. Sabates R, Smith T, Apple DJ. Ocular histopathology in juvenile rheumatoid arthritis. *Ann Ophthalmol* 1979;11:733–737.

217. Kimura SJ, et al. Uveitis and joint disease: A review of 191 cases. *Trans Am Ophthalmol Soc* 1966;64:291.

218. Smiley WK. The eye in juvenile rheumatoid arthritis. *Trans Ophthalmol Soc UK* 1974;94:817.

219. Cassidy JT, et al. A study of classification criteria for a diagnosis of juvenile rheumatoid arthritis. *Arthritis Rheum* 1986;29:274.

220. Chylack LT, et al. Ocular manifestations of juvenile rheumatoid arthritis. *Am J Ophthalmol* 1975;79:1026.

221. Hopkins DJ, Horan E, Burton IL, et al. Ocular disorders in 332 patients with Crohn's disease. *Br J Ophthalmol* 1974;58:732–737.

222. Knox DL, Snip RC, Stark WJ. The keratopathy of Crohn's disease. *Am J Ophthalmol* 1980;90:862–865.

223. Greenstein AJ, et al. The extra-intestinal complications of Crohn's disease and ulcerative colitis: A study of 700 patients. *Medicine* 1976;55:401.

224. Flynn T, Martin J, Green WR. Histopathologic studies of eyes in 13 cases of multiple sclerosis. In: *Ophthalmic pathology: an atlas and textbook*, ed 3. Philadelphia: WB Saunders, 1985.

225. Giles CL. Peripheral uveitis in patients with multiple sclerosis. *Am J Ophthalmol* 1970;70:17.

226. Breger BC, Leopold IH. The incidence of uveitis in multiple sclerosis. *Am J Ophthalmol* 1966;62:540.

227. Font RL, et al. Ocular involvement in Whipple's disease: light and electron microscopic observations. *Arch Ophthalmol* 1978;96: 1431.

228. Gartner J. Whipple's disease of the central nervous system, associated with ophthalmoplegia externa and severe asteroid hyalitis: a clinicopathologic study. *Doc Ophthalmol* 1980;49:155.

229. Selsky EJ, Knox DL, Maumenee AE, et al. Ocular involvement in Whipple's disease. *Retina* 1984;4:103–106.

230. Merriam JC, et al. Early onset pauciarticular juvenile rheumatoid arthritis: a histopathologic study. *Arch Ophthalmol* 1983;101: 1085.

231. Goldberg MF, Erozan YS, Duke JR, et al. Cytopathologic and histopathologic aspects of Fuchs' heterochromic iridocyclitis. *Arch Ophthalmol* 1965;74:604–609.

232. McCartney AC, et al. Fuchs' heterochromic cyclitis: an electron microscopy study. *Trans Ophthalmol Soc UK* 1986;105:324–329.

233. Murray PI, Hoekzema R, Luyendijk L, et al. Analysis of aqueous humor immunoglobulin G in uveitis by enzyme-inked immunosor-

bent assay, isoelectric focusing, and immunoblotting. *Invest Ophthalmol Vis Sci* 1990;31:2129.

234. Aaberg TM. The enigma of pars plantis. *Am J Ophthalmol* 1987; 103:828.

235. Brockhurst RJ, et al. Uveitis. II. Peripheral uveitis: clinical description, complications and differential diagnosis. *Am J Ophthalmol* 1960;49:1257.

236. Brockhurst RJ, et al. Uveitis. III. Peripheral uveitis: pathogenesis, etiology and treatment. *Am J Ophthalmol* 1961;51:19.

237. Brockhurst RJ, Schepens CL. Uveitis. IV. Peripheral uveitis: the complications of retinal detachment. *Arch Ophthalmol* 1968;80: 747.

238. Pederson JE, et al. Pathology pars planitis. *Am J Ophthalmol* 1978; 86:762.

239. Smith RE, et al. Chronic cyclitis. I. Course and visual prognosis. *Trans Am Acad Ophthalmol Otolaryngol* 1973;77:760.

240. Green WR, Kincaid MC. Michels RG, et al. Pars planitis. *Trans Ophthalmol Soc UK* 1981;101:361–367.

241. Gartner J. The vitreous base of the human eye and "pars planitis": Electron microscopic observations. *Mod Prob Ophthalmol* 1972; 10:250.

242. Wetzig RP, et al. Clinical and immunopathological studies of pars planitis in a family. *Br J Ophthalmol* 1988;72:5.

243. Jampol LM, et al. Multiple evanescent white dot syndrome. I. Clinical findings. *Arch Ophthalmol* 1984;102:671.

244. Aaberg TM, Campo RV, Joffe L. Recurrences and bilaterality in the multiple evanescent white-dot syndrome. *Am J Ophthalmol* 1985;100:29–37.

245. Nozik RA, Dorsch W. A new chorioretinopathy associated with anterior uveitis. *Am J Ophthalmology* 1973;76:758–762.

246. Krill AE, Deutman AF. Acute retinal pigment epithelitis. *Am J Ophthalmol* 1972;74:193.

247. Deutman AF. Acute retinal pigment epithelitis. *Am J Ophthalmol* 1974;78:571–578.

248. Gass JDM. Acute posterior multifocal placoid pigment epitheliopathy. *Arch Ophthalmol* 1968;80:177–185.

249. Gass JDM. Acute posterior multifocal placoid pigment epitheliopathy: a long-term follow-up study. In: Fine SL, Owen SL, eds. *Management of retinal vascular and macular disorders*. Baltimore: Williams & Wilkins, 1983:176.

250. Deutman AF, et al. Acute posterior multifocal placoid pigment epitheliopathy: Pigment epitheliopathy or choriocapillaritis. *Br J Ophthalmol* 1972;56:863.

251. Ryan SJ, Maumenee AE. Acute posterior multifocal placoid pigment epitheliopathy. *Am J Ophthalmol* 1972;74:1066.

252. Palestine AG, et al. Progressive subretinal fibrosis and uveitis. *Br J Ophthalmol* 1984;68:667.

253. Palestine AG, et al. Histopathology of the subretinal fibrosis and uveitis syndrome. *Ophthalmology* 1985;92:838–844.

254. Bos JPM, Deutman AF. Acute macular neuroretinopathy. *Am J Ophthalmol* 1975;80:573.

255. Priluck IA, Buettner H, Robertson DM. Acute macular neuroretinopathy. *Am J Ophthalmol* 1978;86:775–778.

256. Gass JDM, et al. Diffuse unilateral subacute neuroretinitis. *Trans Am Acad Ophthalmol Otolaryngol* 1978;85:521–545.

257. Gass JDM. Vitiliginous chorioretinitis. *Arch Ophthalmol* 1981;99: 1778–1787.

258. Gass JDM, Braunstein RA. Further observations concerning the diffuse unilateral subacute neuroretinitis syndrome. *Arch Ophthalmol* 1983;101:1689.

259. Ryan SJ, Maumenee AE. Birdshot retinochoroidopathy. *Am J Ophthalmol* 1980;89:31.

260. Gass JDM. Vitiliginous chorioretinitis. *Arch Ophthalmol* 1981;99: 1778.

261. Kaplan HJ, Aaberg TM. Birdshot retinochoroidopathy. *Am J Ophthalmol* 1980;90:773.

262. Nussenblatt RB, et al. Birdshot retinochoroidopathy associated with HLA-A29 antigen and immune responsiveness to retinal S-antigen. *Am J Ophthalmol* 1982;94:147.

263. Hamilton AM, Bird AC. Geographical choroidopathy. *Br J Ophthalmol* 1974;58:784–97.

264. Laatikainen L, Erkkila H. A follow-up study on serpiginous choroiditis. *Acta Ophthalmol (Copenh)* 1981;59:707–718.

265. Chisholm IH, et al. The late stage of serpiginous (geographic) choroiditis. *Am J Ophthalmol* 1976;82:343–51.

266. Dreyer WB Jr, et al. Sympathetic ophthalmia. *Am J Ophthalmol* 1981;92:816.

267. Puliafito CA, Smith TR, Packer AJ, Albert DM. Sympathetic uveitis. *Ophthalmology* 1980;87:355–358.

268. Duke-Elder WS, Perkins ES. Diseases of the uveal tract. In: Duke-Elder WS, ed. *System of ophthalmology*. Vol. IX. St. Louis: CV Mosby, 1965;295–92,558–93,817–8,852–54.

269. Lubin JR, Albert DM, Weinstein M. Sixty-five years of sympathetic ophthalmia: a clinicopathologic review of 105 cases (1913-1978). *Ophthalmology* 1980;87:109–121.

270. Rao NA, Robin J, Hartmann D, et al. The role of the penetrating wound in the development of sympathetic ophthalmia: experimental observations. *Arch Ophthalmol* 1983;101:102.

271. Lewis ML, et al. Sympathetic uveitis after trauma and vitrectomy. *Arch Ophthalmol* 1978;96:263–7.

272. Muller-Hermelink HK, Kraus-Mackiv E, Daus W. Early stage of human sympathetic ophthalmia: histologic and immunopathologic findings. *Arch Ophthalmol* 1984;102:1353–1357.

273. Gass JDM. Sympathetic ophthalmia following vitrectomy. *Am J Ophthalmol* 1982;93:552–558.

274. Green WR, Maumenee AE, Sanders TE, Smith ME. Sympathetic uveitis following evisceration. *Trans Am Acad Ophthalmol Otolaryngol* 1972;76:625–644.

275. Blodi FC. Sympathetic uveitis as an allergic phenomenon with a study of its association with phacoanaphylactic uveitis and a report of the pathologic findings in sympathizing eyes. *Trans Am Acad Ophthalmol Otolaryngol* 1959;63:642–9.

276. Easom HA, Zimmerman LE. Sympathetic ophthalmia and bilateral phacoanaphylaxis: a clinicopathologic correlation of sympathogenic and sympathizing eyes. *Arch Ophthalmol* 1964;72:9.

277. Pusin SM, et al. Simultaneous bacterial endophthalmitis and sympathetic uveitis after retinal detachment surgery. *Am J Ophthalmol* 1976;81:57–61.

278. Marak GE. Recent advances in sympathetic ophthalmia. *Surv Ophthalmol* 1979;24:141–156.

279. Winter FC. Sympathetic uveitis: a clinical and pathologic study of the visual result. *Am J Ophthalmol* 1955;39:340–347.

280. Font RL, et al. Light and electron microscopic study of Dalen-Fuchs nodules in sympathetic ophthalmia. *Ophthalmology* 1982; 89:66.

281. Marak GE, et al. Histologic variation related to race in sympathetic ophthalmia. *Am J Ophthalmol* 1974;78:935–938.

282. Makley TA, Azra A. Sympathetic ophthalmia. *Arch Ophthalmol* 1978;96:257–262.

283. Ikui H, et al. Histologic investigations of idiopathic uveitis (Vogt-Koyanagi syndrome): Report of two cases. *Acta Soc Ophthalmol Japan* 1952;56:1079.

284. Matsuda H, Sugiura S. Ultrastructural changes of the melanocyte in Vogt-Koyanagi-Harada syndrome and sympathetic ophthalmia. *Jpn J Ophthalmol* 1969;15:69.

285. Snyder DA, Tessler HH. Vogt-Koyangi-Harada syndrome. *Am J Ophthalmol* 1980;90:69.

286. Lubin JR, Ni C, Albert DM. A clinicopathologic study of the Vogt-Koyanagi-Harada syndrome. *Int Ophthalmol Clin* 1982;22: 147.

287. Fine BS, Gilligan JH. The Vogt-Koyanagi syndrome: a variant of sympathetic ophthalmia: report of two cases. *Am J Ophthalmol* 1957;43:433.

288. Ohno S, Char DH, Kimura SJ, et al. Vogt-Koyanagi-Harada syndrome. *Am J Ophthalmol* 1977;83:735–740.

289. Marcus DF, Bovino JA, Burton TC. Sarcoid granuloma of the choroid. *Ophthalmology* 1982;89:1326–1330.

290. Zimmerman LE, Maumenee AE. Ocular aspects of sarcoidosis. *Am Rev Resp Dis* 1961;84(Suppl 5):38.

291. James DG. Ocular sarcoidosis. *Am J Med* 1959;26:331.

292. James DG, Neville E, Langley DA. Ocular sarcoidosis. *Trans Ophthalmol Soc UK* 1976;96:133–139.

293. James DG, et al. Ocular sarcoidosis. *Trans Ophthalmol Soc UK* 1976;96:133.

294. Obenauf CD, et al. Sarcoidosis and its ophthalmic manifestations. *Am J Ophthalmol* 1978;86:648.

295. Mayock RL, Bertrand P, Morrison CE, et al. Manifestations of

sarcoidosis. Analysis of 145 patients, with a review of nine series selected from the literature. *Am J Med* 1963;35:67–89.

296. Olk RJ, et al. Solitary choroidal mass as the presenting sign in systemic sarcoidosis. *Br J Ophthalmol* 1983;67:826,

297. Beardsley T, et al. Eleven cases of sarcoidosis of the optic nerve. *Am J Ophthalmol* 1984;97:62–77.

298. Blain JG, Riley W, Logothetis J. Optic nerve manifestation of sarcoidosis. *Arch Neurol* 1965;13:307–309.

299. Jampol LM, Woodfin W, McLean EB. Optic nerve sarcoidosis. *Arch Ophthalmol* 1972;87:355–360.

300. Kelley JS, Green WR. Sarcoidosis involving the optic nerve head. *Arch Ophthalmol* 1973;89:486–488.

301. Gould H, Kaufman HE. Sarcoid of the fundus. *Arch Ophthalmol* 1961;65:161.

302. Spalton DJ, Sanders MD. Fundus changes in histologically confirmed sarcoidosis. *Br J Ophthalmol* 1981;65:348–358.

303. Zimmerman LE, Maumenee AE. Ocular aspects of sarcoidosis. *Am Rev Resp Dis* 1961;84(Suppl):38.

304. Gass JDM, Olson CL. Sarcoidosis with optic nerve and retinal involvement: a clinicopathologic case report. *Trans Am Acad Ophthalmol Otolaryngol* 1973;77:739–750.

305. Ingestad R, Stigmar G. Sarcoidosis with ocular and hypothalamic-pituitary manifestations. *Acta Ophthalmol* 1971;49:1.

306. Nichols CW, Eagle RC Jr, Yanoff M, Menocal NG. Conjunctival biopsy as an aid in the evaluation of the patient with suspected sarcoidosis. *Ophthalmology* 1980;87:287–291.

307. Muftuoglu U, Yurdakul S, Yazici H, et al. Vascular involvement in Behçet's disease: a review of 129 cases. In: Lehner T, Barnes CG, eds. *Recent advances in Behcet's disease*. London: Royal Society of Medicine Services, 1986:255–260.

308. Mamo JG, Baghdassarian A. Behcet's disease: a report of 28 cases. *Arch Ophthalmol* 1964;71:4.

309. James DG. Behcet's syndrome. *N Engl J Med* 1979;301:431.

310. Ritzmann SW. HLA patterns and disease associations. *JAMA* 1976;236:2305.

311. Michelson JB, Chisari FV. Behcet's disease. *Surv Ophthalmol* 1982;26:190–203.

312. Ohno S, et al. Studies on HLA antigens in American patients with Behçet's disease. *Jpn J Ophthalmol* 1978;22:58.

313. Lehner T, Barnes CG. Criteria for diagnosis and classification of Behcet's syndrome. In: Lehner T, Barnes CG, eds. *Behcet's syndrome: clinical and immunological features. Proceedings of a conference sponsored by the Royal Society of Medicine.* London: Academic Press, 1979:1–9.

314. Evans AD, Pallis C, Spillane J. Involvement of the nervous system in Behcet's syndrome: Report of three cases and isolation of virus. *Lancet* 1957;2:349.

315. Sanders MD. Ophthalmic features of Behcet's disease. In: Lehner T, Barnes CG, eds. *Behcet's syndrome: clinical and immunological features. Proceedings of a conference sponsored by the Royal Society of Medicine.* London: Academic Press, 1979:183–189.

316. Colvard DM, Robertson DM, O'Duffy JD. The ocular manifestation of Behcet's disease. *Arch Ophthalmol* 1977;95:1813–1817.

317. Bietti GB, Bruna R. An ophthalmic report on Behçet's disease. In: *International symposium on Behcet's disease.* Rome: Basel S. Krager, 1966:77.

318. Winter FC, Yukins RE. The ocular pathology of Behcet's disease. *Am J Ophthalmol* 1966;62:257.

319. Fenton RH, Easton HA. Behcet's syndrome: a histopathologic study of the eye. *Arch Ophthalmol* 1984;72:71.

320. Green WR, Koo BS. Behcet's disease: A report of the ocular histopathology of case. *Surv Ophthalmol* 1967;12:324.

321. Dawson CR, et al. Experimental inclusion conjunctivitis in man. III. Keratitis and other complications. *Arch Ophthalmol* 1967;78:341.

322. Dawson CR. Lids conjunctiva and lacrimal apparatus: Eye infection with chlamydia. *Arch Ophthalmol* 1975;93:854.

323. Kanai A, Kaufman HE. The retrocorneal ridge in syphilis and herpetic interstitial keratitis: an electron microscopic study. *Ann Ophthalmol* 1982;14:120–124.

324. Waring GO, et al. Clinical and pathological alterations of Descemet's membrane with emphasis on endothelial metaplasia. *Surv Ophthalmol* 1974;18:325.

325. Waring GO, et al. Alterations of Descemet's membrane in interstitial keratitis. *Am J Ophthalmol* 1976;81:773.

326. Harris DJ, et al. Late bacterial and fungal keratitis after corneal transplantation. *Ophthalmology* 1988;95.1450.

327. Turner L, Stinson I. *Mycobacterium fortuitum* as a cause of corneal ulcer. *Am J Ophthalmol* 1965;60:329.

328. Nagington J, et al. Amoebic infection of the eye. *Lancet* 1974;2:1537.

329. Ashton N, Wirasinha PA. Encephalitozonosis (nosematosis) of the cornea. *Brit J Ophthal* 1973;57:669.

330. Key SN III, et al. Keratitis due to *Acanthamoeba castellani:* a clinicopathologic case report. *Arch Ophthalmol* 1980;98:475.

331. Brincker P, et al. Acanthamoeba keratitis, clinico-pathological report of 2 cases. *Acta Ophthalmol* 1988;66:210.

332. Florakis GJ, et al. Elevated corneal epithelial lines in Acanthamoeba keratitis. *Arch Ophthalmol* 1988;106:1202.

333. Lindquist TD, et al. Clinical signs and medical therapy of early Acanthamoeba keratitis. *Arch Ophthalmol* 1988;106:73.

334. Stehr-Green JK, Bailey TM, Visvesvara GS. The epidemiology of *Acanthamoeba* keratitis in the United States. *Am J Ophthalmol* 1989;107:331.

335. Edwards WC, Reed RE. Mooren's ulcer: a pathologic case report. *Arch Ophthalmol* 1968;80:361–364.

336. Kurz GH. Phacoanaphylactic endophthalmitis. *Arch Ophthalmol* 1963;69:473.

337. Verhoeff FH, Lemoine AN. Endophthalmitis phacoanaphylactica. *Am J Ophthalmol* 1922;5:737.

338. Perlman EM, Albert DM. Clinically unsuspected phacoanaphylaxis after ocular trauma. *Arch Ophthalmol* 1977;95:244–246.

339. Rahi AHS, et al. Immunopathology of the lens. I. Humoral and cellular immune responses to heterologous lens antigens and their roles in ocular inflammation. *Br J Ophthalmol* 1977;61:164.

340. Rahi AHS, et al. Immunopathology of the lens. III. Humoral and cellular immune responses to autologous lens antigens and their roles in ovular inflammation. *Br J Ophthalmol* 1977;61:371.

341. Yanoff M, Scheie HG. Cytology of human lens aspirate: its relationship to phacolytic glaucoma and phacoanaphylactic endophthalmitis. *Arch Ophthalmol* 1968;80:166.

342. Irvine SR, Irvine AR Jr. Lens-induced uveitis and glaucoma. Part II. The "phacotoxic" reaction. *Am J Ophthalmol* 1952;35:370.

343. Engel HM, et al. Diagnostic vitrectomy. *Retina* 1981;1:121.

344. Fenton RH, Zimmerman LE. Hemolytic glaucoma: an unusual cause of acute open-angle secondary glaucoma. *Arch Ophthalmol* 1963;70:236.

345. Kenyon KR, et al. Fibroglial proliferation in pars planitis *Trans Ophthalmol Soc* 1975;95:391.

346. Brinton GS, et al. Idiopathic vitritis. *Retina* 1983;3:95.

347. Wise G. Clinical features of idiopathic preretinal macular fibrosis. *Am J Ophthalmol* 1975;79:349.

348. Yakura H, Wakisaka A, Aizawa M, et al. HLA-D antigen of Japanese origin (LD-Wa) and its association with Vogt-Koyanagi-Harada syndrome. *Tissue Antigens* 1976;8:35–42.

349. Tagawa Y, et al. HLA and Vogt-Koyanagi-Harada syndrome. *Jpn J Ophthalmol* 1977;21:22.

350. Calin A, Fries JF. An extraordinarily high prevalence of "ankylosing spondylitis" (AS) in B27-positive males and females. A controlled study. *Arthritis Rheum* 1975;18:390.

351. Corwin JM, Weiter JJ. Immunology of chorioretinal disorders. *Surv Ophthalmol* 1981;25:287–305.

352. Beck AD, et al. Clinical challenges: optic nerve enlargement and chronic visual loss. *Surv Ophthalmol* 1994;38:55.

353. Percy AK, et al. Optic neuritis and multiple sclerosis: An epidemiologic study. *Arch Ophthalmol* 1972;87:135.

354. Watson PG, Hayreh SS. Scleritis and episcleritis. *Br J Ophthalmol* 1976;60:163.

355. McGavin DDM, Williamson J, Forester JV, et al. Episcleritis and scleritis: a study of their clinical manifestations and association with rheumatoid arthritis. *Br J Ophthalmol* 1976;60:192–226.

356. Edstrom G, Osterlind G. A case of nodular rheumatic episcleritis. *Acta Ophthalmol* 1948;26:1.

357. Ferry AP. The histopathology of rheumatoid episcleral nodules: An extra-articular manifestation of rheumatoid arthritis. *Arch Ophthalmol* 1969;82:77.

358. Friedman AH, Henkind P. Unusual causes of episcleritis. *Trans Am Acad Ophthalmol Otolaryngol* 1974;78:890–895.

359. Cleary PE, et al. Visual loss due to posterior segment disease in scleritis. *Trans Ophthalmol Soc UK* 1974;95:297.

360. Benson WE, et al. Posterior scleritis, a cause of diagnostic confusion. *Arch Ophthalmol* 1979;97:1482.

361. Rao N, Marak GE, Hidayat AA. Necrotizing scleritis: a clinicopathologic study of 41 cases. *Ophthalmology* 1985;92:1542–1549.

362. Jakobiec FA, Jones IS. Orbital inflammations. In: Jones IS, Jakobiec FA, eds. *Diseases of the orbit.* Hagerstown: Harper and Row, 1979;187–262.

363. Jakobiec FA. Orbital inflammations and lymphoid tumors. *Proc N Orleans Acad Med* 1982;30:52.

364. Sisler H, Jakobiec FA, Trokel S. Ocular abnormalities and orbital changes of Graves' disease. In: Duane T, ed. *Clinical ophthalmology.* Philadelphia: JB Lippincott/Harper Medical, 1982:1–30.

365. Trokel SL, Jakobiec FA. Correlation of CT scanning and pathologic features of ophthalmic Graves' disease. *Ophthalmology* 1981;88:553–564.

366. Werner SC. Modification of the classification of the eye changes of Graves' disease. *Am J Ophthalmol* 1977;83:725.

367. Hufnagel TJ, Hickey WF, Cobbs WH, et al. Immunohistochemical and ultrastructural studies on the exenterated orbital tissues of a patient with Graves' disease. *Ophthalmology* 1984;91:1411–1419.

368. Garner A, Klintworth GK. Tumors of the orbit, optic nerve and lacrimal sac. In: Garner A, Klintworth GK, eds. *Pathobiology of ocular disease. A Dynamic Approach. Part A.* New York: Marcel Dekker, 1982;741–821.

369. Campbell RJ. Pathology of Graves' disease. In: Gorman C, Waller R, Dyer J, eds. *The Eye and Orbit in Thyroid Disease.* New York: Raven Press, 1984;25–32.

370. Kroll AJ, Kuwabara T. Dysthyroid ocular myopathy: Anatomy, histology, and electron microscopy. *Arch Ophthalmol* 1966;76:244.

371. Rootman J, Nugent R. The classification and management of acute orbital pseudotumors. *Ophthalmology* 1982;89:1040–1048.

372. Mottow-Lippa L, Jakobiec FA. Idiopathic inflammatory orbital pseudotumor in childhood. I. Clinical characteristics. *Arch Ophthalmol* 1978;96:1410.

373. Mottwo-Lippa L, et al. Idiopathic inflammatory orbital pseudotumor in childhood. II. Results of diagnostic tests and biopsies. *Ophthalmology* 1981;88:565.

374. Blodi FC, Gass JM. Inflammatory pseudotumor of the orbit. *Trans Am Acad Ophthalmol Otolaryngol* 1967;71:303.

375. Kennerdell JS, Dresner SC. The nonspecific orbital inflammatory syndromes. *Surv Ophthalmol* 1984;29:93–103.

376. Kennedy RE. An evaluation of 820 orbital cases. *Trans Am Ophthalmol Soc* 1984;82:134–157.

377. Shields JE. *Diagnosis and management of orbital tumors.* Philadelphia: Saunders, 1989.

378. Aron-Rosa D, et al. Tolosa-Hunt syndrome. *Ann Ophthalmol* 1978;10:1161.

379. Kline LB. The Tolosa-Hunt syndrome. *Surv Ophthalmol* 1982;27:79.

380. Grimson BS, Simona KB. Orbital inflammation, myositis and systemic lupus erythematosus. *Arch Ophthalmol* 1983;101:736.

381. Weinstein GS, Dresner SC, Slamovits TL, Kennerdell JS. Acute and subacute orbital myositis. *Am J Ophthalmol* 1983;96:209.

382. Watters EC, et al. Acute orbital cellulitis. *Arch Ophthalmol* 1976;94:785.

383. Jarrett WH, Gutman FA. Ocular complications of infection in the paranasal sinuses. *Arch Ophthalmol* 1969;683.

384. Chandler JR, et al. The pathogenesis of orbital complications in acute sinusitis. *Laryngoscope* 1970;70:1414.

385. Hornblass A, et al. Orbital abscess. *Surv Ophthalmol* 1984;29:169.

386. Austin P, Dekker A, Kennerdell JS. Orbital aspergillosis: Report of a case diagnosed by fine needle aspiration biopsy. *Acta Cytol* 1983;27:166.

387. Morris FH Jr, Spock A. Intracranial aneurysm secondary to mycotic orbital and sinus infection: Report of a case implicating *Penicillium* as an opportunistic fungus. *Am J Dis Child* 1970;119:356.

388. Margo CE, et al. Subacute zygomycosis of the orbit. *Arch Ophthalmol* 1983;101:1580–1585.

389. Straatsma BR, et al. Phycomycosis: A clinicopathologic study of 51 cases. *Lab Invest* 1962;11:963.

390. Stefani FH, Mehraein P. Acute rhino-orbitocerebral mucormycosis. *Ophthalmologica* 1976;172:38.

391. Blodi FC, et al. Lethal orbitocerebral phycomycosis in otherwise healthy children. *Am J Ophthalmol* 1969;67:698.

392. Ferry AP. Cerebral mucormycosis (phycomycosis): Ocular findings and review of literature. *Surv Ophthalmol* 1961;6:1.

393. Ferry AP, Abedi S. Diagnosis and management of rhino-orbito-cerebral mucormycosis (phycomycosis). A report of 16 personally observed cases. *Ophthalmology* 1983;90:1096.

394. Bullen CL, et al. Ocular complications of Wegener's granulomatosis. *Ophthalmology* 1983;90:279–290.

395. Haynes BF, et al. The ocular manifestation of Wegener's granulomatosis: 15 years experience and review of literature. *Am J Med* 1977;63:131.

396. DeRemee RA, et al. Wegener's granulomatosis: Anatomic correlates, a proposed classification. *Mayo Clin Proc* 1976;51:777.

397. Fauci AS, Wolff SM. Wegener's granulomatosis. Studies in eighteen patients and a review of the literature. *Medicine* 1973;52:535.

398. Koyama T, et al. Wegener's granulomatosis with destructive ocular manifestations. *Am J Ophthalmol* 1984;98:736.

399. Chess J, et al. Serological and immunopathologic findings in temporal arteritis. *Am J Ophthalmol* 1983;96:283–289.

400. Holland GN, et al. Ocular disorders associated with a new severe acquired cellular immunodeficiency syndrome. *Am J Ophthalmol* 1982;93:393.

401. Holland GN, et al. Acquired immune deficiency syndrome. Ocular manifestations. *Ophthalmology* 1983;90:859.

402. Ai E, Wong KL. Ophthalmic manifestations of AIDS. *Ophthalmol Clinics N Am* 1988;1:53–61.

403. Heinemann M-H. Medical management of AIDS patients. *Med Clin N Am* 1992;76:83–97.

404. Jabs DA, Green WR, Fox R, et al. Ocular manifestations of acquired immune deficiency syndrome. *Ophthalmology* 1989;96:1092.

405. Culbertson WW. Infections of the retina in AIDS. *Intl Ophthalmol Clin* 1989;29:108–18.

406. Pepose JS, et al. AIDS. Pathogenic mechanisms of ocular disease. *Ophthalmology* 1985;92:472.

407. Heinemann M-H. Characteristics of cytomegalovirus retinitis in patients with acquired immunodeficiency syndrome. *Am J Med* 1992;92:12S–16S.

408. Khadem M, et al. Ophthalmologic findings in acquired immune deficiency syndrome (AIDS). *Arch Ophthalmol* 1984;102:201–6.

409. Freeman WR, Lerner CW, Mines JA, et al. A prospective study of the ophthalmologic findings in the acquired immune deficiency syndrome. *Am J Ophthalmol* 1984;97:133–142.

410. Lipson BK, Freeman WR, Beniz J, et al. Optic neuropathy associated with cryptococcal arachnoiditis in AIDS patients. *Am J Ophthalmol* 1989;107:523–527.

411. Macher AM, et al. Pneumocystis carinii choroiditis in a male homosexual with AIDS and disseminated pulmonary and extrapulmonary *P. carinii* infection. *N Engl J Med* 1987;1092.

412. Weiss A, et al. Toxoplasmic retinochoroiditis as an initial manifestation of the acquired immune deficiency syndrome. *Am J Ophthalmol* 1986;101:248.

413. Holland GN, et al. Ocular toxoplasmosis in patients with the acquired immunodeficiency syndrome. *Am J Ophthalmol* 1988;106:653–67.

414. Shuler JD, et al. External ocular disease and anterior segment disorders associated with AIDS. *Intl Ophthalmol Clin* 1989;29:98.

415. Cole EL, et al. Herpes zoster ophthalmicus and acquired immune deficiency syndrome. *Arch Ophthalmol* 1984;102:1027.

416. Sandor EV, et al. Herpes zoster ophthalmicus in patients at risk for the acquired immune deficiency syndrome (AIDS). *Am J Ophthalmol* 1986;101:153.

417. Young TL, et al. Herpes simplex keratitis in AIDS patients. *Ophthalmology* 1988;95(Suppl):163.

418. Rosenwasser GOD, Greene WH. Simultaneous herpes simplex types 1 and 2 keratitis in acquired immunodeficiency syndrome. *Am J Ophthalmol* 1992;113:102–103.

419. Nanda M, Pflugfelder C, Holland S. Fulminant pseudomonal keratitis and scleritis in human immunodeficiency virus-infected patients. *Arch Ophthalmol* 1991;109:503–505.

420. Kohn SR. *Molluscum contagiosum* in patients with acquired immunodeficiency syndrome. *Arch Ophthalmol* 1987;105:458.

421. Passo MS, Rosenbaum JT. Ocular syphilis in patients with human immunodeficiency virus infection. *Am J Ophthalmol* 1988;106:1.

422. Friedman DI. Neuro-ophthalmic manifestations of human immunodeficiency virus infection. *Neurol Clin* 1991;9:55.

423. Johns DR, et al. Alterations in the natural history of neurosyphilis by concurrent infection with the human immunodeficiency virus. *N Engl J Med* 1987;316:1569.

424. Tramont EC. Syphilis in the AIDS era. *N Engl J Med* 1987;316:1600.

425. Stoumbos VD, Klein ML. Syphilitic retinitis in a patient with acquired immunodeficiency syndrome-related complex. *Am J Ophthalmol* 1987;103:103.

426. Levy JH, Liss RA, Maguire AM. Neurosyphilis and ocular syphilis in patients with concurrent human immunodeficiency virus infection. *Retina* 1989;9:175.

427. Kurosawa A, Pollock SC, Collins MP, et al. Sporothrix schenckii endophthalmitis in a patient with human immunodeficiency virus infection. *Arch Ophthalmol* 1988;106:376–380.

428. Kreiger AE, Holland GN. Ocular involvement in AIDS. *Eye* 1988;2:496.

429. Newman NJ, Lessell S. Bilateral optic neuropathies with remission in two HIV-positive men. *J Clin Neuro-ophthalmol* 1992;12:1.

430. Newsome DA. Noninfectious ocular complications of AIDS. *Intl Ophthalmol Clin* 1989;29:95.

431. Winward KE, et al. The spectrum of optic nerve disease in human immunodeficiency virus infection. *Am J Ophthalmol* 1989;107:373.

432. Keane JR. Neuro-ophthalmologic signs of AIDS: 50 patients. *Neurology* 1991;41:841.

433. Friedberg DN, Stenson SM, Orenstein JM, et al. Microsporidial keratoconjunctivitis in acquired immunodeficiency syndrome. *Arch Ophthalmol* 1990;108:504–508.

434. Davis RM, et al. Corneal microsporidiosis: a case report including ultrastructural observations. *Ophthalmology* 1990;97:953.

435. Lowder CY, Meisler DM, McMahon JT, et al. Microsporidia infection of the cornea in a man seropositive for human immunodeficiency virus. *Am J Ophthalmol* 1990;109:242–244.

436. Cali A, Meisler DM, Rutherford I, et al. Corneal microsporidiosis in a patient with AIDS. *Am J Trop Med Hyg* 1991;44:463.

437. Crumpacker CS, Heath-Chiozzi M. Overview of cytomegalovirus infections in HIV-infected patients: current therapies and future strategies. *J AIDS* 1991;4:S1.

438. Sison RF, Holland GN, MacArthur LJ. Cytomegalovirus retinopathy as the initial manifestation of the acquired immunodeficiency syndrome. *Am J Ophthalmol* 1991;112:243–249.

439. Culbertson WW. Discussion of Henderly DE, Freeman WR, Casey DM, Rao NA: cytomegalovirus retinitis and response to therapy with ganciclovir. *Ophthalmology* 1987;94:432.

440. O'Donnell JJ, Jacobson MA. Cotton-wool spots and cytomegalovirus retinitis in aids. *Int Ophthalmol Clin* 1989;29:105–107.

441. Grossniklaus HE, Frank KE, Tomask RL. Cytomegalovirus retinitis and optic neuritis in acquired immune deficiency syndrome. *Ophthalmology* 1987;94:1601.

442. Lee S, Ai E. Disc neovascularization in patients with AIDS and cytomegalovirus retinitis. *Retina* 1991;11:305–308.

443. DeVenecia G, et al. Cytomegalic inclusion retinitis in an adult: a clincal, histopathologic, and ultrastructural study. *Arch Ophthalmol* 1971;86:44.

444. Bachman DM, Rodriques MM, Chu FC, et al. Culture-proven cytomegalovirus retinitis in a homosexual man with acquired immunodeficiency syndrome. *Ophthalmology* 1982;89:797–804.

445. Lewis ML, et al. Herpes simplex virus type I. A cause of the ARN syndrome. *Ophthalmology* 1989;96:875.

446. Jabs DA, et al. Presumed varicella zoster retinitis in immunocompromised patients. *Retina* 1987;7:9.

447. Sternberg P Jr, et al. Acute retinal necrosis syndrome. *Retina* 1982;2:145–51.

448. Culbertson WW, et al. The acute retinal necrosis syndrome. II. Histopathology, and etiology. *Ophthalmology* 1982;89:1317.

449. Fisher JP, et al. The acute retial necrosis syndrome. Part 1: clinical manifestations. *Ophthalmology* 1982;89:1309.

450. Margolis TP, Lowder CY, Holland GN, et al. Varicella-zoster virus retinitis in patients with the acquired immunodeficiency syndrome. *Am J Ophthalmol* 1991;112:119–131.

451. Schwartz JN, et al. Necrotizing retinopathy with herpes zoster ophthalmicus: A light and electron microscopical study. *Arch Pathol Lab Med* 1976;100:386.

452. Willerson D Jr, et al. Necrotizing vaso-occlusive retinitis. *Am J Ophthalmol* 1977;84:209.

453. Blumenkranz MS. Discussion of chickenpox-associated ARN syndrome. *Ophthalmology* 1991;98:1645–1646.

454. Culbertson WW, et al. Varicella-zoster virus is a cause of the ARN syndrome. *Ophthalmology* 1986;93:559.

455. Soushi S, et al. Demonstration of varicella-zoster virus antigens in the vitreous aspirates of patients with ARN syndrome. *Ophthalmology* 1988;95:1394.

456. Fox GM, Crouse CA, Chuang EL, et al. Detection of herpesvirus DNA in vitreous and aqueous specimens by the polymerase chain reaction. *Arch Ophthalmol* 1991;109:266–271.

457. Nussenblatt RB, Palestine AG. Human immunodeficiency virus, herpes zoster, and the retina. *Am J Ophthalmol* 1991;112:206.

458. Charles NC, et al. Cryptococcosis of the anterior segment in acquired immune deficiency syndrome. *Ophthalmology* 1992;99:813.

459. Carney MD, et al. Cryptococcal choroiditis. *Retina* 1990;10:27.

460. Denning DW, Armstrong RW, Fishman M, et al. Endophthalmitis in a patient with disseminated cryptococcosis and AIDS who was treated with itraconazole. *Rev Infect Dis* 1991;13:1126–1130.

461. Hiss PW, et al. *Ophthalmology* 1988;95:162–165.

462. Good CB, Leeper HF. Profound papilledema due to cryptococcal meningitis in acquired immunodeficiency syndrome: successful treatment with fluconazole. *Southern Med J* 1991;84:394.

463. Golnik KC, Newman SA, Wispelway B. Cryptococcal optic neuropathy in the acquired immune deficiency syndrome. *J Clin Neuro-ophthalmol* 1991;11:96–103.

464. Johnston SRD, Corbett EL, Foster O, et al. Case report: raised intracranial pressure and visual complications in AIDS patients with cryptococcal meningitis. *J Infect* 1992;24:185–189.

465. Kupfer C, McCrane E. A possible cause of decreased vision in cryptococcal meningitis. *Invest Ophthalmol* 1974;13:801.

466. Rao NA, Zimmerman PL, Boyer D, et al. A clinical, histopathologic, and electron microscopic study of *Pneumocystis carinii* choroiditis. *Am J Ophthalmol* 1989;107:218–228.

467. Shami MJ, et al. A multicenter study of Pneumocystis choroidopathy. *Am J Ophthalmol* 1991;112:15.

468. Foster RE, Lowder CY, Meisler DM, et al. Presumed *Pneumocystis carinii* choroiditis. *Ophthalmology* 1991;98:1360–1365.

469. Friedberg DN, Warren FA, Lee MH, et al. *Pneumocystis carinii* of the orbit. *Am J Ophthalmol* 1992;113:595–596.

470. Freeman WR, et al. *Pneumocystis carinii* choroidopathy: a new clinical entity. *Arch Ophthalmol* 1989;107:863–867.

471. Berenger A, Frezzotti R. Active neuro-ophthalmic toxoplasmosis: a clinical study on 19 patients. *Adv Ophthalmol* 1962;12:265.

472. Holland GN, et al. Choroidal pneumocystosis. *Arch Ophthalmol* 1991;109:1454.

473. Parke DW II, Font RL. Diffuse toxoplasmic retinochoroiditis in a patient with AIDS. *Arch Ophthalmol* 1986;104:571–575.

474. Rehder JR, et al. Acute unilateral toxoplasmic iridocyclitis in an AIDS patient. *Am J Ophthalmol* 1988;106:740.

475. Grossniklaus HE, Specht CS, Allaire G, et al. Toxoplasma gondii retinochoroiditis and optic neuritis in acquired immune deficiency syndrome. *Ophthalmology* 1990;97:1342–1346.

476. Schuman JS, Weinberg RS, Ferry AP, et al. Toxoplasmic scleritis. *Ophthalmology* 1988;95:1399–1403.

477. Macher A, et al. Disseminated bilateral chorioretinitis due to *Histoplasma capsulatum* in a patient with the acquired immunodeficiency syndrome. *Ophthalmology* 1985;92:1159.

478. Specht CS, Mitchell KT, Bauman AE, et al. Ocular histoplasmosis with retinitis in a patient with acquired immune deficiency syndrome. *Ophthalmology* 1991;98:1356–1359.

Ophthalmic Pathology with Clinical Correlations,
edited by Joseph W. Sassani, M.D.
Lippincott-Raven Publishers, Philadelphia © 1997.

CHAPTER 4

Pediatric Ophthalmic Pathology

Harry H. Brown

This chapter highlights opthalmic entities that manifest during infancy and childhood for which clinicopathologic correlation is important for diagnosis, prognosis, and treatment. Neoplasms and conditions simulating them in the pediatric population are emphasized.

For information on common entities for which pathologic tissue examination is rarely if ever indicated, such as strabismus, amblyopia, cataract, or glaucoma, and for comprehensive resources on the genetic bases for opthalmic disorders, see the bibliography at the end of this chapter.

GENETICS

The genetic basis for diagnosing certain congenital and developmental ophthalmologic disorders has advanced rapidly in the past decade with the advent of sophisticated molecular diagnostic tools. Although an understanding of classic Mendelian genetics is required to understand hereditary processes, most diseases are multifactorial, with a combination of polygenetic and environmental influences. Certain disease states, however, have been identified as having a single chromosomal or genetic abnormality. Probably the most well-known example in ophthalmology is the development of retinoblastoma due to an abnormality of both alleles of the retinoblastoma gene at the q14 locus on chromosome 13.

The somatic cells of the human body contain 46 chromosomes: one pair each of 22 autosomal chromosomes and one pair of sex chromosomes. The chromosomes, although paired, are not identical, because normally one is maternal in origin and the other paternal. Each chromosome is composed of two chromatids, joined at a single point called the **centromere.** The chromatids of a specific chromosome are of unequal length; the shorter chromatid (or arm) is labeled ''p'' and the longer ''q.'' Genes are

referenced both according to the chromatid on which they are located and numerically by their distance from the centromere (the higher the number, the greater the distance). For example, the retinoblastoma gene is located at the locus 14 on the long arm of chromosome 13 (13q14). Before mitotic cell division, each chromosome replicates itself, so that at cell division there are two identical sister chromatids per chromosome; in other words, the cell is transiently tetraploid. During metaphase, the centromeres are pulled to opposite sides of the cell and the duplicate chromosomes are separated, one each then populates the resulting two diploid daughter cells.

Meiosis, or the formation of haploid germ cells, differs in that there are two cycles of cell division. The first is identical to mitosis with the formation of two diploid daughter cells. The second is without the duplication of chromosomes prior to division, resulting in four cells each containing one each of the 22 autosomal chromosomes and one sex chromosome. It is during this second cycle of meiosis that nondisjunction may occur. Nondisjunction can result in unequal chromosome numbers within daughter cells. Cells either may contain an entire extra chromosome (**trisomy**) or be missing an entire chromosome (**monosomy**). The most common example of a trisomy is Down's syndrome, in which there is an additional chromosome 21. Trisomies also may involve the sex chromosomes, as in Klinefelter's syndrome (47,XXY). Deletion of an entire autosomal chromosome is lethal in utero; however, monosomy of the X chromosome may be compatible with life (Turner's syndrome; 45,XO). Alterations in chromosome number are easily identified in karyotypic analysis of cells undergoing mitotic division. Table 1 includes the most common chromosomal aberrations and their ophthalmic manifestations.

During either cycle of meiotic cell division, genetic material from one chromosome may cross over to another, resulting in translocations. If both affected chromosomes end up in the same daughter cell, then the translocation is balanced because all the genetic material is retained within each cell, albeit in abnormal position for the trans-

H. H. Brown: Departments of Pathology and Ophthalmology, University of Arkansas for Medical Sciences, Little Rock, Arkansas 72205.

TABLE 1. *Chromosomal defects with ocular findings**

Genetic defect	Karyotype	Incidence	Ocular findings
TRISOMY			
21:Down's syndrome	47,XX or XY,+21	1 in 1000 live births	Oblique palpebral fissures, epicanthal folds, keratoconus, cataract, myopia, Brushfield's spots/iris stromal atrophy, strabismus, increased number of retinal vessels crossing the optic disc margin
18:Edwards' syndrome	47,XX or XY,+18	1 in 5000 live births	Cataract
13:Patau's syndrome	47,XX or XY,+13	1 in 6000 live births	Microphthalmia, coloboma, cataract
XXY:Klinefelter's syndrome	47,XXY	1 in 850 live male births	Myopia, iris coloboma, aniridia, epicanthal folds, strabismus, Brushfield's spots
MONOSOMY			
XO:Turner's syndrome	45,XO	1 in 3000 live female births	Cataract, coloboma, nystagmus, epicanthal folds, keratoconus
PARTIAL DELETION			
13q−	46,XX or XY,13q−		Retinoblastoma, epicanthal folds, ptosis, iris coloboma
11p−:WAGR syndrome	46,XX or XY,11p−		Aniridia, glaucoma, cataract
5p−:cri du chat syndrome	46,XX or XY,5p−	1 in 50,000 live births	Epicanthal folds, strabismus, cataract, oblique palpebral fissure

* For an exhaustive listing of genetic diseases with ocular manifestations, see chapter 1 tables in Harley RD, ed. *Pediatric ophthalmology,* ed 3. Philadelphia: WB Saunders, 1991.

located genes. If, however, the affected chromosomes are pulled in opposite directions, the resultant daughter cells are unbalanced with regard to genetic material.

More subtle alterations in chromosomes, such as deletions or translocations of portions of a chromosome, may be detected by karyotype banding techniques. Only the use of advanced molecular techniques, such as restriction length fragment polymorphisms and polymerase chain reaction amplification, can identify small defects in DNA at the gene level.

Chromosomes in the nucleus of cells are not the only things carrying genetic information. Mitochondria have also been shown to possess DNA (maternally inherited), and alterations of mitochondrial DNA may lead to diseases with ophthalmologic manifestations. Examples of such mitochondrial genetic disorders are Leber's optic neuropathy and Kearns-Sayre syndrome.

EYELID MASSES

Tumoral conditions involving the eyelids in the pediatric population can be divided into inflammatory masses (hordeolum, chalazion, or virally induced masses), vascular masses (hemangioma, lymphangioma, pyogenic granuloma), cystic (epidermal or dermoid cyst) or the rare adnexal neoplasms (pilomatrixoma, syringocystadenoma papilliferom). Some of these entities are discussed in the section on orbital masses. Molluscum contagiosum is presented here due to its distinctive histopathologic appearance.

Molluscum Contagiosum

Molluscum contagiosum is a relatively common tumorous infection of the eyelids in children, caused by a DNA virus of the poxvirus family, and is spread by direct contact. It appears most commonly as a single umbilicated, dome shaped, white-tan mass. Multiple lesions suggest an immunocompromised state. Often located on the lid margin, it may cause a secondary follicular conjunctivitis due to persistent spillage of virus into the tears. The natural history is one of spontaneous resolution over a few months.

Histopathologic examination demonstrates a cup-shaped invagination formed by closely packed lobules of proliferating epidermal squamous cells, with a central crater exuding desquamated keratin and viral particles (Fig. 4-1). There is a characteristic evolutionary sequence identifiable within the lobules. The peripheral lining basal cells of the invagination are unremarkable. As one scans toward the center of the lobule, the infected cells show intracytoplasmic eosinophilic inclusions ("molluscum bodies"), which increase in size and number and compress the nucleus to the periphery of the cell. At the level of the stratum granulosum, the inclusions become basophilic and the nucleus disappears, so that the stratum corneum is filled with large, basophilic spherules that are extruded into the center of the lesion. Involution is characterized by a surrounding and infiltrating mononuclear cell response.

Treatment in many cases is not necessary because the lesions resolve spontaneously; however, in recalcitrant

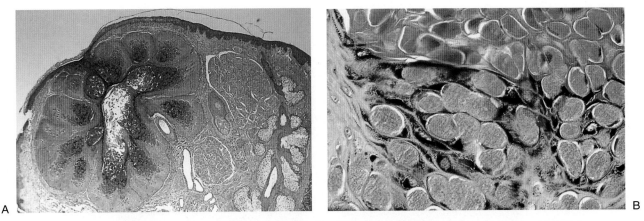

FIG. 4-1. (**A**) Molluscum contagiosum involving the lid margin. (**B**) Note the progressive expansion of the cell by viral particles as it matures toward the center of the lesion.

cases or those with secondary complications, surgical excision or curettage is curative.[1]

Epibulbar masses

The most common growths on the epibulbar surface in children up to age 15, as determined by a review of specimens excised over two to five decades, include nevi, choristomas, epithelial cysts, and papillomas.[2,3] Only five of 584 cases reviewed were malignant—three squamous-cell carcinomas and two rhabdomyosarcomas. Choristomas and viral papillomas are considered here.

Choristoma

Dermoid

Dermoid, as the name implies, is a mass recapitulating dermal tissue on the epibulbar surface. Dermoids typically occur at the limbus inferotemporally. In one third of cases, dermoids are associated with other congenital anomalies; the most well known is Goldenhar's syndrome (oculoauriculovertebral dysplasia). Clinically, they are characterized by a white-tan to pink, circumscribed, dome-shaped configuration usually straddling the limbus, with fine hairs emanating from the surface (Fig. 4-2A). More extensive lesions may reach the pupillary axis and block vision or involve the deep limbal structures and adjacent intraocular tissue.

Histopathologic examination reveals a solid mass covered by keratinizing stratified squamous epithelium, but without obvious rete peg formation, overlying dermal collagen containing pilosebaceous units (Fig. 4-2B). Sweat glands and adipose tissue also have been described in these lesions.

Treatment depends on the extent and depth of the mass. Simple excision by lamellar dissection is optimal, but more extensive lesions in a blind eye may require enucleation for cosmetic reasons.[4]

Dermolipomas

Dermolipomas are distinct from dermoids both clinically and histopathologically. Dermolipomas typically involve the superotemporal conjunctiva, are less well-demarcated, and may extend posteriorly into the orbit. Due to their fat content, they have a more yellow appearance.

Histopathologically, dermolipomas demonstrate nonkeratinizing stratified squamous epithelium overlying dermal-type collagen typically devoid of adnexal structures. There is an abundance of adipose tissue at the deep aspect of the mass, and it is often the predominating histopathologic feature. Surgical resection is for cosmetic benefit only, because these lesions are nonprogressive and do not interfere with vision.

Complex Choristoma

Dermoids or dermolipomas in which other ectopic tissues are demonstrated histopathologically are classified as complex choristomas. Examples of lacrimal gland, brain, cartilage, tooth, and bone have been described (Fig. 4-2C).[5] When one tissue predominates (eg, bone) then that particular tissue assumes nomenclature status (e.g., episcleral osseous choristoma).

Viral Papilloma

Viral papillomas may involve the eyelid or any portion of the conjunctiva, although the fornices seem especially prone to develop them. Those of the conjunctiva in the pediatric population may cause significant cosmetic disfigurement, forming bulky, protuberant masses multifo-

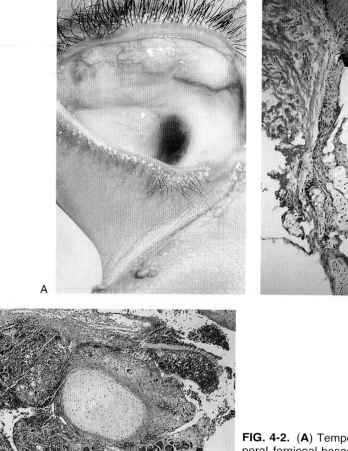

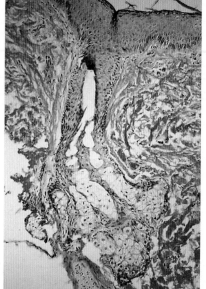

FIG. 4-2. (A) Temporal limbal-based dermoid and superior temporal forniceal-based complex choristoma (Courtesy of Michael C. Brodsky, MD). **(B)** Pilosebaceous structure embedded in dermal collagen beneath keratinizing squamous epithelium in a limbal dermoid. **(C)** Complex choristoma containing lacrimal gland and cartilage (courtesy of Todd Makley, MD).

cally and bilaterally (Fig. 4-3A). The external appearance of conjunctival papillomas resembles the surface of a strawberry, due to the variegated pattern of closely packed, translucent white papillae containing pinpoint central congested vessels. Papillomas can be either sessile or pedunculated.

Histopathologically, viral papillomas of the eyelid are characterized by acanthotic, hyperkeratotic stratified squamous epithelium covering elongated dermal papillae (Fig. 4-3B). Clues to the viral etiology are found in the stratum granulosum, where the cells exhibit cytoplasmic clearing, nuclear hyperchromasia and membrane irregularity, and coarse basophilic keratohyaline granules. Conjunctival papillomas demonstrate nonkeratinizing, stratified conjunctival epithelium containing goblet cells and infiltrated by acute inflammatory cells. Viral cytologic features identifiable in the epidermis of the skin are not as conspicuous within conjunctival lesions; however, human papillomavirus types 6 and 11 have been identified within the epithelium of conjunctival papillomas in the pediatric population.[6] The central fibrovascular cores often contain an acute and chronic inflammatory infiltrate.

Treatment usually consists of excision with an adequate margin and cryotherapy to the base. Recurrences are not uncommon, however. Interferon-alpha has also been used for recurrent lesions, but appears only to suppress rather than prevent growth of the papillomas.[7]

Intraocular Masses: Anterior Segment

Juvenile Xanthogranuloma

Ocular involvement by juvenile xanthogranuloma may be orbital, adnexal, or intraocular, with the latter predominating.[8] The vast majority of cases present before age 2 years, with a male predominance. Patients typically have multifocal skin involvement at the time of ocular presentation, making complete inspection of the skin a necessary part of the physical examination when this diagnosis is suspected.

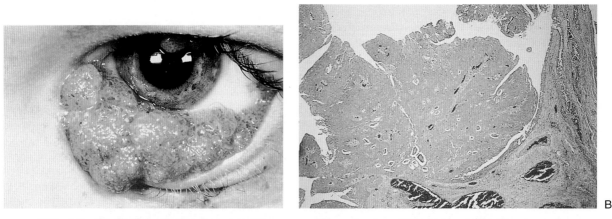

A
B

FIG. 4-3. (**A**) Multiple confluent viral papillomas causing ectropion of the lower eyelid (Courtesy of James R. Patrinely, MD). (**B**) Acanthotic squamous epithelium lining fibrovascular papillae emanating from the conjunctival surface.

The intraocular lesions are almost always unilateral and involve the iris or ciliary body.[9] Clinically, the tumor appears as a highly vascularized tan-yellow–to–brown mass on or within the iris, often associated with a spontaneous hyphema. Diffuse lesions of the iris may produce heterochromia iridis. Cells on the surface may be dispersed into the anterior chamber and simulate anterior uveitis. The masses may regress with time, but complications, such as recurrent bleeding, anterior synechiae, and secondary glaucoma, may supervene.

Histopathologically, there is a histiocytic proliferation within the iris and ciliary body stroma, often accompanied by lymphocytes and occasional eosinophils. Vascularization may be so prominent as to mimic a hemangioma. Histiocytes typically are cytologically bland, with round to oval nuclei and regular nuclear contours. The cytoplasm ranges from eosinophilic to finely vacuolated. Immunohistochemically, they are largely S100-protein negative, in contrast to Langerhans' cell histiocytosis.[10] As the lesions evolve, the histiocytes acquire more lipid within their cytoplasm, and Touton giant cells, with their characteristic rosette of nuclei separating a central area of eosinophilic cytoplasm from an outer finely vacuolated cytoplasm, become more conspicuous (Fig. 4-4).

Because the disease process is self-limited, treatment, when indicated, is aimed at preventing the morbid complications mentioned earlier.

Intraocular Masses: Posterior Segment

Retinoblastoma

Retinoblastoma is the most common childhood intraocular malignancy, estimated to occur in from 1 in 18,000 to 1 in 34,000 live births. This neoplasm can occur from birth to adulthood, but the vast majority manifest before age 3 years, and occurrence is rare beyond the age 5

years. The average age at diagnosis is within the first year of life for bilateral tumors and slightly younger than age 2 years for unilateral cases. Those patients known to be at risk because of a family history of retinoblastoma are typically diagnosed earlier due to neonatal screening.

Two thirds of cases are sporadic and associated with a somatic mutation in the retinoblastoma gene, resulting in a single (and therefore unilateral) neoplasm without the possibility of transmitting the mutation to offspring. In 10% to 15% of sporadic cases, however, the mutation is germline, meaning all the host cells have the mutation. This results, as in hereditary cases, in the potential for multifocal unilateral tumors, bilateral tumors, and the possibility of transmitting the defect to offspring.

Clinically, inherited retinoblastoma resembles an autosomal dominant disorder because more than 90% of persons with the mutation develop retinoblastoma. At the cellular level, however, it is a recessive phenomenon in which both alleles of chromosome 13 must be affected for the neoplasm to develop. Knudsen proposed a "two-hit" hypothesis in which one chromosome, either at the

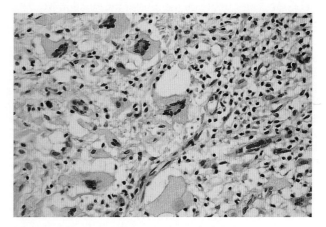

FIG. 4-4. Numerous Touton giant cells within a juvenile xanthogranuloma of the skin.

germline or postzygotic level, has a mutation. Subsequently, a mutation occurs in the second chromosome 13, leading to the formation of a tumor.[11] If the first mutation is germline (either inherited from one parent or a spontaneous mutation), then all cells in the body derived from the affected cell contain that mutation. In such a case, it is likely that more than one cell would experience a mutation in the second chromosome, leading to the formation of multiple tumors. A postzygotic (ie, somatic) first mutation would result in far fewer cells at risk for a second mutation, and consequently, the development of multiple tumors would be extremely remote.

Confirmation of Knudsen's hypothesis and identification and characterization of the retinoblastoma gene have been instrumental in opening a new avenue in cancer genetics—the concept of tumor supressor genes. The normal retinoblastoma gene, located at the 14.2 locus of the long arm of chromosome 13, encodes a nuclear phosphoprotein ($p110^{RB1}$) that binds to and is involved in regulating DNA proliferation.[12] Most mutations of the retinoblastoma gene result in production of truncated, unstable proteins. Mutation of the retinoblastoma gene, therefore, causes deregulation of DNA synthesis and allows the cell to proliferate unchecked, leading to neoplastic growth.

Because more than half of all patients with retinoblastoma have a germline mutation, genetic analysis is important in identifying patients and family members at risk for developing retinoblastoma. These individuals may pass the mutation on to offspring and are at risk for developing other nonocular malignancies, such as osteosarcoma, in which RB1 gene mutations have been identified. With molecular techniques, such as analysis of DNA sequence polymorphisms by restriction enzymes and polymerase chain reaction amplification, direct DNA sequencing can be performed to identify even a single-point mutation in the retinoblastoma gene. It is important to note that fresh tumor tissue is necessary for defining the specific genetic mutation with these techniques. Thus, the pathologist must be forewarned about enucleation in order to handle the specimen appropriately and to take any necessary steps to obtain the utmost information from the specimen.[13]

Retinoblastoma, particularly in sporadic cases, is usually detected when an abnormal coloration of the pupil (eg, **leukocoria,** a white pupil) is noted in the child. Strabismus may also be present. Rarely, the eye may appear inflamed, with tumor cells in the anterior chamber mimicking hypopyon (**pseudohypopyon**). Of course, many other conditions—such as cataract, persistent hyperplastic primary vitreous, retinal detachment as in Coat's disease or retinopathy of prematurity, ocular toxocariasis—also may cause leukocoria. Careful clinical examination and other diagnostic modalities are necessary to narrow the differential diagnosis.[14] Ultrasound and computed tomography (CT) scans may be helpful in determining whether a solid mass is present. The presence of radiodensities consistent with calcifications within the mass is a strong, although not pathognomonic, indicator for retinoblastoma (Fig. 4-5A). CT and magnetic resonance imaging (MRI) also may help in detecting extraocular extension of the tumor.

Retinoblastomas may arise from any retinal cell layer. Therefore, they may be predisposed to either an endophytic growth pattern (ie, growing from the retinal surface toward and seeding the vitreous) or an exophytic pattern resulting in retinal detachment and seeding of the retinal pigment epithelium. A combination of both patterns is typical. The gross appearance of retinoblastoma is that of a variegated white-gray mass (Fig. 4-5B). The variegated appearance is a result of areas of necrosis, presumably due to rapid growth outstripping the vascular supply, surrounding islands of viable tumor containing a central "feeding" vessel (Fig. 4-5C). Tumor-cell aggregates in the vitreous have just the opposite architecture, with the cells located in the center of the aggregate undergoing necrosis and the surrounding peripheral cells retaining a viable appearance (Fig. 4-5D).

Microscopically, retinoblastomas fall under the rubric of "small blue cell tumors of childhood." Tumor cells have hyperchromatic nuclei with coarse chromatin, inconspicuous nucleoli, and scant cytoplasm. These primitive-looking cells typically form solid sheets, but abortive attempts at maturation or differentiation are manifested by the formation of rosettes (Fig. 4-5E). A ring of nuclei surrounding a central core of neurofibrils is termed a **Homer Wright rosette.** Such histologic structures are not unique to retinoblastoma and may be seen in other neuroectodermal tumors such as neuroblastoma and medulloblastoma. More recognizable attempts at retinal differentiation, with tumor cell nuclei surrounding an empty central luminal space formed by tumor cell membranes connected at their apices by terminal bars, (corresponding to the external limiting membrane of the retina), are called **Flexner-Wintersteiner rosettes.** If focal rudimentary photoreceptor inner-segment differentiation is detected as bulbous cytoplasmic projections into the luminal space, the rosette loses its round shape, becomes more elliptical or reniform, and is termed a **fleurette.** Tumors composed entirely of fleurettes are termed **retinocytomas,** to convey their greater morphologic maturation and to predict an excellent outcome for the patient, because such tumors are not recognized to behave in a malignant fashion. Their occurrence, however, is rare.

Histologic parameters indicative of aggressive clinical behavior include lack of differentiation (absence of rosette formation), vitreous seeding, invasion into the choroid, and most importantly, invasion into the optic nerve (Fig. 4-5F). Once the tumor invades through the lamina cribrosa of the optic nerve head, the potential exists for tumor spread into the meninges of the optic nerve sheath and subsequent intracranial central nervous system dissemination. Systemic metastases usually first involve the

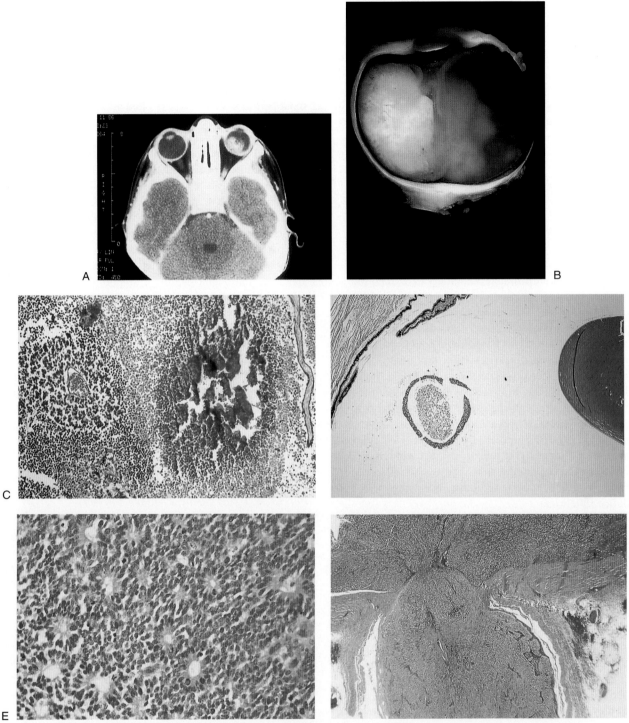

FIG. 4-5. (**A**) CT scan of a retinoblastoma involving the posterior segment of the left eye. (**B**) Gross photomicrograph of an exophytic retinoblastoma with complete retinal detachment. (**C**) Pseudorosette of viable tumor cells surround a central vessel (*left*); necrosis and calcification are present (*right*). Note the basophilic staining of the vessel wall at far right. (**D**) Retinoblastoma seeding the vitreous. Note the central necrosis and viable cells at the periphery. (**E**) Numerous Flexner-Wintersteiner rosettes and rare Homer Wright rosettes within a differentiated area of retinoblastoma. (**F**) Massive invasion of the optic nerve and peripapillary choroid.

lymphatic system before hematogenous spread to visceral organs ensues. Metastatic disease, when it occurs, usually does so within 2 years of the initial diagnosis. Local recurrence almost always is associated with incomplete excision of primary retinoblastomas with extraocular extension.

Enucleation has been the mainstay of therapy, but with earlier diagnosis and more and better treatment modalities available, alternative therapies that may conserve the affected eye and even retain functional vision are being advanced.[15] These modalities include radiotherapy, photocoagulation, and cryotherapy.

Medulloepithelioma

Far less common than retinoblastoma, medulloepithelioma is the only other primary, potentially malignant intraocular neoplasm of childhood with sufficient incidence to merit discussion. Earlier eponyms for this neoplasm include **teratoneuroma** (Verhoeff) and **diktyoma** (Fuchs). In contrast to its retinal neuroepithelial counterpart, medulloepithelioma typically arises from the ciliary epithelium and only rarely originates from the retina or optic nerve. The median age at diagnosis is 2 years, similar to retinoblastoma, although the mean age was from 5 to 7 years in the series of 56 cases reported by Zimmerman[16] and of 16 cases reported by Canning.[17] The higher mean age at diagnosis is due to the occasional occurrence of medulloepithelioma in adults. No bilateral or familial inheritance patterns have been reported for medulloepithelioma.

Most patients present with decreased vision and pain. Leukocoria or a visible mass in the iris or anterior chamber are somewhat less common presenting signs. Leukocoria is much less common as a presenting sign in medulloepithelioma than in retinoblastoma. Rubeosis is seen in 20% to 80% of cases and cataract in 50%.

Medulloepitheliomas are often at least partially cystic, due to production of presumed vitreous humor by the neoplastic cells (Fig. 4-6A). This feature, and also the usual lack of calcification, are helpful clues in differentiating medulloepithelioma from retinoblastoma on CT and ultrasound examination (Fig. 4-6B). Occasionally, small cysts may break off and appear in the anterior chamber or vitreous cavity.

Medulloepitheliomas are composed of primitive neuroectodermal cells forming variable architectural patterns, including cords, membranes, tubules, and sheets of closely packed, columnar epithelial cells forming one or more nuclear layers oriented perpendicular to the long axis of the cord. Where organized into membranes, the cells exhibit some degree of polarization in that the more apical portion of the cells bordering optically clear areas show intercellular junctional complexes similar to the external limiting membrane of the normal retina. In addition,

the opposite side abuts the loose myxoid stroma rich in hyaluronic acid, indicative of primitive vitreous humor (Fig. 4-6C).

Histopathologic examination of medulloepitheliomas can be segregated into those neoplasms with (teratoid) or without (nonteratoid) heterologous differentiation. The most common heterologous element is cartilage. Striated muscle or brain tissue is less commonly recognizable. Heterologous elements are seen in one third to half of all cases and are more frequent in histologically malignant tumors than in benign medulloepitheliomas. The histopathologic criteria for the diagnosis of malignancy is not well defined. Most authors use some combination of mitotic activity, nuclear pleomorphism, solid-growth pattern of either primitive neuroblastic or sarcomatous elements, and invasion of adjacent structures, in making that determination. Broughton reported four deaths due to the spread of malignant medulloepithelioma in 37 histologically diagnosed malignancies, all within 4 years of diagnosis[16]; however, Canning reported no tumor deaths in 16 cases studied, with a minimum of 5 years follow-up in malignant cases.[17]

Although radiation therapy may be a treatment option, as for similar tumors arising within the cranium, the rarity of occurrence and necessity of obtaining tissue for diagnosis make enucleation the primary treatment modality. Small tumors initially treated by iridocyclectomy usually result in subsequent enucleation for persistent or recurrent disease.

Persistent Hyperplastic Primary Vitreous

The term **persistent hyperplastic primary vitreous** describes the presence of a retrolental fibrovascular plaque adherent to the posterior lens capsule and centripetally pulling elongated ciliary processes.[18] The plaque is supplied posteriorly by the hyaloid artery. This condition is usually associated with microphthalmia, and therefore, also demonstrates a shallow anterior chamber. Cataract formation develops after birth, and the swollen lens often precipitates a pupillary block glaucoma.

Persons afflicted with persistent hyperplastic primary vitreous are identified at birth or shortly thereafter because of leukocoria. No genetic, racial, or sexual predilection is known, although a vertical transmission in a family has been documented.[19]

Histopathologic examination of enucleation specimens demonstrates the presence of a fibrovascular tissue proliferation in the retrolental space adherent to the posterior lens capsule, ciliary processes, and peripheral retina. Often, a patent hyaloid artery can be identified emanating posteriorly from the mass. There also may be glial elements within the tissue, and occasionally ectopic tissue such as cartilage is found.[20,21] Depending on the severity and duration of the process before enu-

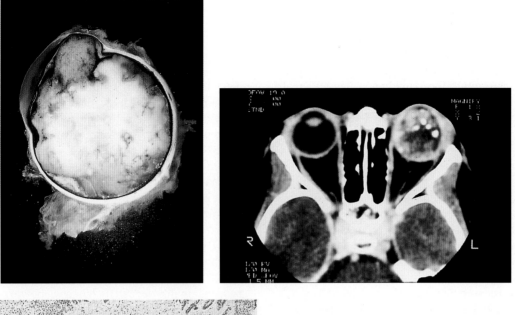

A

B

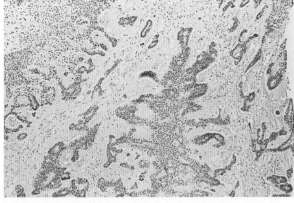

C

FIG. 4-6. (**A**) Malignant medulloepithelioma filling the eye, with extrascleral extension subconjunctivally. (**B**) CT scan demonstrates calcifications within the tumor. (**A,B** Courtesy of Narsing A. Rao, MD). (**C**) Acid mucopolysaccharide between cords of tumor cells (courtesy of William C. Lloyd III, MD).

cleation, associated findings may include tractional or rhegmatogenous retinal detachment, cataract, intraocular hemorrhage, and peripheral anterior synechiae. Contraction of the retrolental tissue is believed to cause tears of the posterior lens capsule and centripetal displacement of ciliary processes (Fig. 4-7).

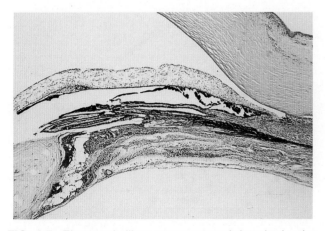

FIG. 4-7. Elongated ciliary processes and detached retina drawn toward retrolental fibrovascular tissue in persistent hyperplastic primary vitreous.

Surgical removal of the lens and retrolental tissue has shown potential for good visual outcome when the principal involvement of the globe is anteriorly located. If the disease involves more posteriorly located tissues, the visual prognosis is much poorer.[22]

Coats' Disease

Coats' disease is a sporadic condition principally occurring in young males without any associated systemic findings.[23] Because a nearly identical clinicopathologic picture can be seen in certain inflammatory states, particularly toxocariasis, the terms **Coats' response** or **Coats' lesion** also may be encountered. The typical age of onset for Coats' disease is in the late first to early second decade of life, but cases from infancy to the seventh decade have been reported. There is no known racial or familial predilection, but males are affected in more than two thirds of cases. The disease is unilateral more than 90% of the time. Symptoms at presentation are often related to either poor vision, strabismus, or leukocoria.

The pathophysiology of Coats' disease is well understood, although the pathogenesis remains a mystery.[23] Abnormal retinal vessels leak plasma constituents into the retina, where the lipid-rich fluid permeates the retina and pools in the subretinal space, causing an exudative detachment of the neurosensory retina (Fig. 4-8A). This process may be unifocal or multifocal and more often affects the temporal retina. The involved vessels are telangiectatic and congested, with saccular dilatation and aneurysm formation. The endothelial cells may become necrotic and slough into the lumen. Areas of nonperfusion develop as demonstrated by fluorescein angiography.

The histopathologic picture of Coats' disease highlights the fluid accumulation within the retina and subretinal space (Fig. 4-8B). Eosinophilic proteinaceous material may be found at all levels of the retina, although the fluid preferentially fills the outer plexiform layer. Similar material expands the subretinal space. Within the proteinaceous fluid are numerous foamy, lipid-laden macrophages and clefts outlining positions occupied by cholesterol crystals that have dissolved in tissue processing. Retinal vessels are dilated, congested, and often hyalinized. Photoreceptors are degenerated in areas of detachment. Subretinal fibrovascular scars, similar to the disciform scars in age-related macular degeneration, may develop in response to longstanding subretinal exudate. Ultrastructurally, the retinal vasculature demonstrates increased separation of endothelial cells and fenestrations destroying the blood–retinal barrier.

The natural history of the disease is one of gradual progression, leading (although not invariably) to total retinal detachment, rubeosis iridis, neovascular glaucoma, cataract, and eventually phthisis bulbi. Treatment is aimed at preventing these sequelae and consists of ablating leaking vessels and draining subretinal fluid. Both laser photocoagulation and transscleral cryopexy have been used to treat Coats' disease. Even with timely intervention, however, the prognosis for good visual function is guarded.[24]

Toxocariasis

The identification of nematode larvae within intraocular tissues was first documented in 1950 by Helenor Wilder, who by scrupulous microscopic examination of eyes enucleated for suspected retinoblastoma, discovered larvae or their capsules in more than half of cases containing intraocular granulomatous inflammation and eosinophil microabscesses.[25] The larvae were subsequently determined to be *Toxocara canis*.

The organism, after ingestion of ova from fecally contaminated soil or fomites, hatches and travels from its point of entry in the mucosa of the small intestine hematogenously, first via the portal system, and subsequently the systemic system. In the natural host, dogs (and especially puppies), the larvae then reach the lumen of the esophagus from the lungs and return to the intestine, where they mature into adult worms and produce ova to be shed in the feces. In humans, however, the larvae do not reach the esophagus and are peripatetic travelers throughout the body, hence the name **visceral larval migrans**.[26] Any visceral organ may be infested, but the usual sites of involvement include the liver, lungs, brain, and eye. Although originally thought to provoke an inflammatory reaction only upon the death of the larvae, more recent studies suggest that an antigen deposited in tissue by the larva is responsible (the *Toxocara* ES antigen).[27]

Ocular involvement may take a variety of forms: posterior or peripheral retinochoroiditis, optic papillitis, endophthalmitis, or anterior segment involvement. Those cases producing a mass effect in the posterior aspect of the eye with associated retinal detachment are most likely to be confused with retinoblastoma (Fig. 4-9A). Several clinical clues and radiologic evaluation may aid in differentiating the two. Toxocariasis typically demonstrates single cells in the vitreous and vitreoretinal traction bands, a cataract secondary to inflammation, and no evidence of

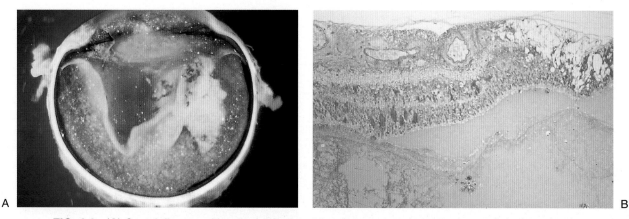

FIG. 4-8. (A) Coats' disease with retinal detachment and numerous cholesterol crystals in the subretinal fluid and also in the other ocular chambers (From Shields JA, et al. Coats' disease as a cause of anterior chamber cholesterolosis. *Arch Ophthalmol* 1995;113:975–977) ©1995 American Medical Association. **(B)** Telangiectatic vessels in the inner retinal layers with intraretinal and subretinal fluid accumulations.

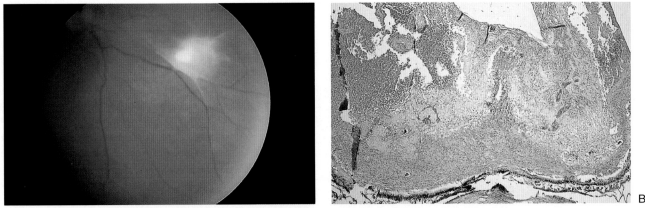

FIG. 4-9. **(A)** White mass in the posterior retina with stellate vitreoretinal traction bands in ocular toxocariasis (Courtesy of Frederick H. Davidorf, MD). **(B)** Foci of necrosis and calcification within the reactive gliotic and inflammatory tissue on the inner retinal surface.

calcifications on CT scan. Retinoblastoma, when involving the vitreous, does so with aggregates of tumor cells, lacks vitreoretinal traction bands, and often contains calcifications. Enzyme-linked immunosorbent assay (ELISA) testing of patient serum to detect antibodies to *T. canis* antigen is the most widely used and reliable laboratory test for the diagnosis of ocular toxocariasis. Titers of 1:8 or greater are considered significant.[26]

Histopathologic study of eyes infested with *T. canis* typically show a severe granulomatous inflammation of the retina and choroid, with an exudative retinal detachment (Fig. 4-9B). Granulomas often have central eosinophilic microabscesses, with degranulated eosinophil contents coating the larva and creating the Splendore-Hoeppli phenomenon. A mixed inflammatory infiltrate of lymphocytes, plasma cells, and eosinophils surrounds the granuloma and infiltrates the uveal tissues. Rarely, one may serendipitously find an intact or degenerating larva within the center of the granuloma or a ''subretinal tube'' lined by inflammatory cells, presumably the track of the larva.

Treatment modalities include antihelmintic therapy, corticosteroids, vitreoretinal surgery to remove traction bands and reattach the retina, and laser therapy if the larva can be visualized directly.

Retinopathy of Prematurity

Since Terry originally described it in 1942, retinopathy of prematurity (ROP) has continued to be a leading cause of blindness in infants in developed countries. Despite advances in understanding the pathogenesis of this potentially devastating condition, technologic advances in neonatal care have problematically compounded what was once thought to be a completely avoidable situation.

ROP, as the name now implies, is a condition that preferentially affects preterm neonates; the greater the degree of prematurity (and correspondingly, the lower the birth weight), the greater the incidence and severity of retinopathy.[28–30] Neonates weighing less than 1250 g are particularly prone to serious complications. The ability of neonatologists to prolong and support the lives of these high-risk neonates has actually created a resurgence in retinopathy of prematurity in recent years, following a period of abrupt decline when the correlation between retinopathy and excessive oxygen exposure was determined in the 1950s. Despite careful monitoring of oxygen therapy and arterial oxygen values, the disease is not yet completely controllable and certainly not yet a matter of only historical interest.

Vascularization of the retina begins during the fourth month of gestation and proceeds from the optic disc peripherally, reaching its most anterior (or peripheral) extent at term. Because the distance from the optic disc to the temporal retina is greater than that to the nasal retina, it naturally follows that insults to the normal progression of vessel growth are first evident in the temporal retina. Furthermore, the earlier in gestation the insult, the greater the area affected, so that in severe cases the condition is circumferential.

At the light microscopic level, vascularization is characterized by a proliferation of spindle cells, which undergo modeling to form solid cords of cells that then canalize, forming arborizing capillaries. Remodeling then produces fully formed arterial and venous systems linked by a capillary bed. The traditional theory of the pathophysiologic events that produce the clinical picture of retinopathy of prematurity is that the developing retinal vasculature is susceptible to excess oxygen exposure, causing retinal vasoconstriction and an arrest of further vessel maturation. Microscopically, there is a disordered ''piling up'' of spindle cells, ultimately forming a ridge (Fig. 4-10). Reduction in oxygen tension is followed by vasodilatation and renewed growth. Unfortunately, this renewed proliferation of vessels may no longer assume

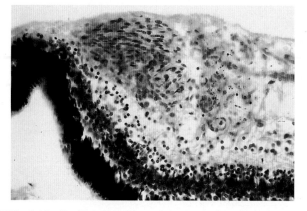

FIG. 4-10. Proliferation of vanguard spindle cells and rearguard endothelial cells in stage 2 retinopathy of prematurity.

an orderly progression as before the arrest, but results in arteriovenous shunting and capillary budding onto the surface of the retina and into the vitreous. The aberrant capillaries are incompetent and prone to bleed, inciting a reparative tissue reaction with cicatrization and contraction. In the worst-case scenario, the end result is a funnel-shaped tractional retinal detachment and blindness. Another theory espouses the role of gap junction formation between spindle cells as a response to stress and hypoxia, inhibiting further migration and maturation of affected spindle cells.[31]

Clinically, the degree of severity of retinopathy of prematurity has been divided into five stages (Table 2). Spontaneous regression may occur at any stage of the disease prior to extensive detachment and is the rule for milder forms of the disease process. Stage 1 ROP shows a sharp delineation between the zones of vascular and avascularized retina as compared with the gradual transition seen in normal development. In stage 2, an elevated ridge separates the two zones. Stage 3 is characterized by the formation of extraretinal vascularization and is subdivided into mild, moderate, and severe vascularization. In addition, if there is vascular tortuosity and congestion in the posterior retina, it is termed **plus disease**. Stage 4 shows a partial tractional

retinal detachment, which may (stage 4B) or may not (stage 4A) involve the macula. In stage 5, the detachment is total with either an open or closed funnel shape. Histopathologic correlates for each stage have been described (Table 2).[32]

Oxygen restriction is often not an option for these immature neonates because it would be incompatible with life. Therefore, retinopathy of prematurity is still an unavoidable iatrogenic complication. Even rigorous continuous monitoring of arterial oxygen partial pressures does not predict which neonates and infants will be affected or the degree to which they will be affected. Preventive therapies, such as vitamin E and other antioxidants, have been proposed, but their efficacy is not uniformly accepted, and the increase in other side effects of the treatment argue against its routine use.[28-30,33] The increase in ambient light in the neonatal intensive care units also has been implicated in the resurgence of ROP, but reports are conflicting.[34,35]

Phakomatoses

The phakomatoses are a diverse collection of syndromes exhibiting hamartomatous proliferations involving multiple organ systems, often including the eye and ocular adnexae. These include neurofibromatosis, tuberous sclerosis complex, Sturge-Weber syndrome, von Hippel-Lindau syndrome, Wyburn-Mason syndrome, and ataxia-telangiectasia, among others. The first four, which may produce a mass in the posterior segment of the eye, are described further.

Neurofibromatosis

Neurofibromatosis, once a unifying term for a disease manifested by multiple tumors of neural origin involving the skin and other sites, is now subdivided into two clinically and genetically distinct subgroups. Neurofibromatosis type 1 (NF-1), also known as **von Recklinghausen's disease** or **peripheral neurofibromatosis,**

TABLE 2. *Clinicopathologic stages of retinopathy of prematurity*

Stage	Clinical findings	Pathologic findings
Stage 1	Sharp demarcation between vascularized and avascular retina	Hyperplasia of vanguard spindle cells
Stage 2	Elevated ridge between vascularized and avascular retina	Hyperplasia of rearguard endothelial cells; vasodilatation
Stage 3	Extraretinal vascularization along ridge	Extraretinal vascularization (placoid, polypoid, or pedunculated)
Stage 4	Partial retinal detachment	Exudative (smooth, dome-shaped) or tractional (irregular, concave) retinal detachment
Stage 5	Complete retinal detachment	Pleated or scroll-like, funnel-shaped tractional retinal detachment

(From Foos RY. Retinopathy of prematurity: pathologic correlation of clinical stages. *Retina* 1987;7:260–276).

occurs in approximately 1 in 4000 births and is 10 times more common than neurofibromatosis type 2 (NF-2), also known as **central neurofibromatosis.** Diagnostic criteria for NF-1 include multiple cafe-au-lait spots or freckles in intertriginous regions of the skin, multiple neurofibromas of the skin and soft tissues, plexiform neurofibroma, Lisch nodules of the iris, unilateral or bilateral optic nerve glioma, dysplasia of the sphenoid, and an immediate family history (first-degree relative) of NF-1. Diagnostic criteria for NF-2 are bilateral acoustic neuromas, unilateral acoustic neuroma with other central nervous system glial or meningothelial neoplasms, peripheral nerve sheath tumors, adolescent-onset posterior subcapsular cataracts, and an immediate family history of NF-2.[36] NF-1 has been mapped to chromosome 17q11; the defective gene in NF-2 has been located on chromosome 22q22.[37]

Ocular and adnexal findings, as might be expected, are more commonly seen in NF-1. These include, in addition to Lisch nodules and optic nerve gliomas, cafe-au-lait spots and neurofibromas of the eyelids, thickened corneal and uveal nerves, neurofibromas and schwannomas of the uveal tract and orbit, melanocytic proliferations of the uvea, including an increased incidence of melanoma,[38] and astrocytomas of the retina identical to those seen in the tuberous sclerosis complex (Fig. 4-11A). Glaucoma in association with ipsilateral eyelid plexiform neurofibromas has been ascribed to either primary anterior chamber angle maldevelopment or to secondary angle closure.

Histopathologic examination of ocular tissues involved by neurofibromatosis reflects either hamartomatous or neoplastic proliferations of cells of melanocytic or peripheral nerve sheath derivation (Fig. 4-11B and C). Neurofibromas of eyelid, orbit, conjunctiva, and uvea are histologically similar. Spindle-cell neoplasms composed of an admixture of Schwann cells, perineural cells, and fibroblasts, form either circumscribed, but not encapsulated, fusiform enlargement of a nerve, ill-defined masses, or a plexiform pattern resembling a ''bag of worms.'' Mast cells and nerve axons are often interspersed throughout the tumor.

Schwannomas may be an adnexal or intraocular manifestation of the syndrome and are distinguished from neurofibromas by certain characteristics: true encapsulation, eccentric formation along a nerve so that axons are not found diffusely throughout the tumor, cellular (Antoni A) and loose myxoid (Antoni B) areas, and distinctive foci of nuclear palisading separated by anuclear eosinophilic zones (Verocay bodies). Melanocytic hyperplasias of the uveal tract may form distinct masses, as in Lisch nodules of the iris, or diffuse hyperplasias admixed with hamartomatous neural elements in the ciliary body and choroid.

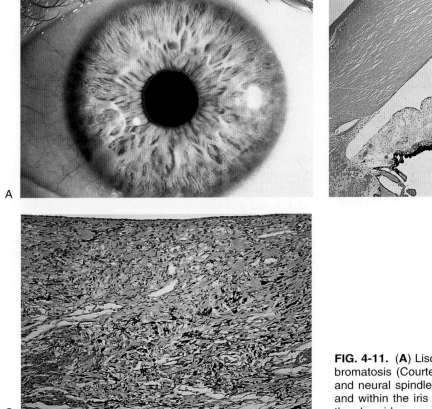

FIG. 4-11. (A) Lisch nodules dotting the iris in neurofibromatosis (Courtesy of Larry Merin). **(B)** Melanocytic and neural spindle cell proliferation on the iris surface and within the iris stroma and **(C)** diffusely expanding the choroid.

Tuberous Sclerosis Complex

The triad of epilepsy, mental retardation, and adenoma sebaceum constitute the principal features of tuberous sclerosis, also known as **Bourneville's syndrome.** Other associated entities include astrocytic hamartomas of the retina and optic disc, angiomyolipomas of the kidney, cysts of the pancreas, and rhabdomyomas of the heart. The hereditary pattern is one of autosomal dominant transmission with variable penetrance resulting in a widely variable clinical picture. Genetic defects have been variously located on chromosomes 9 (9q34) and 16 (16p13.3).[39]

Tuberous sclerosis refers to the multifocal glial tumor nodules within the subependymal and cortex of the cerebrum. These astrocytic hamartomas often display degenerative cystic changes and calcification and are readily detected radiographically or by CT scans. Compression of adjacent brain parenchyma is presumed to be the cause of the epileptic seizures, which are typically grand mal.

Adenoma sebaceum is an incorrect term for the symmetrically arranged, red papular skin lesions seen in this syndrome. Histopathologic examination demonstrates them to be angiofibromas characterized by dermal fibrosis and capillary dilatation. Pilosebaceous units usually are atrophied and surrounded by concentrically arranged collagen fibers. Other skin lesions often seen in tuberous sclerosis include subungual and periungual fibromas that lack the capillary dilatation of angiofibromas, lumbosacral shagreen patches due to increase in dermal collagen, and ash-leaf–shaped areas of depigmentation, seen best under ultraviolet illumination and reported to be the earliest cutaneous manifestation of the syndrome.

The retinal astrocytic hamartomas tend to conform to one of two morphologic types, although intermediate or transitional forms are possible: flat, salmon-to-gray colored translucent masses in the posterior pole and the less common but more easily recognized multinodular, white "mulberry" lesions that may calcify with age and are usually present at the disc margin.[40] Histopathologic examination reveals nodular proliferations of spindle-shaped glial cells arising from the nerve fiber layer in the retina or optic nerve head (Fig. 4-12). Calcospherites may be readily apparent. Individual cells display oval-to-round nuclei without significant pleomorphism or hyperchromasia. The cytoplasm is fibrillary and cell boundaries are indistinct. Cystic degeneration may be present, but necrosis is not a feature of these growths. The astrocytic proliferations have limited growth potential; thus, most remain stationary over long periods of observation.[41] No treatment is necessary unless secondary complications arise.

Sturge-Weber Syndrome

The presence of facial hemangioma, glaucoma with or without buphthalmos, seizures, and intracranial calcifica-

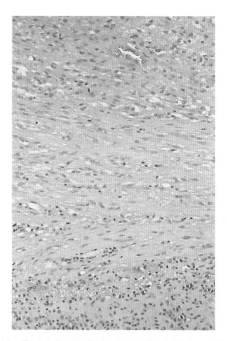

FIG. 4-12. Retinal astrocytoma with spindle cells arising from the nerve fiber layer (*bottom of field*).

tions comprise the Sturge-Weber syndrome, although in most cases only some of these findings are present. No hereditary pattern has been identified for this phakomatosis. The facial hemangioma typically is unilateral and present at birth (termed **nevus flammeus** or **port-wine stain**) and occupies the dermatome distribution of some or all of the divisions of the trigeminal nerve. The skin supplied by the first and second divisions is most commonly affected. If the upper eyelid, which is supplied sensation by cranial nerve V_1, is involved, the likelihood of ipsilateral glaucoma is great.

Histopathologic examination of the cutaneous hemangioma prior to age 10 years is unremarkable. After that age, there is capillary telangiectasia and congestion within the superficial dermis surrounded by collagen fibers in a loose, lamellar configuration. As the patient ages, vessels deeper within the dermis and even in the subcutis also become ectatic.

The seizures associated with this syndrome are usually localized to the side opposite the facial hemangioma. They are believed to be caused by compression and atrophy with dystrophic calcification of the cerebral cortex by leptomeningeal hemangiomas ipsilateral to the facial hemangioma. Glaucoma in these patients may result from congenital abnormal development of the anterior chamber angle, elevated episcleral venous pressure from epibulbar vascular anomalies, or the development of neovascularization of the anterior chamber angle and peripheral anterior synechiae following retinal detachment.

Intraocular components of this syndrome, in addition to glaucoma, include diffuse hemangiomas of the choroid in about half of all cases.[42] Due to their diffuse nature and minimal elevation, they may be difficult to detect clinically, but they often impart a redder appearance to the fundus, creating the so-called "tomato catsup" fundus. Ultrasonography may be helpful in confirming the presence and nature of the lesion.

The histopathologic appearance of the leptomeningeal and choroidal hemangiomas is similar to the cutaneous hemangiomas. In the choroid, the hemangioma occupies the entire thickness of the choroid and merges gradually with the adjacent normal architecture of the choroid (Fig. 4-13A). Secondary degeneration of the retinal pigment epithelium results in drusen formation and fibrous metaplasia. Serous retinal detachment and photoreceptor degeneration are the morbid consequences of choroidal hemangioma (Fig. 4-13B).

Argon laser photocoagulation may allow reattachment, but detachment recurs in half of initially successful cases. Enucleation may be the only recourse when the affected eyes become blind and painful as a result of retinal detachment and glaucoma.

Von Hippel-Landau Syndrome

Hemangiomas of the retina, associated with similar neoplasms of the cerebellum, are the principal findings of von Hippel-Lindau syndrome. Although the discovery of the retinal tumors are credited to von Hippel, their occurrence in association with cerebellar tumors was first described by Lindau in 1927. Other systemic manifestation of the syndrome may include hemangioblastomas in other central nervous system sites, including the medulla and spinal cord, cysts that may involve the pancreas or kidney, pheochromocytomas of the adrenal and sympathetic chain, and renal cell carcinoma.[43] The syndrome is inherited in an autosomal dominant fashion but with incomplete penetrance, and the genetic defect has been isolated to an area on the short arm of chromosome 3 (3p26-p25).[44]

The retinal hemangiomas may be detected in childhood, but more commonly are not observed until early adulthood. They may be single or multiple, unilateral or bilateral, endophytic or exophytic, and may involve the peripheral or juxtapapillary retina (Fig. 4-14A). Early lesions are pinpoint gray tumors often without fluorescein dye leakage. Well-developed endophytic tumors are highly vascular, yellow–to–pink-red masses with a prominent feeder arteriole and draining venule. Exophytic lesions are more subtle and may be overlooked or misdiagnosed on fundoscopy. They may remain stationary for years or enlarge and develop complications including retinal edema, circinate retinopathy, and exudative retinal detachment due to breakdown of the blood–retinal barrier. These complications are directly proportional to the size of the hemangioma and the duration of the neoplasm. Endophytic tumors also may predispose to retinal surface neovascularization with its attendant complications. Neovascular glaucoma may ensue, and phthisis bulbi is a not infrequent end result.

Histopathologic examination of retinal and cerebellar hemangioblastomas reveals closely packed capillaries with intervening cells, believed to be glial in origin, that have abundant foamy cytoplasm (Fig. 4-14B).[45] Occa-

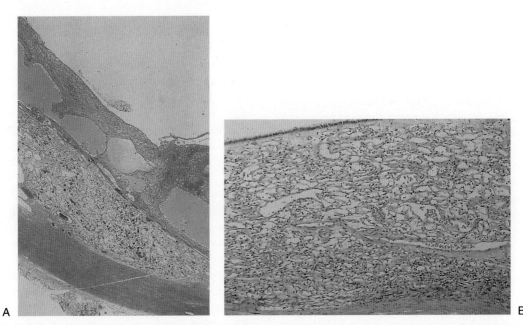

A   B

FIG. 4-13. **(A)** Diffuse choroidal hemangioma with overlying serous retinal detachment. **(B)** Choroidal hemangioma composed of closely packed, thin-walled vascular spaces. (Both courtesy of David Sevel, MD, PhD).

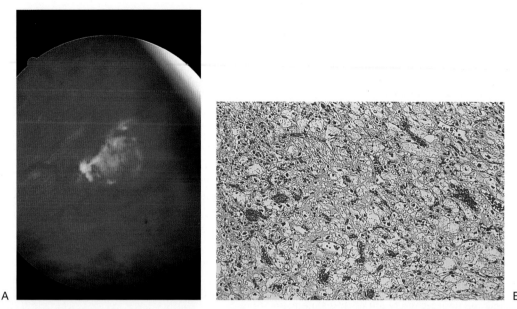

A   B

FIG. 4-14. (A) Retinal angioma with prominent feeder vessels in von Hippel-Lindau syndrome. **(B)** Histopathology demonstrates capillaries separated by cells with clear-to-foamy cytoplasm. (Both courtesy of Careen Y. Lowder, MD, PhD).

sionally more solid-appearing areas are present and may be associated with greater growth potential.

Treatment modalities of the primary tumor have included cryotherapy, diathermy, and laser photocoagulation. Results have been mixed.

Optic Nerve Masses

Optic Nerve Glioma

Gliomas are the most common type of optic nerve tumor in the pediatric population. The median age at diagnosis is 7 years.[46] There is a slight preponderance of females afflicted. Tumors may involve the orbital portion of the nerve alone, intracranial nerve alone, or span both portions of the nerve. The optic chiasm is involved in over half of the cases reported.[46,47] There is a strong association between optic nerve glioma and neurofibromatosis type 1. It is estimated that between 25% and 50% of patients with this neoplasm either have concurrent or subsequent stigmata of neurofibromatosis. Bilateral involvement may occur, but is distinctly uncommon.

As might be expected, vision loss is the predominant presenting symptom, no matter what portion of the nerve involved. Axial proptosis is usually seen in cases with involvement of the orbital portion of the nerve. These neoplasms typically grow slowly, and a significant number may spontaneously stop enlarging. CT and MRI scans are valuable in characterizing the fusiform enlargement of the nerve. The extent of the tumor, however, may be

difficult to determine radiographically because the proximal and distal aspects of the neoplasm taper and blend into normal nerve (Fig. 4-15A). This is also true of histologic examination, making determination of the adequacy of excision by frozen sections difficult if not impossible.

Pathologically, gliomas of the optic nerve are smooth-surfaced, fusiform or dumbbell-shaped if both orbital and intracranial portions are involved (Fig. 4-15B). On cut surface, they demonstrate marked swelling of the nerve proper and may invade into the leptomeninges and expand that space (Fig. 4-15C); however, they almost always are confined by the dura. Secondary meningeal hyperplasia also may occur, contributing to the expansion of the meningeal space and creating a potential pitfall in histologic diagnosis: if only a superficial portion of the neoplasm is biopsied, it might erroneously be interpreted as representative of a meningioma. The occurrence of meningiomas in the pediatric population is well documented, and in this age group, they are often associated with neurofibromatosis type 2.[48]

Microscopically, optic gliomas of childhood are composed of a mildly hypercellular proliferation of pilocytic astrocytes, causing expansion of the bundles of fascicles at the expense of the nerve axons (Fig. 4-15D). Individual astrocytes demonstrate minimal nuclear enlargement and hyperchromasia and typically lack mitotic activity. Often, ribbon-like or globular eosinophilic material known as **Rosenthal fibers** are present within the fibrillary background of these neoplasms and represent intracytoplasmic aggregation of glial filaments. Although useful in charac-

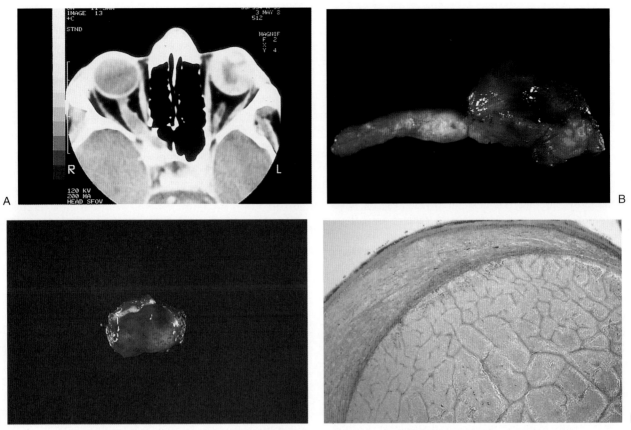

FIG. 4-15. (**A**) CT scan demonstrates fusiform thickening of the right optic nerve with intracranial extension. Note the melanoma in the left eye in this patient with neurofibromatosis (From Antle CM, et al. Uveal malignant melanoma and optic nerve glioma in von Recklinghausen's neurofibromatosis. *Br J Ophthalmol* 1990;74:502–504). (**B**) Appearance externally and (**C**) of transverse section of a resected optic nerve glioma. (**D**) Pilocytic astrocytoma expanding the optic nerve and meningeal space without extradural extension.

terizing the neoplasm as astrocytic, Rosenthal fibers are not pathognomonic for gliomas and can be seen in reactive glial proliferations as well. Hemorrhage and cystic degeneration may supervene in areas. Tumors that have remained in situ for a long period often demonstrate degenerative changes identical to those of "ancient" schwannomas, which include fibrosis, hyalinization of vessel walls, and infiltration by foamy histiocytes.

Treatment decisions are based on the size, growth rate, and location of the tumors. Surgical resection is the treatment of choice when intervention is deemed necessary as for documented posterior extension impinging on the chiasm or hypothalamus. Adjuvant radiation therapy is controversial.[49,50]

Orbital Masses

Space-occupying lesions in the orbit in childhood are quite often benign processes. Inflammatory disorders and vascular and cystic tumors predominate. Malignant tumors of the orbit in the pediatric age are rare; rhabdomyo-sarcoma leads the list of primary orbital malignancies. Metastatic malignancies secondarily involving the orbit, such as neuroblastoma and leukemia, are probably more frequent and must be considered in the differential diagnosis of orbital masses in the young.

Rhabdomyosarcoma

The most common primary malignant process in the orbit in the pediatric population is rhabdomyosarcoma.[51] The mean age at diagnosis is 7 years, and although the range of reported cases is from birth to 78 years, more than 75% of cases occur within the first decade.[51] No racial predilection is known. The neoplasm is slightly more common in males.

Typically, the tumor causes a rapidly progressive exophthalmos, sometimes accompanied by chemosis, ptosis, and ocular congestion. Involvement of the nasal cavity and paranasal sinuses may cause symptoms of nasal stuffiness and epistaxis. Ancillary studies such as CT scans and ultrasonography are helpful in excluding cystic neoplasms from the differential diagnosis and in delineating the extent of disease.

Because the appropriate therapy for rhabdomyosarcoma is a combination of radiation and chemotherapy, the surgical approach is aimed at acquiring sufficient tissue for pathologic confirmation of the clinical diagnosis. Tissue submitted in the fresh state for frozen section diagnosis may be necessary to determine the adequacy and viability of the excised specimen as well as to allow the pathologist latitude in distributing tissue for special procedures, such as electron microscopy, flow cytometry, and cytogenetic and molecular diagnostic studies.

Rhabdomyosarcoma has been subdivided on the basis of cytomorphology and architectural pattern into three categories: embryonal (including the botryoid variant), alveolar, and pleomorphic. **Embryonal rhabdomyosarcoma** is the most common subtype encountered in the orbit and is composed of closely packed, small round-to-spindle cells without any organoid pattern. **Botryoid rhabdomyosarcoma** typically occurs in the genitourinary tract and only rarely in the ocular adnexa. It demonstrates a loose, myxoid appearance beneath mucosal tissue with increased density of tumor cells just beneath the epithelial surface (the so-called "cambium layer"). **Alveolar rhabdomyosarcoma** is the only prognostically significant subtype, in that it conveys a poorer prognosis than the others. Its name comes from the architectural similarity to lung parenchyma in that tumor cells are divided into aggregates by fibrovascular septae. The cells closest to the septae adhere to the wall; those removed from the septae become dyscohesive and float freely in the center of the spaces thus formed (Fig. 4-16A). **Pleomorphic,** or **differentiated rhabdomyosarcoma,** as the name implies, is composed of cells with abundant eosinophilic cytoplasm, with cross striations often found. It is more common in adults.

In all subtypes, pathologic diagnosis of rhabdomyosarcoma is predicated on the identification of some degree of rhabdomyoblastic differentiation within the cytoplasm of tumor cells, often in an otherwise undifferentiated spindle- or small, round-cell neoplasm (Fig. 4-16B). This may be accomplished at the light microscopic level by the presence of cross striations within tumor cells or immunohistochemically by cytoplasmic positivity for muscle-specific actin, myoglobin, or desmin. It may also be accomplished at the ultrastructural level by the presence of thick and thin myofilaments often demonstrating some attempt at sarcomere banding (Fig. 4-16C).[52]

Treatment of rhabdomyosarcoma consists of debulking as much of the tumor as possible without compromising vital structures followed by radiation and chemotherapy. The choice of surgical approach and the amount of tissue procured for histopathologic diagnosis are dictated by the location and extent of the tumor. Those tumors located anteriorly in the orbit are more easily accessible and amenable to resection. Tissue should be submitted for both light and electron microscopy in appropriate fixatives to enhance the chances of obtaining an accurate and specific diagnosis. Prior to adjuvant therapy, the treatment for rhabdomyosarcoma was exenteration, and the mortality rate was on the order of 75% by 3 years. The survival rate now exceeds 90% for the same follow-up period.[53]

Hemangioma

Capillary hemangiomas are the most common neoplasm of the orbit in children. In most cases, they involve the anterior tissues of the orbit.[54,55] Extension into, or involvement solely of, the skin of the eyelids and periorbita cause the typical "strawberry" nevus appearance; however, if it is only subcutaneous, the lesion has a purple-blue discoloration similar to a bruise. Those isolated to the orbit may not be visible and may present with a mass effect in the orbit, causing exophthalmos or extraocular motility disturbance. There is a female predominance, and at least one report has suggested a lower incidence in black children compared with whites.[55]

In approximately one third of cases, the tumors are present at birth, and in the remainder, signs and symptoms are noted by 6 to 12 months of age. At the onset, there may be rapid growth of the neoplasm for weeks to a few months, followed by a time of quiescence and involution measured in years. Complete resolution generally occurs around ages 5 to 6 years, usually without cosmetic deformity; however, both functional deficit (amblyopia, ptosis, strabismus) or physical deformity (residual tumor, fibrosis) may ensue.

The histopathologic appearance of excised tumors reflects the evolutionary sequence noted clinically. In the actively proliferating stage, the neoplasm exhibits marked capillary endothelial proliferation, forming solid nests and cords of plump cells with absent to markedly compressed lumina. The vascular nature of the tumor may thus be difficult to discern, but immunohistochemical stains for endothelial cell markers, such as factor VIII and ULEX Europaeus, identify the cells as vascular in origin. Ultrastructural demonstration of Weibel-Palade bodies within tumor cells also confirms their endothelial nature. Mitotic activity, as would be expected, is evident. Interstitial connective tissue is not well developed. In the quiescent stage, the endothelial cells become flat, and the luminal spaces expand, allowing for a histopathologic diagnosis to be rendered without difficulty (Fig. 4-17). The interstitium is more noticeable and surrounds lobules of capillary proliferation.

In the involutional stage, the capillaries become irregular in outline and progressively obliterated by fibrous tissue. Because the natural history of these neoplasms is one of spontaneous regression, intervention is only required when complications are imminent or likely. These situations would include ptosis due to upper eyelid involvement encroaching upon or obscuring the visual

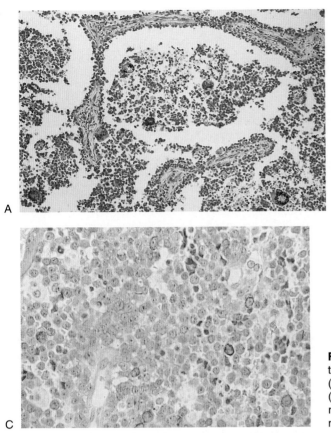

A

B

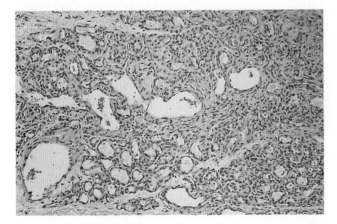

C

FIG. 4-16. (A) Alveolar pattern of rhabdomyosarcoma. Note the multinucleated giant cells within the dyscohesive cells. **(B)** Numerous spindle cells with eosinophilic cytoplasm ("strap" cells). No cross striations are present. **(C)** Immunoreactivity for muscle-specific actin in an embryonal rhabdomyosarcoma. (All courtesy of David J. Wilson, MD.)

axis or creating significant astigmatism by direct pressure on the globe or exophthalmos causing corneal exposure or optic nerve dysfunction.

Intralesional corticosteroid injections are the usual first line of therapy. Alternative therapies include the use of topical and or systemic steroids, interferon-alpha, radiation therapy, laser therapy, and surgical excision.[56]

Lymphangioma

Because lymphoid tissue is not regarded as normally occurring in the orbit, some consider lymphangiomas in

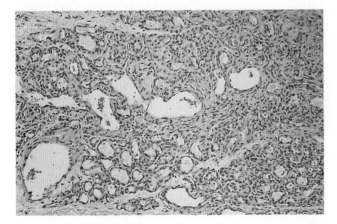

FIG. 4-17. Capillary hemangioma with focally ectatic spaces.

that location to represent choristomas. As with capillary hemangiomas in the same location, approximately one third are present at birth. The remaining cases, however, are detected over a longer span, with most manifesting within the first decade.[57] No sex or racial predilection is evident.

Most cases demonstrate a gradual growth, with waxing and waning especially correlated with onset and resolution of upper respiratory infections. Spontaneous regression is not a clinical characteristic of lymphangioma. Fulminant acute proptosis, however, may occur following infection or trauma due to acute hemorrhage within the tumor, resulting in the so-called "chocolate cyst" when visualized grossly. Such occurrences, if the presenting feature of the tumor, may cause clinical confusion with other causes of rapidly developing proptosis, such as orbital cellulitis or rhabdomyosarcoma. Imaging modalities, particularly MRI, aid in the differentiation. Lymphangiomas demonstrate a multicystic quality with variable intensities corresponding to recent and old hemorrhage.[58]

Histopathologic examination of lymphangioma shows multiple, variably sized, thin-walled cysts lined by flattened endothelial cells that ultrastructurally have an interrupted basal lamina, as opposed to the continuous basal lamina of vascular endothelial cells (Fig. 4-18). Pericytes and smooth muscle are lacking. The neoplasms may be circumscribed, but more commonly are diffusely infiltrative and therefore difficult or impossible to completely

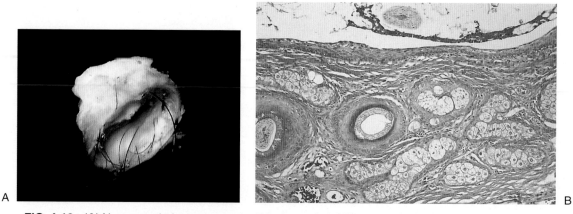

FIG. 4-18. (**A**) Numerous hairs are present within the material filling a dermoid cyst. (**B**) Pilosebaceous structures deep to a stratified squamous epithelial cyst lining.

remove. In pristine spaces without prior hemorrhage, the luminal contents are of a serous nature. Those involved by hemorrhage show partial or complete filling of the lumen by erythrocytes with thrombosis and organization depending on the time of hemorrhage in relation to excision. Fibrosis and hemosiderin deposition within the walls of the cystic spaces are the residual of hemorrhagic episodes. Lymphoid tissue is variable within the interstitium. When present, it may demonstrate germinal center formation.

Due to the diffuse nature of most lymphangiomas, surgical intervention is aimed at alleviating complications of the tumor rather than complete extirpation. Laser therapy may have an adjunctive role.

Choristoma

Dermoid Cyst

Dermoid cysts in the orbit are believed to be a result of entrapment of surface ectoderm within the suture lines of the bony plates of the orbit and craniofacial bones. With time, they enlarge due to cyst formation. The size may change rapidly when the cyst contents are exposed to the immune system and an inflammatory reaction ensues.

Dermoid cysts most frequently occur in the superolateral portion of the orbit. Often they are anterior to the orbital septum and are readily palpable in the upper eyelid. Typically, they are nontender and mobile masses, 1 to 2 cm in greatest dimension. CT scans demonstrate a heterogeneous appearance with molding or a defect of the adjacent bone. Calcification may be present. Surgical exploration may reveal a fibrous stalk attaching the cyst to the adjacent bone. Unless an inflammatory reaction has supervened, the cyst is smooth surfaced and easily excised.

Gross inspection of excised dermoid cysts shows a variably thin-walled cyst containing white-yellow material and hair (Fig. 4-18A). Microscopic examination reveals a cyst lining of keratinizing stratified squamous epithelium containing appendage structures, such as pilosebaceous units, in the wall (Fig. 4-18B). The cyst contents include laminated acellular keratin, hairs, and sebaceous material.

Often there is microscopic evidence of prior rupture of the cyst, with the epithelium destroyed and replaced by a foreign-body granulomatous response to the cyst contents. Rarely, the cyst lining may be completely lost, with the only histologic clue to the etiology of the process being residual hairs, often engulfed by multinucleated giant cells present in an inflammatory mass. Therefore, due to its potent inflammatory stimulus, rupture of the cyst and spillage of its contents during surgical extirpation must be avoided.

Teratoma

Teratomas of the orbit are the ultimate in choristomas in that they recapitulate almost any type of tissue in the body. The vast majority are present at birth or shortly thereafter and often are of massive proportions (Fig. 4-19A).[59] A recognizable eye is usually present anteriorly within the mass. CT, MRI, and ultrasonography of the mass discloses a mixture of solid and cystic elements with the solid-tissue densities ranging from adipose tissue to bone (Fig. 4-19B).

Histopathologically, teratomas contain a veritable treasure trove of tissue types. Cystic areas are typically either dermoid cysts or duplications of luminal structures elsewhere in the body, such as the bronchus or intestine (Fig. 4-19C). Haphazard arrays of adipose tissue, bone, cartilage, and neuroglial tissue are the principal components of the solid areas. All tissues are usually mature histologically. Occasionally, immature neuroblastic foci are present, but only rarely are cases of malignant transformation within an orbital teratoma documented.

In the past, exenteration was typically employed, but

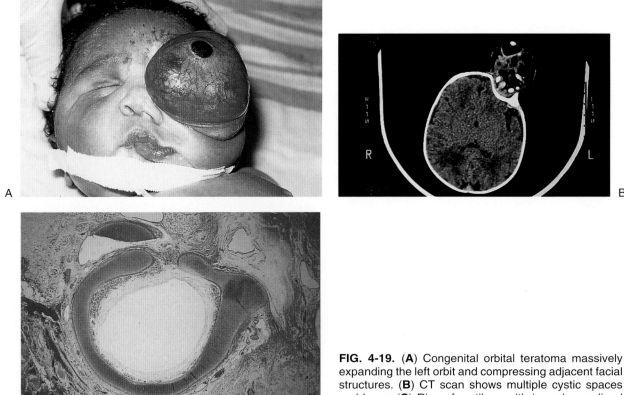

FIG. 4-19. (**A**) Congenital orbital teratoma massively expanding the left orbit and compressing adjacent facial structures. (**B**) CT scan shows multiple cystic spaces and bone. (**C**) Ring of cartilage with inner lumen lined by respiratory epithelium.

more recent attempts to salvage the eye, and possibly even useful vision, have been successful.[59]

REFERENCES

1. Gonnering RS, Kronish JW. Treatment of periorbital molluscum contagiosum by incision and curettage. *Ophthalmic Surg* 1988;19: 325–327.
2. Elsas FJ, Green WR. Epibulbar tumors in childhood. *Am J Ophthalmol* 1975;79:1001–1007.
3. Cunha RP, Cunha MC, Shields JA. Epibulbar tumors in children: a survey of 282 biopsies. *J Pediatr Ophthalmol Strabismus* 1987; 24:249–254.
4. Oakman JH Jr, Lambert SR, Grossniklaus HE. Corneal dermoid: case report and review of classification. *J Pediatr Ophthalmol Strabismus* 1993;30:388–391.
5. Mansour AM, Barber JC, Reinecke RD, Wang FM. Ocular choristomas. *Surv Ophthalmol* 1989;33:339–358.
6. McDonnell PJ, McDonnell JM, Kessis T, Green WR, Shah KV. Detection of human papillomavirus type 6/11 DNA in conjunctival papillomas by in situ hybridization with radioactive probes. *Hum Pathol* 1987;18:1115–1119.
7. Lass JH, Foster CS, Grove AS, et al. Interferon-alpha therapy of recurrent conjunctival papillomas. *Am J Ophthalmol* 1987;103:294–301.
8. Zimmerman LE. Ocular lesions of juvenile xanthogranuloma (nevoxanthoendothelioma). *Trans Am Acad Ophthalmol Otolaryngol* 1965;69:412–442.
9. Hadden OB. Bilateral juvenile xanthogranuloma of the iris. *Br J Ophthalmol* 1975;59:699–702.
10. Tahan SR, Pastel-Levy C, Bhan AK, Mihm MC Jr. Juvenile xanthogranuloma: clinical and pathologic characterization. *Arch Pathol Lab Med* 1989;1057–1061.
11. Knudsen AG Jr. Mutation and cancer: statistical study of retinoblastoma. *Proc Natl Acad Sci USA* 1971;68:820–823.
12. Zhang K, Wang MX, Munier F, et al. Molecular genetics of retinoblastoma. *Int Ophthalmol Clin* 1993;33:53–65.
13. Wiggs JL, Dryja TP. Predicting the risk of hereditary retinoblastoma. *Am J Ophthalmol* 1988;106:346–351.
14. Shields JA, Shields CL, Parsons HM. Differential diagnosis of retinoblastoma. *Retina* 1991;11:232–243.
15. Shields JA. Misconceptions and techniques in the management of retinoblastoma. *Retina* 1992;12:320–330.
16. Broughton WL, Zimmerman LE. A clinicopathologic study of 56 cases of intraocular medulloepithelioma. *Am J Ophthalmol* 1978; 85:407–418.
17. Canning CR, McCartney ACE, Hungerford J. Medulloepithelioma (diktyoma). *Br J Ophthalmol* 1988;72:764–767.
18. Reese AB. Persistence and hyperplasia of the primary vitreous. *Am J Ophthalmol* 1955;40:317–331.
19. Lin AE, Biglan AW, Garver KL. Persistent hyperplastic primary vitreous with vertical transmission. *Ophthalmic Paediatr Genet* 1990;11:121–122.
20. Manschot WA. Persistent hyperplastic primary vitreous. *Arch Ophthalmol* 1958;59:188–203.
21. Duvall J, Miller SL, Cheatle E, Tso MO. Histopathologic study of ocular changes in a syndrome of multiple congenital anomalies. *Am J Ophthalmol* 1987;103:701–705.
22. Pollard ZF. Results of treatment of persistent hyperplastic primary vitreous. *Ophthalmic Surg* 1991;22:48–52.
23. Campbell FP. Coats' disease and congenital vascular retinopathy. *Trans Am Ophthalmol Soc* 1977;74:365–412.
24. Haik BG. Advanced Coats' disease. *Trans Am Ophthalmol Soc* 1991;89:371–476.
25. Wilder HC. Nematode endophthalmitis. *Trans Am Acad Ophthalmol Otolaryngol* 1950;55:99–109.
26. Shields JA. Ocular toxocariasis: a review. *Surv Ophthalmol* 1984; 28:361–381.

27. Gillespie SH, Dinning WJ, Voller A, Crowcroft NS. The spectrum of ocular toxocariasis. *Eye* 1993;7:415–418.
28. Phelps D. Retinopathy of prematurity. *Curr Probl Pediatr* 1992; 22:349–371.
29. Weakley DR Jr, Spencer R. Current concepts in retinopathy of prematurity. *Early Hum Dev* 1992;30:121–138.
30. Hunter DG, Mukai S. Retinopathy of prematurity: pathogenesis, diagnosis, and treatment. *Int Ophthalmol Clin* 1994;34:163–184.
31. Kretzer FL, Hittner HM. Spindle cells and retinopathy of prematurity: interpretations and predictions. *Birth Defects* 1988;24:147–168.
32. Foos RY. Retinopathy of prematurity: pathologic correlation of clinical stages. *Retina* 1987;7:260–276.
33. Pierce EA, Mukai S. Controversies in the management of retinopathy of prematurity. *Int Ophthalmol Clin* 1994;34:121–148.
34. Glass P, Avery GB, Subramanian KN, et al. Effect of bright light in the hospital nursery on the incidence of retinopathy of prematurity. *New Engl J Med* 1985;313:401–404.
35. Ackerman B, Sherwonit E, Williams J. Reduced incidental light exposure: effect on the development of retinopathy of prematurity in low birth weight infants. *Pediatrics* 1989;83:958–962.
36. National Institutes of Health Consensus Development Conference. Neurofibromatosis: conference statement. *Arch Neurol* 1988;45: 575–578.
37. Ragge NK. Clinical and genetic patterns of neurofibromatosis 1 and 2. *Br J Ophthalmol* 1993;77:662–672.
38. Specht CS, Smith TW. Uveal malignant melanoma and von Recklinghausen's neurofibromatosis. *Cancer* 1988;62:812–817.
39. Short MP, Richardson EP Jr, Haines JL, Kwiatkowski DJ. Clinical, neuropathological and genetic aspects of the tuberous sclerosis complex. *Brain Pathol* 1995;5:173–179.
40. Robertson DM. Ophthalmic manifestations of tuberous sclerosis. *Ann NY Acad Sci* 1991;615:17–25.
41. Zimmer-Galler IE, Robertson DM. Long-term observation of retinal lesions in tuberous sclerosis. *Am J Ophthalmol* 1995;119:318–324.
42. Sullivan TJ, Clarke MP, Morin JD. The ocular manifestations of the Sturge-Weber syndrome. *J Pediatr Ophthalmol Strabismus* 1992;29:349–356.
43. Glenn GM, Linehan WM, Hosoe S, et al. Screening for von Hippel-Lindau by DNA polymorphism analysis. *JAMA* 1992;267:1226–1231.
44. Horton WA, Wong V, Eldridge R. Von Hippel-Lindau disease: clinical and pathological manifestations in nine families with 50 affected members. *Arch Intern Med* 1976;136:769–777.
45. Choyke PL, Glenn GM, Walther MM, et al. Von Hippel-Lindau disease: genetic, clinical, and imaging features. *Radiology* 1995; 629–642.
46. Dutton JJ. Gliomas of the anterior visual pathway. *Surv Ophthalmol* 1994;38:427–452.
47. Cohen ME, Duffner PK. Optic pathway tumors. *Neurol Clin* 1991; 9:467–477.
48. Karp LA, Zimmerman LE, Borit A, Spencer W. Primary intraorbital meningiomas. *Arch Ophthalmol* 1974;91:24–28.
49. Wright JE, McNab AA, McDonald WI. Optic nerve glioma and the management of optic nerve tumours in the young. *Br J Ophthalmol* 1989;73:967–974.
50. Levin LA, Jakobiec FA. Optic nerve tumors of childhood: a decision-analytical approach to their diagnosis. *Int Ophthalmol Clin* 1992;32:223–240.
51. Knowles DM, Jakobiec FA, Potter GD, Jones IS. Ophthalmic striated muscle neoplasms: a clinico-pathologic review. *Surv Ophthalmol* 1976;21:219–261.
52. McLean IW, Burnier MN, Zimmerman LE, Jakobiec FA. Tumors of the orbit. In: Rosai J, ed. *Atlas of tumor pathology*, ed 3. Washington: Armed Forces Institute of Pathology, 1994.
53. Wharam M, Beltangady M, Hays D, et al. Localized orbital rhabdomyosarcoma: an interim report of the Intergroup Rhabdomyosarcoma Study Committee. *Ophthalmology* 1987;94:251–254.
54. Holds JB. The spectrum of orbital vascular disease. *Int Ophthalmol Clin* 1992;32:59–72.
55. Haik BG, Karcioglu ZA, Gordon RA, Pechous BP. Capillary hemangioma (infantile periocular hemangioma). *Surv Ophthalmol* 1994; 38:399–426.
56. Bilyk JR, Adamis AP, Mulliken JB. Treatment options for periorbital hemangioma of infancy. *Int Ophthalmol Clin* 1992;32:95–109.
57. Bond JB, Haik BG, Taveras JL, et al. Magnetic resonance imaging of orbital lymphangioma with and without gadolinium contrast enhancement. *Ophthalmology* 1992;99:1318–1324.
58. Harris GJ, Sakol PJ, Bonavolonta G, De Conciliis C. An analysis of thirty cases of orbital lymphangioma: pathophysiologic considerations and management recommendations. *Ophthalmology* 1990; 97:1583–1592.
59. Kivelä T, Tarkkanen A. Orbital germ cell tumors revisited: a clinicopathological approach to classification. *Surv Ophthalmol* 1994; 38:541–554.

BIBLIOGRAPHY

Bateman JB, Punnett HH, Harley RD. Genetics of eye disease. In: Nelson LB, Calhoun JH, Harley RD, eds. *Pediatric ophthalmology*, ed 3. Philadelphia: WB Saunders, 1991;chap 1.

Cotran PR, Bajart AM. Congenital corneal opacities. *Int Ophthalmol Clin* 1992;32:93-105.

Dryja TP. Fundamentals of ophthalmologic genetics. In: Albert DM, Jakobiec FA, eds. *Principles and practice of ophthalmology: basic sciences*. Philadelphia: WB Saunders, 1994;chap 32.

Eller AW, Brown GC. Retinal disorders of childhood. *Pediatr Clin North Am* 1983;30:1087-1101.

Font RL, Ferry AP. The phakomatoses. *Int Ophthalmol Clin* 1972;12: 1-50.

Gayle MO, Kissoon N, Hered RW, Harwood-Nuss A. Retinal hemorrhage in the young child: a review of etiology, predisposed conditions, and clinical implications. *J Emerg Med* 1995;13:233-239.

Mattox C, Walton DS. Hereditary primary childhood glaucomas. *Int Ophthalmol Clin* 1993;33:121-134.

Nelson LB, Wagner RS. Pediatric cataract surgery. *Int Ophthalmol Clin* 1994;34:165-189.

Volpe NJ, Jakobiec FA. Pediatric orbital tumors. *Int Ophthalmol Clin* 1992;32:201-221.

Weiss A. Acute conjunctivitis in childhood. *Curr Probl Pediatr* 1994; 24:4-11.

Wiggs JL. Molecular genetics and ocular disease. *Int Ophthalmol Clin* 1993;33:1-36.

Ophthalmic Pathology with Clinical Correlations,
edited by Joseph W. Sassani, M.D.
Lippincott-Raven Publishers, Philadelphia © 1997.

CHAPTER 5

Cornea and Sclera

Alan D. Proia

CORNEA

Normal Anatomy and Histology

The human cornea is circular when viewed from its posterior surface, but is oval when viewed from the front because of a more prominent limbus superiorly and inferiorly.[1,2] The adult cornea has a horizontal diameter of 11.5 to 12.6 mm and a vertical diameter of 10.5 to 11.7 mm, depending on how the point of transition from the cornea to sclera is defined. The posterior surface of the cornea is more spherical than the anterior surface, so the central cornea is thinner (0.52 mm on average) than the periphery (0.65 mm or greater).

The normal human cornea is composed of five layers: the epithelium, Bowman's layer, stroma, Descemet's membrane, and the endothelium (Fig. 5-1).[1–4] The **epithelium** normally represents 10% of the corneal thickness and is a nonkeratinizing, stratified, squamous epithelium of four to six cell layers. The epithelium contains numerous nerve endings, but these are not visible by routine microscopy. The epithelium is attached to a thin basement membrane (basal lamina), which is most readily recognized by its purple color with periodic acid-Schiff (PAS) stain.

Bowman's layer is an 8- to 14-μm thick acellular band of randomly arrayed collagen fibers and lies along the anterior surface of the stroma. It has a similar degree of eosinophilia as the stroma, does not react positively with PAS stain, and is recognizable by its acellularity. Bowman's layer does not regenerate following injury, and this feature is a useful clue for superficial, well-healed, corneal injuries.

The **stroma** accounts for approximately 90% of the corneal thickness and is composed of stacked lamellae of collagen fibrils with interspersed cells (keratocytes) and extracellular matrix containing glycosaminoglycans and proteoglycans. A rare mononuclear leukocyte or granulocyte is observed in the normal cornea. Blood vessels normally are absent. The keratocytes (stromal fibroblasts) occupy 3% to 5% of the stromal volume and are fusiform with thin nuclei and ill-defined cell borders. The keratocytes synthesize and secrete stromal collagens and extracellular matrix. The extracellular matrix maintains the precise orientation and separation of the collagen fibrils necessary for optical clarity of the cornea. Dehydration of the cornea during processing for paraffin embedding results in artifactual clefts in the stroma due to separation of the collagen lamellae.

Descemet's membrane lies on the posterior surface of the stroma and is the basement membrane secreted by the endothelium. Descemet's membrane is acellular, eosinophilic in hematoxylin-and-eosin (H&E)-stained sections, and stains positively using PAS stain. The anterior portion of Descemet's membrane is sometimes slightly less eosinophilic than the posterior portion. Descemet's membrane is secreted throughout life, and its thickness consequently increases with age. It may thicken further in pathologic conditions such as bullous keratopathy and Fuchs' endothelial dystrophy. The normal and pathologic thickening of Descemet's membrane occurs in the posterior portion of the membrane; the anterior portion remains of relatively constant thickness (approximately 3 μm) throughout life. The posterior portion of Descemet's membrane increases in thickness with age. At 2 years of age it averages 2 μm thick; at age 80 years, it is 10 μm thick.[5]

The **corneal endothelium** is a single layer of cells approximately 4 to 6 μm thick. When viewed from the posterior surface, the endothelial cells are predominantly hexagonal and about 20 μm wide. In histologic cross-sections, the endothelial cells appear rectangular with pale staining, granular to finely vacuolated cytoplasm, and a centrally located round-to-oval nucleus. The number of endothelial cells decreases with age, and the remaining cells flatten to cover Descemet's membrane. The endothelium actively pumps water from the corneal stroma and is essential for normal corneal hydration. The endothelial

A.D. Proia: Departments of Pathology and Ophthalmology Duke University Medical Center, Durham, North Carolina 2771

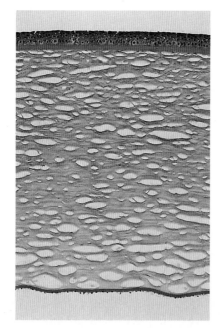

FIG. 5-1. The normal cornea is composed of five cell layers. The epithelium accounts for about 10% of the corneal thickness and the stroma for about 90%. The clefts in the stroma are an artifact resulting from dehydration during histologic processing.

cells are fragile, but they are normally protected by their location in the anterior chamber. Loss of endothelial cells from trauma, such as surgery, or from pathologic conditions, such as Fuchs' endothelial dystrophy, may lead to corneal edema and bullous keratopathy.

Developmental Abnormalities

Developmental abnormalities of the cornea are rare, and often involve other anterior segment structures.[2,6] These conditions are summarized in Table 1, and the reader is referred to the articles by Spencer[2] and Waring and co-workers[6] for a detailed discussion of these entities. An example of Peters' anomaly is shown in Fig. 5-2 because this developmental anomaly most frequently leads to surgical intervention.

Nonspecific Responses of the Cornea to Injury, Disease, and Aging

All layers of the cornea may undergo nonspecific responses to injury, disease, or aging[2,4,7] (Table 2).

The most common nonspecific response of the epithelium is edema, which is almost always accompanied by a reduction in the number of corneal endothelial cells. Epithelial edema is manifest as hydropic swelling of the epithelial cells, which causes clearing (pallor) of the cytoplasm around their nuclei (Fig. 5-3). The basal epithelial

cells often assume a columnar configuration instead of their normal cuboidal profiles. Corneal edema also may result in separation of the epithelium from Bowman's layer (bullae). In cases of chronic epithelial edema, the epithelium above the bullae may thin and rupture. Repeated cycles of this may lead to abnormal epithelial healing with deposition of basement membrane within the epithelium. Sometimes, intraepithelial cysts containing degenerating epithelial cells also form after longstanding edema (Fig. 5-4). The histologic appearance of the intraepithelial basement membrane and cysts resulting from edema is identical to that of map-dot-fingerprint dystro-

TABLE 1. *Development abnormalities of the cornea*

Name of abnormality	Most common anatomic features
Axenfeld's anomaly	Prominent Schwalbe's ring (often displaced anteriorly) with attached strands of tissue from the peripheral iris; termed *Axenfeld's syndrome* when glaucoma is present
Cornea plana congenita	Flat, thin cornea with hazy limbus and stromal clouding; shallow anterior chamber
Keratoglobus	Corneas of normal size but diffusely thinned
Megalocornea	Enlargement of the anterior segment; deep anterior chamber
Microcornea	Corneal diameter less than 10 mm, but histologically unremarkable
Peters' anomaly	Central cornea is opacified in region where Descemet's membrane and endothelium are absent; strands of iris stroma extend from iris collarette region to attach to posterior cornea at edge of defect in Descemet's membrane and endothelium
Posterior keratoconus	Dome-shaped central thinning of the posterior cornea due to loss of stroma
Rieger's anomaly	Anterior chamber angle changes similar to Axenfeld's anomaly but with associated iris abnormalities such as loss of stroma, off-center pupil (corectopia), or slitlike pupil; *Rieger's syndrome* has associated dental and skeletal abnormalities[36]
Sclerocornea	Peripheral or diffuse opacification of the cornea; cornea histologically resembles sclera

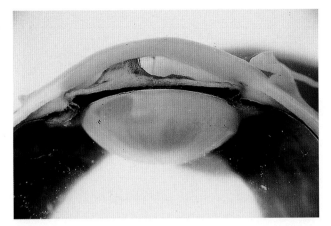

FIG. 5-2. Peters' anomaly demonstrating iris strands attached to a paracentral posterior corneal defect where Descemet's membrane and endothelium are absent.

phy.[8,9] Chronic corneal edema frequently results in accumulation of fibrocollagenous tissue (fibrocollagenous pannus) between the epithelium and Bowman's layer (Fig. 5-5). The pannus sometimes contains blood vessels (fibrovascular pannus), but this finding is more common following penetrating keratoplasty or inflammation of the cornea than in uncomplicated corneal edema (Fig. 5-6).

Keratinization and conjunctivalization are uncommon, but are clinically serious, nonspecific reactions that involve the corneal epithelium. **Keratinization** is a charac-

TABLE 2. Nonspecific responses of the cornea to injury, disease, or aging

Corneal layer	Responses
Epithelium	Hydropic swelling (edema) Bullae Intraepithelial basement membrane Intraepithelial cysts Subepithelial pannus (fibrocollagenous or fibrovascular) Keratinization Conjunctivalization
Bowman's layer	Calcific band keratopathy Chronic actinic keratopathy
Stroma	Lipid accumulation (arcus lipoides) Edema Inflammation Ulceration Scarring Vascularization Amyloid deposition
Descemet's membrane	Diffuse thickening Guttata (guttae) Folds or tears Granulomatous inflammatory reaction
Endothelium	Reduced cell number Increased cell size (spreading) Retrocorneal fibrous membrane

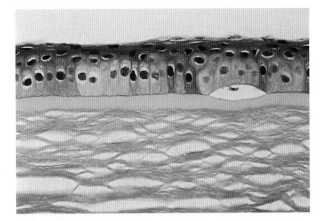

FIG. 5-3. Epithelial edema is manifest as hydropic swelling of the epithelial cells. In this example, the basal cells exhibit pallor and clearing of the perinuclear cytoplasm. The basal epithelial cells have assumed a columnar configuration instead of their normal cuboidal profiles. A subepithelial bulla is between the basal epithelium and Bowman's layer to the right of center.

teristic manifestation of vitamin A deficiency (xerophthalmia), but in developed countries it more commonly reflects keratitis sicca, superior limbic keratoconjunctivitis, or cicatricial pemphigoid. Keratinization is histologically manifest as a thickened corneal epithelium with the superficial layers more flattened and eosinophilic than usual. Conjunctival keratinization almost always occurs together with corneal epithelial keratinization. **Conjunctivalization,** or overgrowth of conjunctival epithelium onto the cornea, occurs after an extensive injury of the corneal surface that extends beyond the limbus. Such damage may result from chemical injury, cicatricial pemphigoid, or Stevens-Johnson syndrome. Conjunctivalization is readily recognized by the presence of goblet cells in the epithelium covering the cornea. The cornea typically is severely scarred and vascularized.

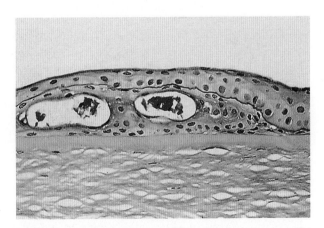

FIG. 5-4. Chronic corneal epithelial edema may result in intraepithelial basement membrane and cysts containing degenerating epithelial cells. The basement membrane is easily visualized using periodic acid-Schiff stain.

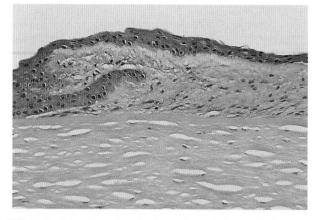

FIG. 5-5. Chronic corneal edema frequently results in accumulation of fibrocollagenous tissue (fibrocollagenous pannus) between the epithelium and Bowman's layer.

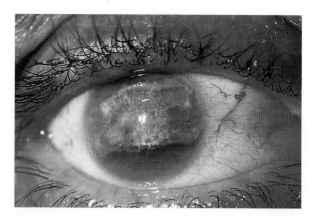

FIG. 5-7. Advanced calcific band keratopathy with opacification extending horizontally across the central cornea in the interpalpebral region (Courtesy of Gary N. Foulks, MD).

Bowman's layer may undergo calcification in the horizontal meridian of the interpalpebral region, most commonly following prolonged, chronic inflammation. Much less frequently, Bowman's layer may become calcified in association with systemic hypercalcemia.[10] The calcification begins at the medial and temporal limbus and may extend to form a band across the central cornea (Fig. 5-7); hence the name **calcific band keratopathy.** In many cases, the calcium appears as discrete basophilic particles within Bowman's layer (Fig. 5-8). The identity of the calcium can be confirmed using histochemical stains such as von Kossa's or alizarin red S. In longstanding cases of calcific band keratopathy, Bowman's layer may be fragmented, and the calcified fragments may be present within fibrocollagenous pannus or scarred anterior stroma.

Chronic actinic keratopathy initially involves the peripheral cornea in the horizontal meridian, and with time, it may extend across the cornea in a fashion resembling calcific band keratopathy (Fig. 5-9). In chronic actinic keratopathy, Bowman's layer and the anterior stroma contain amorphous, extracellular globules (concretions) of protein, which may be pale staining or lightly basophilic.[11] These globules are larger and more irregular than the particles in calcific band keratopathy, and they are not limited to Bowman's layer (Fig. 5-10). The globules are similar to those observed in pingueculae, pterygia, and occasionally in actinic (solar) elastosis of the skin. Clinically, the particles are usually bilateral and are white, gray, or yellow. Chronic actinic keratopathy is most frequent in individuals chronically exposed to excessive ultraviolet light, and its incidence increases with age. Chronic actinic keratopathy is known by several other names, including climatic droplet keratopathy, spheroidal degeneration of the cornea, Labrador keratopathy, and noncalcific band keratopathy. Globules identical to those in chronic actinic keratopathy may accumulate unilaterally in the cornea in association with absolute glaucoma, phthisis bulbi, or chronic corneal inflammation and scarring. Such cases are referred to as spheroidal degeneration

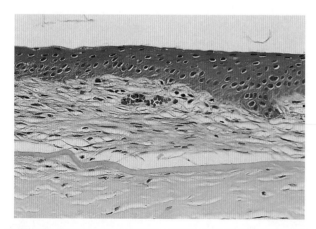

FIG. 5-6. A pannus containing blood vessels (fibrovascular pannus) developed in this patient with chronic corneal edema following a penetrating keratoplasty.

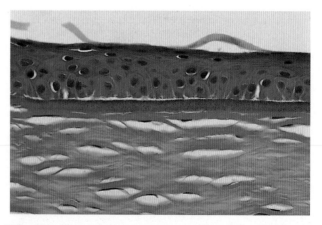

FIG. 5-8. The calcium appears as basophilic stippling of Bowman's layer in this case of calcific band keratopathy, which developed in a patient who received intravitreal silicone oil for reattachment of a large retinal detachment associated with proliferative vitreoretinopathy .

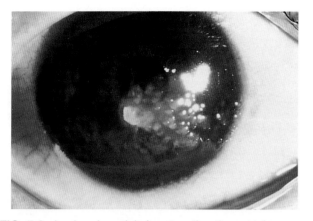

FIG. 5-9. In chronic actinic keratopathy, the proteinaceous deposits may have a nodular pattern against a hazy background. In advanced cases, the deposits may extend across the cornea in a fashion resembling calcific band keratopathy (Courtesy of Gary N. Foulks, MD).

of the cornea, although as noted earlier, some authors use this term to refer to the bilateral condition.

Nonspecific responses of the corneal stroma include lipid accumulation (arcus lipoides), edema, inflammation (discussed later), ulceration, scarring, vascularization, and amyloid deposition.[2,7,12,13] **Arcus lipoides** (also known as arcus senilis or arcus juvenilis) can occur at any age, although it is almost always found in older individuals. In younger individuals, corneal arcus is sometimes, but not always, a reflection of hyperlipidemia.[10] Clinically, arcus senilis is an opaque zone near the corneal periphery that begins superiorly and inferiorly. With time, the zone of lipid infiltration may extend to form a ring around the corneal periphery. The opaque zone is separated from the limbus by a narrow band of clear cornea. Arcus is not apparent in paraffin-embedded tissue sections because of the lipid being dissolved during histologic processing. Using frozen sections stained for lipid (oil red O, Sudan

IV), lipid accumulation is seen in the periphery of Bowman's layer, in the stroma, and within peripheral Descemet's membrane. The lipid accumulation has the cross-sectional appearance of an hourglass.[2]

Edema is another common stromal response and occurs in conjunction with corneal trauma, inflammation, and glaucoma. Stromal edema results in a thickened cornea, and in severe cases, there is a reduction in or absence of the normal artifactual clefts between collagen lamellae. Stromal edema reduces the normal transparency of the cornea.

Corneal ulceration may result from bacterial, viral, or fungal infection, as a consequence of systemic diseases of immunity (especially rheumatoid arthritis), or as a result of chemical or thermal injury. There is a marked inflammatory response when ulceration is due to infection, chemicals, or thermal injury, but stromal ulceration or ''melting'' associated with rheumatoid arthritis may occur with only a mild degree of leukocytic infiltration.[4]

Stromal scarring is recognizable by the loss of normal lamellar architecture and is usually associated with discontinuity in Bowman's layer (Fig. 5-11). Hypercellularity, due to proliferation of keratocytes, and accumulation of lightly basophilic glycosaminoglycans are frequent in early scars, but these changes diminish with time. There is a variable inflammatory infiltrate depending on the time elapsed since corneal injury.

Corneal vascularization is a nonspecific sequela to numerous inflammatory processes involving the cornea. In the United States, it is most frequently a result of infection or accidental trauma or is a complication of penetrating keratoplasty. Corneal vascularization is a major clinical problem because it interferes with vision and predisposes the patient to a much higher incidence of corneal graft failure. It is readily recognized clinically and in histologic sections because the normal cornea is avascular.

Amyloid deposits occur in the corneal stroma as a nonspecific result of longstanding corneal diseases including

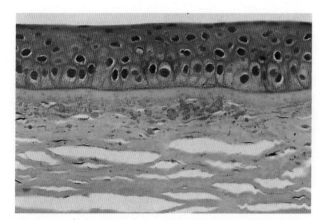

FIG. 5-10. In chronic actinic keratopathy, Bowman's layer and the anterior stroma contain amorphous, extracellular globules of protein, which may be pale staining or lightly basophilic.

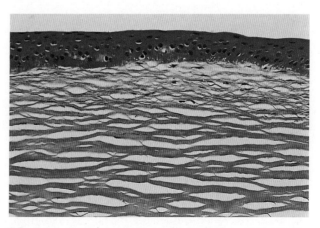

FIG. 5-11. Corneal scarring with loss of normal lamellar architecture, hypercellularity, and absence of Bowman's layer.

trauma, keratoconus, trachoma, chronic actinic keratopathy, and syphilitic interstitial keratitis.[12] The amyloid deposits associated with syphilitic interstitial keratitis may mimic those of lattice corneal dystrophy (LCD) in histologic sections. The deposits following trauma may be massive.

Descemet's membrane may undergo diffuse thickening, formation of guttata, folding or tearing, or development of a granulomatous inflammatory reaction as nonspecific responses to injury. Mild chronic endothelial disease, as seen after cataract surgery, is the most common cause of diffuse thickening of Descemet's membrane. This thickening is often uniform, but may be moderately irregular with an undulating posterior surface, often described clinically as a "beaten metal" appearance. Formation of focal excrescences (guttata or guttae) is ubiquitous in the periphery of Descemet's membrane in adults, and the number increases with age. These peripherally located guttata are referred to as **Hassall-Henle warts.** Guttata involving the central cornea are predominantly seen in individuals with Fuchs' dystrophy (discussed later), but they are also observed as a sequela to syphilitic interstitial keratitis, with macular corneal dystrophy, and rarely as a result of trauma. The secondary guttata in cases of interstitial keratitis and trauma tend to be less uniform than those due to Fuchs' dystrophy (Fig. 5-12).

Irregular folds in Descemet's membrane are almost always the result of stromal edema. In contrast, tears most commonly occur from penetrating injuries and less commonly from keratoconus. Remote tears may be difficult to recognize in histologic sections because the endothelium migrates over the wound site and new Descemet's membrane is deposited. This new Descemet's membrane is thinner than the surrounding membrane, and the edge of the preexisting membrane commonly is visible (Fig. 5-13). PAS stain helps to delineate sites of remote damage

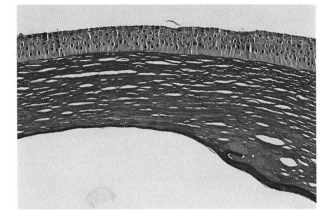

FIG. 5-13. This patient with keratoconus had a remote rupture in Descemet's membrane leading to acute stromal edema (hydrops). By the time the penetrating keratoplasty was performed, a thin layer of new Descemet's membrane had been deposited over the previously bare posterior surface of the stroma. Note the curling of Descemet's membrane at the edge of the rupture site.

to Descemet's membrane. A granulomatous inflammatory reaction to Descemet's membrane is uncommon, but when it does develop, it is usually from chronic herpetic stromal keratitis (Fig. 5-14).

Nonspecific changes in the corneal endothelium result from accidental or surgical trauma (cataract surgery), during failure of corneal grafts, and less commonly from chronic glaucoma. Because the endothelium has no to limited ability to replicate, any insult to the endothelium results in a diminished number of cells. The remaining cells flatten (increase in size) to cover as much as possible of the surface of Descemet's membrane.

Fibrous membranes between Descemet's membrane and the corneal endothelium typically are seen in specimens of failed corneal grafts (Fig. 5-15), and they occur in a small but significant proportion of corneal transplant buttons removed because of aphakic or pseudophakic bul-

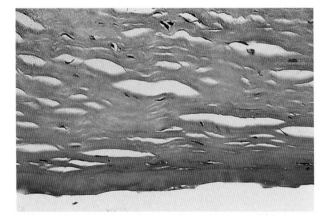

FIG. 5-12. Thickened Descemet's membrane with irregularly shaped and almost confluent guttata resulting from syphilitic interstitial keratitis. Also note the small blood vessel within the posterior stroma.

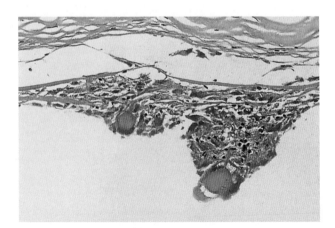

FIG. 5-14. A granulomatous response to Descemet's membrane resulted from herpes simplex virus stromal keratitis.

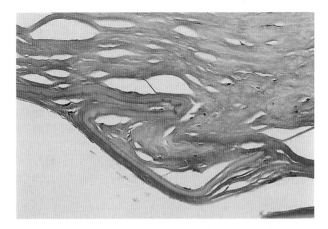

FIG. 5-15. Retrocorneal fibrous membranes are frequently seen in failed corneal grafts, although the extent of the membrane varies widely. A retrocorneal membrane is most commonly observed only in the vicinity of the donor–host interface.

lous keratopathy. Retrocorneal fibrous membranes also may result from vitreous or silicone oil coming into contact with the posterior surface of the cornea.

Inflammation and Infections

The cornea may exhibit acute, chronic, or granulomatous inflammation. *Acute inflammation* is characterized by localized or diffuse edema, infiltration predominantly by neutrophils, hyperemia of the limbal vessels, and iritis. It occurs most commonly following trauma or infection. A mild neutrophilic infiltrate is seen in 5% to 10% of corneal buttons removed during penetrating keratoplasty for chronic bullous keratopathy. Severe acute inflammation may lead to ulceration or perforation. It is important to realize that neutrophils infiltrating the corneal stroma may be difficult to differentiate from lymphocytes because they become distorted during their insinuation between the collagenous lamellae (Fig. 5-16).

Chronic inflammation of the cornea may result from lack of prompt resolution of the stimulus that caused the acute inflammatory response, or it may reflect viral infection or graft failure. The chronic inflammatory infiltrate consists mainly of lymphocytes with fewer macrophages. It is often referred to as a mononuclear leukocytic infiltrate. **Granulomatous inflammation** of the cornea is usually a reaction to a foreign body such as a suture, but also results from injury to Descemet's membrane or to stromal keratitis from herpes simplex virus (HSV) infection. The granulomatous keratitis due to HSV may occur at any level of the stroma but is frequently just beneath Bowman's layer or in the vicinity of Descemet's membrane. Granulomatous keratitis is not specific for HSV infection because it may be observed in patients with juvenile xanthogranuloma, sarcoidosis, and leprosy.[4]

Granulomatous inflammation is histologically defined by an infiltrate of epithelioid histiocytes (recognizable by their large size, abundance of eosinophilic cytoplasm, and indistinct cell borders), lymphocytes, and variable numbers of multinucleated giant cells.

Corneal infection may result from bacteria,[14,15] viruses,[16–18] fungi,[19,20] and parasites.[21,22] The more common organisms causing corneal infection within each category and some of their clinical characteristics are listed in Table 3.

Bacterial infection may result in ulcerative or nonulcerative keratitis. Ulcerative bacterial keratitis is clinically manifest as decreased visual acuity, photophobia, pain, redness, swelling, and discharge. It is rapidly progressive unless promptly and adequately treated. Factors predisposing to the development of ulcerative bacterial keratitis include corneal abrasions with contaminated matter, contact lens use (especially extended wear lenses), ocular surface disease (HSV infection, keratitis sicca, bullous keratopathy, previous surgery, atopic disease), and eyelid disease. The bacteria most frequently isolated from ulcers associated with contact lens use are *Pseudomonas aeruginosa, Staphylococcus* sp., and *Serratia marcescens*. Bacteria most commonly associated with ulcerative keratitis in patients with ocular surface disease are *Staphylococcus* sp., *Pseudomonas aeruginosa, Streptococcus pneumoniae* (pneumococcus), and *Moraxella* sp. Histologically, ulcerative bacterial keratitis exhibits severe acute inflammation with varying degrees of ulceration and stromal necrosis. The stromal necrosis causes basophilia and a smudged appearance to the stromal collagen.

Nonulcerative bacterial keratitis, more commonly referred to as interstitial keratitis, is much less common than ulcerative keratitis in the United States, but remains an important cause of visual impairment in underdeveloped countries. The keratitis results in mildly to severely diminished visual acuity, ocular pain, tearing, and photophobia. It is nonsuppurative, stro-

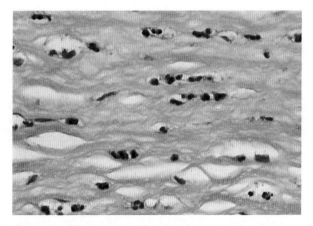

FIG. 5-16. Neutrophils infiltrating the corneal stroma may be difficult to distinguish from lymphocytes because their lobules are often obscured by compression between collagenous lamellae.

TABLE 3. *Some agents causing corneal infections*

Organism	Clinical features
BACTERIA	
Ulcerative keratitis	
Streptococcus pneumoniae	After trauma; rapid spread; hypopyon; fibrin on endothelial side of ulcer; deep stromal abscesses
Staphylococcus sp.	Compromised corneas; tend to stay localized with distinct borders and clear surrounding stroma
Pseudomonas aeruginosa	After trauma; rapid spread; hypopyon; diffuse epithelial edema; ring ulcer if untreated
Moraxella sp.	After trauma in systemically debilitated patients; indolent oval ulcer; inferior cornea; mild anterior chamber reaction
Nonulcerative (interstitial) keratitis	
Treponema pallidum	Congenital syphilis more common; progressive, florid, and regressive stages; bilateral; deep stromal haze with ghost vessels
Borrelia burgdorferi	Lyme disease; mild bilateral decrease in vision; multiple nebular stromal opacities
Mycobacterium leprae	Quite rare in the United States; superficial keratitis; usually begins in superior temporal quadrant
VIRUSES	
Herpes simplex virus	Recurrent disease: infectious, dendritic, ulceration; trophic [metaherpetic] ulceration; viral necrotizing keratitis; interstitial keratitis, immune rings, and limbal vasculitis; disciform keratitis; endotheliitis, trabeculitis, or iridocyclitis.
Varicella-zoster virus	Chickenpox: superficial punctate keratitis, branching dendritic ulcers, immune disciform disease. Herpes zoster ophthalmicus: punctate keratitis, pseudodendrites, anterior stromal infiltrates, etc.
Adenovirus	Epidemic keratoconjunctivitis: punctate keratitis followed by subepithelial infiltrates
FUNGI	
Fusarium sp.	Stromal infiltrates: feathery, hyphate edges; gray, dry, and slightly elevated above corneal surface
Aspergillus sp.	Similar to *Fusarium* sp.
Candida sp.	Stromal keratitis tends to be localized with a "collar button" configuration
Curvularia sp.	Similar to *Fusarium* sp., pigment may be apparent
Acremonium (*Cephalosporium*) sp.	Similar to *Fusarium* sp.
Paecilomyces sp.	Similar to *Fusarium* sp.
PARASITES	
Protozoa	
Acanthamoeba sp.	Contact lens wearers; photophobia; severe pain; dendritiform ulcer; ring infiltrate
Microsporidia	Patients with AIDS; punctate epithelial keratopathy
Hemoflagellates	
Leishmania sp.	Stromal keratitis with vascularization (uncommon)
Trypanosoma brucei	African trypanosomiasis (sleeping sickness); interstitial keratitis
Nematodes	
Onchocerca volvulus	Punctate keratitis; sclerosing keratitis with vascularization
Thelazia callipaeda	Oriental eye worm; superficial scarring of corneal surface from repeated migration of parasites
Thelazia californiensis	Superficial scarring of corneal surface from repeated migration of parasites
Gnathostoma spinigerum	Corneal ulceration (uncommon)

mal, and often results in vascularization. The most common agent causing interstitial keratitis in the United States is *Treponema pallidum;* approximately 90% of the cases result from congenital infection.[15]

HSV is by far the most common virus causing clinically significant corneal disease, and it is the leading infectious cause of corneal blindness in the United States. Approximately 500,000 cases of HSV corneal infection are reported here annually.[18] Ocular HSV infection is caused primarily by type 1 (oral) HSV, although it may result from type 2 (genital) HSV infection. Corneal HSV infection is divided into three groups: congenital and neonatal, primary, and recurrent. Congenital and neonatal disease is extremely rare.[18] Primary ocular HSV infection is usually subclinical, and 60% of children have been infected by age 5 years and are carriers of the latent virus within their trigeminal ganglia and autonomic nervous system. When manifest clinically, primary HSV infection may cause acute follicular conjunctivitis or keratoconjunctivitis. Primary HSV keratitis is usually confined to the epithelium, and it may initially be a nonspecific diffuse punctate keratitis that progresses to multiple microdendritic figures. Recurrent ocular HSV disease is more serious than primary infection because the patients have both cellular and humoral immunity against the virus. The resultant inflammatory response may lead to significant corneal damage. Recurrent disease may primarily involve the epithelium (infectious [dendritic] ulceration; trophic [metaherpetic] ulceration), the stroma (viral necrotizing keratitis; interstitial keratitis, immune rings, and limbal vasculitis due to immune complex hypersensitivity; disciform keratitis due to delayed-type hypersensitivity reaction to antigen in the stroma and on stromal-cell membrane), or it may cause endotheliitis, trabeculitis, or iridocyclitis. The pathogenesis of these latter entities is not well understood.[18] Histopathologic examination of epithelial disease is rarely performed because the clinical manifestations are often considered diagnostic. Viral culture or immunofluorescent staining of epithelial scrapings may be done if necessary. The histologic findings in stromal disease are nonspecific and include pannus, scarring, chronic inflammation, vascularization, and rarely granulomatous inflammation.

Varicella-zoster virus (VZV) causes varicella (chickenpox) and herpes zoster (shingles). Virtually all individuals in the United States have been exposed to and are seropositive for VZV by 60 years of age. Superficial punctate keratitis, branching dendritic ulcers without terminal knobs, or immune disciform disease may occasionally develop in association with chickenpox.[18] Herpes zoster is a recurrent infection with VZV that has been dormant in sensory ganglia. Approximately 300,000 cases of herpes zoster occur annually in the United States, and an estimated 9% to 16% of cases are trigeminal zoster.[18] About one half to two thirds of people with periocular zoster have involvement of ocular structures (conjunctivitis, scleritis, keratitis, iridocyclitis). Corneal involvement with herpes zoster ophthalmicus may be punctate keratitis, pseudodendrites, anterior stromal infiltrates, sclerokeratitis, keratouveitis, peripheral ulcerative keratitis, disciform keratitis, neurotrophic keratitis, or exposure keratitis. The histologic findings in corneas undergoing penetrating keratoplasty are nonspecific and include scarring, chronic inflammation, and vascularization.

Adenoviruses encompass 47 serotypes in six subgroups. Adenoviral ocular infection occurs worldwide, involves many different serotypes, and is probably the most common external ocular viral infection.[17] The cornea is involved in patients with epidemic keratoconjunctivitis (EKC), although the disease only rarely causes permanent damage to the cornea. Most often, EKC causes a punctate keratitis that is due to viral replication in epithelial cells. The keratitis is easily visualized with fluorescein or rose bengal staining. After about 2 weeks, the epithelial involvement has cleared, but there are grayish-white subepithelial infiltrates. Histologic examination of these subepithelial infiltrates has been performed only rarely, but reveals focal collections of lymphocytes and histiocytes in the region of Bowman's layer. This is thought to represent a delayed-type hypersensitivity response to viral antigen that has accumulated in the anterior stroma.

Fungal infections of the cornea result from a bewildering variety of fungi,[19,20] and the fungi prevalent as corneal pathogens vary markedly from one locale to another. Fungal keratitis accounted for about 15% of cases of stromal microbial keratitis at the Bascom Palmer Eye Institute in Miami during a 9-year period ending in 1977.[19] Most cases are caused by opportunistic fungi in a trauma setting in individuals without prior ocular disease or in those using corticosteroids or antibiotics.[19] The more common organisms causing fungal keratitis in the United States include filamentous, nonpigmented fungi such as *Fusarium* sp., *Aspergillus* sp., *Acremonium (Cephalosporium)* sp,, and *Paecilomyces* sp.; dematiacious (brown-pigmented) filamentous fungi such as *Curvularia* sp.; and yeast members of the *Candida* sp. The clinical manifestations of fungal keratitis do not vary markedly among species. In general, mycotic keratitis caused by filamentous fungi features stromal infiltrates with feathery, hyphate edges, and infiltrates that tend to be gray, dry-appearing, and slightly elevated above the corneal surface. Stromal keratitis caused by *Candida* sp. and other yeasts tends to be more localized with a "collar button" configuration resulting from a small ulcer overlying an expanding stromal infiltrate.[19] Fungal keratitis may be an indolent or a rapidly progressing infection. Diagnosis of the specific agent involved requires culture. Histopathologic examination can confirm the presence of fungus, but is not reliable for separating the various species of filamentous fungi because they are all similar in appearance and stain readily using methenamine silver (Fig. 5-17). Yeasts are readily distinguished from the filamentous fungi in histologic sections because of their shape, size, and brilliant purple staining with the PAS technique (Fig. 5-18). Because the vast majority of corneal yeast infections in the United States are due to *Candida* sp., the identification of PAS-positive yeast is a presumptive identification of candidal keratitis.

Parasitic keratitis may result from many different organisms (Table 3), but only infection by *Acanthamoeba* sp. occurs with sufficient frequency in the United States to merit discussion. *Acanthamoeba* are ubiquitous, small, free-living protozoa that have been isolated from fresh, marine, and chlorinated water, soil, vegetable matter,

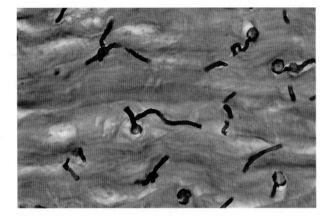

FIG. 5-17. Filamentous fungi cannot be reliably distinguished from each other in histologic sections. This is an example of keratitis resulting from *Fusarium solani*.

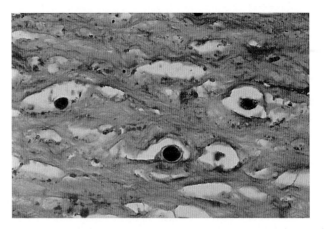

FIG. 5-19. *Acanthamoeba* keratitis with a cyst near the lower center of the photomicrograph and a trophozoite above and to each side in the stroma.

dust, and air.[21] Only 7 of the 22 *Acanthamoeba* sp. cause human keratitis, with *Acanthamoeba castellani* and *Acanthamoeba polyphaga* accounting for most of the reported cases. Epidemiologic studies have implicated contact lens wear and corneal trauma as the first and second most important risk factors for developing amebic keratitis in the United States. Foreign-body sensation, photophobia, and unusually severe pain are the typical symptoms of *Acanthamoeba* keratitis. Early infection causes granular epithelial irregularity with punctate or dendritiform changes. Later, patchy anterior stromal infiltrates develop and slowly merge into a crescentic or annular configuration. A ring infiltrate is a hallmark of *Acanthamoeba* keratitis, although it is not always present and is not pathognomonic. In histologic sections, identification of cysts is necessary to confirm the clinical diagnosis because large, reactive corneal fibroblasts may resemble trophozoites. *Acanthamoeba* cysts are 10 to 25 μm in

diameter and have a double wall; trophozoites range from 15 to 45 μm in diameter.[21] Some authors advocate the use of histochemical stains (such as calcofluor white, PAS, methenamine silver, or Giemsa), immunofluorescent antibody stains, or transmission electron microscopy for identifying organisms, although the cysts are usually recognized easily with routine stain (Fig. 5-19).

Keratoconus

Keratoconus is a noninflammatory disorder with progressive thinning and scarring of the central cornea.[11,23-25] Keratoconus is usually bilateral (approximately 85% of cases) and has its onset in adolescence. Affected corneas assume a conical shape because of thinning and protrusion, and they have decreased tensile strength. The corneal ectasia is most often located in the inferotemporal paracentral cornea. Early clinical manifestations are myopia and astigmatism, while progression of the disease leads to visual impairment from irregular astigmatism and scarring. The frequency of familial keratoconus varies from 6% to 19%, and apparent autosomal dominant and autosomal recessive modes of inheritance have been reported.[11]

Histologic examination of penetrating keratoplasty specimens from patients with keratoconus typically reveals central epithelial thinning, multiple breaks in Bowman's layer, and central stromal thinning (Figs. 5-20 and 5-21). In 20% of corneas, breaks in Bowman's layer are not evident, and there is less central epithelial thinning than in the typical cases.[25] Another finding in approximately 50% of specimens of keratoconus is iron within basal epithelial cells in a circle surrounding the cone (Fleischer's ring). The iron is recognizable grossly by its golden to brown color in formalin fixed tissue, but histologically it can be seen only using special histochem-

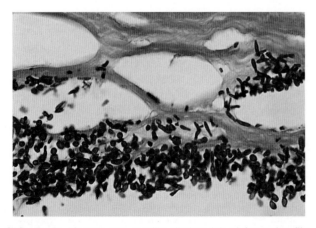

FIG. 5-18. Yeasts are readily distinguished from the filamentous fungi by their shape, size, and brilliant purple staining with the periodic acid-Schiff technique. These yeasts and pseudohyphae were in the deep stroma just anterior to Descemet's membrane in a failed corneal graft.

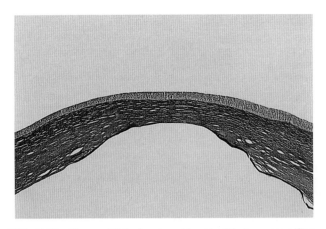

FIG. 5-20. Corneal thinning is evident in this low magnification view of a keratoconus corneal button. This is the same specimen illustrated in Fig. 5-13.

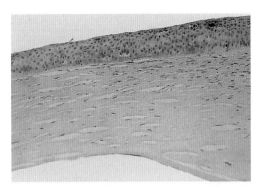

FIG. 5-22. Iron within the epithelium (Fleischer's ring) is evident as blue staining in this keratoconus specimen using Perls' Prussian blue method.

ical staining for iron (Perls' Prussian blue method) (Fig. 5-22).

Corneal Dystrophies

The cornea is affected by many inherited dystrophies that occur bilaterally and may involve any layer of the cornea (Table 4). Many of these dystrophies are rare, and only the more common ones will be discussed further.[2,12,26–29]

Fuchs' dystrophy is by far the most common corneal dystrophy in the United States, with other corneal dystrophies being rare in comparison to it. Approximately 75% of patients are women.[30] Fuchs' dystrophy affects both corneas, although the degree of signs and symptoms is usually asymmetric. In the first stage of the disease, the patient is asymptomatic, but corneal guttata are observed in the central cornea by slit lamp examination. This stage of Fuchs' dystrophy is usually noted between the third and fifth decades of life. In the second stage, there is

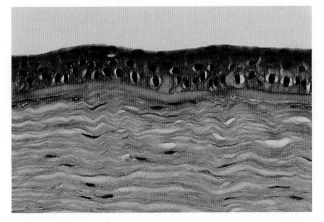

FIG. 5-21. Breaks in Bowman's layer are a typical finding in keratoconus.

development of corneal edema with symptoms of blurred vision, glare, and colored halos around lights. Initially, the blurred vision improves as the day progresses because tear evaporation increases the osmolality of the tears with resultant deturgescence of the cornea. The third clinical stage of Fuchs' dystrophy has pannus formation and severely impaired vision. Progression of the disease is slow and usually spans 10 to 20 years before severe visual impairment develops. Fuchs' dystrophy is considered to be an autosomal dominant disorder, with incomplete penetrance accounting for a lack of familial history in many patients. It is considered to be a primary disorder of the endothelium, with the guttata being a reflection of cellular dysfunction. Histologically, the hallmark of Fuchs' dystrophy is corneal guttata together with thickening of Descemet's membrane and a paucity of endothelial cells (Fig. 5-23). The remaining endothelial cells usually contain scattered melanin granules. In some cases, the guttata are buried within thickened Descemet's membrane and can only be readily visualized using periodic acid-Schiff staining. Penetrating keratoplasty specimens from patients with Fuchs' dystrophy also characteristically exhibit histologic changes of corneal edema, with or without formation of a fibrocollagenous pannus.

Granular dystrophy is an autosomal dominant disorder that clinically has multiple, sharply demarcated, irregularly shaped, white opacities within the stroma, especially in the central and superficial cornea[12,26] (Fig 5-24). The cornea between the deposits and the peripheral cornea remains clear. The deposits usually begin during the first decade of life, and they enlarge and become more numerous with advancing age. In H&E-stained sections, the deposits are brightly eosinophilic, vary widely in size, have irregular borders, and occur at all levels of the stroma. Large deposits appear to be a conglomeration of smaller deposits (Fig. 5-25). The deposits stain bright red using Masson trichrome stain, and this distinguishes them from the deposits of lattice corneal dystrophy (LCD). The uninvolved stroma as well as the epithelium, Descemet's membrane, and endothelium appear unremarkable. The

TABLE 4. *Corneal dystrophies**

Layer/dystrophy	Inheritance	Clinical/pathological features
EPITHELIUM		
Epithelial baseline membrane dystrophy	No specific pattern	Nonspecific reaction; epithelial microcysts and intraepithelial basement membrane
Meesmann's dystrophy	AD	Punctate epithelial opacities; intraepithelial microcysts with "peculiar substance" by transmission electron microscopy
BOWMAN'S LAYER/SUPERFICIAL STROMA		
Familial subepithelial amyloidosis	AR	Gelatinous droplike dystrophy; nodular deposits of amyloid beneath the epithelium
Reis-Bücklers' dystrophy	AD	Reticular opacity with recurrent epithelial erosions; subepithelial "curly" fibers by transmission electron microscopy
STROMA		
Central crystalline dystrophy	AD	Disciform opacity with needle-like crystals; cholesterol crystals in anterior stroma
Fleck dystrophy	AD	Flecks, clouds, snowflake opacities; fibroblasts stain with Alcian blue and for lipids
Granular dystrophy	AD	Discrete spots, central cornea; protein deposits stain red with Masson trichrome stain
Lattice dystrophy		
Type 1	AD	Delicate, interdigitating, linear opacities; fusiform deposits of amyloid
Type 2	AD	Corneal opacities as in type 1 and systemic amyloidosis; fusiform amyloid deposits
Type 3	AR	Thicker lattice lines; larger amyloid deposits than in type 1 or 2
Type 3a	AD	Similar to type 3 but with AD inheritance pattern
Macular dystrophy		
Type 1	AR	Cloudy opacities with indistinct margins; glycosaminoglycan deposits do not react to keratan sulfate antibodies
Type 2	AR	Cloudy opacities with indistinct margins; glycosaminoglycan deposits react to keratan sulfate antibodies
ENDOTHELIUM		
Congenital hereditary endothelial dystrophy	AR/AD	"Ground glass" appearance, thickened corneas; sparse endothelial cells, thickened DM
Fuchs' dystrophy	±AD	Central guttata, corneal edema; guttata, thickened DM
Posterior polymorphous dystrophy	AD	Irregular lesions in region of DM; multilayered epithelial plaques on DM

* AD, autosomal dominant inheritance; AR, autosomal recessive inheritance; ±AD, sometimes autosomal dominant inheritance; DM, Descemet's membrane.

deposits in granular dystrophy are extracellular protein, but its nature and origin are uncertain.

LCDs are four related entities that clinically exhibit a network of interdigitating filaments, especially in the central cornea (Fig. 5-26). The four types of LCD are distinguished by differing modes of inheritance (Table 4), the presence of systemic amyloidosis in lattice dystrophy type 2, and thicker interdigitating filaments in lattice dystrophy types 3 and 3a.[4,12] LCD type 1 usually becomes evident clinically toward the end of the first decade of life. Corneal changes in LCD type 2 become apparent after age 20 years, but LCD types 3 and 3a do not manifest clinically until late in life. All forms of LCD are typically bilateral and slowly progressive. Recurrent epithelial erosions are common in patients with LCD type 1 and result in scarring. Histologically, LCDs all feature amyloid deposits within the corneal stroma (Fig. 5-27). The amyloid deposits are homogeneous and eosinophilic in H&E-stained sections, many are fusiform, and they are orange

when stained with Congo red. The amyloid is birefringent when stained with Congo red and viewed with polarized light. It is important to remember that amyloid deposits in the stroma may occur in other disorders, and the mere presence of such deposits is not sufficient for a diagnosis of LCD (see previous section on nonspecific responses of the cornea).

Two variants of macular corneal dystrophy (MCD) can be differentiated by absent-to-low (type 1) or normal (type 2) levels of keratan sulfate in the serum and by negative (type 1) or positive (type 2) immunostaining for keratan sulfate in the cornea.[4,28] Both forms of MCD clinically begin at about puberty when irregular, poorly defined, cloudy regions develop in both corneas (Fig. 5-28). The cloudy regions enlarge and coalesce with resultant opacification of the cornea, usually before the fifth decade of life.[28] MCD is rare in the general population, but there are isolated, inbred, groups within the United States and other countries where it is common. Histologically, both

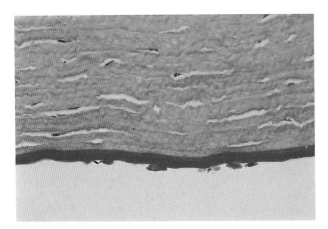

FIG. 5-23. In Fuchs' dystrophy, Descemet's membrane is thickened and has excrescences (guttata). There are also fewer endothelial cells.

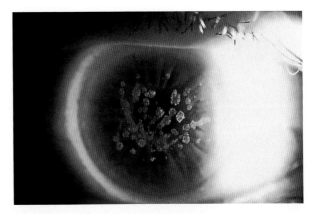

FIG. 5-24. Multiple, sharply demarcated, irregularly shaped white opacities within the stroma, especially in the central and superficial cornea, are clinically characteristic of granular dystrophy (Courtesy of Gary N. Foulks, MD).

forms of MCD exhibit intracytoplasmic accumulation of glycosaminoglycans (mucopolysaccharides) within keratocytes and endothelial cells. Extracellular material may form pools in the region of Bowman's layer and the anterior stroma with lesser amounts of extracellular material elsewhere in the stroma. The extracellular pools of glycosaminoglycans are sometimes recognizable in H&E-stained sections as wispy, faintly basophilic material or as clear spaces. The intracellular glycosaminoglycans are usually visible only with stains such as Alcian blue or colloidal iron (Fig. 5-29). Corneal guttata are a common feature in corneas from patients with MCD.

Pigmentations

Of the numerous forms of corneal pigmentation that have been reported (Table 5), only epithelial iron lines, melanin pigmentation, and blood staining occur relatively frequently.[2,10,31,32]

Iron lines are the most frequent cause of corneal epithelial pigmentation. Most common is the **Hudson-Stähli line,** which is a horizontal brown to brownish-green line at the junction of the middle to lower third of the cornea in individuals with otherwise unremarkable corneas. Hudson-Stähli lines have a maximal incidence at 60 to

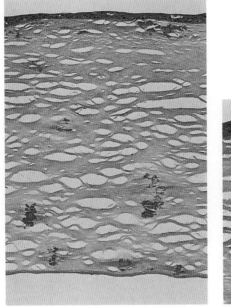

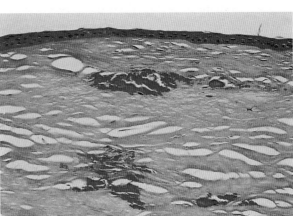

FIG. 5-25. (A) The stromal deposits in granular dystrophy are easily seen in hematoxylin and eosin stained sections because they are brightly eosinophilic. (B) The borders of the deposits are irregular. Note superficial stromal scarring in this example.

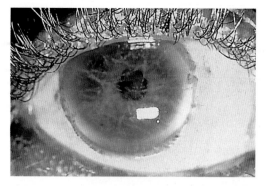

FIG. 5-26. A network of interdigitating filaments, especially in the central cornea, is characteristic of lattice dystrophy. The blue coloration of the lattice lines is due to the illumination (Courtesy of Gary N. Foulks, MD).

70 years of age[31] and are of no clinical significance. A Fleischer's ring, as mentioned and illustrated previously (Fig. 5-22), forms a circle surrounding the cone in approximately 50% of corneas with keratoconus. Less common epithelial iron lines are **Stocker's lines** (or Stocker-Busacca lines), which are vertical lines at the head of a pterygium, and **Ferry's lines,** which are adjacent to filtering blebs used for treating glaucoma. In all types of iron lines, the iron is restricted to the epithelium, and its concentration is greater in the basal cells than in the superficial cells.

Melanin pigmentation of the corneal epithelium is seen in blacks, usually as a result of inflammation or trauma. In histologic sections, the melanin appears as intracytoplasmic, coarse, brown granules, which may be in all layers of the epithelium but is sometimes concentrated in the basal cells. Melanin also may accumulate in endothelial cells and extracellularly on the posterior surface of the cornea. In Fuchs' dystrophy, melanin granules are commonly seen within the cytoplasm of the remaining endothelial cells. Melanin may accumulate in central endothelial cells in a vertical, spindle-shaped configuration termed a **Krukenberg's spindle** in ocular diseases with dispersion of iris pigment throughout the anterior chamber. This may occur in patients with pigment dispersion syndrome (Fig. 5-30), iritis, or diabetic iridopathy. Melanin may also accumulate within fibroblasts in retrocorneal fibrous membranes. A mild degree of melanin pigmentation of retrocorneal fibrous membranes is common in histologic sections of failed corneal grafts.

Blood staining of the cornea results from hemorrhage into the anterior chamber with subsequent passage of hemoglobin globules into the corneal stroma. Corneal blood staining is most frequent in the presence of elevated intraocular pressure, but it may occur with normal or low intraocular pressure, especially if the endothelium has been damaged. Blood-stained corneas are opaque and most often green to greenish-yellow. Histologic sections stained with H&E disclose numerous, small, extracellular, red globules throughout the stroma (Fig. 5-31). The globules are bright red when stained with Masson trichrome stain. Initially, iron is not demonstrable using Perls' Prussian blue technique because it is bound in the hemoglobin. Later, after the hemoglobin is phagocytosed and degraded by keratocytes, iron is seen within their cytoplasm in the

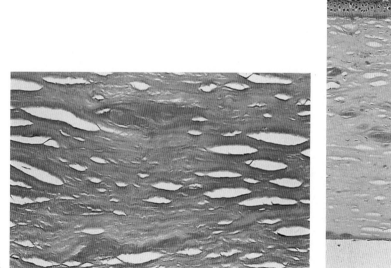

A   B

FIG. 5-27. Deposits of amyloid within the corneal stroma are characteristic of lattice dystrophy. **(A)** They may be difficult to observe in H&E stained sections, **(B)** but they are readily apparent after staining with Congo red because they stain orange.

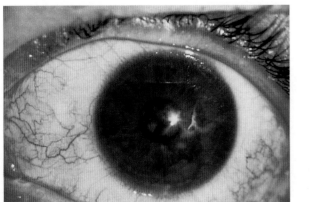

FIG. 5-28. Poorly defined, cloudy regions in the cornea of a patient with macular corneal dystrophy (Courtesy of Gary N. Foulks, MD).

form of hemosiderin (Fig. 5-32). At this stage, the condition can be referred to as **corneal siderosis**.

Neoplasms

Primary neoplasms of the cornea are exceedingly rare.[33,34] Virtually all tumors of the cornea represent direct spread of conjunctival of squamous cell carcinoma or melanoma.

SCLERA

Normal Anatomy and Histology

The sclera is the dense fibrous tunic that constitutes five-sixths of the circumference of the eye.[35,36] It extends from the periphery of the cornea to the optic nerve, aver-

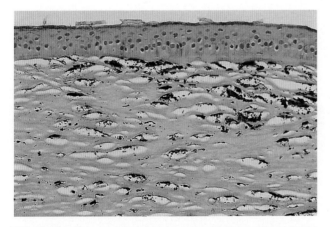

FIG. 5-29. Glycosaminoglycan accumulation within keratocytes in cases of macular corneal dystrophy is well demonstrated using colloidal iron staining which turns the deposits blue. A thin layer of mucin on the epithelial surface is also apparent.

TABLE 5. *Corneal pigmentation*

Main layer involved	Cause of pigmentation
Epithelium	Amiodarone
	Arsenic
	Bismuth
	Chemical dusts (benzoquinone, hydroquinone)
	Chloroquine
	Chlorpromazine keratopathy
	Cytosine arabinoside (cytarabine; Ara-C)
	Fabry's disease
	Hydroxychloroquine (Plaquenil)
	Iron
	Melanin
	Mepacrine (quinacrine)
	Tyrosine crystals
	Urate crystals
Stroma	Adrenochrome (epinephrine)
	Chlorpromazine
	Cystine crystals (cystinosis)
	Gold (chrysiasis)
	Hemoglobin (blood staining)
	Immunoglobulin crystals
	Indomethacin
	Iron (siderosis)
	Ochronosis (alkaptonuria)
	Refsum syndrome
	Thioridazine
	Urethane
Descemet's membrane	Copper
	Mercury
	Silver (argyrosis)
Endothelium	Blood staining (hemoglobin or hemosiderin)
	Melanin

ages 22 mm in diameter, and varies in thickness. It is about 0.8 mm thick near the cornea, approximately 0.3 mm thick near the insertions of the rectus muscles, and about 1 mm thick near the optic nerve.[35]

The sclera has three layers: the episclera, the stroma, and the lamina fusca. The **episclera** is the outermost component of the sclera that is located between Tenon's capsule and the denser scleral stroma. It consists of loose collagenous tissue and is thicker and more vascular anteriorly. The collagen bundles in the deeper episclera are thicker and merge imperceptibly with the scleral stroma.

The **stroma** is by far the largest component of the sclera. It is composed principally of bundles of collagen, which are larger in diameter than those in the episclera. The stroma also contains small amounts of elastic fibers and a few fibroblasts. The collagen bundles vary in thickness and have a complex interdigitating pattern (Fig. 5-33). The variation in size of the collagen bundles, their random array, and a low state of hydration are thought to be responsible for the sclera being opaque. The stroma is relatively avascular except for vessels that penetrate it to supply the uveal tract and optic nerve head or to drain aqueous humor from the region of Schlemm's canal. Nourishment of the stroma is derived from small branches

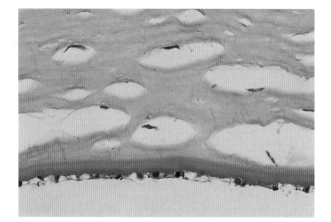

FIG. 5-30. Melanin is seen within endothelial cells in a Krukenberg's spindle in a patient with pigment dispersion syndrome.

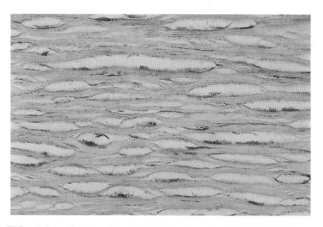

FIG. 5-32. During the evolution of corneal blood staining, hemosiderin within keratocytes stains blue with Perls' Prussian blue method.

of the anterior and posterior ciliary arteries, and to a lesser extent, from the choroidal circulation. The more posterior penetrating vessels are contained within emissarial canals that contain accompanying nerves and scattered melanocytes. In individuals with a heavily pigmented uveal tract, melanocytes within these emissarial canals may make it difficult to identify scleral extension of a choroidal melanoma.

The **lamina fusca** is the transition zone from the scleral stroma to the underlying choroid. Distinguishing it from the choroid is difficult. The lamina fusca is composed of loose collagen bundles derived from the scleral stroma, mixed with melanocytes and connective tissue from the uveal tract.

Developmental Abnormalities

The sclera may develop localized or diffuse melanin pigmentation shortly after birth in congenital melanosis

oculi and oculodermal melanocytosis (nevus of Ota). Scleral pigmentation is more frequent in blacks and Asians but can occur in whites. Diffuse melanin pigmentation also may affect the episclera.[37]

Thinned sclerae, which causes them to appear blue because of the underlying uveal pigment being visible, are a feature of some forms of **osteogenesis imperfecta** (OI). OI is a group of four related disorders in which synthesis of type I collagen is impaired. It is important to remember that blue sclerae are typical in neonates and that only the persistence of blue sclerae beyond the first few months of infancy is pathologic.

Scleral ectasia may occur in association with a coloboma of the choroid and is most common when the coloboma is adjacent to the optic disc.

Aging and Degenerative Changes

The sclera is thin in neonates. During the first decade of life, the sclera progressively thickens and becomes

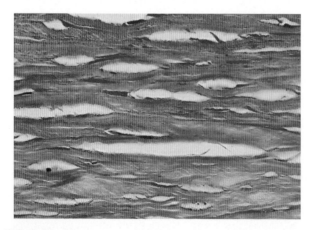

FIG. 5-31. Numerous red globules of hemoglobin are within the stroma in the early stage of corneal blood staining. The globules tend to accumulate within the keratocytes, causing them to appear bright red in hematoxylin-and-eosin–stained sections.

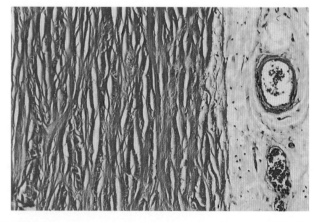

FIG. 5-33. Normal sclera showing the looser connective tissue of the episclera (*right*) and the denser connective tissue of the scleral stroma (*left*). Note the varying diameter of the collagen fibers in the stroma and their interdigitating pattern.

more rigid and opaque. the thinness and distensibility of the sclera in childhood allows the eye to stretch and deform during prolonged episodes of glaucoma. Uncontrolled glaucoma in adults does not cause uniform enlargement and stretching of the sclera, but local areas of ectasia may result, especially anteriorly. If uvea is visible through the ectatic area, then it appears blue and is termed a **staphyloma.**

A consistent finding in the eyes of elderly individuals is scleral calcification. This typically appears as varying degrees of basophilic stippling among the scleral collagen bundles in H&E-stained sections. When sections of eyes are stained histochemically for calcium (eg, to confirm calcific band keratopathy), the scleral calcification may appear prominent. The calcification may be misinterpreted as being pathologic, instead of a normal aging change.

Senile scleral plaques are another common aging-related change. They are almost always located between the limbus and the insertion of the medial or lateral rectus muscles. Clinically, the sclera is translucent, blue gray, and slightly depressed over an area several millimeters in diameter. The lesion may be hard due to calcification. Senile scleral plaques do not require treatment. Histologically, the early lesion has actinic damage with ropy, serpiginous fibers. Calcification often is present, and advanced lesions usually are calcific plaques.

Irregular thickening of the sclera is a ubiquitous finding in eyes with phthisis bulbi. It has no special significance in this process but is part of the overall diffuse degeneration that occurs in phthisical eyes.

Infections

Scleral infections are most commonly the result of trauma, and the agent may be bacterial or fungal. *Pseudomonas aeruginosa* causes the most serious bacterial infection, because the organism produces proteases that rapidly digest the sclera and often cause perforation or endophthalmitis necessitating enucleation. Mycotic infections may be indolent and indistinguishable from a nodular scleritis in their early stages.[37]

Patients with herpes zoster ophthalmicus may develop a nodular episcleritis that spontaneously resolves in 3 to 4 weeks. The patient may present again after 1 to 4 months with nodular scleritis that may be necrotizing. The recurrent lesion is resistant to treatment, may require months to resolve, and may leave an area of scleral thinning or recur.[37] The necrotizing scleritis due to herpes zoster typically exhibits zonal granulomatous inflammation around necrotic sclera. It is similar histologically to the necrotizing scleritis in patients with rheumatoid arthritis.[38]

Inflammatory Disorders

By far, the most important lesions of the sclera are the noninfectious inflammatory disorders episcleritis and scleritis.[36,37,39,40] Though these disorders are the most common scleral problems, they account for only about 0.1% of new patient referrals to eye hospitals.[40] During a 10-year period, 207 patients with episcleritis and 159 patients with scleritis were evaluated at Moorfields Eye Hospital in London.[40]

TABLE 6. *Clinical features of episcleritis and scleritis*

Entity	Age/sex	Onset	Redness	Pain	Photophobia/ lacrimation	Vascular changes	Chemosis	Scleral thinning	Visual acuity
Episcleritis									
Simple	Adult/ M = F	Sudden	Bright red	Slight local	Occasional	Superficial episcleral	Occasional	Rare	Normal
Nodular	Adult/ M = F	Usually sudden	Red	Slight local	Occasional	Superficial episcleral	Rare	Rare	Normal
Anterior scleritis									
Diffuse	Adult/ F > M	Gradual	Bluish red	Moderate local/ referred	Occasional	Superficial/ deep episcleral	Common	Common	Occasional loss
Nodular	Adult/ F > M	Gradual	Dusky red	Moderate local/ referred	Occasional	Superficial/ deep episcleral	Rare	Common	Normal
Necrotizing (with inflammation)	Adult/ F > M	Gradual	Bluish red	Severe local/ referred	Common	Superficial/ deep episcleral	Variable	Common	Common loss
Scleromalacia perforans	Adult/ F	Insidious	Very slight	Slight or absent	None	Avascular area	Absent	Always	Common loss
Posterior scleritis	Adult/ F ≫ M	Gradual	Variable	Severe local/ referred	Uncommon	Superficial/ deep episcleral	Common	Rare	Very common loss

M, male; F, female.

(Adapted from Watson P, Hayreh SS. Scleritis and episcleritis. *Br J Ophthalmol* 1976;60:163–191).

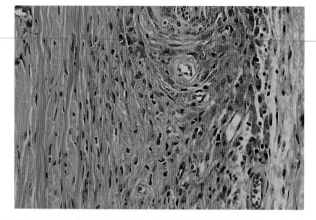

FIG. 5-34. Diffuse anterior scleritis with macrophages laden with granular eosinophilic debris and lymphocytes in the outer sclera near the junction with the episclera.

Watson and Hayreh subclassified these disorders based on an analysis of the clinical features of their patients at Moorfields Eye Hospital[40]:

- Episcleritis
  - Simple episcleritis
  - Nodular episcleritis
- Anterior scleritis
  - Diffuse scleritis
  - Nodular scleritis
  - Necrotizing scleritis (with inflammation)
  - Scleromalacia perforans (necrotizing scleritis without inflammation)
- Posterior scleritis

A summary of some of the most important distinguishing clinical features of these disorders is presented in Table 6.[40]

It is important to emphasize that episcleritis is almost

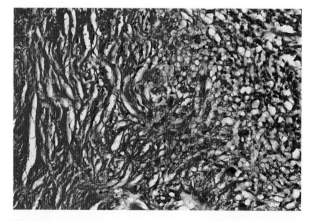

FIG. 5-35. Necrotizing anterior scleritis with ill-defined granulomatous inflammation and collagen necrosis. Collagen necrosis is on the left, bordered by a zone of epithelioid histiocytes with indistinct cell borders. Lymphocytes are to the right of the epithelioid histiocytes.

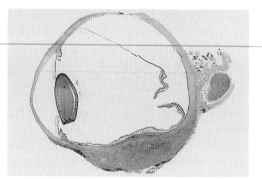

FIG. 5-36. Marked thickening of the sclera in this globe with posterior scleritis due to inflammation, edema, and reactive proliferation of connective tissue.

always a benign inflammatory disorder, usually resolves on its own, and often recurs. Approximately 40% of patients develop episcleritis in both eyes. It is not regularly associated with systemic autoimmune diseases.

In contrast to episcleritis, scleritis is a severe destructive disorder that can lead to loss of an eye from decreased vision, severe and intractable pain, or occasionally perforation of the globe.[37,39,40] The disease was bilateral in 45% of the patients studied by Watson and Hayreh.[40] Scleritis was associated with corneal changes in 29% of patients, and the corneal abnormalities included acute stromal keratitis, sclerosing keratitis, limbal guttering, and keratolysis.[40] Approximately 50% of patients with scleritis have an underlying systemic disorder, most commonly rheumatoid arthritis. Its incidence in individuals presenting with scleritis is approximately 30%, but the incidence of scleritis in patients presenting with rheumatoid arthritis is only about 1%.[39] These numbers reflect the common occurrence of rheumatoid arthritis and the relative rarity of scleritis. Other systemic associations of scleritis include juvenile polyarthritis, systemic lupus erythematosus, Wegener's granulomatosis, polyarteritis nodosa, relapsing polychondritis, and the seronegative spondyloarthropathies such as ankylosing spondylitis and Reiter's disease.[39]

Despite an abundance of clinical information about episcleritis and scleritis, histopathologic examination of specimens from these disorders is uncommon and has contributed little to our understanding of their pathogenesis.[37–39] Specimens of simple and nodular episcleritis typically contain lymphocytes concentrated around vessels, dilated vessels, and extravasated proteinaceous fluid. Diffuse anterior scleritis may have histologic features similar to episcleritis, except that the scleral stroma is involved by the inflammatory process. Macrophages containing ingested tissue debris also are a feature when the case is chronic (Fig. 5-34). Necrotizing scleritis associated with autoimmune diseases is characterized by scleral necrosis surrounded by zonal granulomatous inflammation and vasculitis.[38] Reactive proliferation of connective tissue is

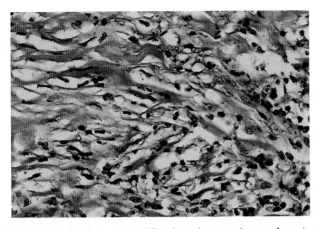

FIG. 5-37. At higher magnification, the specimen of posterior scleritis has an infiltrate of lymphocytes, plasma cells, and macrophages. The inflammatory infiltrate and edema expand the sclera. Over time, fibrous tissue proliferates, contributing to the scleral thickening.

absent. Idiopathic necrotizing scleritis has diffuse infiltration of the sclera with predominantly lymphocytes, no vasculitis, and, in about 25% of cases, ill-defined nonzonal granulomatous inflammation[38] (Fig. 5-35). Reactive proliferation of connective tissue is a prominent feature of idiopathic necrotizing scleritis. Posterior scleritis may have features of idiopathic necrotizing anterior scleritis, or it may lack granulomatous inflammation or necrosis and have only an infiltrate of lymphocytes and plasma cells with reactive proliferation of connective tissue (Figs. 5-36 and 5-37).

Neoplasms

The anterior sclera may occasionally be invaded by squamous cell carcinoma or mucoepidermoid carcinoma arising in the conjunctiva. Conjunctival lymphomas often infiltrate into the episclera. The posterior sclera may be directly invaded by uveal melanoma, or tumor may extend into or through the sclera in the emissary canals which carry the blood vessels and nerves that supply the uveal tract. Primary tumors of the sclera are exceptionally rare and include episcleral osseous choristoma, nodular fasciitis, fibrous histiocytoma, and a melanocytoma.[36]

REFERENCES

1. Klyce SS, Beuerman RW. Structure and function of the cornea. In: Kaufman HE, Barron BA, McDonald MB, Waltman SR, eds. *The Cornea.* New York: Churchill Livingstone, 1988.
2. Spencer WH. Cornea. In: Spencer WH, ed. *Ophthalmic pathology: an atlas and textbook,* ed 3. Philadelphia: WB Saunders, 1985.
3. Kenyon KR. Morphology and pathologic responses of the cornea to disease. In: Smolin G, Thoft RA, eds. *The cornea: scientific foundations and clinical practice,* ed 2. Boston: Little, Brown, 1987.
4. Scroggs MW, Klintworth GK. The eye and ocular adnexa. In: Stern-berg SS, ed. *Diagnostic surgical pathology,* ed 2. New York: Raven Press, 1994.
5. Johnson DH, Bourne WM, Campbell RJ. The ultrastructure of Descemet's membrane. I. Changes with age in normal corneas. *Arch Ophthalmol* 1982;100:1942–1947.
6. Waring GO III, Rodrigues MM, Laibson PR. Anterior chamber cleavage syndrome: a stepladder classification. *Surv Ophthalmol* 1975;20:3–27.
7. Kenyon KR, Chaves HV. Morphology and pathologic response of corneal and conjunctival disease. In: Smolin G, Thoft RA, eds. *The cornea: scientific foundations and clinical practice,* ed 3. Boston: Little, Brown, 1994.
8. Brodrick JD, Dark AJ, Peace GW. Fingerprint dystrophy of the cornea: a histologic study. *Arch Ophthalmol* 1974;92:483–489.
9. Rodrigues MM, Fine BS, Laibson PR, Zimmerman LE. Disorders of the corneal epithelium: a clinicopathologic study of dot, geographic, and fingerprint patterns. *Arch Ophthalmol* 1974;92:475–482.
10. Arffa RC, Eve FR. Systemic associations of corneal deposits. *Int Ophthalmol Clin* 1991;31:89–110.
11. Klintworth GK. Degenerations, depositions, and miscellaneous reactions of the ocular anterior segment. In: Garner A, Klintworth GK, eds. *Pathobiology of ocular disease: a dynamic approach,* ed 2. New York: Marcel Dekker, 1994.
12. Klintworth GK. Proteins in ocular disease. In: Garner A, Klintworth GK, eds. *Pathobiology of ocular disease: a dynamic approach,* ed 2. New York: Marcel Dekker, 1994.
13. Klintworth GK, Font RL. The eye and ocular adnexa. In: Spicer SS, ed. *Histochemistry in pathologic diagnosis.* New York: Marcel Dekker, 1986.
14. Burd EM. Bacterial keratitis and conjunctivitis: bacteriology. In: Smolin G, Thoft RA, eds. *The cornea: scientific foundations and clinical practice,* ed 3. Boston: Little, Brown, 1994.
15. Ogawa GSH, Hyndiuk RA. Bacterial keratitis and conjunctivitis: clinical disease. In: Smolin G, Thoft RA, eds. *The cornea: scientific foundations and clinical practice,* ed 3. Boston: Little, Brown, 1994.
16. Easty DL, Williams C. Viral and rickettsial disease. In: Garner A, Klintworth GK, eds. *Pathobiology of ocular disease: a dynamic approach,* ed 2. New York: Marcel Dekker, 1994.
17. Gordon JS. Viral keratitis and conjunctivitis. Clinical disease: adenovirus and other nonherpetic viral diseases. In: Smolin G, Thoft RA, eds. *The cornea: scientific foundations and clinical practice,* ed 3. Boston: Little, Brown, 1994.
18. Pavan-Langston D. Viral keratitis and conjunctivitis. Clinical disease: herpetic infections. In: Smolin G, Thoft RA, eds. *The cornea: scientific foundations and clinical practice,* ed 3. Boston: Little, Brown, 1994.
19. Forster RK. Fungal keratitis and conjunctivitis: clinical disease. In: Smolin G, Thoft RA, eds. *The cornea: scientific foundations and clinical practice,* ed 3. Boston: Little, Brown, 1994.
20. O'Brien TP, Green WR. Fungus infections of the eye and periocular tissues. In: Garner A, Klintworth GK, eds. *Pathobiology of ocular disease: a dynamic approach,* ed 2. New York: Marcel Dekker, 1994.
21. Osato MS. Parasitic keratitis and conjunctivitis: parasitology. In: Smolin G, Thoft RA, eds. *The cornea: scientific foundations and clinical practice,* ed 3. Boston: Little, Brown, 1994.
22. Wilhelmus KR. Parasitic keratitis and conjunctivitis: clinical disease. In: Smolin G, Thoft RA, eds. *The cornea: scientific foundations and clinical practice,* ed 3. Boston: Little, Brown, 1994.
23. Krachmer JH, Feder RS, Belin MW. Keratoconus and related noninflammatory corneal thinning disorders. *Surv Ophthalmol* 1984;28:293–322.
24. Pouliquen Y. Doyne lecture: keratoconus. *Eye* 1987;1:1–14.
25. Scroggs MW, Proia AD. Histopathological variation in keratoconus. *Cornea* 1992;11:553–559.
26. Klintworth GK. Corneal dystrophies. In: Nicholson EH, ed. *Ocular pathology update.* New York: Masson Publishing, 1980.
27. Klintworth GK. Corneal dystrophies. *Curr Opin Ophthalmol* 1991;2:382–391.
28. Klintworth GK. Disorders of glycosaminoglycans (mucopolysaccharides) and proteoglycans. In: Garner A, Klintworth GK, eds. *Pathobiology of ocular disease: a dynamic approach,* ed 2. New York: Marcel Dekker, 1994.
29. Ross JR, Foulks GN, Sanfilippo FP, Howell DN. Immunohisto-

chemical analysis of the pathogenesis of posterior polymorphous dystrophy. *Arch Ophthalmol* 1995;113:340–345.

30. Wilson SE, Bourne WM. Fuchs' dystrophy. *Cornea* 1988;7:2–18

31. Brodrick JD. Pigmentation of the cornea: review and case history. *Ann Ophthalmol* 1979;11:855–861.

32. Pilger IS. Pigmentation of the cornea: a review and classification. *Ann Ophthalmol* 1983;15:1076–1082.

33. Mizuno K. Squamous cell carcinoma of cornea. *Arch Ophthalmol* 1965;74:807–808.

34. Pierse D, Steele AD McG, Garner A, Tripathi RC. Intraepithelial carcinoma (''Bowen's disease'') of the cornea. *Br J Ophthalmol* 1971;55:664–670.

35. Scroggs MW, Klintworth GK. Normal eye and ocular adnexa. In:

36. Spencer WH. Sclera. In: Spencer WH, ed. *Ophthalmic pathology: an atlas and textbook,* ed 3. Philadelphia: WB Saunders, 1985.

37. Watson P. Diseases of the sclera. In: Tasman W, Jaeger EA, eds. *Duane's clinical ophthalmology.* Philadelphia: JB Lippincott, 1987.

38. Rao NA, Marak GE, Hidayat AA. Necrotizing scleritis: a clinico-pathologic study of 41 cases. *Ophthalmology* 1985;92:1542–1549.

39. Hakin KN, Watson PG. Systemic associations of scleritis. *Int Ophthalmol Clin* 1991;31:111–129.

40. Watson P, Hayreh SS. Scleritis and episcleritis. *Br J Ophthalmol* 1976;60:163–191.

Sternberg SS, ed. *Histology for pathologists.* New York: Raven Press, 1992.

Ophthalmic Pathology with Clinical Correlations,
edited by Joseph W. Sassani, M.D.
Lippincott-Raven Publishers, Philadelphia © 1997.

CHAPTER 6

Disorders of the Crystalline Lens

Curtis E. Margo

The **crystalline lens** is a transparent spheroid of protein suspended in the visual axis by the lens zonules. The primary function of the lens is to converge light onto the neurosensory retina. The structure of the lens is relatively simple, composed of two morphologically distinct cells—lens fibers and lens epithelium—that represent different stages of differentiation. The core of the lens is composed of fibers that comprise more than 99% of the lens by volume. The fibers are capped anteriorly by a parenteral monolayer of epithelium. Both fibers and epithelia are surrounded by a thick basement membrane known as the **lens capsule.**

The lens capsule, although thick, is a typical basement membrane secreted anteriorly by the epithelial cells and posteriorly by cortical fibers. It is composed largely of glycoproteins and type IV collagen.[1] The structure of the capsular matrix is important in maintaining its clarity.[2] The capsule is a dynamic membrane that undergoes constant renewal by the underlying epithelium and fibers.[3] The composition of the lens capsule changes, demonstrating less collagen and heparin sulfate with age.[1] The capsule is a passive tissue with no intrinsic metabolic activity.

The underlying lens epithelium is a monolayer that is firmly attached to the anterior lens capsule. Normally, these low cuboidal cells end at the equator where they transdifferentiate into lens fibers. The lens epithelial cells are mitotically and metabolically active. The greatest amount of epithelial DNA synthesis occurs anterior to the lens equator in a region known as the *germinative zone* in preparation for transformation into lens fibers.

At the region of the lens bow, terminal differentiation into lens fibers is associated with alterations in the macromolecular composition of the cells. Cellular protein increases dramatically as almost all other cellular constituents and organelles diminish. The nucleus of the transformed fibers gradually disappears in the lens cortex.

This life-long process of fiber production begins after formation of the embryonic nucleus. The repetitive production of fibers creates an onion-like structure. The fibers converge in a radiating pattern of axial sutures that have an anterior upright and a posterior inverted ''Y'' pattern when viewed at the slit lamp. The outer lens fibers represent cortex; however, with time, they are compressed centrally to become the **lens nucleus.** Optically distinct zones of lens fibers can be appreciated clinically, but no such distinction can be made with histologic inspection. The crystalline lens has very little extracellular matrix. Fibers fit together with a tongue-and-groove type of arrangement. The lens becomes progressively heavier as it grows, but because of its limited capacity to expand, the fibers become increasingly compressed. The adult crystalline lens has a diameter of 9.6 mm and a thickness of 4.2 mm, about the size of an aspirin tablet.[4]

DEVELOPMENTAL ABNORMALITIES

A common finding in many normal eyes is a **Mittendorf's dot,** an extracapsular remnant of the posterior tunica vasculosa lentis. This embryonic remnant is extralenticular and rarely interferes with visual function.

Coloboma

Coloboma of the lens is characterized by the congenital absence of zonular fibers and not by loss of lens tissue itself. Regional loss of zonular support results in a focal lens notch and concomitant thickening of the lens. The condition is usually an isolated finding.

Lenticonus

Lenticonus is a domelike axial herniation of lens cortex. The disorder can affect either the anterior or posterior lens surface. Anterior lenticonus is associated with **Alport's syndrome,** an inherited metabolic defect of basement

C. E. Margo: Department of Ophthalmology, University of South Florida, Tampa, Florida 33612.

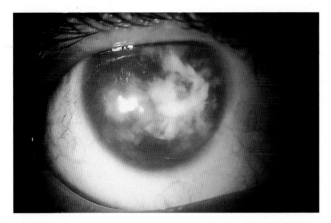

FIG. 6-1. Congential cataract in aniridia. The nucleus is opaque white and surrounded by irregular projections of semitransparent cortex. A corneal opacity is present just temporal to the center.

membrane, and may be the initial manifestation of the disease.[5] One of the earliest signs of lenticonus is an oil-droplet shadow seen with retroillumination. Histologically, the anterior lens capsule is abnormally thin with dehiscence of anterior cortex.

Posterior lenticonus occurs both as a familial abnormality and sporadically.[6] It is usually an isolated ocular finding. Clinically, the earliest changes are detected with retroillumination. By light microscopy, the posterior capsule appears attenuated and thin.[7]

Secondary abnormalities of the lens capsule are found in several disorders. In Down's syndrome, wartlike excrescences of capsular basement membrane project between epithelial cells usually peripherally. These small excrescences are found in several other conditions, including aniridia and Lowe's syndrome, and are probably clinically imperceptible unless associated with nodular proliferations of lens epithelium[8–10] (Figs. 6-1 and 6-2).

CLASSIFICATION OF CATARACTS

There is no universally accepted method of classifying cataracts. The term **cataract** implies both an optical opacity of the lens and interference with visual function, although the term is often used to refer to any detectable opacity regardless of the effects on visual function. Cataracts can be described on the basis of clinical morphology, age of onset, and cause. Since the cause of most cataracts is unknown, classification systems are usually descriptive. **Congenital cataracts** are present at birth. **Acquired cataracts** may have their clinical onset during infancy, childhood, young adulthood, and middle age, i.e., **presenile cataract** or in advanced age, i.e., **senile cataract.**[11–13] Most progressive cataracts involve the nucleus (nuclear cataract), cortex (cortical cataract), or tissue just beneath the lens capsule (anterior and posterior subcapsular cataracts).

CATARACTS IN INFANTS AND CHILDREN

Lens opacities in infants and children are associated with a variety of systemic and ocular conditions (Tables 1 and 2). Classification of cataracts in this age group is most informative when based on cause or a definable associated condition rather than on morphology. Nearly half of pediatric cataracts have an identifiable association or cause are inherited.[13]

Congenital cataracts are found in approximately one in 250 live births. All patterns of inheritance occur, but autosomal dominant is the most common. Although the mechanism of inherited cataract formation is unclear, it is likely that some are due to a mutation in one of the crystalline protein genes.

Congenital anterior polar cataracts can be caused by subclinical inflammation or trauma during gestation, although clinical evidence supporting these possibilities is lacking in most cases. Clinically, they appear as a sharply circumscribed, opaque nodule protruding from the anterior lens surface (Fig. 6-3). They vary in size from several millimeters to a diameter that fills the pupil. Vision loss is roughly proportional to the size of the opacity. Underlying cortex is usually uninvolved. Most congenital anterior polar cataracts demonstrate similar morphologic alterations as anterior subcapsular cataracts in adults (Fig. 6-4). The metaplastic fibrous nodule beneath the lens capsule may become sequestered from the remaining lens cortex by basement membrane. Some congenital anterior

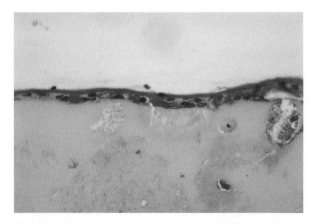

FIG. 6-2. Cataract in aniridia shows wartlike projections of the anterior lens capsule between lens epithelium.

TABLE 1. *Metabolic diseases associated with cataract*

Diabetes mellitus
Galactokinase deficiency
Galactosemia
Homocystinuria
Hypoglycemia
Hypoparathyroidism
Hypophosphatasia
Mannosidosis

TABLE 2. *Inherited syndromes associated with cataract*

Disorder	Inheritance*
Anhidrotic ectodermal dysplasia	AD
Alport's syndrome	XL
Conrodi's syndrome	XL
Conradi-Hunermann syndrome	AR
Crouzon's disease	AD
Fabry's disease	XL
Garcin syndrome	AD
Glucose-6-phosphate dehydrogenase deficiency	XL
Hallermann-Streiff-François syndrome	AR
Hallgren syndrome	AR
Icthyosis	AR
Incontinentia pigmenti	XL
Laurence-Moon-Biedl syndrome	AR
Lowe's disease	XL
Menkes' syndrome	XL
Myotonic dystrophy	AD
Norrie's disease	XL
Osteogenesis imperfecta	AD
Osteopetrosis	AR
Oxycephaly	AD
Pierre Robin syndrome	AD
Refsum's disease	AR
Treacher Collins syndrome	AD
Usher syndrome	AR
Weill-Marchesani syndrome	AD
Werner's syndrome	AR
Wilson's disease	AR
Zellweger syndrome	AR

* AD, autosomal dominant; AR, autosomal recessive; XL, X-linked.

polar opacities represent mesenchymal defects due to abnormalities in lenticulocorneal separation.

Congenital nuclear cataracts display a variety of morphologic patterns. These patterns vary from dotlike opacities clustering around the Y-sutures to uniform opacification of the embryonal and fetal nucleus (Fig. 6-5). Congenital zonular cataracts probably reflect a type of temporal injury occurring at the time new fibers are added

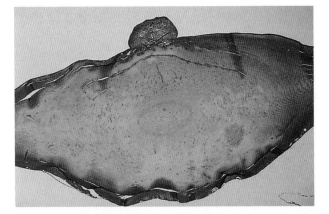

FIG. 6-4. Congenital anterior polar cataract reveals a well-defined nodular proliferation of spindle cells beneath the lens capsule. The fibrous nodule in this case is not sequestered from the underlying lens fibers.

to the growing lens (Figs. 6-6 and 6-7). Usually, the cause of lenticular injury is not determined, but occasionally, cataracts are associated with an identifiable event such as transient hypocalcemia. Histologically, alterations in the lens are nonspecific. Areas of opacification correspond to degenerating fibers and liquefactive necrosis. The **rubella cataract** is caused by viral infection during the first trimester of pregnancy. The systemic teratogenic effects of gestational infection with rubella also include cardiac and auditory anomalies. Postnatal ocular abnormalities in the congenital rubella syndrome other than cataract include microphthalmia, abnormalities of the retinal pigment epithelium, and glaucoma.[14] The clinical appearance of the rubella cataract is variable because both primary and secondary lens fibers can be involved (Fig. 6-8). Nuclear opacification with variable amounts of cortical change are usually observed. Histologically, the lens displays abnormal retention of fiber nuclei (Fig. 6-9). Other signs of

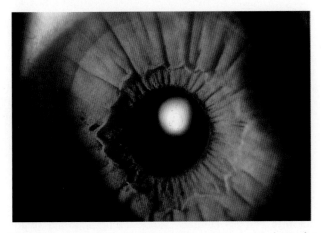

FIG. 6-3. Congenital anterior polar cataract consists of a discrete white nodule resting on clear cortex.

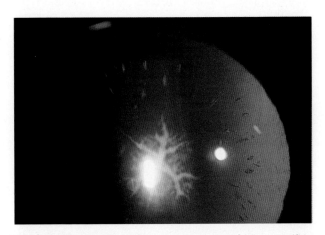

FIG. 6-5. Congenital cataract consisting of white opacification of lens sutures. Dotlike opacities are densely cluster around the Y branching sutures and are less densely scattered peripherally.

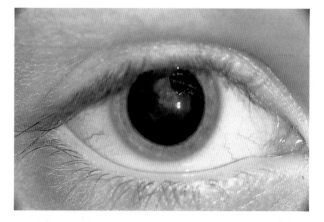

FIG. 6-6. Congenital zonular (lamellar) cataract consisting of a spherical semitransparent opacity with a white opaque center.

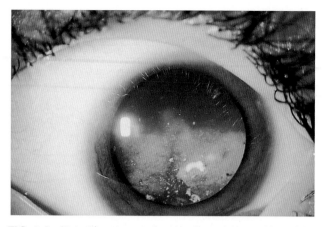

FIG. 6-8. Rubella cataract showing irregular opacities of the lens nucleus and cortex.

lens fiber degeneration can be seen depending on the severity of involvement. Although the retention of lens fiber nuclei is characteristic of rubella cataract, this phenomenon is also found in other conditions such as Lowe's syndrome and trisomy 13.[15,16]

Membranous cataract is an ill-defined entity that probably refers to the end-stage findings that accompany spontaneous adsorption of the lens. Several underlying diseases, including congenital rubella syndrome, are associated with spontaneous absorption of the lens. Membranous cataracts, however, can occur as the consequence of congenital or acquired lenticular disease.

LENS CHANGES ASSOCIATED WITH PERSISTENT HYPERPLASTIC PRIMARY VITREOUS

Although congenital cataract is not a feature of persistent hyperplastic primary vitreous (PHPV), several types

of acquired lens defects are found in PHPV.[17] Failure of the primary vitreous to regress probably stimulates lens epithelium to migrate posteriorly resulting in posterior subcapsular opacification. As the primary vitreous becomes organized, tractional forces on the posterior lens capsule will eventually cause it to tear. Exposure of lens protein induces an inflammatory response (see the section on Lens-Induced Inflammation). Occasionally, mature adipose tissue replaces lens cortex in PHPV. Although the pathogenesis of this anomaly is unclear, it presumably reflects some type of mesenchymal metaplasia.

Acquired Cataracts

Acquired anterior subcapsular cataracts are most often associated with chronic inflammation and trauma, although other types of damage to the lens may result in this pattern of cataract. An injury to lens epithelium from a variety of sources can stimulate cellular and mesenchymal proliferative responses. Thus, lens epithelium can

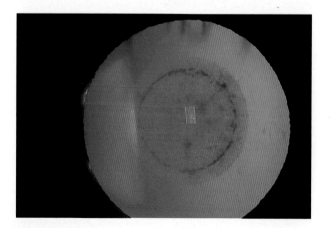

FIG. 6-7. Congenital zonular (lamellar) cataract seen in retroillumination.

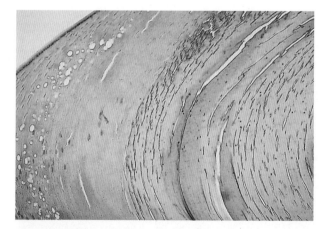

FIG. 6-9. Rubella cataract demonstrating abnormal retension of lens fiber nuclei. The oval basophilic nuclei are present in the lens nucleus.

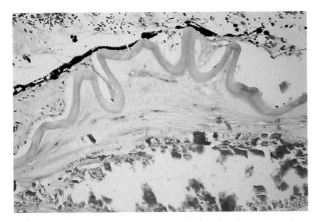

FIG. 6-10. Anterior subcapsular cataract with severe wrinkling of the anterior lens capsule. The basophilic deposits beneath the fibrous plaque are calcified lens fibers.

undergo fibrous metaplasia, and the resulting fibroblastic cells can produce type I and III collagen as well as mucopolysaccharides. Metaplastic tissue eventually may be ''walled off'' from cortical fibers by lens epithelium and thick basement membrane (ie, new lens capsule).[18] Metaplastic epithelium also produces smooth muscle actin, a cytoskeletal protein normally found in myofibroblasts. Secondary wrinkling of the anterior lens capsule is a common finding in anterior subcapsular cataracts and probably reflects the contractile property of the myofibroblast (Fig. 6-10).

Posterior subcapsular cataract is a common pattern of lenticular degeneration in adults. It is often associated with nuclear or cortical cataract, and by itself, may cause considerable visual morbidity because of the tendency of the opacity to be most severe within the visual axis (Fig. 6-11). The opacity corresponds to the aberrant proliferation of lens epithelium along the posterior lens capsule. Several conditions are associated with the disruption of normal meridional migration of lens epithelium at the equator, including prolonged administration of corticosteroids and exposure to ionizing radiation.[19] Normally, lens epithelial cells enter the cortex as new fibers at the equator; however, in posterior subcapsular cataracts, epithelial cells enlarge and migrate along the lens capsule.[20] Cells initially have a spindle shape, but as they reach the posterior polar region, lens epithelia enlarge to five to 10 times their normal size. The cytoplasm of these bloated epithelial cells has a finely granular appearance with hematoxylin-eosin stain and are referred to as **bladder cells** (Fig. 6-12). Bladder cells contain crystalline proteins, few organelles, and abundant cytoskeletal proteins. Bladder cells have prominent interdigitations with neighboring cells and are not associated with aberrant basement membrane. They typically do not produce extracellular matrix, unlike injured epithelial cells beneath the anterior capsule. This poorly understood paradox underscores the fact that the mechanisms that promote and inhibit the equatorial migration of lens epithelium remain unknown.

Cortical cataracts refer to the opacification of lens fibers residing between the nucleus and lens capsule. The resulting white discoloration of cortical fibers is common after age 60 years. It typically begins at the equator and extends circumferentially toward the visual axis, having a wedge or cuneiform shape (Fig. 6-13). The spokelike opacities are often associated with clear spaces or water clefts. Histologically, early wedge-shaped opacities are difficult to detect on hematoxylin-eosin–stained sections. More advanced degenerative changes associated with water clefts correspond to globules of denatured lens protein, or so-called **morgagnian globules** (Fig. 6-14). Cortical cataracts are often associated with nuclear and posterior subcapsular cataracts.

Nuclear degeneration of the lens is the most frequent cause of a clinically significant cataract. Despite the

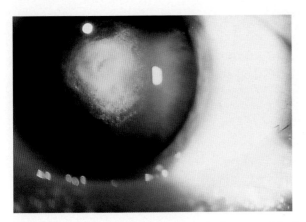

FIG. 6-11. Posterior subcapsular opacity is present in the visual axis. The opacity was considered responsible for the patient's 20/200 visual acuity.

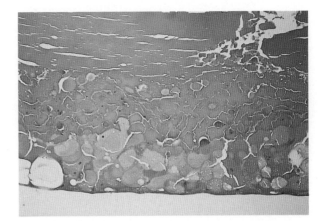

FIG. 6-12. Posterior subcapsular cataract with enlarged bladder cells just beneath the posterior lens capsule. The cells have a small, round nucleus and abundant pale, granular cytoplasm.

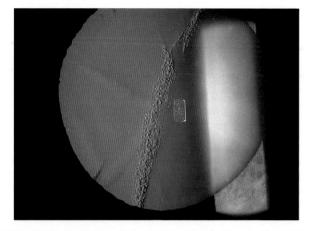

FIG. 6-13. Cortical cataract seen in retroillumination. The spindle-shaped opacity has a granular quality.

frequency of nuclear cataracts in the geriatric population, the pathogenesis of nuclear degeneration is incompletely understood.[21,22] There is no known effective way to prevent or retard the development of nuclear cataracts. Clinically, the lens nucleus normally scatters light giving it a transparent but faint, white appearance even in childhood. With age, the nucleus accumulates a variety of substances that give it even greater light scattering properties. Over decades, the lens fibers become more compact (sclerotic) because they proliferate within the confines of the lens capsule. The sclerotic nucleus slowly and inexorably becomes more visible with colors ranging from lemon yellow to deep mahogany. Histologically, on hematoxylin-eosin–stained sections, even the most advanced nuclear cataract is very bland. Compact lens fibers appear more homogenously pink than in softer, nonsclerotic nuclei, but this change is very subjective. Sclerotic nuclei tend to fracture less on histologic sectioning than softer nuclei, but this

finding is highly variable and depends on the length and type of fixation as well as the sharpness of the microtome blade. Following histologic staining, the most brunescent lens nucleus has tinctorial properties that are similar to a young, noncataractous lens nucleus. Thus, nuclear sclerosis in tissue section is difficult to detect. The presence of nuclear sclerosis is often inferred because of its frequent association with cortical and posterior subcapsular abnormalities that are more readily recognized in tissue section (Fig. 6-15).

The clinical term **mature cataract** refers to a completely white lens that precludes visualization of the posterior pole. In a hypermature cataract, cortical lens fibers have undergone liquefactive degeneration. With the loss of lens volume due to leaching of denatured lens protein, the capsule becomes wrinkled. If the process continues, the indigestible nucleus eventually sinks within the liquefied cortex (morgagnian cataract). In histologic section, the hard nucleus often is dislodged, leaving an empty capsular bag (Fig. 6-16). Morgagnian cataracts are becoming clinically uncommon.

EXTRACAPSULAR CATARACT EXTRACTION

The most common complication of extracapsular cataract extraction (ECCE), with or without the implantation of a posterior chamber intraocular lens (PC-IOL), is posterior capsule opacification. Opacification of the posterior capsule reduces vision by interfering with the passage of light through the visual axis (Fig. 6-17). Posterior capsular opacification may also interfere with vision secondarily when mechanical forces related to lens epithelial fibrous metaplasia displace the PC-IOL from its normal position within the capsular bag. Fibrous contraction of the posterior capsule with the formation of striae is a less frequent cause of mechanically induced vision loss.

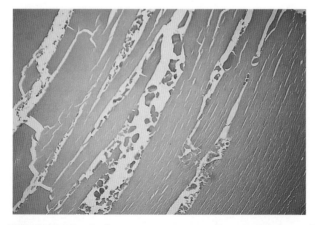

FIG. 6-14. Cortical cataract corresponding to the type of defect seen in Figure 13. Globular clusters of degenerating lens protein separate irregular masses of pink, homogeneous lens fibers.

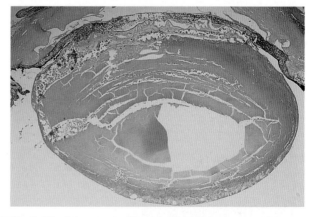

FIG. 6-15. Advanced cataract. This lens demonstrates anterior and posterior subcapsular cataract, cortical cataract, and nuclear sclerosis. The homogenously pink-staining nucleus was fractured during histologic sectioning. A portion of the nucleus is absent on the right.

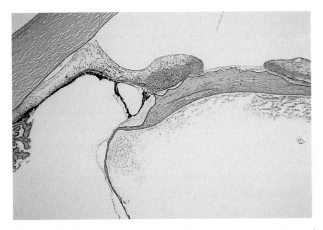

FIG. 6-16. Hypermature cataract (morgagnian cataract) showing liquified lens cortex. The entire lens nucleus fell out during processing, leaving the lens capsule and anterior subcapsular fibrous plaque. The iris is adherent to the anterior lens surface, a condition termed *posterior synechiae*.

The incidence of posterior capsular opacification varies but be as high as 50% after 5 years.[23] Of the many factors that influence posterior capsular opacification, perhaps the two most important are the amount of residual lens material left after cortical clean-up and the age of the patient. Nearly half of all infants and children undergoing extracapsular cataract extraction have opacified capsules 1 year after surgery.[24] Since the likelihood of posterior opacification is so high in infants and children, primary discission at the time of lens extraction is often performed to obviate the need of a second procedure.

The morphologic appearance of posterior capsular opacification is generally similar regardless of the method of lens removal, although there is evidence that certain surgical techniques and IOL designs may reduce the incidence of opacification.[4] The two major components of posterior capsular membranes, fibrous matrix and cellular proliferation, are found in varying proportions. The lens epithelium is the origin of both types of proliferative processes.

After extracapsular cataract extraction, a portion of the anterior capsule, lens equator, and posterior capsule remain in the eye. The residual lens epithelial cells beneath the anterior lens capsule and cells at the equator are the source of postoperative membranes. There is some evidence that epithelial cells beneath the anterior capsule have a propensity toward fibrous metaplasia, although the germinal cells at the equator give rise to pearl formation.[25]

Following extracapsular cataract surgery, lens epithelial cells are stimulated to migrate posteriorly along the capsule and enlarge in cytoplasmic volume. Transformed epithelial cells can become enormous, measuring more than 100 microns in diameter. As in acquired posterior subcapsular cataracts, these abnormal cells are referred to as bladder or Wedl cells. They contain a single small nucleus and abundant pink cytoplasm. The cellular prolif-

eration has a tendency to form spherical nests that, when large enough to identify on clinical examination, are called **pearls** (Hirschberg-Elschnig pearls). They have little clinical significance unless they obstruct the visual axis. On biomicroscopic examination, semitransparent pearls look like clusters of glistening fish eggs.

The related postoperative Soemmering's ring cataract has more historic than practical significance. When first described by Soemmering, this donut-shaped remnant of lens cortex and capsule was often the result of accidental trauma. This configuration of residual lens material is now a natural consequence of routine extracapsular cataract extraction. The donut-shape residuum is often minuscule following a thorough cortical clean-up. Residual lens material; however, can give rise to epithelial proliferation and fibrous metaplasia. These so-called *second cataracts* may demonstrate pearl formation and posterior capsule opacification.

TRAUMATIC INJURY TO THE LENS

Traumatic injury to the eye may result in cataract or other morphologic abnormalities through several different mechanisms. A pigmented ring on the anterior lens capsule (Vossius ring) follows contusion without rupture of the lens capsule. The nature of the pigment is unclear. It is typically believed to represent a melanocytic imprint from the pupillary boarder. The ring may be partial or complete, and it often is transient lasting several days. Occasionally, a residual faint, white ring occurs later and probably corresponds to underlying injury to the lens epithelium or cortical fibers.

Other manifestations of lens fiber injury caused by severe ocular contusion take on a variety of patterns. Generalized lenticular injury can result in a rosette-shaped pat-

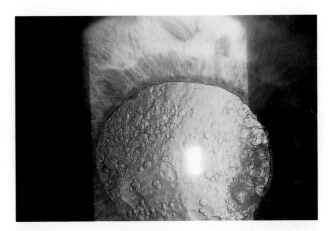

FIG. 6-17. Postoperative proliferation of lens epithelium on posterior lens capsule. The abnormal cellular proliferation following extracapsular cataract extraction with implantation of posterior camber lens has a bubbled appearance in retroillumination.

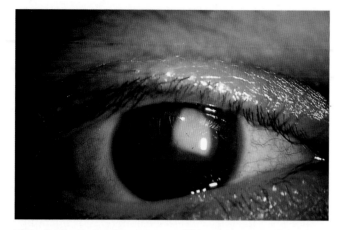

FIG. 6-18. Contusion cataract. This white cortical opacity has remained stable several months after blunt trauma.

tern of fiber whitening beneath the anterior and posterior lens capsule.[26] Opacified fibers have a feather-like appearance radiating peripherally from the suture lines. Sector cataracts reflect regional lenticular injury and consist of fine opacities of the anterior cortex. They tend to develop within weeks of an injury, but can then remain stable (Fig. 6-18).

ABNORMALITIES OF THE LENS CAPSULE

The lens capsule is a passive extracellular tissue that occasionally becomes noticeable when an exogenous material is deposited within it. In Wilson's disease (hepatolenticular degeneration), for example, inorganic copper forms a patelliform discoloration on the anterior and posterior lens capsules.[27] The distinctive faint brown-to-green deposit of copper is known as a **sunflower cataract** and is chemically identical to the deposit found in the peripheral cornea that is known as a **Kaiser-Fleischer ring.** A simi-

lar type of capsular deposit can occur with an intraocular foreign body composed of copper (Fig. 6-19). So-called *chalcosis lentis* was relatively common after World War I because of the prevalence of brass intraocular foreign bodies.

Intraocular silver, gold, and mercury due to iatrogenic or occupational exposures also can be deposited within lens capsule. Phenothiazines have been associated with fine pigment deposits on the anterior lens capsule. Those due to thioridazine give the lens capsule a brown cast, but rarely interfere with vision. Similar deposits are found in the cornea.

Pseudoexfoliation of the Lens Capsule

Pseudoexfoliation of the lens capsule is a systemic abnormality; however, its only clinically recognizable manifestation is the intraocular deposition of dandruff-like material on the lens capsule and iris. Between 20% and 60% of patients with pseudoexfoliation develop glaucoma. Although most patients have open-angle glaucoma, narrowing of the anterior chamber angle has been reported in as many as 30% of persons with pseudoexfoliation. Some use the term **pseudoexfoliation syndrome** for patients with glaucoma. Characteristic capsular findings are present in one eye in 50% to 75% of patients at the time of initial diagnosis. Within 5 to 10 years, approximately 15% of cases become bilateral.[28] Unilateral cases are diagnosed in patients 5 years younger than those with bilateral disease.

The characteristic findings on the anterior lens capsule consist of a subtly gray central disc just larger than the undilated pupil. Complete inspection through a fully dilated pupil reveals an intermediate clear zone and a peripheral zone of grayish granular material (Fig. 6-20). The

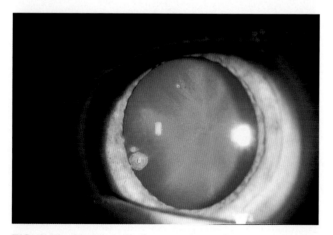

FIG. 6-19. Chalcosis lentis secondary to an intraocular copper foreign body seen in the lower left portion of the lens. The lens capsule has an unusual greenish color.

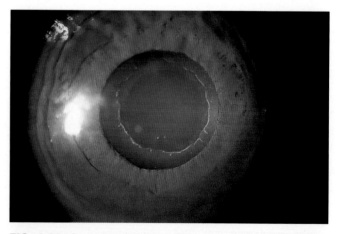

FIG. 6-20. Psuedoexfoliation of the lens capsule showing typical rolled edges and central clear zone. The capsule opacity is easily seen once the pupil is dilated.

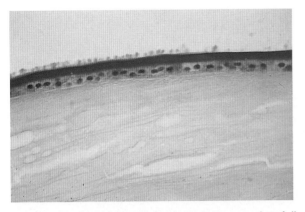

FIG. 6-21. The fine extracellular deposits in pseudoexfoliation appear to be sprinkled on the anterior lens capsule which stains magenta on periodic acid-Schiff reaction.

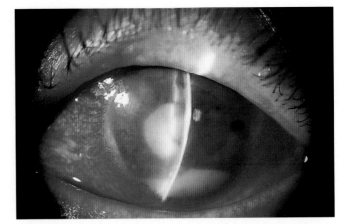

FIG. 6-22. Severe endophthalmitis (sterile) due to rupture of the anterior lens capsule following YAG iridotomy. The large iridotomy was created by a neodymium:YAG laser.

translucent deposits, centrally and peripherally, often curl up giving the impression the material is peeling off the capsular surface.

Histologically, the extracellular material is eosinophilic and rests on the anterior capsular surface like iron filings (Fig. 6-21). Intraocular deposits can be found on the iris, ciliary processes, and anterior hyaloid membrane. Ultrastructurally, the deposit consists of straight and curved fibers with two types of banding patterns.[29] Fibers exist in diameters of both 15 to 20 nm and 40 to 50 nm. This same material has been found in the conjunctiva, orbit, skin, and visceral organs of patients with pseudoexfoliation. Biochemical analysis has demonstrated some similarities between pseudoexfoliative material and the fibrillar units of elastic tissue. The amount of material present in visceral organs is small and usually found near oxytalan or elastic fibers.[30]

ACQUIRED DISORDERS OF LENS EPITHELIUM

The lens epithelium accumulates elemental iron in ocular hemosiderosis and in systemic hemochromatosis. Clinically, intracellular iron gives the epithelium a yellow-brown color. Intracellular iron can be identified in histologic sections using Perls' or Prussian blue stains.

Lens-Induced Inflammation

Accidental or surgical trauma to the lens can be followed by progressively severe inflammation if exposed lens fibers are not adequately removed. This condition, referred to as **phacoanaphylactic endophthalmitis,** is characterized clinically by acute and chronic inflamma-

tion of variable severity (Fig. 6-22). Because the inflammatory response is not mediated by IgE antibodies or mast cells, the term **phacoanaphylactic** is considered inappropriate and has been replaced by the term **phacogenic uveitis.** Although evidence exists that this disorder is an autoimmune response to lens protein, the immunopathogenesis is poorly understood. Histologically, the exposed lens fibers are surrounded by variable proportions of neutrophils and chronic inflammatory cells (Fig. 6-23).[31] Macrophages bloated with lens material are commonly found along the perimeter of residual lens fibers. Epithelioid histiocytes and multinucleated giant cells may be present in large numbers. A chronic inflammatory cell reaction is often found in other portions of the uveal tract. Sympathetic ophthalmia and lens-induced inflammation can coexist as both are caused by penetrating trauma.[32]

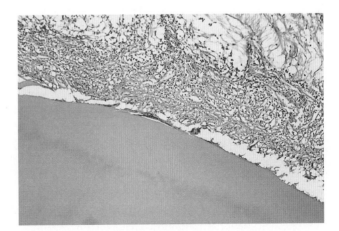

FIG. 6-23. Lens-induced inflammation caused by a retained nuclear fragment following extracapsular cataract extraction. The homogenously pink lens nucleus is surrounded by chronic inflammation cells. The inflammatory reaction is becoming organized. Multinucleated giant cells are present between the nucleus and mantle of chronic inflammatory cells.

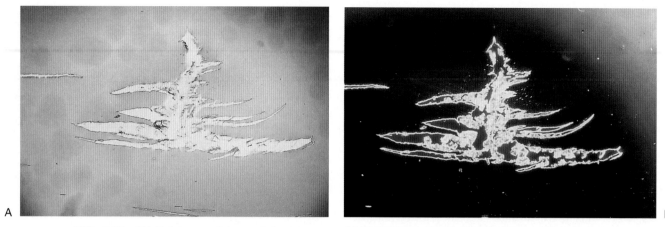

A   B

FIG. 6-24. (A) Calcium oxalate crystals are present in a tree-shaped fracture within the lens nucleus. **(B)** Calcium oxalate crystals under polarized light.

Phacolytic Glaucoma

Phacolytic glaucoma describes the ocular response to escaped denatured lens protein from a hypermature cataract. Unlike phacoanaphylactic endophthalmitis in that a capsular rent must occur to initiate the inflammatory reaction, in phacolytic glaucoma the lens capsule is intact. As denatured lens protein leaches through the capsule, it incites a macrophage response. The mechanism leading to elevated intraocular pressure is not entirely clear. Both denatured lens protein and the cellular reaction may contribute to obstruction of aqueous outflow. The diagnosis of phacolytic glaucoma should be considered when a hypermature cataract is associated with elevated intraocular pressure, open angles, and mild to moderate anterior chamber cell and flare reaction. Cytologic examination of material from an anterior chamber paracentesis typically reveals relatively few cells consisting predominately of macrophages with abundant clear cytoplasm.

Lenticular Crystals

Crystals and crystal-like deposits can occur within the lens. The most common type of crystal found in routine histologic sections is calcium oxalate (Fig. 6-24). These readily polarizable spherical deposits are found in all types of advanced cataracts. They are not associated with any systemic metabolic abnormality and probably represent a local metabolic derangement.

Lenticular crystals have been clinically described in patients with multiple myeloma and cystinosis.

The lens changes in myotonic dystrophy take on several morphologic patterns. The most characteristic finding is small red and green iridescent dots clustering in the most posterior portion of the cortex. They seldom cause visual symptoms, but when present early in the disease, the colorful opacities help establish the clinical diagnosis. The iridescent dots in young patients with myotonic dystrophy are distinguished from the much more common iridescent opacities seen in age-related cataracts by their preferential distribution in the posterior cortex. Iridescent dots probably are caused by reflections from degenerating multilaminated membranes. White punctate lens opacities in patients with myotonic dystrophy can occur in both the anterior and posterior cortical layers. Progression to visually significant opacity is variable.

Secondary Lenticular Calcification

Any longstanding cataract can trap inorganic cations, particularly calcium and phosphorus (Fig. 6-25). Calcified lens fibers appear opaque white and can be misinterpreted on a computed tomogram as a foreign body by radiologists unfamiliar with the clinical history. Spontaneous rupture of the lens capsule of a calcified lens has resulted in dispersion of the calcified material throughout the eye. This condition has been referred to as **calcific phacolysis;** its histologic appearance is striking.[33]

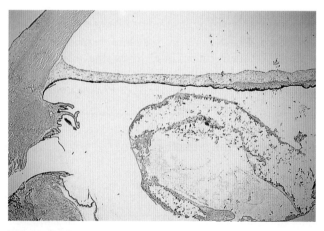

FIG. 6-25. Advanced cataract showing extensive calcification.

REFERENCES

1. Peczon BD, Peczon JD, Cintron C, et al. Changes in chemical composition of anterior lens capsules of cataractous human eyes as a function of age. *Exp Eye Res* 1980;30:155–165.
2. Dische Z, Zelmanis G, Rothschild C. The hexosaminohexuronide of the bovine lens capsule. *Arch Biochem Biophys* 1967;121:685–694.
3. Young RW, Ocumpaugh DE. Autoradiographic studies on the growth and development of the lens capsules in the rat. *Invest Ophthalmol* 1960;5:583–593.
4. Apple DJ, Solomon KD, Tetz MR, et al. Posterior capsule opacification. *Surv Ophthalmol* 1992;37:73–116.
5. Arnott EJ, Crawfurd MA, Toghill PJ. Anterior lenticonus and Alport's syndrome. *Br J Ophthalmol* 1966;50:390–403.
6. Pollard ZF. Familial bilateral posterior lenticonus. *Arch Ophthalmol* 1983;101:1238–1240.
7. Makley TA. Posterior lenticonus: report of a case with histologic findings. *Am J Ophthalmol* 1955;39:308–312.
8. Zimmerman LE, Font RL. Congenital malformations of the eye. *JAMA* 1966;196:684–692.
9. Cogan DG, Kuwabara T. Pathology of cataracts in mongoloid idiocy. *Doc Ophthalmol* 1962;16:73.
10. Margo CE. Congenital aniridia: a histopathologic study of the anterior segment in children. *J Pediatr Ophthalmol Strabismus* 1983;20:192–198.
11. Luntz MH. Clinical types of cataract. In: Tasman W, Jaeger EA, eds. *Duanes's clinical ophthalmology.* Philadelphia: JB Lippincott, 1992:1–20.
12. Silbiger J, Margo CE. Presenile cataracts. In: Margo CE, Hamed LM, Mames RN, eds. *Diagnostic problems in clinical ophthalmology.* Philadelphia: WB Saunders, 1994:273–282.
13. Del Monte MA. Diagnosis and management of congenital and developmental cataracts. *Ophthalmol Clin North Am* 1990;3:205–220.
14. Zimmerman LE. Histopathologic basis for ocular manifestations of congenital rubella syndrome. *Am J Ophthalmol* 1968;65:837–862.
15. Tripathi RC, Cibis GW, Tripathi BJ. Pathogenesis of cataracts in patients with Lowe's syndrome. *Ophthalmology* 1986;93:1046–1051.
16. Hoepner J, Yanoff M. Ocular anomalies in trisomy 13-15: an analysis of 13 eyes with two new findings. *Am J Ophthalmol* 1972;24:729–737.
17. Haddad R, Font RL, Reeser F. Persistent hyperplastic primary vitreous: a clinicopathologic study of 62 cases and review of the literature. *Surv Ophthalmol* 1978;23:123–134.
18. Font RL, Brownstein S. A light and electron microscopic study of anterior subcapsular cataracts. *Am J Ophthalmol* 1974;78:972–984.
19. Greiner JV, Chylack LT. Posterior subcapsular cataracts: histopathologic study of steroid-associated cataracts. *Arch Ophthalmol* 1979;97:135–144.
20. Streeten BW, Eshaghian J. Human posterior subcapsular cataract: a gross and flat preparation study. *Arch Ophthalmol* 1978;96:1653–1658.
21. Lerman S. Evaluation of risk factors in human cataractogenesis. *Dev Ophthalmol* 1991;21:120–132.
22. Schwab IR, Armstrong MA, Friedman GD, et al. Cataract extraction risk factor in an HMO population under 60 years of age. *Arch Ophthalmol* 1988;106:1062–1065.
23. Sterling S, Wood T. Effect of intraocular lens convexity on posterior capsule opacification. *J Cataract Refract Surg* 1986;12:655–657.
24. Metge P, Cohen H, Graff F. Intercapsular intraocular lens implantation in children: 35 cases. *Eur J Implant Refract Surg* 1989;1:169–173.
25. McDonnell PJ, Zarbin MA, Green WR. Posterior capsule opacification in pseudophakic eyes. *Ophthalmology* 1983;90:1548–1553.
26. Cordes FC. *Cataract types: a manual.* Rochester, Minn.: American Academy of Ophthalmology, 1961.
27. Tso MOM, Fine BS, Thorpe HE. Kayser-Fleischer ring and associated cataract in Wilson's disease. *Am J Ophthalmol* 1975;79:479–488.
28. Roth M, Epstein DL. Exfoliation syndrome. *Am J Ophthalmol* 1980;89:477–481.
29. Dark AJ, Streeten BW, Cornwall CC. Pseudoexfoliative disease of the lens: a study in electron microscopy and histochemistry. *Br J Ophthalmol* 1977;61:462–472.
30. Streeten BW, Brookman L, Ritch R, et al. Pseudoexfoliative fibrillopathy in the conjunctiva: a relation to elastic fibers and elastosis. *Ophthalmology* 1987;94:1439–1449.
31. Margo CE, Grossniklaus HE. *Ocular histopathology: a guide to differential diagnosis.* Philadelphia: WB Saunders, 1991;40–44.
32. Eason HA, Zimmerman LE. Sympathetic ophthalmia and bilateral phacoanaphylaxis: a clinicopathologic correlation of the sympathogenic and sympathizing eyes. *Arch Ophthalmol* 1964;72:9.
33. Scroggs MW, Proia AD, Helms HA, et al. Calcific phacolysis: a new clinicopathologic entity. *Ophthalmology* 1993;100:377–383.

Ophthalmic Pathology with Clinical Correlations,
edited by Joseph W. Sassani, M.D.
Lippincott-Raven Publishers, Philadelphia © 1997.

CHAPTER 7

Glaucoma

Joseph W. Sassani

The term **glaucoma** encompasses many ocular disorders characterized by optic nerve and visual field changes. The pathophysiologic thread linking all these entities is an intraocular pressure that exceeds the tolerance of the optic nerve. If one uses these features to define the glaucomas, it is not surprising that this group of optic neuropathies encompasses a wide spectrum of mechanisms and intraocular pressure levels that may damage the optic nerve. For example, a healthy and well-supported optic nerve may require a marked elevation of intraocular pressure before sustaining injury. Conversely, an optic nerve lacking adequate structural support or with intrinsic vascular disease may sustain similar damage at an intraocular pressure within the statistically "normal" range. In fact, at least 30% of patients with glaucoma have normal intraocular pressures when first diagnosed. This type of glaucoma is referred to as **low-tension glaucoma** because it involves intraocular pressures that are seldom above the statistically normal range. A better term for it is **normal-pressure glaucoma.**

In summary, the hallmark of glaucoma is characteristic optic nerve damage that is reflected in typical patterns of visual field loss. Abnormal intraocular pressure is not necessary for the diagnosis of glaucoma.

SIGNIFICANCE OF GLAUCOMA

Approximately 5.2 million people, or 15% of the world's blind population, have lost their sight from glaucoma.[1] The reported prevalence of glaucoma among various populations and nationalities has varied widely from 0.47% to as high as 8.8%.[2-4] Some of this statistical variation may result from differences in sampling techniques; however, the actual incidence and prevalence of glaucoma probably vary widely among various populations and ethnic groups. For example, there are significant racial differences in the reported incidence and prevalence of primary

J. W. Sassani: Department of Ophthalmology, Penn State University, Milton S. Hershey Medical Center, Hershey, Pennsylvania 17033.

open-angle glaucoma (POAG), the most common type in the United States. The Beaver Dam Eye Study, which contained a largely white population, found an overall prevalence of POAG of 3.1%.[5] These findings are consistent with those of the Baltimore Eye Survey, which found a prevalence of POAG among whites ranging from 0.92% at age 40 years to 2.16% at 80 years.[6] The prevalence of POAG among blacks in the Baltimore study, however, was four to five times higher than that of whites, ranging from 1.23% to 11.26% for similar age groups. It is not surprising, therefore, that there is considerable variation worldwide in the distribution of the various forms of glaucoma. More details about these dissimilarities are presented for each type of glaucoma discussed in this chapter.

CLASSIFICATION

The various forms of glaucoma can be classified in many ways. The following is a system that uses both the anatomic configuration of the anterior chamber angle and the specific pathophysiologic mechanisms:

- Normal outflow
  - Hypersecretion glaucoma
- Impaired outflow
  - Congenital (infantile) glaucoma
    - Primary
    - Secondary
  - Primary glaucoma
    - Angle closure with pupillary block
    - Angle closure without pupillary block
    - Open angle
  - Secondary glaucoma
    - Angle closure with pupillary block
    - Angle closure without pupillary block
    - Open angle
- Variable outflow
  - Normal-pressure glaucoma

Normal outflow hypersecretion glaucoma was described by Becker and associates and is included in this classification scheme for the sake of completeness; however, this type of glaucoma is uncommon.[7]

Impaired Outflow: Embryologic Considerations in the Classification of Glaucoma

Neural-crest–derived tissue is now recognized as contributing extensively to the embryologic development of the anterior segment of the globe. In fact, mesenchyme (embryonic connective tissue) originating in neural crest plays the same role in the development of the head and neck as does the middle embryonic layer, mesoderm, in the ontogeny of other regions of the body. Therefore, abnormalities in the migration, maturation, and development of this tissue are of great significance in classifying some forms of glaucoma.[8,9] Extensive reviews of this topic exist elsewhere[10,11]; therefore, only a brief overview is presented here, drawing on these and other sources.[12–17]

The neural crest cells migrate from the crests of the neural folds during the first month of gestation prior to closure of the neural tube. During that period, they surround the developing optic vesicles. Subsequently, neural-crest–derived cells provide much of the anterior ocular segment tissue. Specific ocular tissues that may be neural-crest derived include corneal stroma and endothelium, anterior iris stroma, iris melanocytes, ciliary body, sclera, intraocular vascular pericytes, and portions of trabecular meshwork including endothelium. Table 1 outlines the role of neural crest tissue in ocular embryogenesis. As Kaiser-Kupfer has pointed out, the neural crest provides virtually all of the connective tissue between the lens and the anterior corneal epithelium.[18]

Three waves of neural-crest cell migration, which pass between the surface ectoderm and the lens, contribute to the formation of the anterior segment of the globe. The first wave of cells differentiates into the corneal endothelium and also produces the trabecular meshwork and its endothelium. The corneal endothelium, in turn, produces Descemet's membrane. The second wave infiltrates between corneal epithelium and endothelium to form keratocytes. The third wave produces the iris stroma. Subsequently, the iris pigment epithelium is derived from neural ectoderm. The endothelium of Schlemm's canal and vascular endothelium probably derive from vascular mesoderm and not from neural crest. Neural-crest cells also

contribute to important structures of the orbit and head including the meninges, pituitary gland, bones and cartilage of the upper face, dental papillae, connective tissue supporting cells of the orbit, orbital nerves, and their associated Schwann cells.

The role of the neural crest in ocular development is discussed further in this chapter relative to the pathogenesis of congenital glaucoma and other developmentally related forms of glaucoma. Table 2 presents an overview of these relationships.

CONGENITAL GLAUCOMA

Primary Congenital (Infantile) Glaucoma

Primary congenital (infantile) glaucoma has been reviewed extensively by deLuise and Anderson.[19] It occurs in 1 in 10,000 births[20] and usually is sporadic; however, autosomal inheritance with variable penetrance has been reported.[19,21] Infantile glaucoma is said to be the cause of blindness for 2% to 15% of institutionalized blind individuals.[22] It has an overall prevalence of 0.01% to 0.04%. In the United States, there is a male predominance,[19] and it is bilateral in 65% to 80% of cases.[22,23]

The classic signs and symptoms of congenital glaucoma are epiphora, photophobia/blepharospasm, corneal enlargement, and corneal clouding. Occasionally, stretching of the cornea results in rupture of Descemet's membrane (Fig. 7-1). Nevertheless, Seidman and associates noted that parents reported epiphora in 55%, photophobia in 41%, and both symptoms in only 32% of children with primary infantile glaucoma at the time of presentation.[24] Similarly, parents noted signs of infantile glaucoma in a minority of the children (corneal haze or clouding in 41%; corneal or globe enlargement in 32%) while such signs were noted by a physician in 92% of the children at the time of presentation.[24] Furthermore, 21% of these children had signs of infantile glaucoma but no history of epiphora, blepharospasm, or photophobia.

In any suspected case of congenital glaucoma, the child's corneal diameter should be documented, particularly because such enlargement may not be obvious in bilateral cases.[24] The 95% ranges of normal corneal diameters are as follows: 9.4 to 11 mm at age 1 month; 10.5 to 11.7 mm at age 6 months; and 10.8 to 12 mm at age 12 months.[25] Morin and colleagues found a corneal

TABLE 1. *Ocular neural crest derivatives*

Cornea	Iris	Iridocorneal angle	Sclera	Choroid
Keratocytes	Stromal melanocytes	Trabecular endothelium	Most or all	Melanocytes
Endothelium	Stroma	Meshwork		Vascular pericytes
				Connective tissue cells

(Modified from Beauchamp GR, Knepper PA. Role of the neural crest in anterior segment development and disease. *J Pediatr Ophthalmol Strab* 1984;21:209–214).

TABLE 2. *Classification of anterior segment disorders based on neural crest origin*

Cell abnormality	Secondary disorder
Deficient neural crest formation (brain–eye–face malformations)	
Abnormal crest-cell migration	Congenital glaucoma Posterior embryotoxin Axenfeld's anomaly syndrome Rieger's anomaly and syndrome Peters' anomaly Sclerocornea
Abnormal crest-cell proliferation	Iris nevus syndrome Chandler's syndrome Essential iris atrophy Iridotrabecular dysgenesis–ectropion uveae syndrome
Abnormal crest-cell terminal induction (final differentiation)	Congenital hereditary endothelial dystrophy Posterior polymorphous dystrophy Fuchs' endothelial dystrophy
Acquired abnormalities	Metaplasia Abiotrophy Proliferation

(Modified from Bahn CF, Falls HF, Varley GA, et al. Classification of corneal endothelial disorders based on neural crest origin. *Ophthalmology* 1984;91:558).

diameter of 11 mm or less in only 24% of primary congenital glaucoma patients younger than 3 months and in only 9% of those 3 months or older.[26] Corneal asymmetry is a very helpful sign in unilateral cases.[27]

Table 3 provides a differential diagnosis of the symptoms and signs in primary infantile glaucoma. It should be emphasized that infantile glaucoma is easily overlooked when evaluating the infant with epiphora.

Other Forms of Congenital (Infantile) Glaucoma

Table 4 presents a listing of ocular disorders associated with infantile glaucoma. As might be anticipated based

TABLE 3. *Differential diagnosis of symptoms and signs in primary congenital (infantile) glaucoma*

Conditions with epiphora
  Conjunctivitis
  Nasolacrimal duct obstruction
  Corneal abrasion*
  Ocular inflammation*
Conditions with signs of corneal enlargement
  Axial myopia
  Megalocornea
Conditions with signs of corneal clouding
  Intrauterine corneal inflammation
    Congenital syphilis
    Rubella keratitis
  Infantile corneal inflammation
    Chemical
    Herpes simplex
    Mumps keratitis
    Varicella-herpes zoster
    Vaccinia and variola
    Inclusion conjunctivitis
  Mucopolysaccharidosis
  Birth trauma
  Hereditary corneal dystrophy
  Cystinosis
  Sclerocornea and cornea plana
  Anterior segment cleavage syndromes

* Also with photophobia.

(Modified from deLuise VP, Anderson DR. Primary infantile glaucoma (congenital glaucoma). *Surv Opthalmol* 1983;28:1–19; Nelson LB. *Pediatric ophthalmology.* Philadelphia: WB Saunders, 1984; Seidman DJ, et al. Signs and symptoms in the presentation of primary infantile glaucoma. *Pediatrics* 1986;77:399–401).

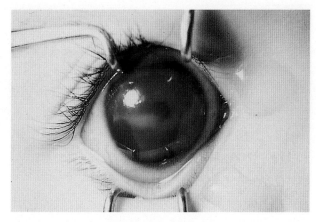

FIG. 7-1. Clinical photograph of congenital glaucoma illustrating horizontal band of prominent corneal edema resulting from rupture of Descemet's membrane.

TABLE 4. *Ocular disorders associated with congenital (infantile) glaucoma*

Corneal anomalies
  Sclerocornea
  Microcornea
  Megalocornea
  Corneal staphyloma

Mesodermal dysgenesis
  Axenfeld's syndrome
  Rieger's syndrome
  Peter's syndrome
  Iridotrabecular dysgenesis–ectropion uveae syndrome

Microphthalmos
  Simple
  Associated

Iris anomalies
  Aniridia
  Colobomata
  Polycoria, microcoria

Lens anomalies
  Congenital aphakia
  Lenticonus
  Lentiglobus
  Spherophakia
  Ectopia lentis
    Homocystinuria
    Marfan's syndrome
    Weill-Marchesani syndrome
    Ehlers-Danlos syndrome

(Modified from Bardelli AM, Hadjistilianou T. Congenital glaucoma associated with other abnormalities in 150 cases. *Glaucoma* 1987;9:10).

TABLE 5. *Systemic disorders associated with congenital (infantile) glaucoma*

Chromosomal defects
  10p–
  Partial trisomy 16q
  Ring chromosome 6
  Trisomy 13

Inborn errors of metabolism
  Homocystinuria
  Hurler's syndrome
  Lowe's syndrome
  Refsum's syndrome

Infection

Rubella

Phakomatoses
  Neurofibromatosis
  Nevus of Ota
  Sturge-Weber syndrome

Pluriformative syndromes
  Coffin-Siris syndrome
  Down's syndrome
  Hallermann-Streiff-François syndrome
  Marfan's syndrome
  Meyer-Schwickerath and Weyers syndrome
  Pierre Robin syndrome
  Rubinstein-Taybi syndrome
  Weill-Marchesani syndrome

(Modified from Bardelli AM, Hadjistilianou T. Congenital glaucoma associated with other abnormalities in 150 cases. *Glaucoma* 1987;9:10).

on the previous discussion of the role of neural crest tissue in ocular embryology, many of the ocular disorders associated with infantile glaucoma involve the ocular anterior segment. Table 5 lists systemic diseases associated with infantile glaucoma. The list is not all-inclusive because isolated reports of glaucoma associated with specific chromosomal abnormalities or with systemic syndromes occur frequently. Rather, this listing is of the better-established infantile glaucoma associations. Some of these entities, such as Sturge-Weber syndrome (Fig. 7-2), occur with sufficient frequency that they may be expected to be observed by the clinician not practicing in a referral setting (see also Chapter 4).

Of particular significance are the mesodermal dysgenesis or anterior-chamber cleavage syndromes, including Axenfeld's, Rieger's, and Peters' syndromes (Table 2). These entities were identified as cleavage syndromes when they were believed to result from failure of the anterior segment to develop properly through a process of cleavage within mesodermal tissue.[28] As has been noted previously, it is recognized currently that these entities represent abnormalities in development of neural-crest–derived tissues.[29] They include a spectrum of ocular and systemic disorders, which should be sought as part of the patient's evaluation. Recently, they have been cited in association with the condition known as bilateral diffuse iris nodular nevi.[30]

Peters' anomaly is associated with abnormalities of the PAX6 gene[31] and as part of the Peters'-Plus syndrome, which includes a typical face, cleft lip and palate, short-limb dwarfism, and developmental retardation.[32,33] It may be found with persistent hyperplastic primary vitreous.

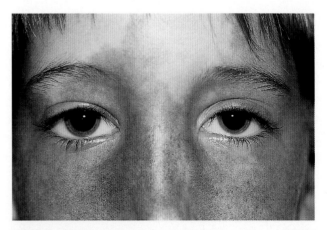

FIG. 7-2. Photograph of a child with bilateral Sturge-Weber angiomas affecting the periocular areas. Upper lid involvement increases the risk of glaucoma.

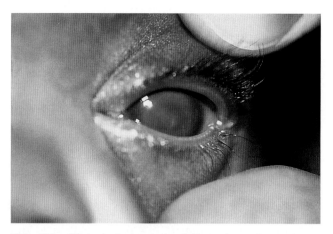

FIG. 7-3. Clinical photograph of Peters' syndrome in an infant with fetal alcohol syndrome. Note the corneal opacification.

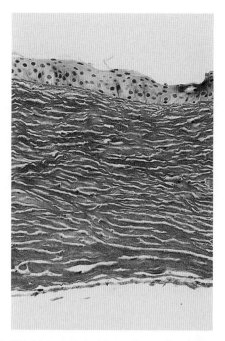

FIG. 7-5. Trichrome-stained specimen illustrating absence of Bowman's and Descemet's membranes in Peters' syndrome.

Many other associations also exist but are beyond the scope of this chapter.[35–37]

Often, Axenfeld's and Rieger's syndromes are considered collectively as the Axenfeld-Rieger syndrome. Ocular findings include anteriorly displaced Schwalbe's line (termed **posterior embryotoxon** when it is an isolated finding), iris processes to Schwalbe's line, other corneal abnormalities, anterior iris insertion at the level of the trabecular meshwork, mild-to-marked iris stromal atrophy with possible hole formation, corectopia, glaucoma, and other infrequent ocular findings.[29] Systemic anomalies may include dental abnormalities, short stature, abnormal external ears, hypertelorism, arachnodactyly, polydactyly, scoliosis, kyphosis, imperforate anus, umbilical hernia, myopathy, and occasionally mental retardation.[38]

Peters' syndrome is characterized by the presence of congenital corneal opacification that usually is bilateral and affects the posterior cornea most severely (Fig. 7-3), but it also can include absence of Bowman's membrane[28,39–43] (Figs. 7-4 and 7-5). It may primarily affect

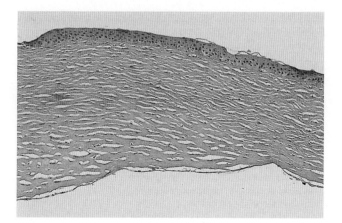

FIG. 7-4. Photomicrograph demonstrating thinning of the central cornea.

the peripheral cornea.[44] Other associated ocular findings include microphthalmos, myopia, aniridia, and cataract.[37] Agenesis of Bowman's layer also has been reported as an isolated finding not associated with Peters' anomaly, inflammation, and so forth.[45] Often the lens has a "top hat" configuration that may mirror the abnormality in the posterior cornea. Immunohistochemical analysis of corneal transplant specimens in Peters' syndrome has suggested a role for extracellular matrix elements, particularly fibronectin, in the disorder.[46]

A recent report of the results of surgery for Peters' anomaly on 30 eyes of 18 patients found that it achieved vision of no better than 20/400 in eyes with concurrent glaucoma.[47] Generally poor results in patients with associated glaucoma also have been reported by others.[48,49]

Recently, these entities have been demonstrated to be part of the **fetal alcohol syndrome** (FAS), which results from maternal alcohol intake early in the first trimester of pregnancy. Typical systemic findings include the following: (1) a characteristic facial appearance including microcephaly, microphthalmia and other ocular abnormalities (see Figs. 7-3–7-5), short palpebral fissures, and poorly developed philtrum, thin upper lip, and flattening of the upper maxillary area; (2) growth retardation; and (3) central nervous system abnormalities, including developmental delay or intellectual impairment.[50,51] According to Stromland, up to 90% of children affected with FAS have eye abnormalities. Most common findings are optic nerve head hypoplasia (up to 48%), tortuosity of the retinal vessels (up to 49%),[52,53] and strabismus (43% to 66%).[52,54] Less frequently reported ocular abnormalities

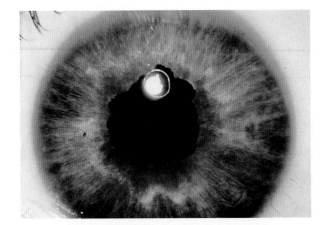

FIG. 7-6. Clinical photograph of ectropion uveae in congenital iridotrabecular dysgenesis ectropion uveae syndrome. (From Dowling JL, Jr., et al. Primary glaucoma associated with iridotrabecular dysgenesis and ectropion uveae. *Ophthalmology* 1985;92:912–921).

are ptosis and microphthalmos.[55] DiGeorge's syndrome also has been reported.[56]

FAS is a devastating public health issue. It is the leading known cause of mental retardation in the United States.[57] The incidence of FAS is 1.9 per 1000 live births worldwide[57]; however, the incidence is as high as 10.3 per 1000 births for native Americans.[58]

Congenital ectropion uvea (CEU) is a rare, nonprogressive anomaly in which iris pigment epithelium migrates onto the anterior iris surface.[59] It may be associated with neurofibromatosis or other ocular anomalies.[59] Ritch and colleagues presented several patients in which it was associated with glaucoma.[59] Other associated findings were neurofibromatosis in three patients, facial hemihypertrophy in two, Rieger's syndrome in one, Prader-Willi syndrome in one, and no systemic disorders in one. Others have reported patients with CEU in association with glaucoma, some of which also had systemic disorders such

as Prader-Willi syndrome.[60–63] Dowling and associates reported CEU with iridotrabecular dysgenesis in 9 patients[64] (Fig. 7-6). These individuals also manifested iris hypoplasia and glaucoma. All patients with congenital ectropion uveae should be followed for the development of glaucoma and for other abnormalities of neural crest origin.[59]

Recently, the heredity of the various forms of childhood glaucoma has been reviewed by Mattox and Walton.[65] These authors restrict the term **secondary childhood glaucoma** to refer to acquired forms of glaucoma related to entities such as trauma, tumors, and uveitis. Tables 6, 7, and 8 are from that review. Table 6 lists the glaucomas that are autosomal dominant in inheritance. Table 7 presents the autosomal recessive and X-linked varieties. Finally, Table 8 lists childhood glaucomas that are sporadic.

Mechanisms and Histopathologic Correlations in Congenital Glaucoma

The exact mechanism(s) and histopathologic correlations underlying trabecular dysfunction in congenital glaucoma have been debated extensively. On gonioscopy, the trabecular meshwork in congenital glaucoma often

TABLE 7. *Primary childhood glaucomas with autosomal recessive or x-linked inheritance*

Autosomal recessive
   Zellweger's (hepatocerebrorenal) syndrome
   Mucopolysaccharidosis (except MPS II)
   Cystinosis
   Warburg's syndrome

X-linked
   Lowe's (oculocerebrorenal) syndrome
   MPS II (Hunter's syndrome)

(From Mattox C, Walton DS. Hereditary primary childhood glaucomas. *Int Ophthalmol Clin* 1993;33:121–134).

TABLE 6. *Primary childhood glaucomas with autosomal dominant inheritance*

Neurofibromatosis type I
Juvenile glaucoma
Stickler syndrome
Oculodental dysplasia
Open-angle glaucoma associated with microcornea and absent frontal sinuses
Osteogenesis imperfecta
Congenital microcornea
Aniridia
Sclerocornea
Familial hypoplasia of the iris
Axenfeld-Rieger syndrome
Posterior polymorphous dystrophy
Marfan's syndrome

(From Mattox C, Walton DS. Hereditary primary childhood glaucomas. *Int Ophthalmol Clin* 1993;33:121–134).

TABLE 8. *Primary childhood glaucomas occurring sporadically*

Primary congenital glaucoma
Juvenile glaucoma
Sturge-Weber syndrome
Rubinstein-Taybi syndrome
Chromosomal trisomies and deletions
Cutis marmorata telangiectasia congenita
Microcornea
Aniridia
Congenital ocular melanosis
Sclerocornea
Peter's anomaly
Iridodysgenesis with ectropion uveae
Elevated episcleral venous pressure
Anterior corneal staphyloma
Congenital lens-iris-angle membrane

(From Mattox C, Walton DS. Hereditary primary childhood glaucomas. *Int Ophthalmol Clin* 1993;33:121–134).

has a peculiar sheen, which led to the hypothesis that an imperforate layer of tissue (Barkan's membrane) covers the trabeculum of affected children. Clinical support for this theory comes from the fact that the surgical procedure goniotomy, which involves incising the superficial face of the trabecular meshwork, usually is curative as might be anticipated if the procedure were disrupting a membranous covering. Nevertheless, histopathologic examination of specimens from individuals with congenital glaucoma has produced conflicting results. Some authors believe they have found the elusive membrane and others have denied its existence.

It is known that the anterior chamber angle in children with congenital glaucoma has a characteristic configuration (Fig. 7-7), as summarized by DeLuise and Anderson[19]:

1. There is an anterior insertion of the iris on the ciliary body but an open angle.
2. The trabecular meshwork is present and perforate, but trabecular beams are thicker than normal.
3. Intertrabecular spaces are patent internally, but more externally located sheets are compressed and lack intertrabecular spaces.
4. An amorphous material is present in the subendothelial region of Schlemm's canal.
5. There are decreased numbers of Holmberg vacuoles on the endothelium of Schlemm's canal.
6. Iris processes (pectinate ligaments) are present.
7. Scleral spur is poorly developed. As a result, longitudinal fibers of ciliary muscle pass through to insert directly onto the trabecular meshwork.
8. Ciliary processes are anteriorly displaced and pulled inward secondary to an enlarging globe but a static-sized lens.

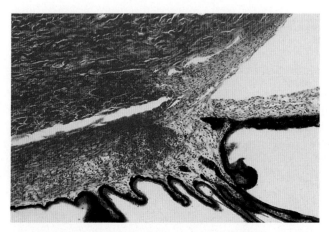

FIG. 7-7. Photomicrograph of immature anterior chamber angle illustrating anterior displacement of ciliary processes and iris root on the ciliary body and redundant tissue in anterior chamber angle. It is not possible to say with certainty whether the histologic appearance of this specimen confirms the diagnosis of congenital glaucoma or merely represents tissue from a normal immature angle.

9. Most observers have found a compact mass of compressed trabecular tissue near the anterior chamber surface of the trabecular meshwork. This tissue may appear imperforate at the resolution level of light microscopy.

Although these findings are characteristic of congenital glaucoma, many are observed, at least at the light microscopic level, in age-matched control specimens from normal infant eyes. Thus, they may partly reflect early stages in the maturation process of the trabecular region.

Primary Angle-Closure Glaucoma

The epidemiology of primary angle-closure glaucoma (PACG) has been reviewed extensively. Although POAG is the most prevalent form of glaucoma among white populations (75% to 95%), PACG is found in approximately the same percentage of Eskimos and Asians.[66] For example, Arkell and associates noted a prevalence of 0.65% for angle-closure glaucoma among 1686 Alaskan Eskimos, which rose to 2.65% in those older than 40 years of age.[67] Women were affected four times more frequently than men. Seventeen percent of individuals older than 50 years had occludable angles. Similar findings were noted in other Eskimo populations.[68] A high incidence of angle-closure glaucoma also is associated with the mixed racial population of South Africa.[69,70]

PACG can be subdivided on the basis of pathophysiologic mechanism into those cases involving a pupillary block mechanism and those lacking such a mechanism (plateau iris syndrome). The most common form of primary angle-closure in white populations results from pupillary block in which the relative resistance to aqueous flow between the iris and lens causes the iris to bow forward (iris bombe) until it contacts the trabecular meshwork thereby obstructing aqueous outflow. Typically, such patients note a sudden onset of ocular pain, blurred vision, and halos around lights. The ocular manifestations may be accompanied by severe systemic signs and symptoms, which may simulate a cardiac or gastrointestinal emergency. In contrast, symptomatic acute angle-closure is much less frequently seen in American blacks. Rather, such individuals often develop subacute or chronic angle-closure, which may be misdiagnosed as POAG.[71]

The common clinical finding in patients predisposed to primary angle-closure is a narrow anterior chamber angle (Fig. 7-8), which can be predicted by pen-light or slit-lamp examination[72] and which must be confirmed gonioscopically. Various authors have attempted to correlate abnormal dimensions of the eye with a predisposition to angle-closure. In general, eyes that develop angle-closure have a smaller corneal diameter, smaller radius of corneal curvature, shorter axial length, and decreased anterior chamber depth compared with normal eyes.[73-79] Some of these parameters are not independent variables, but rather

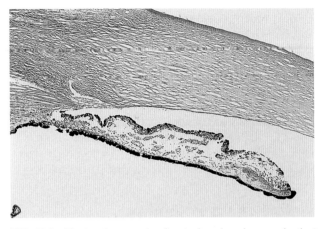

FIG. 7-8. Photomicrograph of anterior chamber angle that would appear narrow on clinical gonioscopic examination. Note the uniformity of the narrow angle compared with a plateau iris as shown in Fig. 7-9.

reflect the overall smaller dimensions of involved eyes. The ratio of lens thickness to ocular axial length reflects the relation between two key variables.[79-81] It has been demonstrated that an increased lens thickness/ocular axial length ratio is found in angle-closure patients and presumably indicates disproportionate lens growth in these patients.[79-81]

An important variant of PACG is the **plateau iris syndrome** in which angle-closure occurs on pupillary dilation in the presence of a patent iridectomy/iridotomy.[82,83] Typically, these patients have relatively deep central anterior chambers and a flat iris contour in that area; however, the peripheral anterior chamber is made shallow by an anterior displacement of the iris in this region (Fig. 7-9). Wand and associates have distinguished the syndrome from the similar appearing plateau configuration. The latter entity responds favorably to iridotomy.[84] Ultrasound

biomicroscopy has disclosed that the distinguishing feature of eyes with plateau iris syndrome is anteriorly placed ciliary processes, which support the peripheral iris in an anteriorly displaced location even after iridotomy is performed.[85,86]

PACG has been associated with several ocular and systemic diseases. Only a few of these are discussed here. (Also see the section on Secondary Angle-Closure Glaucoma in this chapter). Of particular importance to clinicians is the association between PACG and **pseudoexfoliation syndrome** (PXE) (Fig. 7-10), which recently was reviewed extensively by Ritch.[87] Gross and colleagues noted occludable angles in 9.3% of 54 patients with PXE.[88] These findings were supported by Brusini and associates who found an even higher prevalence of occludable angles (21.5%).[89] It has been postulated that the weakened zonules found in association with PXE permit anterior subluxation of the lens thereby contributing to pupillary block in these patients.[90] Other mechanisms also are possible.[88] Ritch has noted that PXE patients may exhibit extremely elevated intraocular pressure in the absence of angle-closure, and that the clinician must be careful to correctly diagnose the glaucoma mechanism in these patients.[87] For a further discussion of PXE, see the section on Secondary Open-Angle Glaucoma.

PACG is found in association with iridoschisis (Fig. 7-11).[91] Salmon and Murray noted a statistically significant similarity in anterior chamber depth and axial length between iridoschisis patients with PACG and other PACG patients.[91] They postulated that the iridoschisis was a manifestation of iris stromal atrophy resulting from intermittent or acute intraocular pressure elevation.

Pitts and Jay reported a series of 24 patients with Fuchs' dystrophy who had axial hypermetropia and shallow anterior chamber.[92] Their data was confirmed by Lowenstein and associates who proposed that there was no causal relationship between Fuchs' dystrophy and the high inci-

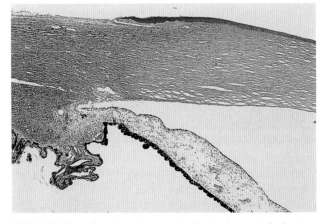

FIG. 7-9. Anterior chamber angle photomicrograph demonstrating a plateau appearance. Note that the central anterior chamber is deep; however, the angle becomes narrow as one examines the anterior chamber periphery. See Fig. 7-8.

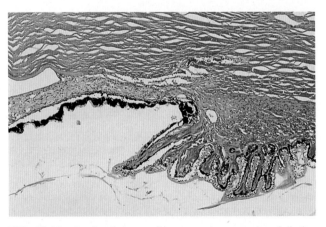

FIG. 7-10. Angle-closure glaucoma in pseudoexfoliation (PXE). The "corrugations" in the pigment epithelium on the posterior iris are characteristic of PXE.

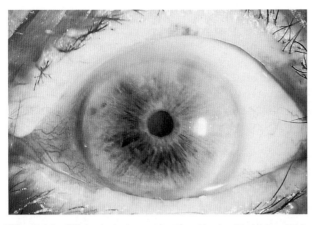

FIG. 7-11. Clinical photograph of patient with iridoschisis. Note iridotomies that were performed for narrow angles.

dence of axial hyperopia and shallow anterior chambers, but rather, the association arose through a common genetic linkage.[93]

PACG in childhood cystinosis is believed to be caused by the accumulation of cystine in the iris stroma.[94] Hagan and Lederer have described a kinship with spontaneous lens subluxation, myopia, and PACG.[95,96] Other associations of angle-closure glaucoma are discussed in the section Secondary Angle-Closure Glaucoma.

PACG affects many ocular structures and shares pathologic findings with other forms of glaucoma particularly secondary angle-closure glaucoma. A significant reduction in corneal endothelial cells compared with unaffected fellow eyes or to individuals who have had prophylactic iridectomy has been reported.[97,98] This decrease in endothelial cells has been postulated to predispose these eyes to corneal decompensation and edema, especially after subsequent surgical procedures such as cataract surgery.[97] Markowitz and Morin noted that endothelial cell loss in primary angle-closure was most likely to occur in association with visual field loss, cup/disk ratio greater than 0.5, previous acute attack, and surgery, in addition to peripheral iridectomy.[99] Bigar and Witmer reported that the degree of endothelial cell loss correlates with the intraocular pressure increase in primary angle-closure.[100] They also found a high incidence (35%) of bilateral corneal guttata. Damage to anterior lens epithelium results in localized opacities termed **glaukomflecken** (Fig. 7-12).

Panda and Jonas studied the photoreceptor count in 23 eyes with secondary angle-closure glaucoma.[101] The retinas demonstrated significantly decreased numbers of photoreceptors compared with 14 eyes with choroidal melanomas. Similarly, Jonas and colleagues have documented thinning of the outer and inner retinal layers and loss of pigment epithelial cells in the parapapillary region in eyes with secondary angle-closure glaucoma.[102] Nevertheless, Kendell and colleagues failed to detect significant photoreceptor loss in primary open-angle glaucoma.[103] Choroidal thinning has been demonstrated in these eyes

and has been postulated to contribute to photoreceptor loss.[104] Thinning of the lamina cribrosa, optic disc cupping, and decreased numbers of corpora amylacea also have been described in eyes with secondary angle-closure glaucoma.[105]

Laser iridotomy is the treatment of choice for angle-closure secondary to pupillary block once the acute attack has been managed medically[106] (see Fig. 7-11). Similarly, prophylactic iridotomy usually should be performed in the fellow eye because up to 50% of such eyes eventually develop angle-closure even while on miotic therapy.[107,108] One also should consider prophylactic iridotomy in patients with severely narrow angles who have not yet suffered an acute attack of angle-closure.[109,110] Nevertheless, laser iridotomy should not be performed without due consideration, as significant complications, including malignant glaucoma,[111] have been reported from the procedure.[106]

Rodrigues and associates examined surgical iridectomy specimens obtained from 3 hours to 10 weeks after YAG iridotomy.[112] Early effects included mild hemorrhages and fibrinous exudates. There was a striking absence of inflammatory cells. Later (up to 2 months after the procedure), there was irregular thickness of the iris pigment epithelium at the iridotomy margins. Tissue atrophy was limited to the immediate iridotomy site. The untreated surrounding iris was intact.

Tetsumoto and colleagues studied sector iridectomy specimens obtained 3 to 5 years after YAG laser iridotomy. The edges of the laser sites were composed of loosely arranged melanocytes, fibrocytes, and blood vessels. Numerous pigment-laden cells were present in the iris stroma. There were no fibrinous aggregates, and no inflammatory response or scarring was noted. Blood vessels appeared intact, and there were no signs of pigment epithelial proliferation. They concluded that the wound healed without fibrous scar formation and with little tendency to closure.[113]

Argon laser peripheral iridoplasty (ALPI) (laser ge-

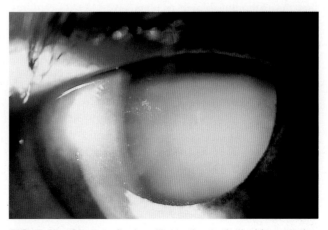

FIG. 7-12. Glaukomflecken illustrating typical white anterior cortical opacities.

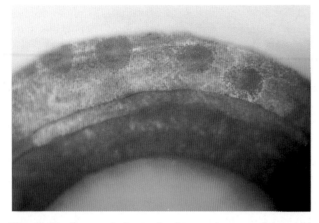

FIG. 7-13. Gross photograph of argon laser peripheral iridoplasty scars at iris periphery.

nioplasty) (Fig. 7-13) is a worthwhile alternative or complement to iridotomy. It is useful in the treatment of peripheral anterior synechias and plateau iris syndrome or when it is not possible to perform iridotomy.[114–116] Light and scanning- and transmission-electron microscopic examination of ALPI-treated iris revealed contraction furrow formation and the proliferation of fibroblast-like cells on the anterior iris surface[117] (Fig. 7-14). Collagen deposition was noted on the iris surface and stromal collagen was denatured. These findings were accompanied by coagulative necrosis within the anterior two thirds of the stroma. The authors postulated that heat shrinkage of collagen as a response to laser thermal effects or the contraction of fibroblastic membranes on the iris surface might be mechanisms for the long-term iris contraction effects resulting from ALPI.[117]

PRIMARY OPEN-ANGLE GLAUCOMA

POAG is a diagnosis made by exclusion. In other words, examination of the optic nerve and visual field confirm the presence of glaucoma; however, establishing that the pathophysiologic mechanism is POAG requires the systematic exclusion of an angle-closure mechanism and the subsequent exclusion of the secondary open-angle glaucomas, most of which have characteristic findings. There are no characteristic slit-lamp or gonioscopic findings in POAG. Only when all other glaucomas have been excluded can one diagnose POAG.

POAG afflicts approximately 2% to 3% of American adults but increases in prevalence with age so that approximately 5% of those 75 years or older are affected.[5] Prevalence estimates vary considerably among nationalities.[3,4,118–120] Even in the United States, the incidence and severity of POAG varies significantly among the races. The Baltimore Eye Survey found that black Americans have a four to five times higher prevalence of POAG than do whites, so that by age 80 years 11.26% of blacks

manifested the disease. POAG also tends to be diagnosed at a later age and to be more advanced at the time of diagnosis in black patients.[121] Sommer and associates found that POAG-associated blindness was six times more frequently encountered in blacks than in whites, began an average 10 years earlier, and accounted for 19% of all blindness among blacks.[122] Other studies have confirmed the increased severity of POAG among black individuals.[123–129]

POAG is a familial disorder.[130] Shin et al found a positive family history in 50% of POAG patients and in 43% of ocular hypertensive patients.[131] A later study, however, concluded that family history is more significantly related to ocular hypertension than to POAG, although it is a significant factor in both diseases.[132] Rosenthal and Perkins noted that the prevalence of raised intraocular pressure was almost four times higher in individuals with a family history of POAG compared with controls.[133]

Recently, a gene associated with juvenile-onset dominantly inherited open-angle glaucoma has been linked to the long arm of chromosome 1.[134,135] Similarly, a common gene for a form of juvenile- and adult-onset POAG was mapped to the same region of chromosome 1 in a study of 142 members of a large multigenerational French Canadian family.[136]

As stated previously, there are no slit-lamp or gonioscopic findings characteristic of POAG. Even at the light microscopic level, the findings in POAG are subtle (Fig. 7-15). Fine and associates examined eight eyes from POAG patients and compared them with control specimens. The POAG eyes were characterized by an exaggerated scleral spur, accretion and compaction of the overlying uveal meshwork, hyalinization and atrophy of the adjacent ciliary muscle, and atrophy of the iris root.[137] They concluded that these findings represented an acceleration of normal aging changes. Others have supported that conclusion.[138]

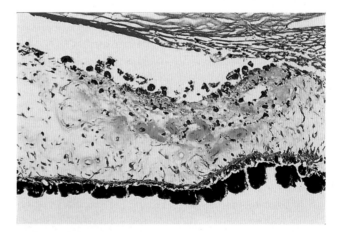

FIG. 7-14. Photomicrograph of argon laser peripheral iridoplasty demonstrating disruption of anterior iris surface and iris contraction resulting in widened anterior chamber angle.

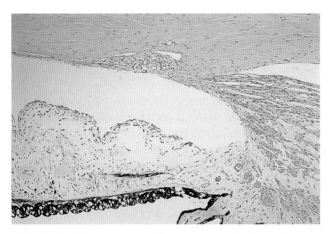

FIG. 7-15. Photomicrograph of open anterior chamber angle. Unless one knew the age of the patient and had experience examining age-matched control specimens, one would not be able to predict whether the example was from a patient with primary open-angle glaucoma.

At the ultrastructural level, the traditional dictum has localized the main obstruction of aqueous outflow in POAG to the juxtacanalicular tissue adjacent to Schlemm's canal[139–144]; however, various authors have found other abnormalities throughout the trabecular region. Rohen noted three types of extracellular deposits within the cribriform layer of the trabecular meshwork in a study of 400 trabeculectomy specimens.[145] It was concluded that these deposits contain glycoproteins that were believed to be secreted by cribriform layer cells. Others have cited various extracellular materials as contributing to decreased aqueous outflow in POAG.[146,147]

Decreased cellularity of the trabecular meshwork compared with age-matched controls was noted in POAG trabecular specimens examined by Alvarado and colleagues and others.[138,148] This decrease in cells was most marked in the inner trabecular tissue and least prominent in the outermost tissue. Alvarado and associates also noted an increased amount of an electron-dense material in the trabecular meshwork of POAG patients.

The endothelial cells lining Schlemm's canal contain pores that have been cited as contributing to aqueous outflow resistance in human eyes.[149] There are fewer of these pores in POAG eyes.[150] Unfortunately, when one evaluates such studies, it is difficult to know if the findings are part of the pathophysiology of POAG or are merely secondary to it. Additionally, significant artifacts can be introduced as a result of regional variations in trabecular anatomy[103,151] or by the techniques used to obtain tissue specimens particularly during trabeculectomy.[152]

The traditional paradigm for POAG treatment consists of medical therapy, followed by laser surgery, and culminating in filtration surgery if medical and laser surgical treatment prove inadequate to prevent the progression of optic nerve damage. Several authors have suggested earlier intervention with laser or filtration surgery. One basis

for these suggestions is the thesis that chronic medical therapy alters the conjunctiva and decreases the success of subsequent filtration surgery. Based on histologic, immunohistochemical, and ultrastructural studies, Nuzzi and associates concluded that individuals treated for a medium or long term with topical ocular glaucoma medications demonstrate changes in the conjunctiva including increased thickness and numbers of epithelial cells, increased fibroblast density in both the subepithelial and deep connective tissue, and more compact connective tissue.[153] They also found evidence of chronic inflammation.

SECONDARY ANGLE-CLOSURE GLAUCOMA

Secondary angle-closure glaucoma (SACG), like POAG, can be subdivided into that with and that without pupillary block. **SACG with pupillary block** involves a hydraulic force causing iris bombe and secondary angle-closure. **SACG without pupillary block** most frequently results from the proliferation of a membrane on the iris and trabecular surface, resulting in peripheral anterior synechias, or from a mass effect displacing the iris-lens diaphragm anteriorly, producing secondary angle-closure. The causes of SACG can be further categorized as follows:

- SACG with pupillary block
  - Untreated PACG
  - Phacogenic
    - Phacomorphic
    - Secondary to lens subluxation or dislocation
  - Posterior synechia-induced
    - Inflammatory
    - Aphakic or pseudophakic pupillary block
    - Ciliary block (malignant glaucoma)
- SACG without pupillary block
  - Secondary to sheetlike cellular or vascular proliferations within the anterior segment
    - Neovascular glaucoma (rubeosis iridis)
    - Iridocorneal endothelial (ICE) syndrome
    - Epithelial downgrowth
    - Stromal ingrowth
    - Endothelialization of the anterior chamber angle
  - Secondary to anterior displacement of anterior segment structures
    - Postoperative failure of formation of the anterior chamber
    - Tumor or cyst related
    - Retinopathy of prematurity
    - Persistent hyperplastic primary vitreous
- Iridoschisis

SACG with Pupillary Block

SACG Resulting from Untreated Primary Angle-Closure Glaucoma

Chronic progressive angle-closure glaucoma (as is frequently seen in blacks) or intermittent subclinical attacks

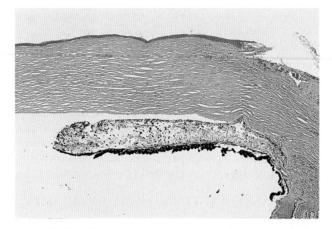

FIG. 7-16. Photomicrograph of peripheral anterior synechia.

of PACG may result in SACG through the formation of **peripheral anterior synechiae** (PAS), which are adhesions between the posterior cornea and the peripheral iris (Fig. 7-16). Even if PAS do not form, repeated subclinical attacks of PACG may result in trabecular damage and scarring, and secondary chronic pressure elevation.

Phacogenic SACG

Phacomorphic SACG

As discussed in the section on PACG, increased lens size in relation to ocular size is typical of PACG. For that reason, most PACG is, to some extent, phacogenic. In its extreme form, however, phacomorphic phacogenic SACG is seen in the final stages of cataract development, which may be characterized by precipitous lens swelling accompanied by anterior displacement of the iris (Fig. 7-17). Asymmetric cataract development may result in significant anterior chamber depth asymmetry.

Phacogenic Glaucoma Secondary to Lens Subluxation or Dislocation

Lens subluxation and dislocation are most frequently seen in one of several clinical settings (Figs. 7-18 and 7-19). The angle-closure associated with PXE already has been discussed as being secondary to abnormal mobility of the lens secondary to lax zonules. In the extreme form, zonular laxity or fragility can result in lens dislocation as is seen in homocystinuria, Marfan's syndrome, and Weill-Marchesani syndrome (microspherophakia). Nelson and Maumenee reviewed ectopia lentis in 1982.[154] Several of the ectopia lentis syndromes have been reported since that review, including ectopic pupil which may be associated with axial myopia, poor vision, retinal detachment, enlarged corneal diameters, pupillary membranes, iris processes in the chamber angle, cataract, and other iris abnormalities.[96,155-166] Ectopia lentis also may be found in up to 56% of patients with aniridia although lens-related glaucoma in aniridia probably is uncommon.[167]

Nagata and associates examined a lens from a woman with Weill-Marchesani syndrome who underwent cataract extraction.[168] The lens was only 6 mm in equatorial diameter and 4.8 mm in anteroposterior diameter. Such relatively small, round lenses are particularly prone to luxate into the anterior chamber resulting in an odd form of "inverse" pupillary block angle-closure. The inverse aspect of the mechanism is due to the iris bowing anteriorly against the lens as opposed to the more common mechanism in which the lens moves anteriorly against the posterior iris surface to obstruct aqueous flow through the pupil. Other lens-related causes of glaucoma besides pupillary block and secondary angle-closure include phacolytic glaucoma, lens-induced uveitis, and vitreous obstruction of the trabecular meshwork.[169] Andrews and associates reported an unusual case of Marfan's syndrome in which G-forces during a roller-coaster ride disrupted the vitreous gel and damaged the lens capsule in a dislo-

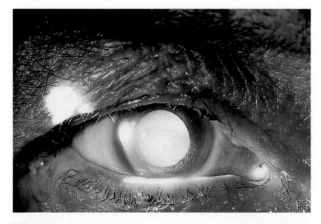

FIG. 7-17. Clinical photograph of a mature cataract. Precipitous lens swelling in the final stages of this cataract's development may result in secondary angle-closure glaucoma (Courtesy of Ali Aminlari, MD).

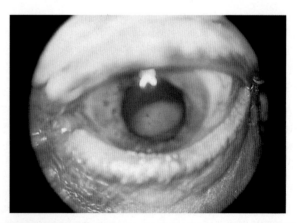

FIG. 7-18. Clinical photograph of a lens dislocated inferiorly. Anterior displacement of a dislocated lens may result in SACG (Courtesy of Ali Aminlari, MD).

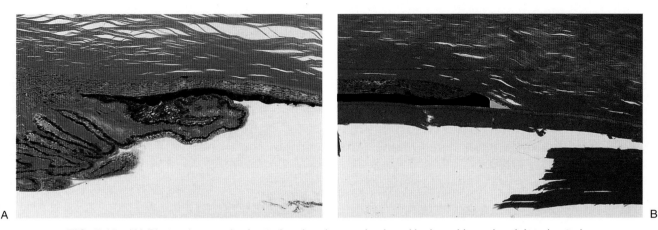

FIG. 7-19. **(A)** Photomicrograph of anterior chamber angle closed by broad-based peripheral anterior synechia. **(B)** Appearance of central anterior segment demonstrating lens remnant pressing iris anteriorly causing angle closure. Such findings would be expected in angle closure secondary to lens dislocation or to lens displacement. The latter might be secondary to intraocular tumor or to failure of anterior chamber reformation following intraocular surgery.

cated lens resulting in glaucoma secondary to uveitis and phacolysis.[169]

The first signs of lens subluxation may be fluctuating visual acuity. The patient may contact the clinician for such visual complaints, thereby permitting the clinician to assist in the diagnosis of one of the ectopia lentis syndromes. The cataract surgeon must be sensitive to the possibility of such systemic disorders because they may present increased surgical risks for ocular and even fatal complications.[170-173] This danger is particularly relevant to homocystinuria patients who are at increased risk from life-threatening thromboembolic and hypoglycemic complications at the time of surgical anesthesia.[174] Lowe and colleagues have suggested that perioperative measures to prevent thromboembolic events include diet therapy to lower serum methionine and homocystine levels, adequate preoperative hydration, maintenance of intraoperative cardiac output, and the use of pneumatic stockings to prevent peripheral stagnation of blood.[174] Hypoglycemia is thought to be due to alterations in insulin release associated with high levels of circulating sulfur-containing amino acids such as methionine. Perioperative measures include normalization of serum methionine and administration of exogenous glucose during periods of fasting.[161]

Kielty and colleagues have found microfibrillar abnormalities in a family with Marfan's syndrome and suggested that structural weakness in the zonules was probably responsible for lens dislocation in these individuals.[175] Mutations in the gene coding for fibrillin on chromosome 15 have been reported to cause Marfan's syndrome.[176] Kainulainen and colleagues have reported 10 novel mutations in this region that result in very different phenotypic expressions.[177]

Homocystinuria is due to deficiency of the enzyme cystathionine-beta-synthetase, and appropriate dietary treatment and vitamin supplementation can significantly reduce its ocular complications if therapy is begun within 6 weeks of birth.[178]

Various techniques have been reported for lens extraction of subluxated or dislocated lenses.[179-183] Children with dislocated lenses who are rendered aphakic either spontaneously or by lensectomy may show gradual improvement in vision and visual potential if properly treated.[184]

Posterior Synechia-Induced Angle-Closure Glaucoma

Posterior synechias are adhesions between the iris (usually at the pupillary margin) and a structure posterior to it (usually the lens). They are significant because they block access of aqueous to the anterior chamber (seclusio pupillae) resulting in iris bombe. Posterior synechias also may form between the iris and a posterior chamber intraocular lens giving rise to pseudophakic pupillary-block glaucoma. In the setting of aphakia, such synechias may form to the vitreous face producing aphakic pupillary-block glaucoma.

Posterior synechias usually are secondary to inflammation (iritis). Such adhesions are particularly devastating in sarcoidosis and other severe forms of anterior uveitis because the iris bombe quickly produces severe PAS formation. These PAS may further compromise aqueous outflow through a trabecular meshwork already damaged by inflammatory exudates.

The treatment of posterior synechias is wide dilation of the pupil, provided an iris plane intraocular lens is not present. Iridotomy may serve as a "safety valve" should recurrent iritis eventuate in recurrent seclusio pupillae and iris bombe.

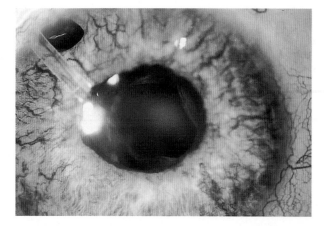

FIG. 7-20. Clinical photograph of iris neovascularization. Note superior temporal tube from seton procedure performed to control intraocular pressure. Although the vascular component of the fibrovascular membrane is more easily seen, it is myofibroblasts of the fibrous component that distort anterior segment anatomy resulting in peripheral anterior synechia formation.

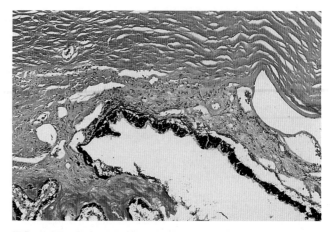

FIG. 7-22. Photomicrograph of iris neovascular membrane and peripheral anterior synechia. Iris pigment epithelial "corrugations" suggest that this patient also had PXE syndrome. The iris neovascularization may have been secondary to central retinal vein occlusion following primary angle closure in PXE or secondary to open-angle glaucoma in PXE. Similarly, the peripheral anterior synechia may have formed as a result of PACG or secondary to iris neovascularization.

SACG Without Pupillary Block

SACG Secondary to Sheetlike Cellular or Vascular Proliferations Within the Anterior Segment

Neovascular Glaucoma

Neovascular glaucoma (NVG) clinically is termed **rubeosis iridis** after the appearance of the anterior iris surface (Fig. 7-20). The underlying process is the proliferation of a fibrovascular membrane on the anterior iris surface (Fig. 7-21) and onto the trabecular meshwork (Fig. 7-22). Initially the anterior chamber angle is open gonioscopically, and secondary open-angle glaucoma may be produced by the membranous covering of the trabecular meshwork (Fig. 7-23). Ultimately, myofibroblasts within the membrane cause it to contract re-

sulting in the characteristic **ectropion uveae,** which is anterior movement of the pupillary "frill" onto the anterior iris surface (Fig. 7-24), and PAS formation (secondary angle-closure glaucoma).[185]

NVG is a final common pathophysiologic pathway re-

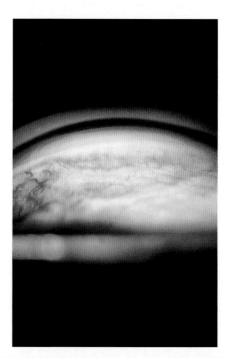

FIG. 7-23. Goniophotograph of neovascularization within the anterior chamber angle. Initially, such neovascular membranes mechanically obstruct aqueous outflow without angle closure. Later, contraction of the myofibroblastic component of the neovascular membrane results in peripheral anterior synechia formation.

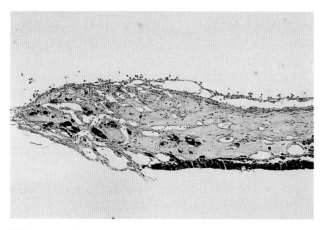

FIG. 7-21. Photomicrograph of neovascular membrane on anterior iris surface near pupillary border.

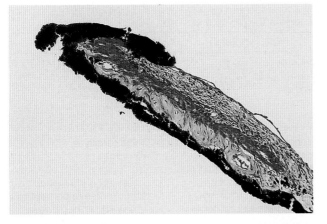

FIG. 7-24. Photomicrograph of iris neovascular membrane resulting in ectropion uveae as iris pigment epithelium is pulled onto anterior iris surface.

sulting from ocular (retinal) ischemia. Brown and associates evaluated 208 patients with NVG. The most common underlying causes for ocular ischemia were retinal venous obstruction in 36%, diabetic retinopathy in 32%, and carotid artery disease in 13%.[186] The authors found associated systemic hypertension in 51% and diabetes in 46% of their patients. They concluded that 97% of their patients had a disease process that produced extensive retinal ischemia preceding the onset of iris neovascularization. Other causes of NVG include intraocular tumors, iritis, and central retinal artery obstruction.

Iridocorneal Endothelial Syndrome

The iridocorneal endothelial (ICE) syndrome represents the confluence of three clinical entities: Chandler's syndrome, iris nevus (Cogan Reese) syndrome, and essential iris atrophy[187–191] (Fig. 7-25). These three clinical syndromes share the characteristics of being unilateral, associated with SACG, affecting middle-aged women, and resulting from endothelial proliferation over the iris and trabecular region. Accompanying manifestations include varying degrees of endothelial dystrophy, iris holes, pupillary distortion, and iris surface tissue clusters.[192–194] One or more of these features predominates in each of the three syndromes; however, considerable overlap exists and a given patient may display features typical of more than one of them. Specular microscopy is helpful in documenting the endothelial changes clinically.[195,196] Table 2 compares and classifies the ICE syndromes and other entities related to abnormalities in neural crest embryology. Table 9 compares the ICE syndromes to the anterior chamber cleavage syndromes and to posterior polymorphous corneal dystrophy.

In their study of 37 consecutive patients with ICE syndrome, Wilson and Shields found that Chandler's syndrome was more common (21 cases) than essential iris

atrophy or iris nevus syndrome (8 cases each).[197] Alterations in endothelial cell size, shape, and apical characteristics are prominent in these eyes, and there is evidence of chronic inflammation.[198] Based on the composition of Descemet's membrane in ICE syndrome, Alvarado and colleagues postulated that the abnormal Descemet's membrane first appeared in postnatal life, years before its clinical recognition, and they speculated a viral origin for the disorder.[199]

In **Chandler's syndrome,** the most prominent finding is corneal dystrophy, which may result in corneal edema even with a modest rise in intraocular pressure.[200,202] Pupillary distortion is minimal and the other more severe manifestations of ICE syndrome, such as iris stromal thinning and iris surface distortion, usually are not present. Patel and colleagues noted diffuse endothelial attenuation and the presence of a posterior collagenous layer in their study of four keratoplasty specimens.[203,204] Based on immunohistochemical studies of a corneal specimen from a 55-year-old woman, Denis and associates proposed an epithelial origin for the cells lining the endothelial cell layer of Descemet's membrane in Chandler's syndrome.[205] A similar conclusion was drawn by Hirst and colleagues based on their findings of intracytoplasmic filaments, desmosomes, microvillus projections, and positive staining for keratin.[206]

Rodrigues and associates compared the endothelium in Chandler's syndrome with that in posterior polymorphous dystrophy.[207] They concluded that these two disorders not only differed in the morphology of the dystrophy, their hereditary transmission, laterality, and rate of progression, but also in the nature of the endothelial pathology. They believed that posterior polymorphous cells exhibited epithelial characteristics whereas the cells in Chandler's syndrome were endothelial in nature.[207] Buxton and Lash have reported a favorable experience with corneal transplantation in a small series of these patients.[208]

Essential iris atrophy (EIA) is the most striking of

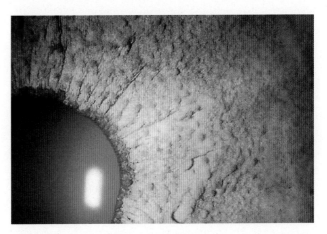

FIG. 7-25. Clinical photograph of iris nevus syndrome. Note multiple nevi on iris surface (Courtesy of Ali Aminlari, MD and George Rosenwasser, MD).

TABLE 9. *Distinctions between Axenfeld-Rieger (A-R) and iridocorneal endothelial (ICE) syndromes and posterior polymorphous dystrophy (PPMD)*

Characteristics	A-R syndrome	ICE syndrome	PPMD
Laterality	Bilateral	Unilateral	Bilateral
Age of presentation	Birth	Young adult	Birth
Sex predilection	None	Women	None
Familial	Frequently	Rarely	Typically
Associated nonocular disorders	Frequently	No	No
Corneal edema	No	Frequently	Occasionally
Corneal endothelium	Normal	Abnormal	Abnormal
Origin of membrane	Retention of primordial issue	Proliferation from abnormal corneal endothelium	Proliferation from abnormal corneal endothelium
Mechanism of secondary glaucoma	Maldevelopment of aqueous outflow system	Outflow obstruction by membrane or peripheral synechiae	Either maldevelopment (as in A-R) or membrane induced (as in ICE)

(Modified from Shields MB, Buckley E, Klintworth GK, et al. Axenfeld-Rieger syndrome: a spectrum of developmental disorders. *Surv Ophthalmol* 1985;29:387).

the ICE entities.[188] Initially, a focal PAS develops in one quadrant. With time, progression of the PAS occurs and iris thinning, sometimes resulting in a full-thickness hole, develops in the quadrant opposite the initial PAS.[209] Pupillary distortion is progressive and ectropion uveae is common. The cause of the iris holes is not known. The holes tend to develop in the iris segment not covered by the proliferating endothelial membrane, which has been suggested to act as a protective "splint" for the iris it covers. Nevertheless, a simple tractional effect of the endothelial membrane as a cause for hole formation is unlikely because iris stromal holes do not develop even in other severe cases of iris traction secondary to surgical and nonsurgical trauma. Therefore, some authors have suggested a vascular cause for iris hole formation,[210] but others dispute this theory.[211,212] The iris distortion may lead to a misdiagnosis of iris melanoma. Such an error occurred was made by the referring physicians in 5.7% of the 200 cases referred to Shields and associates as iris melanomas.[213]

Progression of the PAS results in severe angle-closure glaucoma. Iris nodules sometimes are noted late in the clinical course. On histologic examination, the iris stroma may be severely atrophic, and an endothelial membrane covers the nonatrophic iris. Extensive deposits of basement membrane material often are present beneath the endothelial membrane. A posterior collagenous layer has been noted on Descemet's membrane; however, the endothelial cells displayed normal junctional complexes and lacked desmosomal junctions or increased microvillus projections.[214] Similarly Eagle and Shields failed to find tonofilaments or abundant apical microvilli in the eye involved with EIA in a woman who had guttate dystrophy in the fellow eye.[215]

Bilateral EIA and keratoconus have been reported in a patient who also displayed features of posterior polymorphous dystrophy.[216] DeBroff and Thoft have given a poor prognosis for corneal transplantation in essential iris atrophy because of their findings of chronic anterior uveitis (100%) and immunologic graft failure (83.3%) among six eyes operated on over 21 years.[217] Kidd and colleagues were more optimistic for the success of filtration surgery in these patients and recommended additional filtration surgery even when the initial procedure fails.[218] Their success rates for first, second, and third trabeculectomies were 64%, 79%, and 63%, respectively. Endothelialization of the filtration bleb in iris nevus syndrome has been reported.[219]

In **iris nevus (Cogan-Reese) syndrome,** PAS formation and stromal atrophy also are found, but to a much less severe degree than is seen in essential iris atrophy. The characteristic manifestation, however, is the presence of iris surface nodules and a whorl-like or matted appearance to the iris surface.[194,220,221] The latter changes are accompanied by the loss of surface crypts. The iris nodules seem to poke through holes in the iris surface endothelial membrane. Other findings include ectropion uveae, heterochromia, and secondary glaucoma.

Epithelial Downgrowth

Epithelial downgrowth occurs infrequently following anterior segment surgery and trauma. Terry and associates found an incidence of 0.06% in their review of 45,500 surgical procedures from the Massachusetts Eye and Ear Infirmary in 1939.[222] In 1989, the experience of the same institution was reviewed. The overall incidence was 0.12%; however, it had decreased to 0.08% over the last 10 years of the study.[223] Eighty-two percent of the patients presented within 1 year of their initial surgical procedure, and most commonly complained of blurred vision, red eye, and pain. The most common presenting findings were retrocorneal membrane (45%), glaucoma (43%), corneal edema (21%), and positive Seidel test (23%). A fistulous tract that may or may not filter aqueous is a frequent means of entry of the epithelium into the eye.[224-226]

Epithelial downgrowth is a devastating surgical complication. Although useful vision is salvaged on occasion, often it results in corneal opacification, intractable glaucoma, and may even require enucleation.[223,227-229] Retinal detachment secondary to epithelial downgrowth also has been reported.[230] Numerous surgical treatments have been proposed. Although some successes have been reported, many of the procedures require radical surgery, and overall treatment results remain poor.[231-237] Costa and Katz reported two cases in which intraocular pressure was controlled with a double-plate Molteno implant and useful vision restored with penetrating keratoplasty.[238] It has been successfully treated in two of three cases following excision of iris inclusion cysts.[239]

The clinical diagnosis of epithelial downgrowth may be difficult although its clinical hallmark is the inferior progression of a horizontal line of vanguard epithelium down the posterior cornea.[240] Other common findings are ocular hypotony and chronic inflammation. Corneal striae and vascularization may be present overlying the area of corneal involvement. Iris surface effacement also may be found.

Specular microscopy can help in making the diagnosis,[241,242] and laser photocoagulation of the anterior iris surface can help delineate the extent of iris involvement. Cytologic examination of intraocular fluids or of scrapings from the corneal endothelial or iris surface may provide a definitive diagnosis.

Glaucoma can result from epithelial downgrowth through several mechanisms. Desquamated epithelial cells can obstruct the trabecular meshwork resulting in a secondary open-angle glaucoma. The epithelial sheet may overgrow the pupil producing occlusio pupillae, iris bombe, and SACG. Ultimately, SACG secondary to PAS results. Weiner and associates found SACG

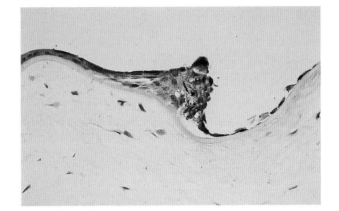

FIG. 7-27. Surface epithelium meeting corneal endothelium in experimental model of epithelial downgrowth. Over the short term, endothelium contact inhibits migration of the epithelium. Eventually and gradually, however, the epithelium progressively covers the posterior cornea and even the anterior ocular structures.

from PAS in 87% of the enucleated specimens they studied.[223]

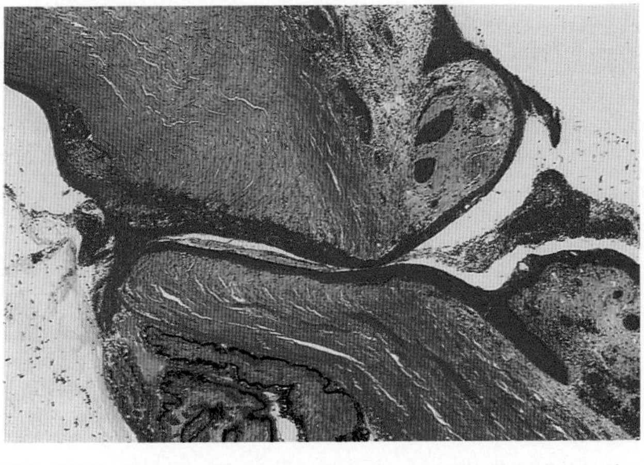

Histopathologic examination reveals sheets of ocular surface epithelium lining the posterior cornea and growing more luxuriantly on the iris surface (Fig. 7-26). Although corneal endothelium has the ability to contact inhibit the migration of corneal epithelium, eventually, endothelial cell death occurs[243-248] (Fig. 7-27). Ultimately, PAS develop and occlude the anterior chamber angle.[249] A thin sheet of epithelium may be present on the iris surface well before it is apparent clinically.[250]

The clinical progression of epithelial downgrowth is difficult to predict. The clinician must weigh the extensive surgery usually required to extirpate the epithelium with the prognosis for useful vision in these cases.

Stromal Ingrowth

Stromal ingrowth represents a proliferation of keratocytes as a retrocorneal membrane on the posterior corneal surface and other anterior segment structures (Fig. 7-28). Usually, continuity with a previous surgical wound can be demonstrated. It is most frequently seen in the setting of failed corneal transplants.[251,252] Kremer and colleagues found such proliferations in 54% of 170 failed corneal transplant grafts.[253] They noted a high correlation between the occurrence of the membrane and the presence of PAS or vitreous adherent to the wound. A high correlation also was found between tube-shunt operations and the presence of diffuse retrocorneal fibrous membranes in failed grafts. Stromal ingrowth may be seen in other surgical procedures such as following cataract surgery.[254,255]

FIG. 7-26. Photomicrograph of surface epithelium lining the limbal wound to gain access to the anterior chamber.

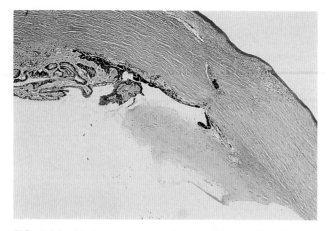

FIG. 7-28. Photomicrograph of stromal ingrowth extending from limbal wound onto posterior cornea and other ocular structures.

Allen noted stromal ingrowth in 18/50 eyes enucleated after cataract surgery and in 26/237 eyes removed after trauma.[256]

All retrocorneal fibrous membranes probably are not of stromal origin. Snip and associates have postulated that corneal endothelial cells can undergo fibrous metaplasia to produce retrocorneal fibrous membranes in the vitreous touch syndrome.[257] The ability of corneal endothelium to give rise to retrocorneal fibrous membranes also was demonstrated by Michels and colleagues.[258]

Endothelialization of the Anterior Chamber Angle

Endothelialization of the anterior chamber angle was present in 20% of 100 enucleated eyes in a study by Colosi et al.[259] It may progress to cover most of the anterior segment structures (Fig. 7-29) and may also cover PAS if present. Endothelialization is believed to be a reactive process. It frequently accompanies iris neovascularization.

SACG Secondary to Anterior Displacement of Anterior Segment Structures

Postoperative Failure of Anterior Chamber Reformation

Flat anterior chamber is a well-known complication following glaucoma filtration surgery[260] and seton procedures,[261,262] particularly if adjunctive antimetabolites are employed.[263–265] In this setting, it usually is the result of overfiltration or wound leak[266]; however, malignant glaucoma also must be excluded.[267–270] Newer trabeculectomy procedures, particularly those employing releasable sutures, and viscoelastic agents have reduced the incidence of flat anterior chamber.[271–277] Particularly dangerous is the presence of corneal-lens touch, which may result in cataract formation and which requires surgical correction if anterior chamber reformation does not occur promptly.[278–280] Decreased intraocular pressure also may result in choroidal detachment.[281] Persistent flat anterior chamber may result in peripheral anterior synechia formation (see Fig. 7-19).

Tumors, and Iris and Ciliary Body Cysts

Shields pointed out that most primary iris cysts are stationary[282]; however, cysts of the iris and ciliary body, particularly if they are multiple, may produce SACG by anteriorly displacing the iris–lens diaphragm.[283] Secondary cysts arising from surgical or nonsurgical trauma are more likely to cause complications.[282,284] Bron and associates reported an unusual ring-shaped primary cyst of the

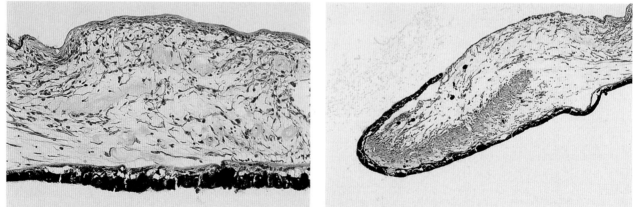

A   B

FIG. 7-29. (A) Endothelialization of anterior iris. **(B)** Endothelialized membrane has contributed to ectropion uveae.

iris pigment epithelium, which produced SACG and was treated by argon laser photocoagulation.[285]

Intraocular Tumors

Intraocular tumors may produce SACG through a mass effect similar to that of iris and ciliary body cysts. The resulting anterior displacement of the iris closes the angle (see Fig. 7-19). The mass effect is compounded by the presence of a retinal detachment.

Retinopathy of Prematurity

Retinopathy of prematurity (ROP) remains a significant cause of childhood blindness worldwide. Merritt and Kraybill found 10 cases of grade 5 cicatricial ROP in 565 premature infants, 110 of which developed ROP during a 5-year period.[286] ROP accounted for 80% of the perinatal blindness and severe visual impairment in Chile in a recent study.[287] Unsuspected glaucoma may be the cause of decreased visual acuity in ROP, particularly if surgical reattachment surgery has been performed; the glaucoma may be reversible.[288]

Hartnett and associates evaluated the mechanism of glaucoma in 27 eyes of 17 individuals with ROP.[289] Of these, 26 had received no previous surgery or treatment. They found angle-closure of greater than 180 degrees in three of the 26 eyes. In 18 eyes, they noted the appearance of a ''Barkan-type'' membrane in the angles. Halperin and Schoch have reported angle-closure following scleral buckling in ROP.[290] The presence of a large lens and shallow anterior chamber may contribute to the development of SACG in ROP even in the absence of a retrolental mass.[291] Progressive anterior chamber shallowing in ROP has been documented.[292] Hittner and colleagues have emphasized the need for careful follow-up examinations because such patients may progress to angle-closure glaucoma. Similarly, otherwise stable adult patients with cicatricial ROP may be at risk for acute angle-closure glaucoma.[293] These patients appear to respond to traditional methods of treating the angle-closure. Ciliary block glaucoma also has been reported.[294]

Persistent Hyperplastic Primary Vitreous

Persistent hyperplastic vitreous (PHPV) is a congenital ocular disorder that most commonly presents with leukocoria, microphthalmos, and cataract[295] (Fig. 7-30) (see also Chapter 4). PHPV may be mistaken for an intraocular neoplasm. Histopathologic and cytopathologic examination of vitrectomy specimens may be helpful in making the correct diagnosis.[296] Pollard has shown that lensectomy alone prevents glaucoma in PHPV; however, membranectomy may be required to achieve visual function.[297]

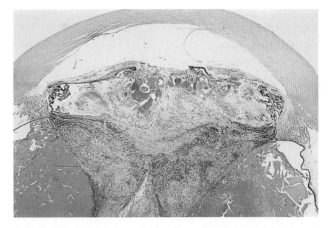

FIG. 7-30. Photomicrograph of persistent hyperplastic primary vitreous demonstrating the ciliary processes and retina drawn centrally by a vascularized mass posterior to and adherent to the lens.

Iridoschisis

Iridoschisis has been discussed previously in association with PACG, in which it may be a secondary finding (see Fig. 7-11).[91] Another frequently cited association is with ocular trauma. Glaucoma develops in 50% of those affected. It may result in unsuspected corneal endothelial cell loss.[298] Iridoschisis has been reported accompanying keratoconus,[299,300] syphilitic interstitial keratitis,[301,302] and microphthalmos.[303,304] Familial iridoschisis in association with narrow anterior chamber angle and presenile cataract also has been reported.[305]

Histopathologic examination of iridoschisis has revealed marked iris stromal atrophy without evidence of vascular or neural abnormalities.[306]

SECONDARY OPEN-ANGLE GLAUCOMA

Secondary open-angle glaucoma (SOAG) is characterized by an open anterior chamber angle on clinical gonioscopic examination, but one which functions poorly for reasons other than POAG. The following classification scheme for SOAG is somewhat arbitrary; nevertheless, it may be helpful for conceptualizing these entities at least in their pure form.

SOAG can be subclassified as follows:

- SOAG caused by cells or debris in the anterior chamber angle
  - Hyphema
  - Uveitis
  - Pigmentary glaucoma
  - Pseudoexfoliation
  - Hemolytic glaucoma
  - Phacolytic glaucoma
  - Nondenatured lens material-induced glaucoma
  - Melanomalytic glaucoma

- Tumor seeding of the trabecular meshwork
- SOAG caused by damaged outflow channels
  - Previous uveitis
  - Blunt trauma
  - Repeated hyphema
  - Siderosis and hemosiderosis oculi
  - Repeated attacks of acute angle-closure glaucoma
  - Early rubeosis or other anterior segment cellular pro-liferative disorder
- SOAG caused by corneoscleral and extraocular disease
  - Interstitial keratitis
  - Orbital venous thrombosis
  - Encircling element following retinal disease
  - Retrobulbar mass
  - Leukemia
  - Mediastinal mass
- SOAG secondary to miscellaneous causes
  - Steroid-induced glaucoma
  - Alpha-chymotrypsin glaucoma
  - Glaucomatocyclitic crisis (Posner-Schlossman syn-drome)
  - Fuchs heterochromic iridocyclitis

It is beyond the scope of this chapter to discuss all of the causes of SOAG cited. Selected topics are described.

SOAG Caused by Cells or Debris in the Anterior Chamber Angle

Hyphema

Hyphema refers to blood in the anterior chamber (see Fig. 9-26, Chapter 9). It most frequently results from blunt trauma or rubeosis iridis. DeRespinis and colleagues found that ocular trauma accounted for 15% of eye injuries at one medical center, and hyphema was the most common admitting diagnosis.[307] Hyphema also was the most common diagnosis among ocular trauma admissions reported by others.[308] Schein and associates reviewed 3184 patients examined in the emergency ward of the Massachusetts Eye and Ear Infirmary over a 6-month period.[309] Sports injuries accounted for only 3.4% of all injuries, but for 60% of hyphemas. Other authors have found a similar high incidence of sports injuries associated with hyphema.[310]

When the globe is struck during blunt trauma, the force of the blow compresses the cornea. The corneal compression sets up a shock wave, which is transmitted throughout the globe and which may damage any ocular structure. When the shock wave impacts the anterior chamber angle, it may lacerate into the face of the ciliary body, rupturing the anterior arterial circle and causing the hemorrhage that becomes a hyphema. Most frequently, the bleeding stops spontaneously as the artery goes into spasm, permitting a clot to occlude the rupture in the arterial wall. Within several days after the initial trauma, a very danger-

ous period ensues during which the clot is most vulnerable to being dislodged from the arterial wall and the wall itself is not yet healed. During this period, there is the greatest danger of spontaneous rebleeding, which may be more severe than at the initial injury. Rebleeding is associated with a poorer visual result especially in children.[311] In unusual cases, Schlemm's canal may be the source of recurrent bleeding.[312]

Volpe and associates found a 5% to 8% rate of spontaneous rebleeding in patients examined within 1 day of the initial injury, and a 15% to 38% rate in those examined more than 1 day after the initial injury.[313,314] A similar low rate of rebleeding was cited by others.[315,316] Other authors believe these rates underestimate the frequency of rebleeding, particularly among black patients.[317–323] These and other authors have suggested aminocaproic acid or steroids as useful in decreasing the incidence of rebleeding.[324,325] Some authors have suggested an association between age younger than 6 years rather than race as a risk factor for rebleeding.[326] Others have cited a relation between aspirin ingestion and recurrent bleeding,[327–329] but this was refuted in a study by Marcus and colleagues.[330]

After the initial injury is healed, the region of the ciliary face laceration can be seen gonioscopically as an area of anterior chamber angle recession characterized by a falling back of the inner aspect of the ciliary body producing an anterior chamber angle that appears deeper than a typical angle. A much higher incidence of corneal endothelial cell loss has been documented in eyes with significant angle recession compared with uninjured fellow eyes.[331] Angle recession is further discussed in the Blunt Trauma section (see also Fig. 9-25 in Chapter 9). A more severe blow may detach the ciliary body from its insertion at the scleral spur, a condition termed **cyclodialysis** (Fig. 7-31). Such hallmarks of previous trauma, including traumatic cataract (Fig. 7-32), should alert the clinician to a possible predisposition to the eventual development of glaucoma.

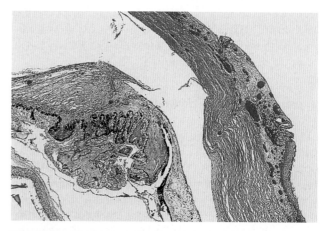

FIG. 7-31. Photomicrograph of detachment of ciliary body from its insertion at the scleral spur, known as **cyclodialysis.**

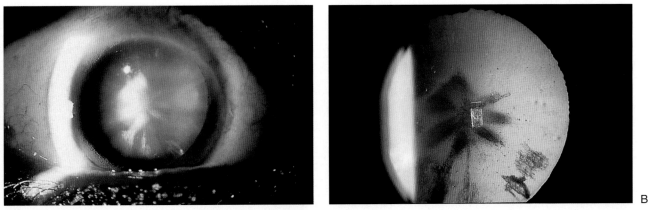

FIG. 7-32. (A) Slit-lamp photograph of the typical petal-shaped appearance of a traumatic cataract. (B) Same cataract seen against the red reflex.

It should be emphasized that a "spontaneous" hyphema in a child most frequently results from blunt trauma, including child abuse.[332,333] Other causes that must be excluded in children include juvenile xanthogranuloma,[334] retinoblastoma,[335–337] and medulloepithelioma[338] (see also Chapter 4).[338] In adults who have had ocular surgery, wound vascularization[339] and the uveitis, glaucoma, hyphema (UGH) syndrome may cause spontaneous hyphema.

Neovascular glaucoma already has been discussed as a cause for SACG. In its initial stages; however, neovascular glaucoma represents a SOAG. In this setting, the fragile vessels within the membrane are easily torn producing hyphema. Such vessels are the source for the spontaneous hyphemas cited earlier as typical of retinoblastoma and medulloepithelioma.

Hyphema may eventuate in SOAG through several mechanisms. The mass of blood generated at the time of the initial injury or during a rebleeding episode may mechanically obstruct the trabecular meshwork. Later, the dissolving clot liberates red blood cell debris, which may further compromise trabecular function. Degenerating "ghost" red blood cells, particularly from the vitreous, are quite rigid and pass through the trabecular meshwork with much more difficulty then typical red blood cells (see Figs. 9-6 and 9-7 in Chapter 9).[340] Macrophages, which move into the area to phagocytose the debris, further compromise aqueous outflow. If rebleeding does occur, the entire cycle repeats.

It should be noted that red blood cells in sickle cell disease are poorly pliable and likely to cause a disproportionate rise in intraocular pressure.[341–343] Optic nerve damage is particularly likely to occur in individuals with sickle cell disease or trait and may do so at a lower pressure than that in unaffected individuals.[344]

Histologically, hyphema is characterized initially by the presence of red blood cells and a fibrin clot (Fig. 7-33). Later, degenerating red blood cells, macrophages, and debris predominate. If ghost cells are present, the macrophages also may contain hemosiderin.

The most severe form of hyphema is the **black ball** in which the blood assumes a characteristic dark color (see Fig. 9-27, Chapter 9). Caprioli and Sears demonstrated the clots in such hyphemas are composed of concentric fibrin layers forming a cohesive internal structure.[345] The surface of the clot consisted of fibrin lacking attachments to intraocular structures. No fibroblastic or neovascular activity was found, and no true organization appeared to occur within the first 7 days after formation of the hyphema.

In the presence of elevated intraocular pressure or corneal endothelial damage, red blood cell fragments and hemoglobin may enter the posterior cornea resulting in corneal blood staining (see Figs. 9-3 and 9-4 in Chapter 9). McDonnell and associates have postulated that porphyrin-induced photosensitivity may contribute to corneal damage secondary to blood staining from hyphema.[346] Although blood staining usually is associated

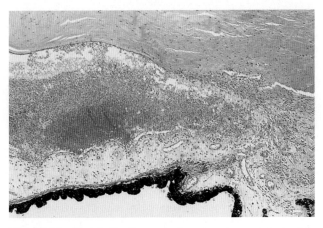

FIG. 7-33. Blood fills the anterior chamber angle in this photomicrograph of hyphema.

with raised intraocular pressure, it has been reported at low pressures.[347]

Uveitis

Aqueous production frequently is reduced in uveitis, which may serve to delay the diagnosis of mechanisms contributing to the development of glaucoma. Later, as inflammation is controlled, normal aqueous production may resume, presenting the picture of a severe glaucoma in a patient with advanced aqueous outflow compromise.

Uveitis may produce glaucoma through several mechanisms. Posterior synechias leading to pupillary block was discussed earlier in the section on SACG. Inflammatory cells and debris may mechanically obstruct the trabecular meshwork (Fig. 7-34). The inflammation may center, in part, on the trabecular meshwork. The ensuing trabeculitis, particularly that seen in herpes zoster and sarcoid associated uveitis, may be very responsive to steroid therapy (Fig. 7-35). On the other hand, individuals already at risk for POAG may respond to steroid therapy with a marked rise in intraocular pressure. The final common pathway for glaucoma associated with repeated episodes of uveitis may be trabecular scarring resulting in further outflow compromise.

Two uveitis syndromes of significance are the syndrome of glaucomatocyclitic crises (Posner-Schlossman syndrome) and Fuchs' heterochromic iridocyclitis. Both of these entities may pose significant diagnostic and therapeutic problems. They will be discussed further, later in this chapter.

Pigment Dispersion Syndrome

Pigment dispersion syndrome (PDS) recently has been reviewed extensively.[348] Typically, it is found in young

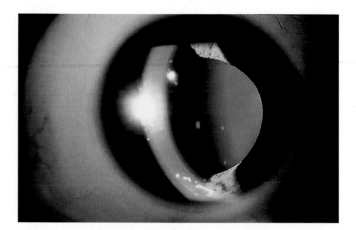

FIG. 7-35. Clinical photograph of granulomatous precipitates on the inferior endothelium. Such findings may indicate the presence of sarcoidosis, which may produce glaucoma through several mechanisms.

adult, white, male myopes,[349] although Becker and Shin reported PDS in 10% of white and black individuals with and without glaucoma.[350] Characteristic clinical findings include midperipheral iris transillumination areas (Fig. 7-36), marked trabecular pigmentation, and the presence of a vertical line of pigment on the corneal endothelium (Krukenberg spindle) (Fig. 7-37). In contrast, a form of pigment-dispersion-syndrome–pigmentary-glaucoma (PDS–PGL) has been described in older, hyperopic, black women who do not display typical iris transillumination areas.[351]

Another version of PDS also has been reported to occur in patients with posterior chamber intraocular lenses.[352,353] In one study, PDS was found in 16% of pseudophakic patients, and 2% developed pigmentary glaucoma, particularly diabetic individuals.[354] PDS and pseudoexfoliation syndrome have been reported in the same individuals.[355]

Mechanical abrasion of the iris pigment epithelium on zonule packets is believed to cause pigment release in

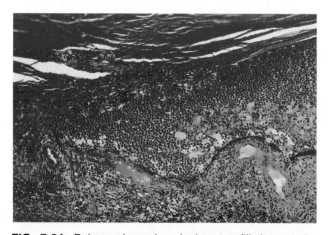

FIG. 7-34. Polymorphonuclear leukocytes fill the anterior chamber angle in this severe case of acute inflammation due to bacterial infection. In the typical case of iritis the findings are much more subtle and may not be visible gonioscopically.

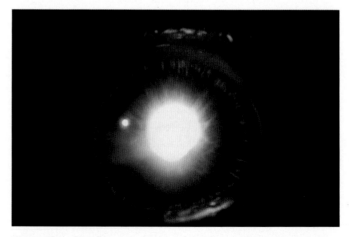

FIG. 7-36. Slit-lamp photograph of midperipheral iris transillumination in pigment dispersion syndrome.

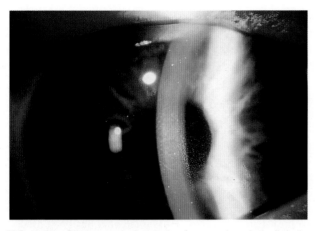

FIG. 7-37. Slit-lamp photograph of corneal endothelial pigment line (Krukenberg spindle).

PDS–PGL.[356] It has been postulated that the apposition of the iris to the zonules is precipitated by a form of inverse pupillary block. The validity of this mechanism and its reversal by laser iridotomy has been supported by studies using the ultrasound biomicroscope.[356–359] The ultrasound biomicroscope also has documented worsening of inverse pupillary block during exercise.[360] This finding may explain the rise in intraocular pressure that is frequently observed in PDS and PGL patients following exercise.[361] It is interesting to note that development of increased traditional pupillary block secondary to progressive cataract has been demonstrated to bow the iris forward and to reduce signs of PDS.[362] Individuals with PDS have been demonstrated to have deeper anterior chambers than can be accounted for by age, sex, or refractive error.[363]

The cause of the intraocular pressure elevation in PGL is not known for certain, but has been assumed to be mechanical obstruction of the trabecular meshwork by pigment and debris. Richter and associates prospectively studied 55 PDS patients and demonstrated that active pigment dispersion was clinically detectable, was correlated with elevation of intraocular pressure, and continued to occur in older patients.[364] Nevertheless, Epstein and colleagues infused pigment granules into monkey eyes and failed to demonstrate decreased outflow facility even with repeated infusions although pigment phagocytosis by trabecular endothelial cells was demonstrated by transmission electron microscopy.[365] The authors postulated that factors other than, or in addition to, pigment particle accumulation in the trabecular meshwork must be involved in the mechanism of PGL. Similarly, Murphy and associates studied tissue from 13 eyes of which 6 had PGL, 2 had PDS, 3 had POAG, and 2 were from normal eyes. They concluded that the aqueous outflow obstruction could not be attributed to pigment accumulation in the juxtacanalicular tissue.[366] No differences in cellularity or morphology were found between pigmented and nonpigmented

areas of trabecular meshwork in each of nine normal eye bank eyes, suggesting that pigment per se does not induce trabecular damage.[367] Alvarado and Murphy performed a morphometric study on 33 trabecular meshwork specimens from 27 patients.[368] They proposed three concepts: (1) Cul-de-sacs in which aqueous outflow channels terminate provide a major portion of normal aqueous outflow resistance; (2) The cul-de-sac area is markedly reduced in PGL and POAG, thereby accounting for a significant amount of the increased outflow resistance; (3) Macrophages are the major cell type responsible for trabecular meshwork clearance of pigment and debris.

Histologic and ultrastructural examination of four eyes in PDS revealed disruption of the cell membranes of the iris pigment epithelium and extrusion of pigment granules.[369] The regions demonstrating these findings corresponded to the course taken by the zonule packets and to areas of peripheral iris transillumination. Within the trabecular meshwork, pigment was found free, within macrophages, and within endothelial cells.

Although PDS and PGL are associated with a **Krukenberg spindle,** in which pigment is deposited on and is found within corneal endothelial cells, no significant difference in endothelial cell count was found between patients with PGL, PDS, or control eyes.[370,371]

There is an increased risk of retinal detachment in PDS–PGL with a reported incidence of 6% among 407 PDS patients from one glaucoma population.[372] An increased incidence of lattice degeneration and full-thickness retinal breaks was found in PDS patients and may, in part, account for the increase in retinal detachment found in this syndrome.[373]

Pseudoexfoliation Syndrome

Pseudoexfoliation (PXE) syndrome is characterized clinically by the presence of deposits on the lens capsule and other anterior segment structures (Figs. 7-38 and 7-39). Other significant clinical findings include pupillary

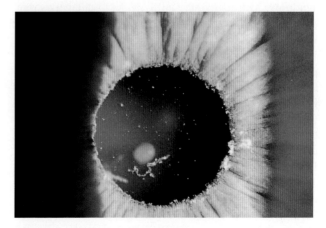

FIG. 7-38. "Frosting" of fine deposits at the pupillary margin in pseudoexfoliation syndrome.

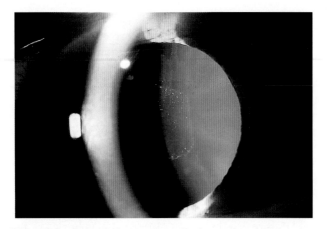

FIG. 7-39. Central circular deposit of pseudoexfoliation material on the anterior lens surface.

ruff defects, iris sphincter transillumination, a characteristic whorl-like pattern of particulate pigment deposition on the iris sphincter, particulate pigment deposition on the peripheral iris and trabecular meshwork, and PXE material on the zonules and ciliary body.[374]

PXE was found in 1.6% of 2121 patients examined in two clinics in southeastern United States, and this group comprised 6% of those with open-angle glaucoma.[375] Henry and associates noted that elevated intraocular pressure developed in 5.3% of PXE syndrome eyes in 5 years and 15.4% in 10 years.[376] Furthermore, they noted the probability of a normal fellow eye developing PXE syndrome was 6.8% in 5 years and 16.8% in 10 years.

Kozart and Yanoff evaluated 100 consecutive patients with PXE found incidentally during ocular examinations in a private, general ophthalmology practice.[377] Of 124 eyes with PXE, 78% had normal intraocular pressure, 15% had ocular hypertension, and 7% demonstrated glaucoma. A subsequent study found the probability of developing elevated intraocular pressure was 5.3% in 5 years and 15.4% in 10 years.[378] In a study of 1941 individuals in Norway, the overall prevalence of open-angle glaucoma was 8.3%. Approximately 30% of those with PXE syndrome had glaucoma and 4.2% had ocular hypertension compared with 4% and 0.8%, respectively, of those who did not have PXE.[379]

Although traditionally associated with northern Europeans, PXE affects diverse populations. According to Forsius, the prevalence of PXE syndrome varies from 0% in Eskimos to 21% in Finns older than 60 years.[380] PXE was found in 7.2% of persons 50 years or older and increased to 11.2% in those 60 years or older among 1356 persons examined in the Eastern Mediterranean area of Turkey.[381] In France the prevalence of PXE syndrome is 5.5%.[382] The percentage of glaucoma among those with PXE was 34.3% and accounted for 46.9% of those with glaucoma. PXE accounted for 53% of the glaucoma among 656 patients with glaucoma or PXE in eastern Algeria.[383] It represented 87.8% of the glaucoma in patients undergoing

trabeculectomy for open-angle glaucoma in Northern Greece.[384] A higher incidence of PXE has been reported in Navajo Indians compared with the general US population.[385]

Individuals with PXE appear to develop glaucomatous damage at lower intraocular pressure than do other individuals.[386,387] Nevertheless, this predisposition to optic nerve damage may be compounded by the finding that intraocular pressure at the time of diagnosis is reportedly higher in PXE than in POAG.[387,388] The glaucoma in PXE is reported to be particularly difficult to treat.[389]

The incidence of glaucoma in patients with PXE syndrome has been reported to be increased 7-fold with blood group K1 in Norway.[390] PXE glaucoma has been associated with goniodysgenesis[391] and with pigment dispersion syndrome.[356] Psilas and associates have suggested a decreased incidence of PXE among diabetic people with background diabetic retinopathy and an even lower incidence in those with proliferative retinopathy.[392] PXE has also been associated with unilateral retinitis pigmentosa.[393]

Of particular significance is the fact that PXE has been associated with anatomically occludable angles, which was discussed in the earlier section on PACG. Gross and associates found such angles in 9.3% of 54 PXE patients.[88] Weakened lens zonules predisposing to anterior shift of the lens has been cited as one mechanism contributing to such angle-closure.[394] Ciliary block angle-closure also has been reported.[90] Weakened zonular support also has been cited as contributing to intraoperative complications during cataract extraction in PXE patients.[395] Naumann found a frequency of vitreous loss in extracapsular cataract surgery of 1.8% in patients without PXE and 9% in those with the disorder.[396]

Henke and Naumann found histologic evidence of pseudoexfoliation in 3.4% of 323 unselected eyes with secondary glaucoma enucleated as blind and painful.[397] Nevertheless, they found only one case among 132 eyes with intraocular tumors.

PXE deposits have most frequently been postulated to be composed of abnormal basement membrane material. Schlotzer-Schrehardt and colleagues studied deposits from 30 anterior lens capsules by immunofluorescence and electron microscopic immunogold techniques. They demonstrated heparan sulfate and chondroitin sulfate proteoglycans, laminin, entactin/nidogen, fibronectin, and amyloid P protein.[398] Type IV collagen was restricted to a microfibrillar layer between the capsule surface and typical PXE material. Elastin also was noted. The authors postulated that PXE represents a multicomponent expression of a disordered extracellular matrix synthesis including the incorporation of the major noncollagenous basement membrane components with an overproduction and abnormal metabolism of glycosaminoglycans. Another study demonstrated that alpha-mannosyl, beta-galactosyl, *N*-acetyl-D-glucosaminyl, and *N*-acetylneuraminic acid residues are present in glycoconjugates of exfoliative material and neighboring tissues.[399]

PXE material can be produced throughout the anterior segment and is not only produced by the lens (Figs. 7-40 and 7-41). In fact, PXE syndrome has developed and material has been found on intraocular lenses years after extracapsular cataract extraction and intraocular lens implantation.[400] Eagle and associates noted the presence of abundant PXE material on the ciliary and iris epithelium but not on the surface of a lens with necrotic epithelium. They characterized it as filamentous basement membrane material of 500-A periodicity.[401] Furthermore, their finding of the material in the wall of a short posterior ciliary artery in the orbit documented an extraocular locus for it.

PXE appears to reflect a systemic disorder. Extraocular deposits of PXE material have been reported in the eyelid skin,[402] extraocular rectus and oblique muscles, vortex veins, and optic nerve sheaths.[403,404] Other nonocular sites for PXE material have included skin, heart, lungs, liver, kidney, and cerebral meninges.[405,406] In the latter study, the PXE material was most frequently associated with the connective tissue components of the organs particularly fibroblasts, and collagen and elastic fibers, myocardial tissue, and heart muscle cells.

Richardson and Epstein failed to demonstrate PXE material within trabecular meshwork cells, and the trabecular spaces were mostly free of it.[407] Rather, the material was concentrated in the juxtacanalicular region with accompanying destruction of Schlemm's canal. Other authors have confirmed the marked deposition of PXE material in the juxtacanalicular tissue adjacent to the inner and outer walls of Schlemm's canal and in the uveal meshwork.[408] They concluded that this material was produced by endothelial and connective cells in the region of its deposition; however, they believed that the material in the uveal trabeculum was derived partially from the aqueous humor. Accumulation of PXE material in the juxtacanalicular

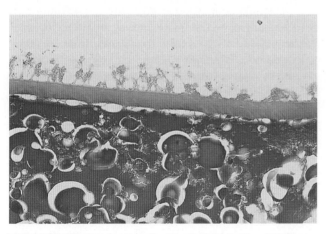

FIG. 7-40. Photomicrograph of typical deposits of PXE material resembling iron filings on the anterior lens capsule.

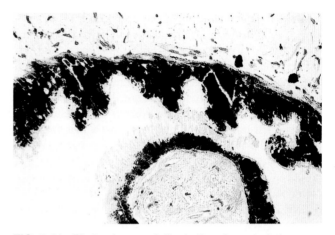

FIG. 7-41. Photomicrograph illustrating characteristic corrugations or clumping of pigment epithelium on the posterior iris surface. Also shown are deposits of pseudoexfoliation material on the ciliary process.

area followed by endothelial cell dysfunction and disorganization of the juxtacanalicular tissue and Schlemm's canal were cited as probable causative factors in the development of PXE glaucoma. Lutjen-Drecoll and colleagues found increased deposition of sheath-derived plaque material in the cribriform layer of the trabecular meshwork of patients with POAG but not those with PXE glaucoma.[409]

Examination of iris blood vessels from specimens obtained at trabeculectomy for PXE glaucoma revealed fluffy, fine filaments with a diameter of 20 to 30 nm and a length of 100 to 700 nm located beneath a thinned vascular endothelium.[410] These deposits narrowed and sometimes occluded the vessel lumen. The authors concluded that the material was produced by vascular endothelial cells, pericytes, and stromal pigmented cells. Konstas and colleagues concluded that PXE material in iris vessels is produced primarily by vascular supporting cells.[411] Decreased vascular integrity may be reflected in abnormal blood-aqueous barrier function, which has been demonstrated in PXE patients compared with normal and POAG patients using the laser flare-cell meter.[412] This lack of vascular integrity may contribute to the fibrin reaction that is more frequently seen following intraocular surgery in PXE patients.[413,414] Further evidence for iris abnormalities in PXE is their decreased response to mydriatic and miotic medications.[415] Poor pupillary dilatation also has been cited as contributing to intraoperative complications during cataract extraction in PXE patients.[395]

Krukenberg spindle,[416] increased anterior chamber angle pigmentation,[417] and increased iris transillumination[418] have been reported as common in PXE syndrome. Pigmentation at or anterior to Schwalbe's line is termed a **Sampaolesi line.**[419] Repo and colleagues have suggested that the iris transillumination at least partially reflects extracranial cerebrovascular disease and have suggested that hypoperfusion contributes to the development of PXE syndrome.[420]

Clinical examination of 48 patients with PXE demonstrated significantly lower corneal endothelial cell counts, accompanied by increased corneal thickness and increased endothelial cell polymegathism.[421] Ultrastructural examination of three corneas from enucleated glaucomatous eyes with PXE revealed large deposits of typical PXE material adhering to the corneal endothelium and incorporated into the posterior Descemet's membrane.[422] In involved areas, the endothelial layer was irregular and discontinuous. Loosely adherent degenerating cells that produced PXE fibers and fibroblastic cells were covering the denuded Descemet's membrane.

PXE is associated with abnormal composition of the connective tissue of the optic nerve head region. Netland and colleagues found marked and widespread elastosis of the lamina cribrosa of four optic nerve heads from two patients with PXE syndrome and glaucoma compared with age-matched controls with and without open-angle glaucoma; however, no typical PXE fibers were noted.[423] Other findings were similar to those with POAG and included a decrease in collagen fiber density, the presence of basement membranes not associated with cell surfaces, and abundant bundles of microfibrils not labeled with elastin antibody. Elastic fibers in other areas of the optic nerve appeared normal in the PXE patients.

Hemolytic Glaucoma

The term **hemolytic glaucoma** was suggested by Fenton and Zimmerman.[424] In its pure form, hemolytic glaucoma results from dissolution of red blood cells and is characterized by the presence of macrophages and red blood cell debris.[425] In ghost-cell glaucoma (see Fig. 9-6 in Chapter 9), red blood cells degenerate in the vitreous taking on a khaki color and pass through a break in the hyaloid face into the anterior chamber where their more rigid structure obstructs the trabecular meshwork.[426-428] In clinical practice, however, both forms of glaucoma frequently are found concurrently, and the terminology in the published literature is muddled. Ghost-cell glaucoma is particularly likely to occur following closed vitrectomy in which vitreous red blood cell debris is incompletely removed.[427] The cells of ghost-cell glaucoma are best seen by phase-contrast microscopy of anterior chamber aspirates.[426]

Phacolytic Glaucoma

In phacolytic glaucoma, usually a mature or hypermature cataract (Fig. 7-42) leaks soluble lens protein into the anterior chamber, although it has been reported as late as 65 years after congenital cataract surgery.[429] The resulting inflammatory response is associated with a severe rise in intraocular pressure, which may be severe enough to suggest acute angle-closure as the mecha-

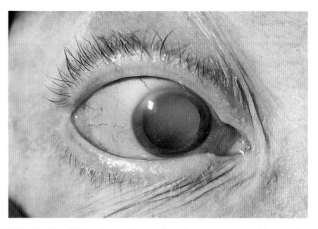

FIG. 7-42. Clinical photograph of a mature cataract that resulted in phacolytic glaucoma. (Courtesy of Ali Aminlari, MD).

nism.[430] There is a prominent anterior chamber flare; however, the cellular response is variable. Macrophages and particulate matter may be seen floating in the anterior chamber. Although intracapsular cataract extraction was traditionally recommended for phacolytic glaucoma, Lane and associates demonstrated that extracapsular cataract extraction with posterior chamber intraocular lens implantation is a safe and effective treatment for this entity.[431]

Flocks and colleagues have shown that the inflammatory cells in phacolytic glaucoma are almost all macrophages.[432] Polychromatic hyperrefringent granules are seen in this entity and have been demonstrated to be cholesterol crystals.[433] Calcium oxalate crystals also have been demonstrated in the aqueous in phacolytic glaucoma.[434] Cytologic examination of material obtained from anterior chamber aspirate may be helpful in making the diagnosis in questionable cases[435]; however, Epstein has cautioned that macrophages are not an invariable finding.[430]

Electron microscopic examination of material obtained from anterior chamber aspirate in a patient with phacolytic glaucoma demonstrated primarily free-floating lens material and numerous macrophages that had digested lens material.[436] Trabeculectomy material from the same patient demonstrated the intertrabecular spaces to be obstructed by phagocytic cells, melanin-laden macrophages, cell debris, and free-floating degenerated lens material.

Epstein has postulated that heavy molecular weight protein (MW greater than 150×10^6), which he believes is of lens origin, may be as responsible for decreasing aqueous outflow in phacolytic glaucoma as is obstruction of the trabecular meshwork by macrophages.[430,437] Similarly, Yanoff and Scheie have emphasized the role of lens protein in causing elevated intraocular pressure in the formerly used lens needling and aspiration procedure.[438] Rosenbaum and colleagues have demonstrated chemotactic activity for lens proteins from sonicated lenses and have associated this activity with the gamma crystallin fraction.[439]

Melanomalytic Glaucoma

The term **melanomalytic glaucoma** was first used by Yanoff and Scheie to describe secondary open-angle glaucoma that they concluded was caused by mechanical blockage of the trabecular meshwork by macrophages laden with melanin pigment released by a necrotic ciliary body malignant melanoma.[440] They drew an analogy between this entity and phacolytic glaucoma. Subsequently, ultrastructural studies have confirmed that the cells obstructing the trabecular meshwork in this entity are macrophages[441]; however, Van Buskirk and Leure-duPree also noted detached, phagocytic trabecular endothelial cells.[442]

Other open-angle glaucoma mechanisms associated with malignant melanoma include seeding of tumor into the anterior chamber angle and invasion of the angle structures by a ring melanoma[443,444] (Fig. 7-43).

SOAG Caused by Damaged Outflow Channels

Blunt Trauma

Hyphema is associated with concurrent direct, gonioscopically detectable injury to the anterior chamber angle region. The anterior chamber angle recession from blunt ocular trauma presumably occurs as the force of the concussive blow is transmitted through the aqueous and slaps up against the anterior chamber angle (see also Chapter 9). The force lacerates into the face of the ciliary body and usually tears the anterior arterial circle, resulting in hyphema.[445] Gonioscopically and histologically, the injury results in an apparent deepening of the anterior chamber angle and a widening of the exposed area of the ciliary

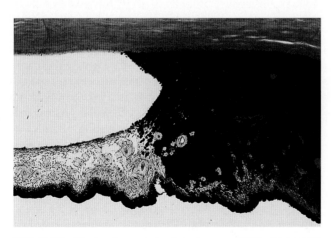

FIG. 7-43. Photomicrograph of melanoma infiltrating angle structures.

body face, resulting in the appearance of anterior chamber angle recession.[445,446]

Blanton found angle recession in 71% of 182 eyes that had traumatic hyphema; however, only 7% developed glaucoma.[447] He also noted that the onset of the glaucoma may be delayed for 10 or more years after the initial injury. Although infrequent, the delayed onset of the glaucoma associated with angle recession also was noted by Kaufman and Tolpin.[448] Canavan and Archer examined the anterior segments of 212 eyes of 205 patients at 1 to 14 years after blunt ocular trauma. Anterior chamber angle recession was noted in 80.5%; however, only one patient developed ocular hypertension.[449]

Salmon and associates found angle recession in 14.6% of 987 people during a population-based glaucoma survey in South Africa.[450] The prevalence of glaucoma in those with angle recession was 5.5% and was 8% in those with 360 degrees of angle recession. Not surprisingly, angle recession was strongly associated with excessive alcohol consumption. Sihota and associates noted a positive association between traumatic glaucoma and traumatic cataracts, angle recession of more than 180 degrees, significant injuries to the iris, and a displacement of the lens.[451] Alper found a particularly high prevalence of glaucoma in eyes with 240 degrees or more of angle recession.[446]

SOAG Secondary to Miscellaneous Causes

The Syndrome of Glaucomatocyclitic Crises (Posner-Schlossman Syndrome)

Posner and Schlossman described the syndrome that bears their names in 1948.[452] In one article, they called it the **syndrome of glaucomatocyclitic crises** to emphasize the recurring nature of episodes of impressive intraocular pressure rise.[453] **Posner-Schlossman syndrome** (PSS) typically affects one eye in individuals in their third to fifth decade of life. During the attacks, the intraocular pressure may rise as high as 90 mmHg.[454] Patients may note symptoms of corneal edema such as halos around lights; however, symptoms of pain and signs of inflammation usually are minimal. Mild pupillary dilation may be found during the acute episode. Although the syndrome has been described as self-limited, attacks may last from hours to weeks in duration. Corneal endothelial cell density may be reduced after repeated attacks.[455] Evidence of optic nerve damage or visual field loss may require filtration surgery.[397]

As noted previously, clinical signs of uveitis usually are mild. Slit-lamp examination may reveal a few fine keratic precipitates, which eventually may assume a more ''mutton fat'' appearance. Anterior chamber reaction characteristically is mild. Aqueous outflow facility is decreased during acute attacks, and aqueous production may be elevated.[456] After the acute episode, intraocular pressure may remain elevated; however, it is often below normal.[457]

The cause of PSS is not known. Abnormal reactivity of the ciliary blood vessels has been suggested,[457] as has a developmental abnormality of the anterior chamber angle.[458] Yamamoto and associates have postulated that herpes simplex virus plays some role in causing the syndrome based on their study of amplified genomic fragments from anterior chamber aspirates.[459] Hirose and colleagues cited an increased prevalence of HLA-Bw54-Cw1 haplotype in involved individuals.[460] A form of protein-induced glaucoma was reported in one patient with PSS and periphlebitis.[461] Abnormal prostaglandin production has been postulated.[462] Some authors have suggested an association between this entity and POAG.[457,463]

Numerous mononuclear cells and erythrocytes have been found in the trabecular meshwork in a trabeculectomy specimen examined by light and electron microscopy.[464] In this specimen, the presence of the erythrocytes was believed to be surgically related. It is interesting to note that giant vacuoles were not noted on the inner wall of Schlemm's canal although the intraocular pressure was considerably elevated preoperatively.

Fuchs' Heterochromic Iridocyclitis

Fuchs' heterochromic iridocyclitis syndrome (FHI) accounted for 6.2% of the uveitis cases for which a specific diagnosis was made in the Uveitis Clinic at the Hospital Jules Gonin over a 3-year period.[465] FHI usually is unilateral, but was reported to be bilateral in 7.8% of cases in one series.[466] It is characterized by the early development of cataract (seen in 80% of cases), which often precedes the development of glaucoma (seen in about 26% of cases),[466,467] and responds reasonably well to cataract surgery[468–472] (Fig. 7-44). Intractable glaucoma has been reported following YAG capsulotomy in FHI.[473]

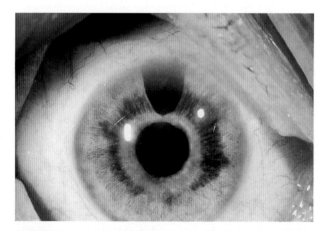

FIG. 7-44. Clinical photograph of Fuchs' heterochromic iridocyclitis. Note the presence of characteristic iris stromal atrophy. This patient has had surgery for the cataract and glaucoma typical of this disorder.

The risk of developing glaucoma in FHI has been estimated to be 0.5% per year.[474] The glaucoma may be particularly difficult to control. In one study of 30 patients with secondary glaucoma from FHI, medical therapy failed to adequately control intraocular pressure in 73%.[475] Nevertheless, they tended to respond to modern filtration techniques,[475] although one author reported a failure rate of 55.5% and recommended antimetabolites as an adjunct to filtration. The glaucoma found in the disorder may be secondary to anterior chamber angle neovascularization, lens-induced angle closure, peripheral anterior synechias, and recurrent hyphema, although chronic open-angle glaucoma is the most common mechanism.[474]

In a recent study, the most common presenting symptom (96.1%) was decreased vision.[476] Only 56.6% of cases were correctly diagnosed at the time of presentation in this study. The disorder may be particularly difficult to diagnose in blacks because of the frequent lack of heterochromia and presence of iris nodules.[477,478] It has been associated with HLA-B27 in one study[479]; however, Munoz and associates found only a negative association with HLA-A2.[480]

The involved eye may be hypochromic early in the disorder but may be the darker eye if iris stroma atrophy renders the pigment epithelium more visible. Iris stromal atrophy may be a more constant finding than heterochromia.[467] Other findings include mild iritis accompanied by fine keratic precipitates, iris muscle atrophy, and mydriasis.

Fluorescein angiography has documented the presence of iris vascular abnormalities including leakage and perfusion defects and has supported the belief that the syndrome results from anterior segment ischemia.[481,482] Fine iris neovascularization is a common finding and may involve the anterior chamber angle; however, extensive PAS usually do not develop. A filiform hemorrhage is a fine stream of bleeding from the neovascularization that may be precipitated by pressure on the globe or from a sudden reduction in intraocular pressure such as at the time of intraocular surgery. It is of no clinical significance. Recently, recurrent subconjunctival hemorrhages have been reported in FHI.[483]

Histopathologic findings include hyalinization of iris blood vessels, which lends credence to a vascular cause for the syndrome. Immune deposits also have been reported in iris blood vessel walls in FHI; however, no evidence of an active inflammatory vascular process was found.[484] Electron microscopic examination of irides of two patients revealed abnormal melanocyte melanin production, abundance of plasma cells, and membranous degeneration of nerve fibers.[485] The authors postulated abnormal adrenergic innervation, either primary or secondary to inflammation, as a possible cause for the abnormal melanin production. Decreased numbers of stromal melanocytes and abnormal melanosomes has been documented by others.[486] In another histologic study from a patient with FHI for 17 years, findings included keratic precipitates, discontinuous anterior chamber angle rubeosis, chronic nongranulomatous iridocyclitis, and trabeculitis.[487]

Chorioretinal lesions have been found in association with FHI.[488,489] Therefore, an association between toxoplasmosis and FHI has been suggested by some,[490] but disputed by others.[491] Increased immunoreactivity to S-antigen has been found in FHI.[492] FHI has been reported in association with sarcoidosis in several patients.[493] Other immunologic abnormalities have also been reported.[494–500] Nevertheless, Murray has questioned whether the immunologic findings in FHI are the cause or the side effects of the underlying disease process.[501]

FHI has been reported in association with congenital Horner's syndrome.[502] A hereditary association also has been cited including a family with retinitis pigmentosa.[503,504]

VARIABLE OUTFLOW: NORMAL-PRESSURE GLAUCOMA

Normal- or low-pressure glaucoma is characterized by glaucomatous optic nerve cupping and visual field loss in individuals demonstrating intraocular pressures within the statistically normal range.[505–508] Some authors have suggested that the visual field defects in NTG patients tend to have a steeper slope, to be located closer to fixation, and to have a greater depth.[509,510] Such findings have suggested different mechanisms between the optic nerve damage in NTG and that in POAG.[510] Other authors did not believe that such differences exist if the degree of optic nerve cupping is held constant.[511]

Normal-pressure glaucoma is probably a more accurate descriptive term than low-pressure glaucoma because intraocular pressure is not below the normal range. De Vivero and colleagues were unable to demonstrate a difference in mean diurnal intraocular pressure range in NTP patients compared with that reported for normal individuals.[512] Similarly, Larsson and colleagues found no difference in aqueous humor dynamics in NTG and normal controls.[513] Although intraocular pressure lowering is one therapeutic modality used in NTG, these patients tend to have a more inexorable course than do those with POAG.[514] The role of intraocular pressure in this disorder is more tenuous than in POAG[515]; however, when there is intraocular pressure asymmetry between two eyes in NTG, the eye with the higher pressure usually suffers the greater damage.[515,516] Another finding associated with NTG includes an increased prevalence of peripapillary pigmentary abnormalities,[517] although Jonas and Xu did not find abnormally large parapapillary atrophy in NTG compared with POAG.[518]

A vascular-related mechanism is most often cited as the proposed pathophysiology of NTG. Based on magnetic resonance imaging studies, Stroman and colleagues proposed that cerebral small-vessel ischemia was more common in NTG patients and may indirectly reflect a vascular cause for the ocular nerve damage in these patients.[519] Other authors have been unable to find consistent abnormalities in coagulation tests and rheologic profiles in NTG patients,[520] although Klaver and associates noted elevated plasma viscosity values and packed cell volumes in NTG patients compared with controls.[521] A significant increase in the vascular resistive index of both the ophthalmic artery and central retinal artery has been demonstrated in NTG patients compared with age-matched controls.[522] NTG patients have been shown to have a decrease in pulsatile ocular blood flow under conditions of temporarily increased intraocular pressure.[523] These findings are consistent with decreased autoregulation of blood flow possibly on a myogenic basis. Others also have cited poor autoregulation of optic nerve blood flow in NTG.[524] Ravalico and associates and others found pulsatile ocular blood flow abnormalities in NTG.[525,526] One mechanism for such poor autoregulation has been postulated to involve abnormalities in the production of vascular endothelium-derived relaxing factors such as nitric oxide, prostacyclin, and a putative hyperpolarizing factor.[527] Abnormal endothelin levels also have been cited in NTG.[528] Using clinical and ultrasound studies of the extracranial carotid arteries, however, Muller and colleagues found no evidence supporting a hemodynamic origin of NTG.[529]

Compression of the optic nerve near the intracranial opening of the optic canal by abnormal segments of the intracavernous carotid arteries has been proposed as another cause of NTG in many cases.[530] An autoimmune process also has been suggested.[531,532] Brierley and associates were unable to demonstrate abnormalities of the mitochondrial respiratory chain in NTG.[533]

Disc hemorrhages are more common in NTG than in POAG[534–537] and may indicate progressive optic nerve damage.[538] Acquired pits of the optic nerve also are more common in NTG patients.[539]

The calcium-channel blocking agent, nifedipine, may be helpful in the treatment of NTG,[540–542] although others have questioned its effectiveness.[543] Positive effects achieved by calcium channel blocking agents may be mediated through the inhibition of vasospasm.[544,545] Argon laser trabeculoplasty[546–548] and filtration surgery aimed at lowering intraocular pressures also may be helpful.[549–551]

PATHOPHYSIOLOGIC MECHANISMS OF OCULAR INJURY IN GLAUCOMA

With the exception of injury to the optic nerve, ocular damage in glaucoma relates directly to the degree of intraocular pressure elevation, if any. This fact is exemplified by the response of the cornea to glaucoma. If intraocular pressure remains within the normal range, there is no

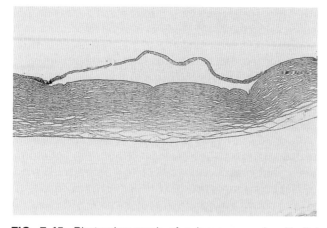

FIG. 7-45. Photomicrograph of a large corneal epithelial bulla.

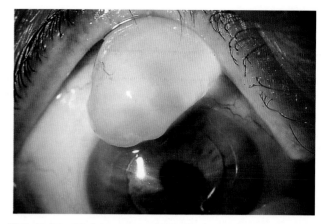

FIG. 7-47. Clinical photograph of a large, overhanging filtering bleb causing chronic irritation and decreased vision.

reason to expect glaucoma to have a significant effect on the cornea. Corneal clarity, however, depends on the ability of its endothelium to maintain it in a relatively dehydrated state. The endothelium, in turn, must work against the pressure gradient produced by the intraocular pressure. As the intraocular pressure rises, endothelial work increases until its function is compromised and the cornea becomes edematous. This edema is reflected histologically in a loss of the usual stromal clefting artifact and by edema of the basal cells. At some point, the ability of the epithelium to remain attached to its basal lamina is compromised and bullae develop (Fig. 7-45). Such chronic edema results in many cycles of epithelial injury and healing. During this process, aberrant basement membrane material often is produced within the epithelium. As these cycles continue, a fibrous pannus may form between epithelium and Bowman's membrane. More significantly, rupture of epithelial bullae are a source of great pain when corneal nerve endings become exposed. Additionally, the resulting breach of the epithelial barrier exposes the cornea to invasion by pathogenic organisms. It

is not surprising, therefore, that intractable pain from corneal ulceration or corneal perforation secondary to such an ulcer are final common pathways often leading to enucleation of glaucomatous eyes.

Persistent elevation of intraocular pressure may result in stretching of the sclera at the limbus particularly in the eyes of children. Such thinned areas are *limbal ectasias* if they are not lined by uvea and are *limbal staphylomas* when uvea lines them. If the ocular coat thinning is located overlying the ciliary body, *intercalary staphyloma* is the appropriate term. Extensive thinning and stretching of the sclera may lead to a blue-black appearance as the uvea is viewed through the sclera. This appearance may be misinterpreted as scleral invasion of a uveal melanoma; however, the simple clinical test of ocular transillumination usually reveals the correct diagnosis of scleral thinning.

Chronically elevated intraocular pressure produces ciliary body atrophy, resulting in ocular hypotony, and initiating a process that concludes with ocular phthisis (Fig. 7-46). This process is described further in Chapter 9.

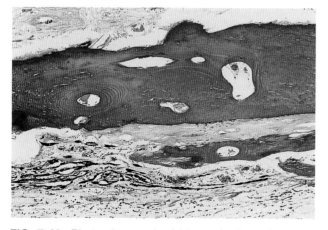

FIG. 7-46. Photomicrograph of intraocular bone formation in an eye undergoing degeneration to phthisis.

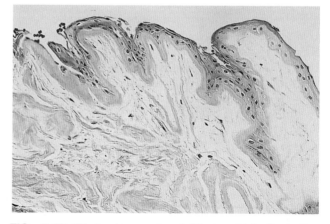

FIG. 7-48. Photomicrograph of filtering bleb illustrating edema of connective tissue and epithelial bullae.

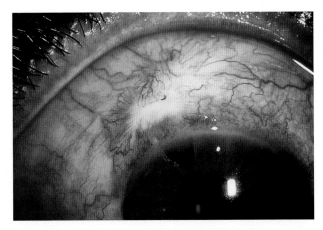

FIG. 7-49. Clinical photograph of blebitis in which infection is localized to the filtering bleb (Courtesy of Ali Aminlari, MD).

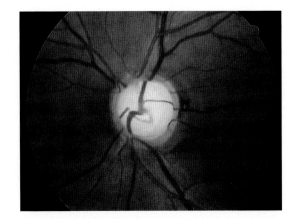

FIG. 7-51. Fundus photograph of extensive glaucomatous optic nerve cupping.

Surgery for glaucoma may result in secondary changes and complications. Cataract is a frequent complication of filtration surgery. Other complications from such procedures are the production of exuberant filtration blebs that may overhang the cornea or cause ocular irritation[552] (Figs. 7-47 and 7-48). Exceptionally thin or leaking filtering blebs, particularly those associated with antimetabolite use, may be a source of blebitis (Fig. 7-49) or endophthalmitis (Fig. 7-50).[553]

The sine qua non of glaucomatous ocular damage is optic nerve injury, characterized by increased optic nerve cupping (Fig. 7-51) and decreased optic nerve rim area.[554–556] Such changes may be partially reversible when intraocular pressure is lowered,[557,558] particularly in children.[560] In experimental primate glaucoma, in animals with an initial C/D ratio of 0.2 to 0.3, Varma and colleagues have associated an increase in C/D ratio of 0.1 with a 10% loss of optic nerve fibers.[560] Clinically detectable nerve fiber layer loss has been cited as preceding

glaucomatous visual field loss.[561] As many as 50% of all retinal ganglion cells may be lost before there is detectable visual field loss.[562] Optic disc hemorrhages may be the harbinger of progression of glaucomatous optic nerve damage.[563,564]

Ultimately, damage to optic nerve axons leads to loss of retinal ganglion cells (Fig. 7-52), some of which may undergo apoptosis.[565] Larger ganglion cells and larger optic nerve fibers appear to be more sensitive to glaucomatous damage.[566–569] It also has been suggested that the corpora amylacea count of retinal ganglion cells decreases with increasing glaucomatous damage to the optic nerve in glaucoma.[570] Nerve fibers are preferentially lost at the superior and inferior segments of the disc in early glaucoma, although astrocytes are relatively resistant to damage.[571] The pore sizes and connective tissue distribution in the lamina cribrosa at the superior and inferior optic disc may predispose to nerve fiber damage in these areas.[572] Changes in pore size and shape in response to glaucoma may exacerbate the tendency to further damage.[573] The direct pathophysiologic mechanism through which intraocular pressure is related to optic nerve dam-

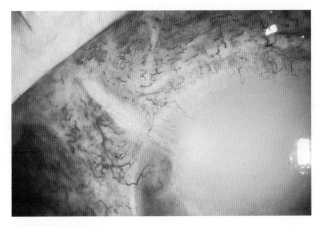

FIG. 7-50. Clinical photograph of endophthalmitis, resulting from dehiscence in the conjunctiva, comprising the filtering bleb in a seton procedure for glaucoma (Courtesy of Ali Aminlari, MD).

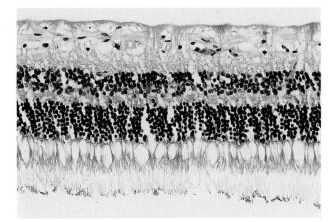

FIG. 7-52. Photomicrograph of retina showing extensive ganglion cell loss from glaucoma.

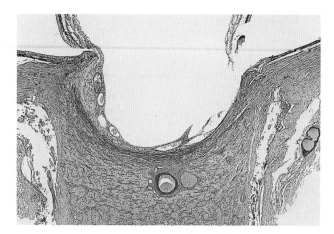

FIG. 7-53. Photomicrograph of extensively cupped optic nerve head in glaucoma, illustrating posterior bowing of plates in the lamina cribrosa.

age remains a matter of chronic discussion, examination, and experimentation. In general, two such mechanisms are most often cited.

The **vascular theory** postulates that compromise of the blood supply secondary to ocular pressure results in ischemia at the level of the optic nerve head.[574,575] The **mechanical theory** holds that the intraocular pressure distorts the conformation of the cribriform plates resulting in obstruction to axoplasmic flow at the level of the optic nerve head[576–586] (Fig. 7-53). It is obvious that these two theories are not mutually exclusive. Rather, there are many instances in which they may be complementary. Nevertheless, in any given glaucoma disorder, one may predominate.

In glaucomatous eyes, alterations in the connective tissue elements in the optic nerve head have been described secondary to elevated intraocular pressure.[574,583–586] It has been suggested that in glaucoma there is a stiffening of the mechanical support of the optic nerve.[587] How these changes relate to the pathophysiology of optic nerve injury in glaucoma is not clear.

Parapillary chorioretinal atrophy accompanies optic nerve damage in glaucoma. The findings are related to atrophy and irregularities in retinal pigment epithelium, and loss of pigment epithelium and photoreceptors.[588,589]

Recently, the lamina cribrosa of rodents has been demonstrated to be similar in composition to that of primates, and may prove useful in helping to delineate the pathophysiology of optic nerve damage in glaucoma.[590]

REFERENCES

1. Thylefors B, Negrel AD. The global impact of glaucoma. *Bull World Health Organ* 1994;72:323–326.
2. Bengtsson B. The prevalence of glaucoma. *Br J Ophthalmol* 1981; 65:46–49.
3. Bengtsson BO. Incidence of manifest glaucoma. *Br J Ophthalmol* 1989;73:483–487.
4. Hollows FC, Graham PA. Intra-ocular pressure, glaucoma, and glaucoma suspects in a defined population. *Br J Ophthalmol* 1966; 50:570–586.
5. Klein BE, Klein R, Sponsel WE, et al. Prevalence of glaucoma: the beaver dam eye study. *Ophthalmology* 1992;99:1499–1504.
6. Tielsch JM, Sommer A, Katz J, et al. Racial variations in the prevalence of primary open-angle glaucoma: the Baltimore eye survey. *JAMA* 1991;266:369–374.
7. Becker B, Keskey GG, Christensen RE. Hypersecretion glaucoma. *Arch Ophthalmol* 1956;56:180–187.
8. Kupfer C, Kaiser-Kupfer MI. New hypothesis of developmental anomalies of the anterior chamber associated with glaucoma. *Trans Ophthalmol Soc UK* 1978;98:213–215.
9. Kupfer C, Kaiser-Kupfer MI. Observations on the development of the anterior chamber angle with reference to the pathogenesis of congenital glaucomas. *Am J Ophthalmol* 1979;88:424–426.
10. Tripathi B, Tripathi R. Embryology of the anterior segment of the human eye. In: Ritch R, Shields MB, Krupin T, eds. *The glaucomas*. St. Louis: CV Mosby, 1989.
11. Ozanics V, Jakobiec FA. Prenatal development of the eye and its adnexa. In: Tasman W, ed. Duane's foundations of clinical ophthalmology, vol 1. Philadelphia: JB Lippincott, 1994.
12. Johnston MC, Noden DM, Hazelton RD, et al. Origins of avian ocular and periocular tissues. *Exp Eye Res* 1979;29:27–43.
13. Beauchamp GR, Knepper PA. Role of the neural crest in anterior segment development and disease. *J Pediatr Ophthalmol Strabismus* 1984;21:209–214.
14. Cook CS. Experimental models of anterior segment dysgenesis. *Ophthalmic Paediatr Genet* 1989;10:33–46.
15. Tripathi BJ, Tripathi RC. Neural crest origin of human trabecular meshwork and its implications for the pathogenesis of glaucoma. *Am J Ophthalmol* 1989;107:583–590.
16. Doran RM. Anterior segment malformations: aetiology and genetic implications [editorial]. *Br J Ophthalmol* 1991;75:579.
17. Williams DL. A comparative approach to anterior segment dysgenesis. *Eye* 1993;7:607–616.
18. Kaiser-Kupfer MI. Neural crest origin of trabecular meshwork cells and other structures of the anterior chamber [editorial]. *Am J Ophthalmol* 1989;107:671–672.
19. deLuise VP, Anderson DR. Primary infantile glaucoma (congenital glaucoma). *Surv Ophthalmology* 1983;28:1–19.
20. Miller SJH. Genetic aspects of glaucoma. *Trans Ophthalmol Sopc U K* 1962;81:425–434.
21. Ritch R, Shields MB, Krupin T, eds. *The glaucomas*. St. Louis: CV Mosby, 1989.
22. Duke-Elder S. Congenital Deformities. In: Duke-Elder S, ed. *System of ophthalmology*. St. Louis: CV Mosby, 1969:548–565.
23. Moller PM. Goniotomy and congenital glaucoma. *Acta Ophthalmologica* 1977;55:436–442.
24. Seidman DJ, Nelson LB, Calhoun JH, Spaeth GL, Harley RD. Signs and symptoms in the presentation of primary infantile glaucoma. *Pediatrics* 1986;77:399–404.
25. Kiskis AA, Markowitz SN, Morin JD. Corneal diameter and axial length in congenital glaucoma. *Can J Ophthalmol* 1985;20:93–97.
26. Morin JD, Merin S, Sheppard RW. Primary congenital glaucoma—a survey. *Can J Ophthalmol* 1974;9:17–28.
27. Walton DS. Primary congenital open angle glaucoma: a study of the anterior segment abnormalities. *Trans Am Ophthalmol Soc* 1979;77:746–768.
28. Waring GO, Rodrigues MM, Laibson PR. Anterior chamber cleavage syndrome: a stepladder classification. *Surv Ophthalmol* 1975; 20:3–27.
29. Shields MB, Buckley E, Klintworth GK, Thresher R. Axenfeld-Rieger syndrome: a spectrum of developmental disorders. *Surv Ophthalmol* 1985;29:387–409.
30. Ticho BH, Rosner M, Mets MB, Tso MO. Bilateral diffuse iris nodular nevi: clinical and histopathologic characterization. *Ophthalmology* 1995;102:419–425.
31. Hanson IM, Fletcher JM, Jordan T, et al. Mutations at the PAX6 locus are found in heterogeneous anterior segment malformations including Peters' anomaly. *Nat Genet* 1994;6:168–173.
32. van Schooneveld MJ, Delleman JW, et al. Peters'-plus: a new syndrome. *Ophthalmic Paediatr Genet* 1984;4:141–145.

33. Hennekam RC, Van Schooneveld MJ, Ardinger HH, et al. The Peters'-Plus syndrome: description of 16 patients and review of the literature. *Clin Dysmorph* 1993;2:283–300.
34. Myles WM, Flanders ME, Chitayat D, et al. S. Peters' anomaly: a clinicopathologic study. *J Pediatr Ophthalmol Strabismus* 1992; 29:374–381.
35. Traboulsi EI, Maumenee IH. Peters' anomaly and associated congenital malformations. *Arch Ophthalmol* 1992;110:1739–1742.
36. Heon E, Barsoum-Homsy M, Cevrette L, et al. Peters' anomaly: the spectrum of associated ocular and systemic malformations. *Ophthalmic Paediatr Genet* 1992;13:137–143.
37. Mayer UM. Peters' anomaly and combination with other malformations (series of 16 patients). *Ophthalmic Paediatr Genet* 1992; 13:131–135.
38. Summitt RL, Hiatt RL, Duenas D, Johnson WW. Mesoectodermal dysplasia of the iris and cornea, mental retardation and myopathy: a sporadic case. *Birth Defects* 1971;7:129–135.
39. Nakanishi I, Brown SI. The histopathology and ultrastructure of congenital, central corneal opacity (Peters' anomaly). *Am J Ophthalmol* 1971;72:801–812.
40. Townsend WM. Congenital corneal leukomas. 1. Central defect in Descemet's membrane. *Am J Ophthalmol* 1974;77:80–86.
41. Townsend WM, Font RL, et al. LE. Congenital corneal leukomas. 2. Histopathologic findings in 19 eyes with central defect in Descemet's membrane. *Am J Ophthalmol* 1974;77:192–206.
42. Kuper C, Kuwabara T, Stark WJ. The histopathology of Peters' anomaly. *Am J Ophthalmol* 1975;80:653–660.
43. Stone DL, Kenyon KR, Green WR, et al. Congenital central corneal leukoma (Peters' anomaly). *Am J Ophthalmol* 1976;81:173–193.
44. Fogle JA, Green WR, Kenyon KR, et al. J. Peripheral Peters' anomaly: a histopathologic case report. *J Pediatr Ophthalmol Strabismus* 1978;15:71–76.
45. Kasner L, Mietz H, Green WR. Agenesis of Bowman's layer: a histopathological study of four cases. *Cornea* 1993;12:163–170.
46. Lee CF, Yue BY, Robin J, Sawaguchi S, et al. Immunohistochemical studies of Peters' anomaly. *Ophthalmology* 1989;96:958–964.
47. Gollamudi SR, Traboulsi EI, Chamon W, et al. Visual outcome after surgery for Peters' anomaly. *Ophthalmic Genet* 1994;15:31–35.
48. Parmley VC, Stonecipher KG, Rowsey JJ. Peters' anomaly: a review of 26 penetrating keratoplasties in infants. *Ophthalmic Surg* 1993;24:31–35.
49. Erlich CM, Rootman DS, Morin JD. Corneal transplantation in infants, children and young adults: experience of the Toronto Hospital for Sick Children, 1979–88. *Can J Ophthalmol* 1991;26:206–210.
50. Rosett H. A clinical perspective of the fetal alcohol syndrome. *Alcohol Clin Exp Res* 1980;4:119–122.
51. Miller M, Israel J, Cuttone J. Fetal alcohol syndrome. *J Pediatr Ophthalmol Strabismus* 1981;18:6–15.
52. Stromland K. Ocular abnormalities in the fetal alcohol syndrome. *Acta Ophthalmol (Copenh)* 1985;171(suppl):1–50.
53. Stromland K. Ocular involvement in the fetal alcohol syndrome. *Surv Ophthalmol* 1987;31:277–284.
54. Altman B. Fetal alcohol syndrome. *J Pediatr Ophthalmol* 1976; 13:255–258.
55. Weiss AH, Kousseff BG, Ross EA, Longbottom J. Simple microphthalmos. *Arch Ophthalmol* 1989;107:1625–1630.
56. Ammann AJ, Wara DW, Cowan MJ, et al. The DiGeorge syndrome and the fetal alcohol syndrome. *Am J Dis Child* 1982;136:906–908.
57. Abel EL, Sokol RJ. Incidence of fetal alcohol syndrome and economic impact of FAS-related anomalies. *Drug Alcohol Depend* 1987;19:51–70.
58. May PA, Hymbaugh KJ, Aase JM, Samet JM. Epidemiology of fetal alcohol syndrome among American Indians of the Southwest. *Soc Biol* 1983;30:374–387.
59. Ritch R, Forbes M, Hetherington J Jr., et al. Congenital ectropion uveae with glaucoma. *Ophthalmology* 1984;91:326–331.
60. Hertzberg R. Congenital ectropion uveae and glaucoma. *Aust N Z J Ophthalmol* 1985;13:45–48.
61. Levin H, Ritch R, Barathur R, Dunn MW, et al. Aniridia, congeni-

tal glaucoma, and hydrocephalus in a male infant with ring chromosome 6. *Am J Med Genet* 1986;25:281–287.
62. Futterweit W, Ritch R, Teekhasaenee C, Nelson ES. Coexistence of Prader-Willi syndrome, congenital ectropion uveae with glaucoma, and factor XI deficiency. *JAMA* 1986;255:3280–3282.
63. Candaele C, Lefebvre A, Meire F, et al. Congenital ectropion uveae with glaucoma. *Bull Soc Belge Ophthalmol* 1993;249:131–137.
64. Dowling JL Jr., Albert DM, Nelson LB, Walton DS. Primary glaucoma associated with iridotrabecular dysgenesis and ectropion uveae. *Ophthalmology* 1985;92:912–921.
65. Mattox C, Walton DS. Hereditary primary childhood glaucomas. *Int Ophthalmol Clin* 1993;33:121–134.
66. Congdon N, Wang F, Tielsch JM. Issues in the epidemiology and population-based screening of primary angle-closure glaucoma. *Surv Ophthalmol* 1992;36:411–423.
67. Arkell SM, Lightman DA, Sommer A, Taylor HR, Korshin OM, Tielsch JM. The prevalence of glaucoma among Eskimos of northwest Alaska. *Arch Ophthalmol* 1987;105:482–485.
68. Van RG, Arkell SM, Charlton W, Doesburg W. Primary angle-closure glaucoma among Alaskan Eskimos. *Doc Ophthalmol* 1988; 70:265–276.
69. Salmon JF, Mermoud A, Ivey A, et al. The prevalence of primary angle closure glaucoma and open angle glaucoma in Mamre, western Cape, South Africa. *Arch Ophthalmol* 1993;111:1263–1269.
70. Salmon JF, Martell R. The role of ethnicity in primary angle-closure glaucoma. *S Afr Med J* 1994;84:623–626.
71. Alper MG, Laubach JL. Primary angle-closure glaucoma in the American Negro. *Arch Ophthalmol* 1968;79:663–668.
72. Van Herick W, Shaffer RN, Schwartz A. Estimation of width of angle of anterior chamber. Incidence and significance of the narrow angle. *Am J Ophthalmol* 1969;68:626–629.
73. Lowe RF. Central corneal thickness. Ocular correlations in normal eyes and those with primary angle-closure glaucoma. *Br J Ophthalmol* 1969;53:824–826.
74. Lowe RF. Corneal radius and ocular correlations. *Am J Ophthalmol* 1969;67:864–868.
75. Lowe RF. Anterior lens curvature: comparisons between normal eyes and those with primary angle-closure glaucoma. *Br J Ophthalmol* 1972;56:409–413.
76. Lowe RF. Acute angle closure glaucoma and the crystalline lens. *Aust J Ophthalmol* 1973;1:89–94.
77. Lowe RF, Clark BA. Radius of curvature of the anterior lens surface: correlations in normal eyes and in eyes involved with primary angle-closure glaucoma. *Br J Ophthalmol* 1973;57:471–474.
78. Lowe RF, Clark BA. Posterior corneal curvature: correlations in normal eyes and in eyes involved with primary angle-closure glaucoma. *Br J Ophthalmol* 1973;57:464–470.
79. Panek WC, Christensen RE, Lee DA, et al. Biometric variables in patients with occludable anterior chamber angles. *Am J Ophthalmol* 1990;110:185–188.
80. Markowitz SN, Morin JD. Angle-closure glaucoma: relation between lens thickness, anterior chamber depth and age. *Can J Ophthalmol* 1984;19:300–302.
81. Markowitz SN, Morin JD. The ratio of lens thickness to axial length for biometric standardization in angle-closure glaucoma. *Am J Ophthalmol* 1985;99:400–402.
82. Godel V, Stein R, Feiler-Ofry V. Angle-closure glaucoma: postoperative acute glaucoma after phenylephrine eyedrops. *Am J Ophthalmol* 1968;65:552–554.
83. Lowe RF. Plateau iris. *Aust J Ophthalmol* 1981;9:71–73.
84. Wand M, Grant WM, Simmons RJ, et al. Plateau iris syndrome. *Trans Am Acad Ophthalmol Otolaryngol* 1977;83:122–130.
85. Pavlin CJ, Ritch R, Foster FS. Ultrasound biomicroscopy in plateau iris syndrome. *Am J Ophthalmol* 1992;113:390–395.
86. Wand M, Pavlin CJ, Foster FS. Plateau iris syndrome: ultrasound biomicroscopic and histologic study [letter]. *Ophthalmic Surg* 1993;24:129–131.
87. Ritch R. Exfoliation syndrome and occludable angles. *Trans Am Ophthalmol Soc* 1994;92:845–944.
88. Gross FJ, Tingey D, Epstein DL. Increased prevalence of occludable angles and angle-closure glaucoma in patients with pseudoexfoliation. *Am J Ophthalmol* 1994;117:333–336.

89. Brusini P, Tosoni C, Miani P. Increased prevalence of occludable angles and angle-closure glaucoma in patients with pseudoexfoliation [letter; comment]. Am J Ophthalmol 1994;118:540.

90. von der Lippe I, Kuchle M, Naumann GO. Pseudoexfoliation syndrome as a risk factor for acute ciliary block angle closure glaucoma. Acta Ophthalmol 1993;71:277–279.

91. Salmon JF, Murray AD. The association of iridoschisis and primary angle-closure glaucoma. Eye 1992;6:267–272.

92. Pitts JF, Jay JL. The association of Fuchs's corneal endothelial dystrophy with axial hypermetropia, shallow anterior chamber, and angle closure glaucoma. Br J Ophthalmol 1990;74:601–604.

93. Loewenstein A, Geyer O, Hourvitz D, Lazar M. The association of Fuch's corneal endothelial dystrophy with angle closure glaucoma [letter; comment]. Br J Ophthalmol 1991;75:510.

94. Wan WL, Minckler DS, et al. Pupillary-block glaucoma associated with childhood cystinosis. Am J Ophthalmol 1986;101:700–706.

95. Hagan JCD, Lederer CM Jr. Primary angle closure glaucoma in a myopic kinship. Arch Ophthalmol 1985;103:363–365.

96. Hagan JCD, Lederer CM Jr. Genetic spontaneous late subluxation of the lens previously reported as a myopic kinship with primary angle closure glaucoma [letter]. Arch Ophthalmol 1992;110:1199–1200.

97. Malaise-Stals J, Collignon-Brach J, Weekers JF. Corneal endothelial cell density in acute angle-closure glaucoma. Ophthalmologica 1984;189:104–109.

98. Brooks AM, Gillies WE. Effect of angle closure glaucoma and surgical intervention on the corneal endothelium. Cornea 1991;10:489–497.

99. Markowitz SN, Morin JD. The endothelium in primary angle-closure glaucoma. Am J Ophthalmol 1984;98:103–104.

100. Bigar F, Witmer R. Corneal endothelial changes in primary acute angle-closure glaucoma. Ophthalmology 1982;89:596–599.

101. Panda S, Jonas JB. Decreased photoreceptor count in human eyes with secondary angle-closure glaucoma. Invest Ophthalmol Vis Sci 1992;33:2532–2536.

102. Jonas JB, Konigsreuther KA, Naumann GO. Optic disc histomorphometry in normal eyes and eyes with secondary angle-closure glaucoma. II. Parapapillary region. Graefes Arch Clin Exp Ophthalmol 1992;230:134–139.

103. Kendell KR, Quigley HA, Kerrigan LA, Pease ME, Quigley EN. Primary open-angle glaucoma is not associated with photoreceptor loss. Invest Ophthalmol Vis Sci 1995;36:200–205.

104. Kubota T, Jonas JB, Naumann GO. Decreased choroidal thickness in eyes with secondary angle closure glaucoma: an aetiological factor for deep retinal changes in glaucoma? Br J Ophthalmol 1993;77:430–432.

105. Jonas JB, Konigsreuther KA, Naumann GO. Optic disc histomorphometry in normal eyes and eyes with secondary angle-closure glaucoma. I. Intrapapillary region. Graefes Arch Clin Exp Ophthalmol 1992;230:129–133.

106. Am Acad Ophthalmol. Laser peripheral iridotomy for pupillary-block glaucoma. Ophthalmology 1994;101:1749–1758.

107. Lowe RF. Acute angle-closure glaucoma, the second eye: an analysis of 200 cases. Br J Ophthalmol 1962;46:641–650.

108. Wishart PK, Batterbury M. Ocular hypertension: correlation of anterior chamber angle width and risk of progression to glaucoma. Eye 1992;6:248–256.

109. Schwartz GF, Steinmann WC, Spaeth GL, Wilson RP. Surgical and medical management of patients with narrow anterior chamber angles: comparative results. Ophthalmic Surg 1992;23:108–112.

110. Wilensky JT, Kaufman PL, et al. Follow-up of angle-closure glaucoma suspects. Am J Ophthalmol 1993;115:338–346.

111. Aminlari A, Sassani JW. Simultaneous bilateral malignant glaucoma following laser iridotomy. Graefes Arch Clin Exp Ophthalmol 1993;231:12–14.

112. Rodrigues MM, Spaeth GL, Moster M, Thomas G, Hackett J. Histopathology of neodymium: YAG laser iridectomy in humans. Ophthalmology 1985;92:1696–1700.

113. Tetsumoto K, Kuchle M, Naumann GO. Late histopathological findings of neodymium: YAG laser iridotomies in humans. Arch Ophthalmol 1992;110:1119–1123.

114. Wand M. Argon laser gonioplasty for synechial angle closure. Arch Ophthalmol 1992;110:363–367.

115. Weiss HS, Shingleton BJ, Goode SM, Bellows AR, Richter CU. Argon laser gonioplasty in the treatment of angle-closure glaucoma. Am J Ophthalmol 1992;114:14–18.

116. Lim AS, et al. Laser iridoplasty in the treatment of severe acute angle closure glaucoma. Int Ophthalmol 1993;17:33–36.

117. Sassani JW, et al. Histopathology of argon laser peripheral iridoplasty. Ophthalmic Surg 1993;24:740–745.

118. Shiose Y. Intraocular pressure: new perspectives. Surv Ophthalmol 1990;34:413–435.

119. Shiose Y, et al. Epidemiology of glaucoma in Japan—a nationwide glaucoma survey. Jpn J Ophthalmol 1991;35:133–155.

120. Dielemans I, Vingerling JR, et al. The prevalence of primary open-angle glaucoma in a population-based study in The Netherlands: the Rotterdam study. Ophthalmology 1994;101:1851–1855.

121. Martin MJ, Sommer A, Gold EB, Diamond EL. Race and primary open-angle glaucoma. Am J Ophthalmol 1985;99:383–387.

122. Sommer A, Tielsch JM, Katz J, et al. Racial differences in the cause-specific prevalence of blindness in east Baltimore. N Engl J Med 1991;325:1412–1417.

123. Wallace J, Lovell HG. Glaucoma and intraocular pressure in Jamaica. Am J Opthalmol 1969;67:93–100.

124. Sasovetz D. Open-angle glaucoma in blacks: a review. J Natl Med Assoc 1977;69:705–708.

125. Wilensky JT, Gandhi N, Pan T. Racial influences in open-angle glaucoma. Ann Ophthalmol 1978;10:1398–1402.

126. Coulehan JL, et al. Racial differences in intraocular tension and glaucoma surgery. Am J Epidemiol 1980;111:759–768.

127. Leske MC, Connell AM, Kehoe R. A pilot project of glaucoma in Barbados. Br J Ophthalmol 1989;73:365–369.

128. Mason RP, Kosoko O, Wilson MR, et al. National survey of the prevalence and risk factors of glaucoma in St. Lucia, West Indies. Part I. Prevalence findings. Ophthalmology 1989;96:1363–1368.

129. Leske MC, Connell AM, et al. The Barbados eye study: prevalence of open angle glaucoma. Arch Ophthalmol 1994;112:821–829.

130. Tielsch JM, Katz J, Sommer A, Quigley HA, Javitt JC. Family history and risk of primary open angle glaucoma: the Baltimore eye survey. Arch Ophthalmol 1994;112:69–73.

131. Shin DH, Becker B, Kolker AE. Family history in primary open-angle glaucoma. Arch Ophthalmol 1977;95:598–600.

132. Uhm KB, Shin DH. Positive family history of glaucoma is a risk factor for increased IOP rather than glaucomatous optic nerve damage (POAG vs OH vs normal control). Korean J Ophthalmol 1992;6:100–104.

133. Rosenthal AR, Perkins ES. Family studies in glaucoma. Br J Ophthalmol 1985;69:664–667.

134. Lichter PR. Genetic clues to glaucoma's secrets: the L Edward Jackson memorial lecture: part 2. Am J Ophthalmol 1994;117:706–727.

135. Richards JE, Lichter PR, Boehnke M, et al. Mapping of a gene for autosomal dominant juvenile-onset open-angle glaucoma to chromosome Iq. Am J Hum Genet 1994;54:62–70.

136. Morissette J, Cote G, Anctil JL, et al. A common gene for juvenile and adult-onset primary open-angle glaucomas confined on chromosome 1q. Am J Hum Genet 1995;56:1431–1442.

137. Fine BS, Yanoff M, Stone RA. A clinicopathologic study of four cases of primary open-angle glaucoma compared to normal eyes. Am J Ophthalmol 1981;91:88–105.

138. Grierson I. What is open angle glaucoma? Eye 1987;1:15–28.

139. Teng CC, Paton RT, Katzin HM. Primary degeneration in the vicinity of the chamber angle as an etiologic factor in wide-angle glaucoma. Am J Ophthalmol 1955;40:619–631.

140. Teng CC, Katzin HM, Chi HH. Primary degeneration in the vicinity of the chamber angle as an etiologic factor in wide-angle glaucoma: Part II. Am J Ophthalmol 1957;43.

141. Ashton N. Doyne memorial lecture: The exit pathway of the aqueous. Trans Ophthalmol Soc UK 1960;80:397–421.

142. Fine BS. Observations on the drainage angle in man and rhesus monkey: A concept of the pathogenesis of chronic simple glaucoma: A light and electron microscopic study. Invest Ophthalmol 1964;3:609–646.

143. Tripathi RC. Aqueous outflow pathway in normal and glaucomatous eyes. B J Ophthalmol 1972;56:157–174.

144. Alvarado JA, Yun AJ, Murphy CG. Juxtacanalicular tissue in primary open angle glaucoma and in nonglaucomatous normals. Arch Ophthalmol 1986;104:1517–1528.

145. Rohen JW. Why is intraocular pressure elevated in chronic simple glaucoma? Anatomical considerations. *Ophthalmology* 1983;90:758–765.

146. Tawara A, Varner HH, Hollyfield JG. Distribution and characterization of sulfated proteoglycans in the human trabecular tissue. *Invest Ophthalmol Vis Sci* 1989;30:2215–2231.

147. Yun AJ, Murphy CG, Polansky JR, Newsome DA, Alvarado JA. Proteins secreted by human trabecular cells: glucocorticoid and other effects. *Invest Ophthalmol Vis Sci* 1989;30:2012–2022.

148. Alvarado J, Murphy C, Juster R. Trabecular meshwork cellularity in primary open-angle glaucoma and nonglaucomatous normals. *Ophthalmology* 1984;91:564–579.

149. Johnson M, Shapiro A, et al. Modulation of outflow resistance by the pores of the inner wall endothelium. *Invest Ophthalmol Vis Sci* 1992;33:1670–1675.

150. Allingham RR, de Kater AW, Ethier CR, et al. The relationship between pore density and outflow facility in human eyes. *Invest Ophthalmol Vis Sci* 1992;33:1661–1669.

151. Tschumper RC, Johnson DH. Trabecular meshwork cellularity. *Invest Ophthalmol Vis Sci* 1990;31:1327–1331.

152. Maglio M, McMahon C, Hoskins D, Alvarado J. Potential artifacts in scanning electron microscopy of the trabecular meshwork in glaucoma. *Am J Ophthalmol* 1980;90:645–653.

153. Nuzzi R, Vercelli A, Finazzo C, et al. Conjunctiva and subconjunctival tissue in primary open-angle glaucoma after long-term topical treatment: an immunohistochemical and ultrastructural study. *Graefes Arch Clin Exp Ophthalmol* 1995;233:154–162.

154. Nelson LB, Maumenee IH. Ectopia lentis. *Surv Ophthalmol* 1982;27:143–160.

155. Goldberg MF. Clinical manifestations of ectopia lentis et pupillae in 16 patients. *Trans Am Ophthalmol Soc* 1988;86:158–177.

156. al-Salem M. Autosomal recessive ectopia Lentis in two Arab family pedigrees. *Ophthal Paediatr Genet* 1990;11:123–127.

157. Colley A, Lloyd IC, Ridgway A, Donnai D. Ectopia lentis et pupillae: the genetic aspects and differential diagnosis. *J Med Genet* 1991;28:791–794.

158. Bjerrum K, Kessing SV. Congenital ectopia lentis and secondary buphthalmos likely occurring as an autosomal recessive trait. *Acta Ophthalmol* 1991;69:630–634.

159. Meire FM. Hereditary ectopia lentis. A series of 10 cases of ectopia lentis et pupillae. *Bull Soc Belge Ophtalmol* 1991;241:25–36.

160. Reichel E, Wiggs JL, Mukai S, et al. Oxycephaly, bilateral ectopia lentis, and retinal detachment. *Ann Ophthalmol* 1992;24:97–98.

161. Verloes A, Hermia JP, Galand A, et al. Glaucoma-lens ectopia-microspherophakia-stiffness-shortness (GEMSS) syndrome: a dominant disease with manifestations of Weill-Marchesani syndromes. *Am J Med Genet* 1992;44:48–51.

162. Bawle E, Quigg MH. Ectopia lentis and aortic root dilatation in congenital contractual arachnodactyly. *Am J Med Genet* 1992;42:19–21.

163. Noble KG, Bass S, Sherman J. Ectopia lentis, chorioretinal dystrophy and myopia: a new autosomal recessive syndrome. *Doc Ophthalmol* 1993;83:97–102.

164. Lonnqvist L, Child A, Kainulainen K, Davidson R, Puhakka L, Peltonen L. A novel mutation of the fibrillin gene causing ectopia lentis. *Genomics* 1994;19:573–576.

165. Edwards MJ, Challinor CJ, Colley PW, et al. Clinical and linkage study of a large family with simple ectopia lentis linked to FBN1. *Am J Med Genet* 1994;53:65–71.

166. Cruysberg JR, Pinckers A. Ectopia lentis et pupillae syndrome in three generations. *Br J Ophthalmol* 1995;79:135–138.

167. Nelson LB, Spaeth GL, Nowinski TS, Margo CE, Jackson L. Aniridia: a review. *Surv Ophthalmol* 1984;28:621–642.

168. Nagata M, Takagi S, Yamasaki A, et al. Histopathological study of microspherophakia in the Weill-Marchesani syndrome. *Jpn J Ophthalmol* 1995;39:89–95.

169. Andrews RM, Bell RW, Jayamanne DG, Basanquet RC, Cottrell DG. "Roller-coaster glaucoma": an unusual complication of Marfan's syndrome [letter]. *Eye* 1994;8:358–360.

170. Regenbogen L, Ilie S, Elian I. Homocystinuria—a surgical and anaesthetic risk. *Metab Pediat Ophthalmol* 1980;4:209–211.

171. Favre JP, Becker F, Lorcerie B, et al. Vascular manifestations in homocystinuria. *Ann Vasc Surg* 1992;6:294–297.

172. Lieberman ER, Gomperts ED, Shaw KN, Landing BH, Donnell GN. Homocystinuria: clinical and pathologic review, with emphasis on thrombotic features, including pulmonary artery thrombosis. *Perspect Pediatr Pathol* 1993;17:125–147.

173. Mandel H, Brenner B, Berant M, et al. Coexistence of hereditary homocystinuria and factor V Leiden—effect on thrombosis. *N Engl J Med* 1996;334:763–768.

174. Lowe S, Johnson DA, Tobias JD. Anesthetic implications of the child with homocystinuria. *J Clin Anesth* 1994;6:142–144.

175. Kielty CM, Davies SJ, Phillips JE, et al. Marfan syndrome: fibrillin expression and microfibrillar abnormalities in a family with predominant ocular defects. *J Med Genet* 1995;32:1–6.

176. Tsipouras P, Del Mastro R, Sarfarazi M, et al. Genetic linkage of the Marfan syndrome, ectopia lentis, and congenital contractual arachnodactyly to the fibrillin genes on chromosomes 15 and 5: the international Marfan syndrome collaborative study. *N Engl J Med* 1992;326:905–909.

177. Kainulainen K, Karttunen L, Puhakka L, Sakai L, Peltonen L. Mutations in the fibrillin gene responsible for dominant ectopia lentis and neonatal Marfan syndrome. *Nat Genet* 1994;6:64–69.

178. Burke JP, M OK, Bowell R, et al. Ocular complications in homocystinuria—early and late treated. *Br J Ophthalmol* 1989;73:427–431.

179. Reese PD, Weingeist TA. Pars plana management of ectopia lentis in children. *Arch Ophthalmol* 1987;105:1202–1204.

180. Syrdalen P. Pars plana technique for removal of congenital subluxated lenses in young patients. *Acta Ophthalmol* 1987;65:585–588.

181. Behki R, Noel LP, et al. Limbal lensectomy in the management of ectopia lentis in children. *Arch Ophthalmol* 1990;108:809–811.

182. Haymet BT. Removal of a dislocated hypermature lens from the posterior viteous. *Austral N Zeal J Ophthalmol* 1990;18:103–106.

183. Adank AM, Hennekes R. Phacoemulsification of the subluxated or atopic lens. *Bull Soc Belge Ophtalmol* 1993;249:33–39.

184. Speedwell L, Russell-Eggitt I. Improvement in visual acuity in children with ectopia lentis. *J Pediatr Ophthalmol Strabismus* 1995;32:94–97.

185. John T, Sassani JW, Eagle RCJ. The myofibroblastic component of rubeosis iridis. *Ophthalmology* 1983;90:721–728.

186. Brown GC, Magargal LE, Schachat A, Shah H. Neovascular glaucoma: etiologic considerations. *Ophthalmology* 1984;91:315–320.

187. Campbell DG, Shields MB, Smith TR. The corneal endothelium and the spectrum of essential iris atrophy. *Am J Ophthalmol* 1978;87:317–324.

188. Shields MB, Campbell DG, Simmons RJ. The essential iris atrophies. *Am J Ophthalmol* 1978;85:749–759.

189. Eagle RJ, Font RL, Yanoff M, et al. Proliferative endotheliopathy with iris abnormalities. The iridocorneal endothelial syndrome. *Arch Ophthalmol* 1979;97:2104–2111.

190. Shields MB. Proliferative endotheliopathy with iris abnormalities: the iridocorneal endothelial syndrome. *Arch Ophthalmol* 1979;97:2104–2111.

191. Shields MB. Progressive essential iris atrophy, Chandler's syndrome, and the iris nevus (Cogan-Reese) syndrome: a spectrum of disease. *Surv Ophthalmol* 1979;24:3–20.

192. Quigley HA, Forster RF. Histopathology of cornea and iris in Chandler's syndrome. *Arch Ophthalmol* 1978;96:1878–1882.

193. Shields MB, McCracken JS, et al. Corneal edema in essential iris atrophy. *Ophthalmology* 1979;86:1533–1550.

194. Eagle RJ, Font RL, Yanoff M, Fine BS. The iris naevus (Cogan-Reese) syndrome: light and electron microscopic observations. *Br J Ophthalmol* 1980;64:446–452.

195. Setala K, Vannas A. Corneal endothelial cells in essential iris atrophy. A specular microscopic study. *Acta Ophthalmol* 1975;57:1020–1029.

196. Hirst LW, Quigley HA, Stark WJ, Shields NB. Specular microscopy of irido-corneal endothelial syndrome. *Aust J Ophthalmol* 1980;8:139–146.

197. Wilson MC, Shields MB. A comparison of the clinical variations of the iridocorneal endothelial syndrome. *Arch Ophthalmol* 1989;107:1465–1468.

198. Alvarado JA, Murphy CG, Maglio M, Hetherington J. Pathogenesis of Chandler's syndrome, essential iris atrophy and the Cogan-Reese syndrome. I. Alterations of the corneal endothelium. *Invest Ophthalmol Vis Sci* 1986;27:853–872.

199. Alvarado JA, Murphy CG, Juster RP, Hetherington J. Pathogenesis

of Chandler's syndrome, essential iris atrophy and the Cogan-Reese syndrome. II. Estimated age at disease onset. *Invest Ophthalmol Vis Sci* 1986;27:873–882.

200. Rodrigues MM, Streeten BW, Spaeth GL. Chandler's syndrome as a variant of essential iris atrophy. A clinicopathologic study. *Arch Ophthalmol* 1978;96:643–652.

201. Hetherington J Jr. The spectrum of Chandler's syndrome. *Ophthalmology* 1978;85:240–244.

202. Lichter PR. The spectrum of Chandler's syndrome: an often overlooked cause of unilateral glaucoma. *Ophthalmology* 1978;85:245–251.

203. Richardson TM. Corneal decompensation in Chandler's syndrome: a scanning and transmission electron microscopic study. *Arch Ophthalmol* 1979;97:2112–2119.

204. Patel A, Kenyon KR, Hirst LW, et al. Clinicopathologic features of Chandler's syndrome. *Surv Ophthalmol* 1983;27:327–344.

205. Denis P, Baudrimont M, Nordmann JP, et al. Immunohistochemical and ultrastructural study of the cornea in Chandler's syndrome: report of a case. *Ophthalmologica* 1994;208:289–293.

206. Hirst LW, Green WR, Luckenbach M, de la Cruz Z, Stark WJ. Epithelial characteristics of the endothelium in Chandler's syndrome. *Invest Ophthalmol Vis Sci* 1983;24:603–611.

207. Rodrigues MM, Phelps CD, Krachmer JH, et al. Glaucoma due to endothelialization of the anterior chamber angle: a comparison of posterior polymorphous dystrophy of the cornea and Chandler's syndrome. *Arch Ophthalmol* 1980;98:688–696.

208. Buxton JN, Lash RS. Results of penetrating keratoplasty in the iridocorneal endothelial syndrome. *Am J Ophthalmol* 1984;98:297–301.

209. Wittebol-Post D, van Bijsterveld OP. Essential progressive iris atrophy: report of two cases. *Ophthalmologica* 1979;178:303–310.

210. Scheie HG, Yanoff M, Kellogg WT. Essential iris atrophy: report of a case. *Arch Ophthalmol* 1976;94:1315–1320.

211. Kaiser-Kupfer M, Kuwabara T, Kupfer C. Progressive bilateral essential iris atrophy. *Am J Ophthalmol* 1977;83:340–346.

212. Kupfer C, Kaiser-Kupfer M, Kuwabara T. Progressive bilateral essential iris atrophy. *Trans Am Ophthalmological Soc* 1977;74:341–356.

213. Shields JA, Sanborn GE, Augsburger JJ. The differential diagnosis of malignant melanoma of the iris: a clinical study of 200 patients. *Ophthalmology* 1983;90:716–720.

214. Rodrigues MM, Jester JV, Richards R, Rajagopalan S, Stevens G. Essential iris atrophy: a clinical, immunohistologic, and electron microscopic study in an enucleated eye. *Ophthalmology* 1988;95:69–78.

215. Eagle RC Jr., Shields JA. Iridocorneal endothelial syndrome with contralateral guttate endothelial dystrophy: a light and electron microscopic study. *Ophthalmology* 1987;94:862–870.

216. Blair SD, Seabrooks D, Shields WJ, Pillai S, Cavanagh HD. Bilateral progressive essential iris atrophy and keratoconus with coincident features of posterior polymorphous dystrophy: a case report and proposed pathogenesis. *Cornea* 1992;11:255–261.

217. DeBroff BM, Thoft RA. Surgical results of penetrating keratoplasty in essential iris atrophy. *J Refract Corneal Surg* 1994;10:428–432.

218. Kidd M, Hetherington J, Magee S. Surgical results in iridocorneal endothelial syndrome. *Arch Ophthalmol* 1988;106:199–201.

219. Yanoff M, Scheie HG, et al. Endothelialization of filtering bleb in iris nevus syndrome. *Arch Ophthalmol* 1976;94:1933–1936.

220. Scheie HG, Yanoff M. Iris nevus (Cogan-Reese) syndrome. A cause of unilateral glaucoma. *Arch Ophthalmol* 1975;93:963–970.

221. Khalil MK, Finlayson MH. Electron microscopy in iris nevus syndrome. *Can J Ophthalmol* 1980;15:44–48.

222. Terry TL, Chisholm JF, Schonberg AL. Studies on surface-epithelium invasion of the anterior segment of the eye. *Am J Ophthalmol* 1939;22:1083–1110.

223. Weiner MJ, Trentacoste J, et al. Epithelial downgrowth: a 30-year clinicopathological review. *Br J Ophthalmol* 1989;73:6–11.

224. Sidrys LA, Demong T. Epithelial downgrowth after penetrating keratoplasty. *Can J Ophthalmol* 1982;17:29–31.

225. Soong HK, Meyer RF, Wolter JR. Fistula excision and peripheral grafts in the treatment of persistent limbal wound leaks. *Ophthalmology* 1988;95:31–36.

226. Schaffer AR, Nalbandian RM, et al. Epithelial downgrowth following wound dehiscence after extracapsular cataract extraction and posterior chamber lens implantation: surgical management. *J Cataract Refract Surg* 1989;15:437–441.

227. Avni I, Blumenthal M, Belkin M. Epithelial invasion of the anterior chamber following repeated keratoplasty. *Metab Pediatr System Ophthalmol* 1982;6:337–341.

228. McAllister IL, Meyers SM, Meisler DM, et al. Epithelial downgrowth. *Ophthalmic Surg* 1988;19:713–714.

229. Anseth A, Dohlman CH, Albert DM. Epithelial downgrowth—fistula repair and keratoplasty. *J Refract Corneal Surg* 1991;7:23–27.

230. McDonnell JM, Liggett PE, McDonnell PJ. Traction retinal detachment due to preretinal proliferation of surface epithelium. *Retina* 1992;12:248–250.

231. Maumenee AE, Paton D, et al. Review of 40 histologically proven cases of epithelial downgrowth following cataract extraction and suggested surgical management. *Am J Ophthalmol* 1970;69:598–603.

232. Brown SI. Treatment of advanced epithelial downgrowth. *Trans Am Acad Ophthalmol Otolaryngol* 1973;77:OP618–22.

233. Friedman AH. Radical anterior segment surgery for epithelial invasion of the anterior chamber: report of three cases. *Trans Am Acad Ophthalmol Otolaryng* 1977;83:216–223.

234. Brown SI. Results of excision of advanced epithelial downgrowth. *Ophthalmology* 1979;86:321–331.

235. Burris TE, Nordquist RE, Rowsey JJ. Cryopexy of epithelial downgrowth. *Cornea* 1986;5:173–180.

236. Weinreb RN. Adjusting the dose of 5-fluorouracil after filtration surgery to minimize side effects. *Ophthalmology* 1987;94:564–570.

237. Loane ME, Weinreb RN. Glaucoma secondary to epithelial downgrowth and 5-fluorouracil. *Ophthalmic Surg* 1990;21:704–706.

238. Costa VP, Katz LJ, Cohen EJ, Raber IM. Glaucoma associated with epithelial downgrowth controlled with Molteno tube shunts. *Ophthalmic Surg* 1992;23:797–800.

239. Orlin SE, Raber IM, Laibson PR, Shields CL, Brucker AJ. Epithelial downgrowth following the removal of iris inclusion cysts. *Ophthalmic Surg* 1991;22:330–335.

240. Feder RS, Krachmer JH. The diagnosis of epithelial downgrowth after keratoplasty. *Am J Ophthalmol* 1985;99:697–703.

241. Smith RE, Parrett C. Specular microscopy of epithelial downgrowth. *Arch Ophthalmol* 1978;96:1222–1224.

242. Holliday JN, Buller CR, Bourne WM. Specular microscopy and fluorophotometry in the diagnosis of epithelial downgrowth after a sutureless cataract operation [letter]. *Am J Ophthalmol* 1993;116:238–240.

243. Cameron JD, Flaxman BA, Yanoff M. In vitro studies of corneal wound healing: epithelial-endothelial interactions. *Invest Ophthalmol* 1974;13:575–579.

244. Yanoff M, Cameron JD. Human cornea organ cultures: epithelial-endothelial interactions. *Invest Ophthalmol Vis Sci* 1977;16:269–273.

245. Iwamoto T, Srinivasan BD, DeVoe AG. Electron microscopy of epithelial downgrowth. *Ann Ophthalmol* 1977;9:1095–1110.

246. Yamaguchi T, Polack FM, Valenti J. Electron microscopic study of epithelial downgrowth after penetrating keratoplasty. *Br J Ophthalmol* 1981;65:374–382.

247. Sassani JW, John T, Cameron JD, Yanoff M, Eagle RCJ. Electron microscopic study of corneal epithelial-endothelial interactions in organ culture. *Ophthalmology* 1984;91:553–557.

248. Burris TE, Rowsey JJ, Nordquist RE. Model of epithelial downgrowth: II. Scanning and transmission electron microscopy of corneal epithelialization. *Cornea* 1984;3:141–151.

249. Sun WR, Shi ZR, Ju MC. Histopathological observation of phacolytic glaucoma: report of 5 cases. *Chin Med J* 1986;99:931–934.

250. Burris TE, Nordquist RE, Rowsey JJ. Model of epithelial downgrowth: III. Scanning and transmission electron microscopy of iris epithelialization. *Cornea* 1985;4:249–255.

251. Hales RH, Spencer WH. Unsuccessful penetrating keratoplasties. Correlation of clinical and histologic findings. *Arch Ophthalmol* 1963;70:805–810.

252. Kurz GH, D'Amico RA. Histopathology of corneal graft failures. *Am J Ophthalmol* 1968;66:184–199.

253. Kremer I, Rapuano CJ, et al. Retrocorneal fibrous membranes in failed corneal grafts. *Am J Ophthalmol* 1993;115:478–483.

254. Friedman AH, Henkind P. Corneal stromal overgrowth after cataract extraction. *Br J Ophthalmol* 1970;54:528–534.

255. Swan KC. Fibroblastic ingrowth following cataract surgery. *Arch Ophthalmol* 1973;89:445–449.

256. Allen JC. Epithelial and stromal ingrowths. *Am J Ophthalmol* 1968;65:179–182.

257. Snip RC, Kenyon KR, et al. Retrocorneal fibrous membrane in the vitreous touch syndrome. *Am J Ophthalmol* 1975;79:233–244.

258 Michels RG, Kenyon KR, Maumence AE. Retrocorneal fibrous membrane. *Invest Ophthalmol* 1972;11:822–831.

259. Colosi NJ, Yanoff M. Reactive corneal endothelialization. *Am J Ophthalmol* 1977;83:219–224.

260. Raitta C, Lehto I, et al. A randomized, prospective study on the use of sodium hyaluronate (Healon) in trabeculectomy. *Ophthal Surg* 1994;25:536–539.

261. Smith MF, Doyle JW, Sherwood MB. Comparison of the Baerveldt glaucoma implant with the double-plate Molteno drainage implant. *Arch Ophthalmol* 1995;113:444–447.

262. Freedman J, Rubin B. Molteno implants as a treatment for refractory glaucoma in black patients [see comments]. *Arch Ophthalmol* 1991;109:1417–1420.

263. Perkins TW, Cardakli UF, et al. Adjunctive mitomycin C in Molteno implant surgery. *Ophthalmology* 1995;102:91–97.

264. Susanna R Jr, Nicolela MT, Takahashi WY. Mitomycin C as adjunctive therapy with glaucoma implant surgery. *Ophthalmic Surgery* 1994;25:458–462.

265. Chihara E, Nishida A, Kodo M, et al. Trabeculotomy ab externo: an alternative treatment in adult patients with primary open-angle glaucoma [Review]. *Ophthalmic Surg* 1993;24:735–739.

266. Tomlinson CP, Belcher CD, et al. Management of leaking filtration blebs. *Ann Ophthalmol* 1987;19:405–408, 411.

267. Lockie P. Ciliary-block glaucoma treated by posterior capsulotomy. *Austral N Zeal J Ophthalmol* 1987;15:207–209.

268. Tomey KF, Senft SH, et al. Aqueous misdirection and flat chamber after posterior chamber implants with and without trabeculectomy. *Arch Ophthalmol* 1987;105:770–773.

269. Epstein DL, Steinert RF, Puliafito CA. Neodymium-YAG laser therapy to the anterior hyaloid in aphakic malignant (ciliovitreal block) glaucoma. *Am J Ophthalmol* 1984;98:137–143.

270. Weber PA, Henry MA, et al. Argon laser treament of the ciliary processes in aphakic glaucoma with flat anterior chamber. *Am J Ophthalmol* 1984;97:82–85.

271. Wada Y, Nakatsu A, Kondo T. Long-term results of trabeculotomy ab externo. *Ophthalmic Surg* 1994;25:317–320.

272. Kolker AE, Kass MA, Rait JL. Trabeculectomy with releasable sutures. *Arch Ophthalmol* 1994;112:62–66.

273. Kolker AE, Kass MA, Rait JL. Trabeculectomy with releasable sutures. *Trans Am Ophthalmol Soc* 1993;91:131–145.

274. Blok MD, Greve EL, Dunnebier EA, Muradin F, Kijlstra A. Scleral flap sutures and the development of shallow or flat anterior chamber after trabeculectomy. *Ophthalmic Surgery* 1993;24:309–313.

275. Raitta C, Setala K. Trabeculectomy with the use of sodium hyaluronate. A prospective study. *Acta Ophthalmol* 1986;64:407–413.

276. Luntz MH, Berlin MS. Combined trabeculectomy and cataract extraction. Advantages of a modified technique and review of current literature. *Trans Ophthalmol Soc UK* 1980;100:533–541.

277. Blondeau P, Phelps CD. Trabeculectomy vs thermosclerostomy. A randomized prospective clinical trial. *Arch Ophthalmol* 1981;99:810–816.

278. Fourman S. Management of cornea-lens touch after filtering surgery for glaucoma. *Ophthalmology* 1990;97:424–428.

279. Veldman E, Greve EL. Glaucoma filtering surgery, a retrospective study of 300 operations. *Doc Ophthalmol* 1987;67:151–170.

280. Koerner FH. Anterior pars plana vitrectomy in ciliary and iris block glaucoma. *Albrecht Von Graefes Archiv Klin Exper Ophthalmol* 1980;214:119–127.

281. Burney EN, Quigley HA, Robin AL. Hypotony and choroidal detachment as late complications of trabeculectomy. *Am J Ophthalmol* 1987;103:685–688.

282. Shields JA. Primary cysts of the iris. *Trans Am Ophthalmol Soc* 1981;79:771–809.

283. Chandler PA, Braconier HE. Spontaneous intra-epithelial cysts of the iris and ciliary body with glaucoma. *Am J Ophthalmol* 1958;45:64–74.

284. Farmer SG, Kalina RE. Epithelial implantation cyst of the iris. *Ophthalmology* 1981;88:1286–1289.

285. Bron AJ, Wilson CB, Hill AR. Laser treatment of primary ring-shaped epithelial iris cyst. *Br J Ophthalmol* 1984;68:859–865.

286. Merritt JC, Kraybill EN. Retrolental fibroplasia: a five-year experience in a tertiary perinatal center. *Ann Ophthalmol* 1986;18:65–67.

287. Gilbert CE, Canovas R, Hagan M, Rao S, Foster A. Causes of childhood blindness: results from west Africa, south India and Chile. *Eye* 1993;7:184–188.

288. Hartnett ME, Gilbert MM, Hirose T, et al. Glaucoma as a cause of poor vision in severe retinopathy of prematurity. *Graefes Arch Clin Exp Ophthalmol* 1993;231:433–438.

289. Hartnett ME, Gilbert MM, Richardson TM, Krug JH Jr, Hirose T. Anterior segment evaluation of infants with retinopathy of prematurity. *Ophthalmology* 1990;97:122–130.

290. Halperin LS, Schoch LH. Angle closure glaucoma after scleral buckling for retinopathy of prematurity: case report. *Arch Ophthalmol* 1988;106:453.

291. Ueda N, Ogino N. Angle-closure glaucoma with pupillary block mechanism in cicatricial retinopathy of prematurity. *Ophthalmologica* 1988;196:15–18.

292. Hittner HM, Rhodes LM, McPherson AR. Anterior segment abnormalities in cicatricial retinopathy of prematurity. *Ophthalmology* 1979;86:803–816.

293. Smith J, Shivitz I. Angle-closure glaucoma in adults with cicatricial retinopathy of prematurity. *Arch Ophthalmol* 1984;102:371–372.

294. Kushner BJ. Ciliary block glaucoma in retinopathy of prematurity. *Arch Ophthalmol* 1982;100:1078.

295. Haddad R, Font RL, Reeser F. Persistent hyperplastic primary vitreous: a clinicopathologic study of 62 cases and review of the literature. *Surv Ophthalmol* 1978;23:123–134.

296. Engel HM, Green WR, Michels RG, Rice TA, Erozan YS. Diagnostic vitrectomy. *Retina* 1981;1:121–149.

297. Pollard ZF. Results of treatment of persistent hyperplastic primary vitreous. *Ophthalmic Surg* 1991;22:48–52.

298. Weseley AC, Freeman WR. Iridoschisis and the corneal endothelium. *Ann Ophthalmol* 1983;15:955–959, 963–964.

299. Eiferman RA, Law M, Lane L. Iridoschisis and keratoconus. *Cornea* 1994;13:78–79.

300. Hersh PS. Iridoschisis following penetrating keratoplasty for keratoconus [letter; comment]. *Cornea* 1994;13:545–546.

301. Salvador F, Linares F, Merita I, Amen M. Unilateral iridoschisis associated with syphilitic interstitial keratitis and glaucoma. *Ann Ophthalmol* 1993;25:328–329.

302. Foss AJ, et al. Interstitial keratitis and iridoschisis in congenital syphilis. *J Clin Neuro-Ophthalmol* 1992;12:167–170.

303. Summers CG, Doughman DJ, et al. Juvenile iridoschisis and mircophthalmos. *Am J Ophthalmol* 1985;100:437–439.

304. Johnson MR, Bachynski BN. Juvenile iridoschisis and microphthalmos [letter]. *Am J Ophthalmol* 1986;101:742–744.

305. Mansour AM. A family with iridoschisis, narrow anterior chamber angle, and presenile cataract. *Ophthalmic Paediat Genet* 1986;7:145–149.

306. Rodrigues MC, Spaeth GL, et al. Iridoschisis associated with glaucoma and bullous keratopathy. *Am J Ophthalmol* 1983;95:73–81.

307. DeRespinis PA, Caputo AR, et al. A survey of severe eye injuries in children. *Am J Dis Child* 1989;143:711–716.

308. Maltzman BA, Pruzon H, Mund ML. A survey of ocular trauma. *Surv Ophthalmol* 1976;21:285–290.

309. Schein OD, Hibberd PL, Shingleton BJ, et al. The spectrum and burden of ocular injury. *Ophthalmology* 1988;95:300–305.

310. Littlewood KR. Blunt ocular trauma and hyphaema. *Australian Journal of Ophthalmology* 1982;10:263–266.

311. Agapitos PJ, Noel LP, Clarke WN. Traumatic hyphema in children. *Ophthalmology* 1987;94:1238–1241.

312. Kelman JP, Dobbie JG, Constantaras AA. Recurrent traumatic hyphema: a sequel of injury to the Schlemm canal. *Arch Ophthalmol* 1977;95:484–485.

313. Volpe NJ, Larrison WI, et al. Secondary hemorrhage in traumatic hyphema. *Am J Ophthalmol* 1991;112:507–513.

314. Fong LP. Secondary hemorrhage in traumatic hyphema: predictive factors for selective prophylaxis. *Ophthalmology* 1994;101:1583.

315. Kennedy RH, Brubaker RF. Traumatic hyphema in a defined population. *Am J Ophthalmol* 1988;106:123–130.

316. Witteman GJ, Brubaker SJ, et al. The incidence of rebleeding in traumatic hyphema. *Ann Ophthalmol* 1985;17:525–529.

317. Crouch ER, Jr., Frenkel M. Aminocaproic acid in the treatment of traumatic hyphema. *Am J Ophthalmol* 1976;81:355–360.

318. McGetrick JJ, Jampol LM, et al. Aminocaproic acid decreases secondary hemorrhage after traumatic hyphema. *Arch Ophthalmol* 1983;101:1031–1033.

319. Cassel GH, Jeffers JB, Jaeger EA. Wills Eye Hospital traumatic hyphema study. *Ophthalmic Surg* 1985;16:441–443.

320. Palmer DJ, Goldberg MF, et al. A comparison of two dose regimens of epsilon aminocaproic acid in the prevention and management of secondary traumatic hyphemas. *Ophthalmology* 1986;93:102–108.

321. Spoor TC, Kwitko GM, JM OG, Ramocki JM. Traumatic hyphema in an urban population. *Am J Ophthalmol* 1990;109:23–27.

322. Lawrence T, Wilison D, et al. The incidence of secondary hemorrhage after traumatic hyphema. *Ann Ophthalmol* 1990;22:276–278.

323. Crouch ER Jr, Williams PB. Secondary hemorrhage in traumatic hyphema [letter; comment]. *Am J Ophthalmol* 1992;113:344–346.

324. Ng CS, Strong NP, Sparrow JM, Rosenthal AR. Factors related to the incidence of secondary haemorrhage in 462 patients with traumatic hyphema. *Eye* 1992;6:308–312.

325. Farber MD, Fiscella R, Goldberg MF. Aminocaproic acid versus prednisone for the treatment of traumatic hyphema: a randomized clinical trial. *Ophthalmology* 1991;98:279–286.

326. Romano PE, Hope GM. The effect of age and ethnic background on the natural rebleed rate in untreated traumatic hyphema in children. *Metab Pediat Sys Ophthalmol* 1990;13:26–31.

327. Crawford JS, Lewandowski RL, Chan W. The effect of aspirin on rebleeding in traumatic hyphema. *Am J Ophthalmol* 1975;80:543–545.

328. Gorn RA. The detrimental effect of aspirin on hyphema rebleed. *Ann Ophthalmol* 1979;11:351–355.

329. Ganley JP, Geiger JM, Clement JR, Rigby PG, Levy GJ. Aspirin and recurrent hyphema after blunt ocular trauma. *Am J Ophthalmol* 1983;96:797–801.

330. Marcus M, Biedner B, et al. Aspirin and secondary bleeding after traumatic hyphema. *Ann Ophthalmol* 1988;20:157–158.

331. Slingsby JG, Forstot SL. Effect of blunt trauma on the corneal endothelium. *Arch Ophthalmol* 1981;99:1041–1043.

332. Marcus DM, Albert DM. Recognizing child abuse. *Arch Ophthalmol* 1992;110:766–767.

333. Tseng SS, Keys MP. Battered child syndrome simulating congenital glaucoma. *Arch Ophthalmol* 1976;94:839–840.

334. Zimmerman LE. Ocular lesions of juvenile xanthogranuloma: nevoxanthoedothelioma. *Am J Ophthalmol* 1965;60:1011–1035.

335. Yoshizumi MO, Thomas JV, Smith TR. Glaucoma-inducing mechanisms in eyes with retinoblastoma. *Arch Ophthalmol* 1978;96:105–110.

336. Margo CE, Zimmerman LE. Retinoblastoma: the accuracy of clinical diagnosis in childern treated by enucleation. *J Pediatr Ophthalmol Strabismus* 1983;20:227–229.

337. Mansour AM, Greenwald MJ, et al. Diffuse infiltrating retinoblastoma. *J Pediatr Ophthalmol Strabismus* 1989;26:152–154.

338. Canning CR, McCartney AC, Hungerford J. Medulloepithelioma (diktyoma). *Br J Ophthalmol* 1988;72:764–767.

339. Swan KC. Late hyphema due to wound vascularization. *Trans Am Acad Ophthalmol Otolaryngol* 1976;81:OP138–OP144.

340. Campbell DG. Ghost cell glaucoma following trauma. *Ophthalmology* 1981;88:1151–1158.

341. Greenwald MJ, Crowley TM. Sickle cell hyphema with secondary glaucoma in a non-black patient. *Ophthalmic Surg* 1985;16:170.

342. Kobayashi H, Honda Y. Intraocular hemorrhage in a patient with hemophilia. *Metab Ophthalmol* 1984;8:27–30.

343. Friedman AH, Halpern BL, et al. Transient open-angle glaucoma associated with sickle cell trait: report of 4 cases. *Br J Ophthalmol* 1979;63:832–836.

344. Wax MB, Ridley ME, et al. Reversal of retinal and optic disc ischemia in a patient with sickle cell trait and glaucoma secondary to traumatic hyphema. *Ophthalmology* 1982;89:845–851.

345. Caprioli J, Sears ML. The histopathology of black ball hyphema: a report of two cases. *Ophthalmic Surg* 1984;15:491–495.

346. McDonnell PJ, Gritz DC, McDonnell JM, Zarbin MA. Fluorescence of blood-stained cornea. *Cornea* 1991;10:445–449.

347. Beyer TL, Hirst LW. Corneal blood staining at low pressures. *Arch Ophthalmol* 1985;103:654–655.

348. Farrar SM, Shields MB. Current concepts in pigmentary glaucoma. *Surv Ophthalmol* 1993;37:233–252.

349. Farrar SM, Shields MB, Miller KN, Stoup CM. Risk factors for the development and severity of glaucoma in the pigment dispersion syndrome. *Am J Ophthalmol* 1989;108:223–229.

350. Becker B, Shin DH, Cooper DG, Kass MA. The pigment dispersion syndrome. *Am J Ophthalmol* 1977;83:161–166.

351. Semple HC, Ball SF. Pigmentary glaucoma in the black population. *Am J Ophthalmol* 1990;109:518–522.

352. Samples JR, Van Buskirk EM. Pigmentary glaucoma associated with posterior chamber intraocular lenses. *Am J Ophthalmol* 1985;100:385–388.

353. Smith JP. Pigmentary open-angle glaucoma secondary to posterior chamber intraocular lens implantation and erosion of the iris pigment epithelium. *J Am Intra-Ocul Implant Soc* 1985;11:174–176.

354. Mastropasqua L, Lobefalo L, Gallenga PE. Iris chafing in pseudophakia. *Doc Ophthalmol* 1994;87:139–144.

355. Layden WE, Ritch R, King DG, Teekhasaenee C. Combined exfoliation and pigment dispersion syndrome. *Am J Ophthalmol* 1990;109:530–534.

356. Lagreze WD, Funk J. Iridotomy in the treatment of pigmentary glaucoma: documentation with high resolution ultrasound. *Ger J Ophthalmol* 1995;4:162–166.

357. Pavlin CJ, Macken P, Trope G, Feldman F, Harasiewicz K, Foster FS. Ultrasound biomicroscopic features of pigmentary glaucoma. *Can J Ophthalmol* 1994;29:187–192.

358. Pavlin CJ. Ultrasound biomicroscopy in pigment dispersion syndrome [letter; comment]. *Ophthalmology* 1994;101:1475–1477.

359. Potash SD, Tello C, et al. Ultrasound biomicroscopy in pigment dispersion syndrome. *Ophthalmology* 1994;101:332–339.

360. Jensen PK, Nissen O, Kessing SV. Exercise and reversed pupillary block in pigmentary glaucoma. *Am J Ophthalmol* 1995;120:110–112.

361. Haynes WL, Johnson AT, Alward WL. Effects of jogging exercise on patients with the pigmentary dispersion syndrome and pigmentary glaucoma. *Ophthalmology* 1992;99:1096–1103.

362. Ritch R, Chaiwat T, Harbin TS Jr. Asymmetric pigmentary glaucoma resulting from cataract formation. *Am J Ophthalmol* 1992;114:484–488.

363. Davidson JA, Brubaker RF, Ilstrup DM. Dimensions of the anterior chamber in pigment dispersion syndrome. *Arch Ophthalmol* 1983;101:81–83.

364. Richter CU, Richardson TM, Grant WM. Pigmentary dispersion syndrome and pigmentary glaucoma. A prospective study of the natural history. *Arch Ophthalmol* 1986;104:211–215.

365. Epstein DL, Freddo TF, Anderson PJ, et al. Experimental obstruction to aqueous outflow by pigment particles in living monkeys. *Invest Ophthalmol Vis Sci* 1986;27:387–395.

366. Murphy CG, Johnson M, Alvarado JA. Juxtacanalicular tissue in pigmentary and primary open angle glaucoma: the hydrodynamic role of pigment and other constituents. *Arch Ophthalmol* 1992;110:1779–1785.

367. Johnson DH. Does pigmentation affect the trabecular meshwork? *Arch Ophthalmol* 1989;107:250–254.

368. Alvarado JA, Murphy CG. Outflow obstruction in pigmentary and primary open angle glaucoma. *Arch Ophthalmol* 1992;110:1769.

369. Kampik A, Green WR, Quigley HA, Pierce LH. Scanning and transmission electron microscopic studies of two cases of pigment dispersion syndrome. *Am J Ophthalmol* 1981;91:573–587.

370. Lehto I, Ruusuvaara P, Setala K. Corneal endothelium in pigmentary glaucoma and pigment dispersion syndrome. *Acta Ophthalmol* 1990;68:703–709.

371. Murrell WJ, Shihab Z, Lamberts DW, Avera B. The corneal endothelium and central corneal thickness in pigmentary dispersion syndrome. *Arch Ophthalmol* 1986;104:845–846.

372. Scheie HG, Cameron JD. Pigment dispersion syndrome: a clinical study. *Br J Ophthalmol* 1981;65:264–269.

373. Weseley P, Liebmann J, Walsh JB, Ritch R. Lattice degeneration of the retina and the pigment dispersion syndrome. *Am J Ophthalmol* 1992;114:539–543.

374. Prince AM, Ritch R. Clinical signs of the pseudoexfoliation syndrome. *Ophthalmology* 1986;93:803–807.

375. Cashwell LF, Jr, Shields MB. Exfoliation syndrome in the southeastern United States. I. Prevalence in open-angle glaucoma and non-glaucoma populations. *Acta Ophthalmol* 1988;184(suppl):99.

376. Henry JC, Krupin T, Schmitt M, et al. Long-term follow-up of pseudoexfoliation and the development of elevated intraocular pressure. *Ophthalmology* 1987;94:545–552.

377. Kozart DM, Yanoff M. Intraocular pressure status in 100 consecutive patients with exfoliation syndrome. *Ophthalmology* 1982;89:214–218.

378. Yanoff M. Intraocular pressure in exfoliation syndrome. *Acta Ophthalmol* 1988;184(suppl):59–61.

379. Ringvold A, Blika S, Elsas T, et al. The middle-Norway eye-screening study. II. Prevalence of simple and capsular glaucoma. *Acta Ophthalmol* 1991;69:273–280.

380. Forsius H. Exfoliation syndrome in various ethnic populations. *Acta Ophthalmol* 1988;184(suppl):71–85.

381. Yalaz M, Othman I, Nas K, et al. The frequency of pseudoexfoliation syndrome in the eastern Mediterranean area of Turkey. *Acta Ophthalmol* 1992;70:209–213.

382. Colin J, Le Gall G, Le Jeune B, Cambrai MD. The prevalence of exfoliation syndrome in different areas of France. *Acta Ophthalmol* 1988;184(suppl):86–89.

383. Lahlou-Boukoffa OS, Douadi F, Saadni F, Flament J. Pseudoexfoliative glaucoma in eastern Algeria: clinical study. *Bull Soc Ophthalmol France* 1989;89:1073–1079.

384. Konstas AG, Allan D. Pseudoexfoliation glaucoma in Greece. *Eye* 1989;3:747–753.

385. Friederich R. Eye disease in the Navajo Indians. *Ann Ophthalmol* 1982;14:38–40.

386. Davanger M, Ringvold A, Blika S. The frequency distribution of the glaucoma tolerance limit. *Acta Ophthalmol* 1991;69:782–785.

387. Davanger M, Ringvold A, Blika S. Pseudo-exfoliation, IOP and glaucoma. *Acta Ophthalmol* 1991;69:569–573.

388. Tezel G, Tezel TH. The comparative analysis of optic disc damage in exfoliative glaucoma. *Acta Ophthalmol* 1993;71:744–750.

389. Crittendon JJ, Shields MB. Exfoliation syndrome in the southeastern United States. II. Characteristics of patient population and clinical course. *Acta Ophthalmologica* 1988;184(suppl):103–106.

390. Ringvold A, Blika S, Elsas T, et al. The middle-Norway eye-screening study. III. The prevalence of capsular glaucoma is influenced by blood-group antigens. *Acta Ophthalmol* 1993;71:207–213.

391. Jerndal T, Lind A. New aspects on the heredity of open angle glaucoma. *Acta Ophthalmol* 1979;57:826–831.

392. Psilas KG, Stefaniotou MJ, Aspiotis MB. Pseudoexfoliation syndrome and diabetes mellitus. *Acta Ophthalmol* 1991;69:664–666.

393. Paolo de Felice G, Bottoni F, Orzalesi N. Unilateral retinitis pigmentosa associated with exfoliation syndrome. *Int Ophthalmol* 1988;11:219–226.

394. Franks WA, Miller MH, Hitchings RA, Jeffrey MN. Secondary angle closure in association with pseudoexfoliation of the lens capsule. *Acta Ophthalmol* 1990;68:350–352.

395. Lumme P, Laatikainen L. Exfoliation syndrome and cataract extraction [see comments]. *Am J Ophthalmol* 1993;116:51–55.

396. Naumann GO. Exfoliation syndrome as a risk factor for vitreous loss in extracapsular cataract surgery (preliminary report): Erlanger-Augenblatter-Group. *Acta Ophthalmol* 1988;184(suppl):129–131.

397. Henke V, Naumann GO. Incidence of the pseudo-exfoliation syndrome in enucleated eyes. *Klin Monatsbl Augenheilkd* 1987;190:173–175.

398. Schlotzer-Schrehardt U, Dorfler S, Naumann GO. Immunohistochemical localization of basement membrane components in pseudoexfoliation material of the lens capsule. *Curr Eye Res* 1992;11:343–355.

399. *Hietanen J, Tarkkanen A. Glycoconjugates in exfoliation syndrome: a lectin histochemical study of the ciliary body and lens. Acta Ophthalmol 1989;67:288–294.*

400. Chen V, Blumenthal M. Exfoliation syndrome after cataract extraction. *Ophthalmology* 1992;99:445–447.

401. Eagle RJ, Font RL, Fine BS. The basement membrane exfoliation syndrome. *Arch Ophthalmol* 1979;97:510–551.

402. Schlotzer-Schredhardt U, Kuchle M, Dorfler S, Naumann GO. Pseudoexfoliative material in the eyelid skin of pseudoexfoliation-suspect patients: a clinico-histopathological correlation. *Ger J Ophthalmol* 1993;2:51–60.

403. Kuchle M, Schlotzer-Schrehardt U, Naumann GO. Occurrence of pseudoexfoliative material in parabulbar structures in pseudoexfoliation syndrome. *Acta Ophthalmol* 1991;69:124–130.

404. Schlotzer-Schrehardt U, Kuchle M, Naumann GO. Electron-microscopic identification of pseudoexfoliation material in extrabulbar tissue. *Arch Ophthalmol* 1991;109:565–570.

405. Schlotzer-Schrehardt UM, Koca MR, Naumann GO, Volkholz H. Pseudoexfoliation syndrome: ocular manifestation of a systemic disorder? *Arch Ophthalmol* 1992;110:1752–1756.

406. Streeten BW, Dark AJ, Wallace RN, Li ZY, Hoepner JA. Pseudoexfoliative fibrillopathy in the skin of patients with ocular pseudoexfoliation. *Am J Ophthalmol* 1990;110:490–499.

407. Richardson TM, Epstein DL. Exfoliation glaucoma: a quantitative perfusion and ultrastructural study. *Ophthalmology* 1981;88:968–980.

408. Schlotzer-Schrehardt U, Naumann GO. Trabecular meshwork in pseudoexfoliation syndrome with and without open-angle glaucoma: a morphometric, ultrastructural study. *Invest Ophthalmol Vis Sci* 1995;36:1750–1764.

409. Lutjen-Drecoll E, Shimizu T, Rohrbach M, Rohen JW. Quantitative analysis of 'plaque material' in the inner- and outer wall of Schlemm's canal in normal- and glaucomatous eyes. *Exp Eye Res* 1986;42:443–455.

410. Shimizu T. Changes of iris vessels in capsular glaucoma: three-dimensional and electron microscopic studies. *Jpn J Ophthalmol* 1985;29:434–452.

411. Konstas AG, Marshall GE, Cameron SA, Lee WR. Morphology of iris vasculopathy in exfoliation glaucoma. *Acta Ophthalmol* 1993;71:751–759.

412. Kuchle M, Nguyen NX, Horn F, Naumann GO. Quantitative assessment of aqueous flare and aqueous "cells" in pseudoexfoliation syndrome. *Acta Ophthalmol* 1992;70:201–208.

413. Zetterstrom C, Olivestedt G, Lundvall A. Exfoliation syndrome and extracapsular cataract extraction with implantation of posterior chamber lens. *Acta Ophthalmol* 1992;70:85–90.

414. Walinder PE, Olivius EO, et al. Fibrinoid reaction after extracapsular cataract extraction and relationship to exfoliation syndrome. *J Cataract Refrac Surg* 1989;15:526–530.

415. Lundvall A, Zetterstrom C. Exfoliation syndrome and the effect of phenylephrine and pilocarpine on pupil size. *Acta Ophthalmol* 1993;71:177–180.

416. Hietanen J, Kivela T, et al. Exfoliation syndrome in patients scheduled for cataract surgery. *Acta Ophthalmol* 1992;70:440–446.

417. Rouhiainen H, Terasvirta M. Pigmentation of the anterior chamber angle in normal and pseudoexfoliative eyes. *Acta Ophthalmol* 1990;68:700–702.

418. Repo LP, Terasvirta ME, Tuovinen EJ. Generalized peripheral iris transluminance in the pseudoexfoliation syndrome. *Ophthalmology* 1990;97:1027–1029.

419. Sampaolesi R, Zarate J, Croxato O. The chamber angle in exfoliation syndrome: clinical and pathological findings. *Acta Ophthalmol* 1988;184(suppl):48–53.

420. Repo LP, Terasvirta ME, Koivisto KJ. Generalized transluminance of the iris and the frequency of the pseudoexfoliation syndrome in the eyes of transient ischemic attack patients. *Ophthalmology* 1993;100:352–355.

421. Stefaniotou M, Kalogeropoulos C, Razis N, Psilas K. The cornea in exfoliation syndrome. *Doc Ophthalmol* 1992;80:329–333.

422. Schlotzer-Schrehardt UM, et al. Corneal endothelial involvement in pseudoexfoliation syndrome. *Arch Ophthalmol* 1993;111:666–674.

423. Netland PA, Ye H, Streeten BW, Hernandez MR. Elastosis of the lamina cribrosa in pseudoexfoliation syndrome with glaucoma. *Ophthalmology* 1995;102:878–886.

424. Fenton RH, Zimmerman LE. Hemolytic glaucoma: an unusual cause of acute open-angle secondary glaucoma. *Arch Ophthalmol* 1963;70:236–239.

425. Phelps CD, Watzke RC. Hemolytic glaucoma. *Am J Ophthalmol* 1975;80:690–695.

426. Campbell DG, Simmons RJ, Grant WM. Ghost cells as a cause of glaucoma. *Am J Ophthalmol* 1976;81:441–450.

427. Campbell DG, Simmons RJ, Tolentino FI, et al. Glaucoma occurring after closed vitrectomy. *Am J Ophthalmol* 1977;83:63–69.

428. Campbell DG, Essigmann EM. Hemolytic ghost cell glaucoma. Further studies. *Arch Ophthalmol* 1979;97:2141–2146.

429. Barnhorst D, Meyers SM, Myers T. Lens-induced glaucoma 65 years after congenital cataract surgery. *Am J Ophthalmol* 1994;118:807–888.

430. Epstein DL. Diagnosis and management of lens-induced glaucoma. *Ophthalmology* 1982;89:227–230.

431. Lane SS, Kopietz LA, Lindquist TD, Leavenworth N. Treatment of phacolytic glaucoma with extracapsular cataract extraction. *Ophthalmology* 1988;95:749–753.

432. Flocks M, Littwin CS, Zimmerman LE. Phacolytic glaucoma. *Arch Ophthalmol* 1955;54:37–45.

433. Brooks AM, Grant G, Gillies WE. Comparison of specular microscopy and examination of aspirate in phacolytic glaucoma. *Ophthalmology* 1990;97:85–89.

434. Bartholomew RS, Rebello PF. Calcium oxalate crystals in the aqueous. *Am J Ophthalmol* 1979;88:1026–1028.

435. Goldberg MF. Cytological diagnosis of phacolytic glaucoma utilizing millipore filtration of the aqueous. *Br J Ophthalmol* 1967;51:847–853.

436. Ueno H, Tamai A, Iyota K, Moriki T. Electron microscopic observation of the cells floating in the anterior chamber in a case of phacolytic glaucoma. *Japanese Journal of Ophthalmology* 1989;33:103–113.

437. Epstein DL, Jedziniak JA, Grant WM. Identification of heavy-molecular-weight soluble protein in aqueous humor in human phacolytic glaucoma. *Invest Ophthalmol Vis Sci* 1978;17:398–402.

438. Yanoff M, Scheie HG. Cytology of human lens aspirate: its relationship to phacolytic glaucoma and phacoanaphylactic endophthalmitis. *Arch Ophthalmol* 1968;80:166–170.

439. Rosenbaum JT, Samples JR, Seymour B, Langlois L, David L. Chemotactic activity of lens proteins and the pathogenesis of phacolytic glaucoma. *Arch Ophthalmol* 1987;105:1582–1584.

440. Yanoff M, Scheie HG. Melanomalytic glaucoma: report of a case. *Arch Ophthalmol* 1970;84:471–473.

441. McMenamin PG, Lee WR. Ultrastructural pathology of melanomalytic glaucoma. *Br J Ophthalmol* 1986;70:895–906.

442. Van Buskirk EM, Leure-duPree AE. Pathophysiology and electron microscopy of melanomalytic glaucoma. *Am J Ophthalmol* 1978;85:160–166.

443. Yanoff M. Glaucoma mechanisms in ocular malignant melanomas. *Am J Ophthalmol* 1970;70:898–904.

444. Yanoff M. Mechanisms of glaucoma in eyes with uveal malignant melanomas. *Int Ophthalmol Clin* 1972;12:51–62.

445. Wolff SM, Zimmerman LE. Chronic secondary glaucoma associated with retrodisplacement of iris root and deepening of the anterior chamber angle secondary to contusion. *Am J Ophthalmol* 1962;54:547–563.

446. Alper MG. Contusion angle deformity and glaucoma. *Arch Ophthalmol* 1963;69:455–467.

447. Blanton FM. Anterior chamber angle recession and secondary glaucoma. *Arch Ophthalmol* 1964;72:39–43.

448. Kaufman JH, Tolpin DW. Glaucoma after traumatic angle recession: a ten-year prospective study. *Am J Ophthalmol* 1974;78:648–654.

449. Canavan YM, Archer DB. Anterior segment consequences of blunt ocular injury. *Br J Ophthalmol* 1982;66:549–555.

450. Salmon JF, Mermoud A, Ivey A, et al. The detection of post-traumatic angle recession by gonioscopy in a population-based glaucoma survey. *Ophthalmology* 1994;101:1844–1850.

451. Sihota R, Sood NN, Agarwal HC. Traumatic glaucoma. *Acta Ophthalmol Scand* 1995;73:252–254.

452. Posner A, Schlossman A. Syndrome of unilateral recurrent attacks of glaucoma with cyclitic symptoms. *Arch Ophthalmol* 1948;39:517–535.

453. Posner A, Schlossman A. Further observations on the syndrome of glaucomatocyclitic crises. *Trans Am Acad Ophthalmol Otolaryngol* 1953;57:531–536.

454. Setala K, Vannas A. Endothelial cells in the glaucomato-cyclitic crisis. *Adv Ophthalmol* 1978;36:218–224.

455. Hung PT, Chang JM. Treatment of glaucomatocyclitic crises. *Am J Ophthalmol* 1974;77:169–172.

456. Spivey BE, Armaly MF. Tonographic findings in glaucomatocyclitic crises. *Am J Ophthalmol* 1963;55:47–51.

457. Raitta C, Vannas A. Glaucomatocyclitic crisis. *Arch Ophthalmol* 1977;95:608–612.

458. Hart CT, Weatherill JR. Gonioscopy and tonography in glaucomatocyclitic crises. *Br J Ophthalmol* 1968;52.682–687.

459. Yamamoto S, Pavan-Langston D, Tada R, et al. Possible role of herpes simplex virus in the origin of Posner-Schlossman syndrome. *Am J Ophthalmol* 1995;119:796–798.

460. Hirose S, Ohno S, Matsuda H. HLA-Bw54 and glaucomatocyclitic crisis. *Arch Ophthalmol* 1985;103:1837–1839.

461. Naveh-Floman N, Spierer A, et al. Protein glaucoma as a possible mechanism in a case of glaucomatocyclitic crisis and periphlebitis. *Metab Pediat Sys Ophthalmol* 1983;7:85–88.

462. Masuda K, Izawa Y, Mishima S. Prostaglandins and uveitis. *Jpn J Ophthalmol* 1973;17:166–170.

463. Kass MA, Becker B, et al. Glaucomatocyclitic crisis and primary open-angle glaucoma. *Am J Ophthalmol* 1973;75:668–673.

464. Harstad HK, Ringvold A. Glaucomatocyclitic crises (Posner-Schlossman syndrome): a case report. *Acta Ophthalmol* 1986;64:146–151.

465. Tran VT, Auer C, Guex-Crosier Y, Pittet N, Herbort CP. Epidemiological characteristics of uveitis in Switzerland. *Int Ophthalmol* 1994;18:293–298.

466. Jones NP. Fuchs' heterochromic uveitis: a reappraisal of the clinical spectrum. *Eye* 1991;5:649–661.

467. La Hey E, Baarsma GS, et al. Clinical analysis of Fuchs' heterochromic cyclitis. *Doc Ophthalmol* 1991;78:225–235.

468. Gee SS, Tabbara KF. Extracapsular cataract extraction in Fuchs' heterochromic iridocyclitis. *Am J Ophthalmol* 1989;108:310–314.

469. Sherwood DR, Rosenthal AR. Cataract surgery in Fuchs' heterochromic iridocyclitis. *Br J Ophthalmol* 1992;76:238–240.

470. Daus W, Schmidbauer J, et al. Results of extracapsular cataract extraction with intraocular lens implantation in eyes with uveitis and Fuchs' heterochromic iridocyclitis. *Germ J Ophthalmol* 1992;1:399–402.

471. Jones NP. Cataract surgery using heparin surface-modified intraocular lenses in Fuchs' heterochromic uveitis. *Ophthalmic Surg* 1995;26:49–52.

472. Ram J, Jain S, et al. Postoperative complications of intraocular lens implantation in patients with Fuchs' heterochromic cyclitis. *J Cataract Refract Surg* 1995;21:548–551.

473. Roussel TJ, Coster DJ. Fuchs's heterochromic cyclitis and posterior capsulotomy. *Br J Ophthalmol* 1985;69:449–451.

474. Jones NP. Glaucoma in Fuchs' heterochromic uveitis: aetiology, management and outcome. *Eye* 1991;5:662–667.

475. La Hey E, de Vries J, Langerhorst CT, Baarsma GS, Kijlstra A. Treatment and prognosis of secondary glaucoma in Fuchs' heterochromic iridocyclitis. *Am J Ophthalmol* 1993;116:327–340.

476. Fearnley IR, Rosenthal AR. Fuchs' heterochromic iridocyclitis revisited. *Acta Ophthalmol Scand* 1995;73:166–170.

477. Tabbut BR, Tessler HH, Williams D. Fuchs' heterochromic iridocyclitis in blacks. *Arch Ophthalmol* 1988;106:1688–1690.

478. Rothova A, La Hey E, et al. Iris nodules in Fuchs' heterochromic uveitis. *Am J Ophthalmol* 1994;118:338–342.

479. Smit RL, Baarsma GS, de Vries J. Classification of 750 consecutive uveitis patients in the Rotterdam Eye Hospital. *Int Ophthalmol* 1993;17:71–76.

480. Munoz G, Lopez-Corell MP, Taboada JF, Ferrer E, Diaz-Llopis M. Fuch's heterochromic cyclitis and HLA histocompatibility antigens. *Int Ophthalmol* 1994;18:127–130.

481. Saari M, Vuorre I, Nieminen H. Fuchs's heterochromic cyclitis: a simultaneous bilateral fluorescein angiographic study of the iris. *Br J Ophthalmol* 1978;62:715–721.

482. Berger BB, Tessler HH, et al. Anterior segment ischemia in Fuchs' heterochromic cyclitis. *Arch Ophthalmol* 1980;98:499–501.

483. Noda S, Hayasaka S. Recurrent subconjunctival hemorrhages in patients with Fuchs' heterochromic iridocyclitis. *Ophthalmologica* 1995;209:289–291.

484. La Hey E, Mooy CM, Baarsma GS, et al. Immune deposits in

iris biopsy specimens from patients with Fuchs' heterochromic iridocyclitis. *Am J Ophthalmol* 1992;113:75–80.

485. Melamed S, Lahav M, Sandbank U, Yassur Y, Ben-Sira I. Fuch's heterochromic iridocyclitis: an electron microscopic study of the iris. *Invest Ophthalmol Vis Sci* 1978;17:1193–1199.

486. McCartney AC, Bull TB, Spalton DJ. Fuchs' heterochromic cyclitis: an electron microscopy study. *Trans Ophthalmological Soc UK* 1986;105:324–329.

487. Perry HD, Yanoff M, Scheie HG. Rubeosis in Fuchs' heterochromic iridocyclitis. *Arch Ophthalmol* 1975;93:337–339.

488. Arffa RC, Schlaegel TF Jr. Chorioretinal scars in Fuchs' heterochromic iridocyclitis. *Arch Ophthalmol* 1984;102:1153–1155.

489. Saraux H, Laroche L, Le Hoang P. Secondary Fuchs's heterochromic cyclitis: a new approach to an old disease. *Ophthalmologica* 1985;190:193–198.

490. Schwab IR. The epidemiologic association of Fuchs' heterochromic iridocyclitis and ocular toxoplasmosis. *Am J Ophthalmol* 1991;111:356–362.

491. La Hey E, Rothova A, Baarsma GS, de Vries J, van Knapen F, Kijlstra A. Fuchs' heterochromic iridocyclitis is not associated with ocular toxoplasmosis. *Arch Ophthalmol* 1992;110:806–811.

492. La Hey E, Broersma L, van der Gaag R, et al. Does autoimmunity to S-antigen play a role in Fuchs' heterochromic cyclitis? *Br J Ophthalmol* 1993;77:436–439.

493. Goble RR, Murray PI. Fuchs' heterochromic uveitis and sarcoidosis. *Br J Ophthalmol* 1995;79:1021–1023.

494. Hammer H, Olah M. Hypersensitivity towards alpha-crystalline in the heterochromia syndrome. *Albrecht Von Graefes Archiv Klini Exper Ophthamol* 1975;197:61–66.

495. Jakobiec FA, Lefkowitch J, Knowles D. B- and T-lymphocytes in ocular disease. *Ophthalmology* 1984;91:635–654.

496. Murray PI, Rahi AH. New concepts in the control of ocular inflammation. *Trans Ophthalmol Soc UK* 1985;104:152–158.

497. la Hey E, Baarsma GS, Rothova A, et al. High incidence of corneal epithelium antibodies in Fuch's heterochromic cyclitis. *Br J Ophthalmol* 1988;72:921–925.

498. van der Gaag R, Broersma L, Rothova A, Baarsma S, Kijlstra A. Immunity to a corneal antigen in Fuchs' heterochromic cyclitis patients. *Invest Ophthalmol Vis Sci* 1989;30:443–448.

499. Murray PI, Hoekzema R, et al. Aqueous humour analysis in Fuchs' heterochromic cyclitis. *Current Eye Research* 1990;9:53–57.

500. Murray PI, Hoekzema R, et al. Aqueous humor interleukin-6 levels in uveitis. *Invest Ophthalmol Vis Sci* 1990;31:917–920.

501. Murray PI. Fuchs' heterochromic cyclitis: an immunological disease or an immunological response? *Int Ophthalmol* 1994;18:313.

502. Regenbogen LS, Naveh FN. Glaucoma in Fuchs' heterochromic cyclitis associated with congenital Horner's syndrome. *Br J Ophthalmol* 1987;71:844–849.

503. Saari M, Vuorre I, Tiilikainen A, et al. Genetic background of Fuchs' heterochromic cyclitis. *Can J Ophthalmol* 1978;13:240–246.

504. Vuorre I, Saari M, Tiilikainen A, Rasanen O. Fuchs' heterochromic cyclitis associated with retinitis pigmentosa: a family study. *Can J Ophthalmol* 1979;14:10–16.

505. Sugar HS. Low tension glaucoma: a practial approach. *Ann Ophthalmol* 1979;11:1155–1171.

506. Levene RZ. Low tension glaucoma: a critical review and new material. *Surv Ophthalmol* 1980;24:621–664.

507. Levene RZ. Low tension glaucoma. Part II. Clinical characteristics and pathogenesis [editorial]. *Ann Ophthalmol* 1980;12:1383.

508. Grosskreutz C, Netland PA. Low-tension glaucoma. *Int Ophthalmol Clin* 1994;34:173–185.

509. Hitchings RA, Anderton SA. A comparative study of visual field defects seen in patients with low-tension glaucoma and chronic simple glaucoma. *Br J Ophthalmol* 1983;67:818–821.

510. Caprioli J, Spaeth GL. Comparison of visual field defects in the low-tension glaucomas with those in the high-tension glaucomas. *Am J Ophthalmol* 1984;97:730–737.

511. Motolko M, Drance SM, Douglas GR. Visual field defects in low-tension glaucoma. Comparison of defects in low-tension glaucoma and chronic open angle glaucoma. *Arch Ophthalmol* 1982;100:1074–1077.

512. De Vivero C, et al. Diurnal intraocular pressure variation in low-tension glaucoma. *Eye* 1994;8:521–523.

513. Larsson LI, Rettig ES, et al. Aqueous humor dynamics in low-tension glaucoma. *Am J Ophthalmol* 1993;116:590–593.

514. Gliklich RE, Steinmann WC, Spaeth GL. Visual field change in low-tension glaucoma over a five-year follow-up. *Ophthalmology* 1989;96:316–320.

515. Crichton A, Drance SM, Douglas GR, Schulzer M. Unequal intraocular pressure and its relation to asymmetric visual field defects in low-tension glaucoma. *Ophthalmology* 1989;96:1312–1314.

516. Cartwright MJ, Anderson DR. Correlation of asymmetric damage with asymmetric intraocular pressure in normal-tension glaucoma (low-tension glaucoma). *Arch Ophthalmol* 1988;106:898–900.

517. Buus DR, Anderson DR. Peripapillary crescents and halos in normal-tension glaucoma and ocular hypertension. *Ophthalmology* 1989;96:16–19.

518. Jonas JB, Xu L. Parapapillary chorioretinal atrophy in normal-pressure glaucoma. *Am J Ophthalmol* 1993;115:501–505.

519. Stroman GA, Stewart WC, Golnik KC, Cure JK, Olinger RE. Magnetic resonance imaging in patients with low-tension glaucoma. *Arch Ophthalmol* 1995;113:168–172.

520. Carter CJ, Brooks DE, Doyle DL, Drance SM. Investigations into a vascular etiology for low-tension glaucoma. *Ophthalmology* 1990;97:49–55.

521. Klaver JH, Greve EL, Goslinga H, Geijssen HC, Heuvelmans JH. Blood and plasma viscosity measurements in patients with glaucoma. *Br J Ophthalmol* 1985;69:765–770.

522. Butt Z, McKillop G, COB, Allan P, Aspinall P. Measurement of ocular blood flow velocity using colour Doppler imaging in low tension glaucoma. *Eye* 1995;9:29–33.

523. Quaranta L, Manni G, Donato F, Bucci MG. The effect of increased intraocular pressure on pulsatile ocular blood flow in low tension glaucoma. *Surv Ophthalmol* 1994;38:S177–S182.

524. Pillunat LE, Stodtmeister R, Wilmanns I. Pressure compliance of the optic nerve head in low tension glaucoma. *Br J Ophthalmol* 1987;71:181–187.

525. Ravalico G, Pastori G, et al. Visual and blood flow responses in low-tension glaucoma. *Surv Ophthalmol* 1994;38:S173–S176.

526. James CB, Smith SE. Pulsatile ocular blood flow in patients with low tension glaucoma. *Br J Ophthalmol* 1991;75:466–470.

527. Haeffliger IO, Meyer P, Flammer J, Luscher TF. The vascular endothelium as a regulator of the ocular circulation: a new concept in ophthalmology? *Surv Ophthalmol* 1994;39:123–132.

528. Sugiyama T, Moriya S, Oku H, Azuma I. Association of endothelin-1 with normal tension glaucoma: clinical and fundamental studies. *Surv Ophthalmol* 1995;39:S49–S56.

529. Muller M, Kessler C, Wessel K, et al. Low-tension glaucoma: a comparative study with retinal ischemic syndromes and anterior ischemic optic neuropathy. *Ophthalmic Surg* 1993;24:835–838.

530. Gutman I, Melamed S, Ashkenazi I, Blumenthal M. Optic nerve compression by carotid arteries in low-tension glaucoma. *Graefes Arch Clin Exp Ophthalmol* 1993;231:711–717.

531. Wax MB, Barrett DA, Pestronk A. Increased incidence of paraproteinemia and autoantibodies in patients with normal-pressure glaucoma. *Am J Ophthalmol* 1994;117:561–568.

532. Romano C, Barrett DA, Li Z, Pestronk A, Wax MB. Antirhodopsin antibodies in sera from patients with normal-pressure glaucoma. *Invest Ophthalmol Vis Sci* 1995;36:1968–1975.

533. Brierley EJ, Griffiths PG, Weber K, Johnson MA, Turnbull DM. Normal respiratory chain function in patients with low-tension glaucoma. *Arch Ophthalmol* 1996;114:142–146.

534. Kitazawa Y, Shirato S, Yamamoto T. Optic disc hemorrhage in low-tension glaucoma. *Ophthalmology* 1986;93:853–857.

535. Hoyng PF, de Jong N, et al. Platelet aggregation, disc haemorrhage and progressive loss of visual fields in glaucoma. A seven year follow-up study on glaucoma. *Intern Ophthalmol* 1992;16:65–73.

536. Hendrickx KH, van den Enden A, Rasker MT, Hoyng PF. Cumulative incidence of patients with disc hemorrhages in glaucoma and the effect of therapy. *Ophthalmology* 1994;101:1165–1172.

537. Jonas JB, Xu L. Optic disk hemorrhages in glaucoma. *Am J Ophthalmol* 1994;118:1–8.

538. Chumbley LC, Brubaker RF. Low-tension glaucoma. *Am J Ophthalmol* 1976;81:761–767.

539. Javitt JC, Spaeth GL, Katz LJ, Poryzees E, Addiego R. Acquired pits of the optic nerve: increased prevalence in patients with low-tension glaucoma. *Ophthalmology* 1990;97:1038–1044.

540. Kitazawa Y, Shirai H, Go FJ. The effect of Ca2(+)-antagonist on visual field in low-tension glaucoma. *Graefes Arch Clinic Exper Ophthalmol* 1989;227:408–412.

541. Netland PA, Chaturvedi N, Dreyer EB. Calcium channel blockers in the management of low-tension and open-angle glaucoma. *Am J Ophthalmol* 1993;115:608–613.

542. Gaspar AZ, Flammer J, Hendrickson P. Influence of nifedipine on the visual fields of patients with optic-nerve-head diseases. *Eur J Ophthalmol* 1994;4:24–28.

543. Lumme P, Tuulonen A, et al. Neuroretinal rim area in low tension glaucoma: effect of nifedipine and acetazolamide compared to no treatment. *Acta Ophthalmol* 1991;69:293–298.

544. Gasser P. Ocular vasospasm: a risk factor in the pathogenesis of low-tension glaucoma. *Intern Ophthalmol* 1989;13:281–290.

545. Gasser P, Flammer J, Guthauser U, Mahler F. Do vasospasms provoke ocular diseases? *Angiology* 1990;41:213–220.

546. Schwartz AL, Perman KI, Whitten M. Argon laser trabeculoplasty in progessive low-tension glaucoma. *Ann Ophthalmol* 1984;16: 560–562, 566.

547. Ticho U, Nesher R. Laser trabeculoplasty in glaucoma. Ten-year evaluation [see comments]. *Arch Ophthalmol* 1989;107:844–846.

548. Eendeback GR, Boen-Tan TN, Bezemer PD. Long-term follow-up of laser trabeculoplasty. *Doc Ophthalmol* 1990;75:203–214.

549. Simmons RJ, Kimbrough RL. Shell tamponade in filtering surgery for glaucoma. *Ophthal Surg* 1979;10:17–34.

550. de Jong N, Greve EL, et al. Results of a filtering procedure in low tension glaucoma. *Int Ophthalmol* 1989;13:131–138.

551. Wilson RP, Steinmann WC. Use of trabeculectomy with postoperative 5-fluorouracil in patients requiring extremely low intraocular pressure levels to limit further glaucoma progression. *Ophthalmology* 1991;98:1047–1052.

552. Sugar HS. Complications, repair and reoperation of antiglaucoma filtering blebs. *Am J Ophthalmol* 1967;63:825–833.

553. Wolner B, Liebmann JM, Sassani JW, Ritch R, Speaker M, Marmor M. Late bleb-related endophthalmitis after trabeculectomy with adjunctive 5-fluorouracil. *Ophthalmology* 1991;98:1053–60.

554. Balazsi AG, Drance SM, et al. Neuroretinal rim area in suspected glaucoma and early chronic open-angle glaucoma. Correlation with parameters of visual function. *Arch Ophthalmol* 1984;102: 1011–1014.

555. Quigley HA. Early detection of glaucomatous damage. II. Changes in the appearance of the optic disk. *Surv Ophthalmol* 1985;30: 111, 117–126.

556. Jonas JB, Fernandez MC, Sturmer J. Pattern of glaucomatous neuroretinal rim loss. *Ophthalmology* 1993;100:63–68.

557. Katz LJ, Spaeth GL, Cantor LB, Poryzees EM, Steinmann WC. Reversible optic disk cupping and visual field improvement in adults with glaucoma. *Am J Ophthalmol* 1989;107:485–492.

558. Funk J. Increase of neuroretinal rim area after surgical intraocular pressure reduction. *Ophthalmic Surg* 1990;21:585–588.

559. Quigley HA. The pathogenesis of reversible cupping in congenital glaucoma. *Am J Ophthalmol* 1977;84:358–370.

560. Varma R, Quigley HA, Pease ME. Changes in optic disk characteristics and number of nerve fibers in experimental glaucoma. *Am J Ophthalmol* 1992;114:554–559.

561. Sommer A, Katz J, Quigley HA, et al. Clinically detectable nerve fiber atrophy precedes the onset of glaucomatous field loss. *Arch Ophthalmol* 1991;109:77–83.

562. Quigley HA, Hohman RM, Addicks EM, Massof RW, Green WR. Morphologic changes in the lamina cribrosa correlated with neural loss in open-angle glaucoma. *Am J Ophthalmol* 1983;95:673–691.

563. Drance SM. Disc hemorrhages in the glaucomas. *Surv Ophthalmology* 1989;33:331–337.

564. Diehl DL, Quigley HA, Miller NR, Sommer A, Burney EN. Prevalence and significance of optic disc hemorrhage in a longitudinal study of glaucoma. *Arch Ophthalmol* 1990;108:545–550.

565. Quigley HA, Nickells RW, Kerrigan LA, Pease ME, Thibault DJ, Zack DJ. Retinal ganglion cell death in experimental glaucoma and after axotomy occurs by apoptosis. *Invest Ophthalmol Vis Sci* 1995;36:774–786.

566. Quigley HA, Sanchez RM, et al. Chronic glaucoma selectively damages large optic nerve fibers. *Invest Ophthalmol Vis Sci* 1987; 28:913–920.

567. Quigley HA, Dunkelberger GR, Green WR. Chronic human glaucoma causing selectively greater loss of large optic nerve fibers. *Ophthalmology* 1988;95:357–363.

568. Glovinsky Y, Quigley HA, Dunkelberger GR. Retinal ganglion cell loss is size dependent in experimental glaucoma. *Invest Ophthalmol Vis Sci* 1991;32:484–491.

569. Glovinsky Y, Quigley HA, Pease ME. Foveal ganglion cell loss is size dependent in experimental glaucoma. *Invest Ophthalmol Vis Sci* 1993;34:395–400.

570. Kubota T, Naumann GO. Reduction in number of corpora amylacea with advancing histological changes of glaucoma. *Graefes Arch Clin Exp Ophthalmol* 1993;231:249–253.

571. Quigley HA, Green WR. The histology of human glaucoma cupping and optic nerve damage: clinicopathologic correlation in 21 eyes. *Ophthalmology* 1979;86:1803–1830.

572. Quigley HA, Addicks EM. Regional differences in the structure of the lamina cribrosa and their relation to glaucomatous optic nerve damage. *Arch Ophthalmol* 1981;99:137–143.

573. Miller KM, Quigley HA. The clinical appearance of the lamina cribrosa as a function of the extent of glaucomatous optic nerve damage. *Ophthalmology* 1988;95:135–138.

574. Minckler DS, Spaeth GL. Optic nerve damage in glaucoma. *Surv Ophthalmol* 1981;26:128–148.

575. Flammer J. The vascular concept of glaucoma. *Surv Ophthalmol* 1994;38:S3–S6.

576. Minckler DS, Tso Mo, Zimmerman LE. A light microscopic, autoradiographic study of axoplasmic transport in the optic nerve head during ocular hypotony, increased intraocular pressure, and papilledema. *Am J Ophthalmol* 1976;82:741–757.

577. Gaasterland D, Tanishima T, Kuwabara T. Axoplasmic flow during chronic experimental glaucoma. 1. Light and electron microscopic studies of the monkey optic nervehead during development of glaucomatous cupping. *Invest Ophthalmol Vis Sci* 1978;17:838–846.

578. Quigley HA, Hohman RM, et al. Blood vessels of the glaucomatous optic disc in experimental primate and human eyes. *Invest Ophthalmol Vis Sci* 1984;25:918–931.

579. Quigley HA, Addicks EM. Chronic experimental glaucoma in primates. II. Effect of extended intraocular pressure elevation on optic nerve head and axonal transport. *Invest Ophthalmol Vis Sci* 1980; 19:137–152.

580. Quigley HA, Flower RW, et al. The mechanism of optic nerve damage in experimental acute intraocular pressure elevation. *Invest Opthalmol Vis Sci* 1980;19:505–517.

581. Quigley HA, Addicks EM, Green WR, Maumenee AE. Optic nerve damage in human glaucoma. II. The site of injury and susceptibility to damage. *Arch Ophthalmol* 1981;99:635–649.

582. Hollander H, Makarov F, et al. Evidence of constriction of optic nerve axons at the lamina cribrosa in the normotensive eye in humans and other mammals. *Ophthalmic Res* 1995;27:296–309.

583. Morrison JC, Dorman-Pease ME, Dunkelberger GR, Quigley HA. Optic nerve head extracellular matrix in primary optic atrophy and experimental glaucoma. *Arch Ophthalmol* 1990;108:1020–1024.

584. Quigley HA, Brown A, Dorman-Pease ME. Alterations in elastin of the optic nerve head in human and experimental glaucoma. *Br J Ophthalmol* 1991;75:552–557.

585. Quigley HA, Dorman-Pease ME, et al. Quantitative study of collagen and elastin of the optic nerve head and sclera in human and experimental monkey glaucoma. *Curr Eye Res* 1991;10:877–888.

586. Fukuchi T, Sawaguchi S, Hara H, Shirakashi M, Iwata K. Extracellular matrix changes of the optic nerve lamina cribrosa in monkey eyes with experimentally chronic glaucoma. *Graefes Arch Clin Exp Opthalmol* 1992;230:421–427.

587. Zeimer RC, Ogura Y. The relation between glaucomatous damage and optic nerve head mechanical compliance. *Arch Ophthalmol* 1989;107:1232–1234.

588. Jonas J. Biomorphometry and histomorphometry of the optic disc with special reference to the parapapillary region. *Bull Soc Belge Ophthalmol* 1992;244:45–60.

589. Kubota T, Jonas JB, Naumann GO. Direct clinico-histological correlation of parapapillary chorioretinal atrophy. *Br J Ophthalmol* 1993;77:103–106.

590. Morrison J, Farrell S, Johnson E, Deppmeier L, Moore CG, Grossmann E. Structure and composition of the rodent lamina cribrosa. *Exp Eye Res* 1995;60:127–135.

Ophthalmic Pathology with Clinical Correlations,
edited by Joseph W. Sassani, M.D.
Lippincott-Raven Publishers, Philadelphia © 1997.

CHAPTER 8

Ophthalmic Pathology of Diabetes

David J. Wilson and W. Richard Green

Diabetes is the leading cause of **blindness** in young patients, so it is not surprising that it produces numerous pathologic effects in ocular tissues. **Diabetes,** at its basic level, is a disorder of carbohydrate metabolism, and it has recently been shown that many of the end-organ effects of diabetes can be markedly delayed or prevented by correction of the abnormal glucose metabolism that characterizes diabetes.[1] The pathophysiology of the disordered carbohydrate metabolism is quite complex and is not reviewed here. The interested reader is referred to more thorough reviews of that subject.[2,3]

In the eye, the pathologic features of diabetes arise through two basic and partly interrelated mechanisms— **thickening of basement membranes** and **ischemia**. The thickening of the basement membrane that occurs in numerous diabetic tissues appears to be due to the activation of **aldose reductase** by persistently elevated glucose levels.[4,5] Ischemia is the hallmark of diabetic retinopathy and may result from the pathologic thickening of the basement membrane of the retinal capillary endothelium. This chapter discusses how these two pathologic mechanisms affect the various ocular tissues. The most severely affected are the retina, vitreous, choroid, and corneal epithelium.

RETINA AND VITREOUS

Diabetic involvement of the retina is the major cause of vision loss in diabetes. Diabetic retinopathy is principally a disorder of the retinal vasculature characterized by thickening of the endothelial basement membrane, loss of pericytes, microaneurysm formation, capillary closure, and **neovascularization.** The clinical features of diabetic retinopathy—edema, exudates, hemorrhage, and cottonwool spots—are secondary to these retinovascular changes.

D. J. Wilson: Department of Ophthalmology, Oregon Health Sciences University, Casey Eye Institute, Portland, Oregon 97202.
W. R. Green: Department of Ophthalmology and Pathology, Johns Hopkins University, School of Medicine, Baltimore, Maryland 21287.

Primary Retinal Changes

Basement Membrane Thickening

One of the earliest and most dramatic changes in the retinal vessels is thickening of the basement membrane **capillary endothelium.**[6] Figure 8-1 is a preparation in which India ink was injected into the retinal blood vessels of a postmortem diabetic eye. The basement membrane thickening is evident by the narrowing of the lumen of the vessel. Figure 8-2 demonstrates the ultrastructure of a capillary from a diabetic patient. There is prominently thickened basement membrane material and lipid vacuoles present. Ashton, who contributed a great deal to our knowledge of diabetic retinopathy, believed that pathologic thickening of the retinal capillary basement membrane was of great importance in the pathogenesis of diabetic retinopathy. He believed that obstruction of the precapillary arterioles by pathologically thickened basement membrane resulted in capillary closure and the subsequent retinal ischemia that characterizes diabetic retinopathy.[6] Studies in experimental animals have supported this hypothesis.[5,7,8] Galactosemic animals develop marked thickening of the capillary basement membrane. This thickening is preventable by the administering aldose reductase inhibitors, suggesting that the excess basement membrane production is due to the activation of aldose reductase by the elevated sugar levels. Nevertheless, a clinical trial of aldose reductase inhibitors in humans with diabetes failed to demonstrate any beneficial effect on clinically detectable retinopathy.[9]

Loss of Pericytes

Trypsin digestion is a pathologic technique that provides a striking representation of the retinal vasculature. This allows the clinician to dramatically correlate pathologic changes with retinovascular abnormalities that are evident with fluorescein angiography (Fig. 8-3). Using trypsin digestion, two types of cells can be identified in

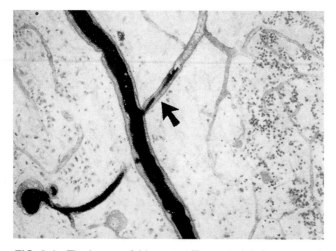

FIG. 8-1. The lumen of this precapillary arteriole is narrowed by basement membrane thickening. From ref. 6, published courtesy of British Medical Association.

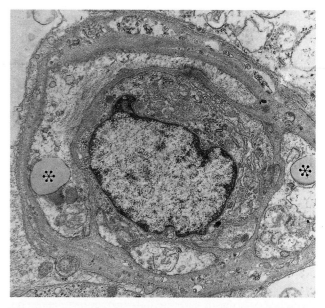

FIG. 8-2. Transmission electron photomicrograph showing basement membrane thickening and lipid vacuoles within the capillary wall. From Green WR, Wilson DJ. Histopathology of diabetic retinopathy. In: Franklin MR, ed. *Retina and Vitreous*. New York: Kugler, 1993;63–81.

retinal capillaries: endothelial cells, which have oval, pale-staining nuclei, and pericytes, which have round darker-staining nuclei (Fig. 8-4). Normally, there is an equal number of endothelial cells and pericytes.

Cogan et al[10] and Kuwabara and Cogan[11] observed that there was a relative loss of the pericyte compared with the endothelial cells in trypsin digest preparations of retinas from diabetic patients (Fig. 8-5).

The exact function of the pericyte is not known; however, it is a contractile cell that forms intercellular junctions with the retinal capillary endothelial cell. It has been shown in vitro to inhibit retinal capillary endothelial cell proliferation.[12] It is possible that loss of the pericyte in diabetic patients permits the formation of hypercellular microaneurysms.

Microaneurysms

Microaneurysms are, perhaps, the earliest recognizable clinical feature of diabetic retinopathy. They occur most abundantly in the posterior pole and particularly surrounding acellular capillary beds. They are important clinically because they are a potential site for plasma leakage, which can accumulate within the retina producing macular edema and lipid exudates. Microaneurysms consist of fusiform or saccular dilations at the capillary level, generally measuring 50 to 100 microns in size. Histopathologically, microaneurysms appear to undergo progression from a hypercellular endothelially lined state to an acellular hyalinized state[13] (Fig. 8-6). The walls of microaneurysms may break down, producing **intraretinal hemorrhages** (Fig. 8-7). Under electron microscopy, microaneurysms have an endothelial lining with some of the

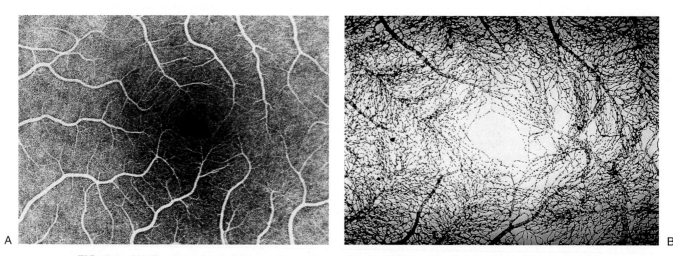

FIG. 8-3. (**A**) Fluorescein angiogram of macular capillaries. (**B**) Trypsin digest preparation of macular capillaries.

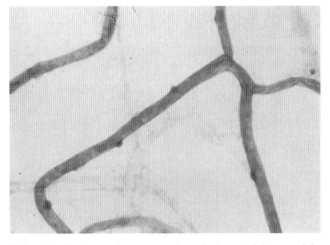

FIG. 8-4. Pericytes have rounder, darker staining nuclei, whereas endothelial cells have more oval, pale staining nuclei.

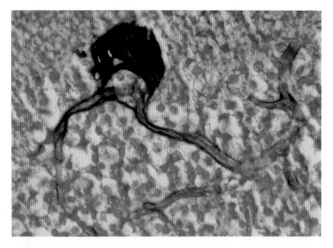

FIG. 8-6. Acellular hyalinized retinal capillary microaneurysm. From Green WR, Wilson DJ. Histopathology of diabetic retinopathy. In: Franklin MR, ed. *Retina and vitreous.* New York: Kugler, 1993;63–81.

cells showing evidence of proliferation. The endothelial junctional complexes appear normal, but the presence of degenerated platelets, fibrin, and lipid in the wall of microaneurysms is evidence of plasma constituents extravasating through the microaneurysm's wall.[14,15]

Acellular Capillaries

Trypsin digest preparations of the retina in diabetes reveal that portions of the capillary bed consist of **acellular basement membrane tubes** (Fig. 8-8). Clinical correlation of these areas with fluorescein angiograms[13] and injection of India ink into digest preparations have demonstrated that these acellular capillary beds are not perfused. Electron microscopy of the acellular capillaries has demonstrated that **Mueller cell processes** gain access to

the inside of these acellular tubes and obliterate the lumen of the vessel[16] (Fig. 8-9).

Intraretinal Microvascular Abnormalities

Intraretinal microvascular abnormalities (IRMA) is a term used clinically to describe flat, intraretinal vessels that have an architecture different from the normal architecture of the retinal vasculature (see Fig. 8-8). Correlation of trypsin digest preparations and fluorescein angiograms shows that IRMAs are vessels that extend from the terminal arterioles and venules toward zones of acellular capillaries. These vessels have a markedly increased number of endothelial cells.[13] They may be single vessels or may be arranged in branching patterns or arcades.

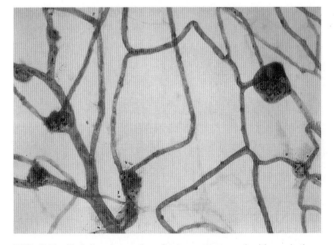

FIG. 8-5. Relative loss of pericytes compared with endothelial cells. Numerous hypercellular microaneurysms are also present. From Green WR, Wilson DJ. Histopathology of diabetic retinopathy. In: Franklin MR, ed. *Retina and vitreous.* New York: Kugler, 1993;63–81.

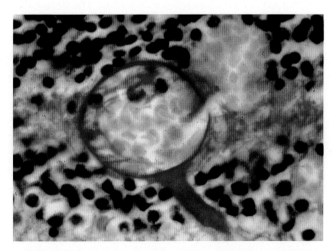

FIG. 8-7. Intraretinal hemorrhage due to rupture in the wall of a microaneurysm. From Green WR, Wilson DJ. Histopathology of diabetic retinopathy. In: Franklin MR, ed. *Retina and vitreous.* New York: Kugler, 1993;63–81.

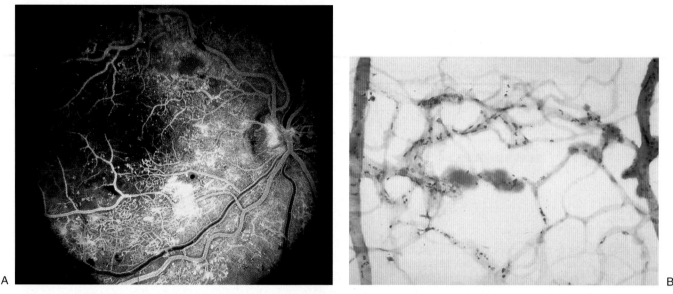

FIG. 8-8. (**A**) Capillary nonperfusion temporal to the fovea. Intraretinal microvascular abnormalities are present along the inferotemporal vessels. (**B**) Intraretinal microvascular abnormalities and acellular capillary beds between two larger retinal vessels.

Neovascularization

Neovascularization is the defining characteristic of proliferative diabetic retinopathy. High-risk proliferative diabetic retinopathy is associated with severe vision loss.[17] Therefore, recognizing the presence of neovascularization is critical in treating diabetic patients.

Neovascularization may develop intraretinally, preretinally, or on the optic nerve head. Neovascularization of the optic nerve head and preretinal neovascularization are most important clinically because these are the sites where vitreous traction on the neovascularization may occur and subsequently result in hemorrhage.

Angiogenesis, or the formation of blood vessels, is a complex process involving basement membrane lysis and endothelial cell proliferation and migration. The stimulus to these events in diabetic retinopathy is hypoxia due to closure of the retinal capillary bed. This stimulus is probably mediated by various growth factors and inhibitors present in the retina and vitreous. Factors potentially playing a role in neovascularization in diabetes are vascular endothelial growth factor, basic fibroblast growth factor, acidic fibroblast growth factor, platelet-derived growth factor, insulin-like growth factor, endothelial stimulating angiogenic factor, transforming growth factor-beta, and various inhibitors of neovascularization[18] (Fig. 8-10).

Neovascularization in diabetics typically originates from the venules and extends into the preretinal space (Fig. 8-11). The new blood vessels become intimately associated with the collagen of the cortical vitreous[19] (Fig. 8-12). The adherence of the adventitia of the new blood vessels to the vitreous collagen promotes preretinal and vitreous hemorrhage at the time of posterior vitreous detachment.

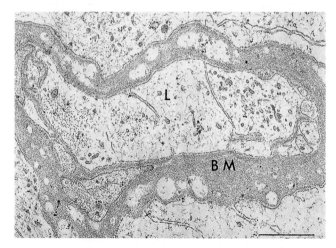

FIG. 8-9. Electron microscopy of this occluded capillary reveals a thickened basement membrane (BM) and lumen (L) have been filled by Mueller cell processes.

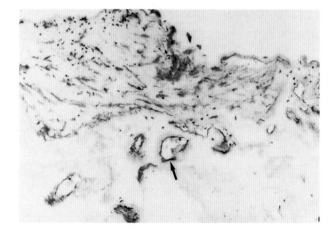

FIG. 8-10. Vitreous neovascularization immunostained for platelet-derived growth factor–beta chain. There is marked staining of the neovascular vessels within the membrane.

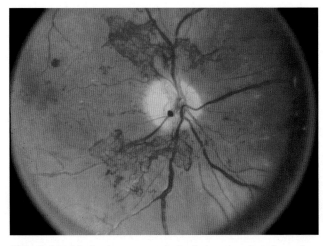

FIG. 8-11. Marked neovascularization extending from the optic nerve head.

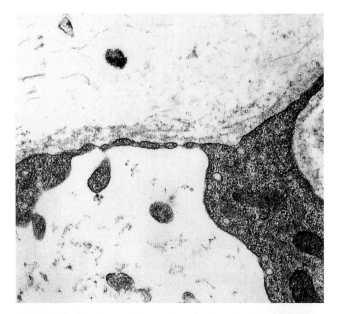

FIG. 8-13. Electron microscopy of neovascular vessel removed from the vitreous showing fenestrated endothelium. From Green WR, Wilson DJ. Histopathology of diabetic retinopathy. In: Franklin RM, ed. *Retina and vitreous.* New York: Kugler, 1993;63–81.

Initially, the new blood vessels lack well-developed intercellular junctions and may have a fenestrated endothelium (Fig. 8-13). These features explain the striking ''leakage'' of fluorescein from these vessels on fluorescein angiography.[20] As the neovascularization develops, the endothelial cells acquire some junctional complexes. In addition, the blood vessel growth is accompanied by the migration of other cellular elements into the vitreous cavity. Many of these other cellular elements contain intracytoplasmic actin and are capable of cell-mediated contraction.[21] Because the neovascular complex being tethered at one end by the retina and to the vitreous at the other, cell-mediated contraction can result in traction retinal detachments.

Secondary Retinal Changes

Edema and Exudates

Leakage of plasma through microaneurysms and other diabetic vascular abnormalities produces retinal edema (Fig. 8-14). Some components of the leakage, water and

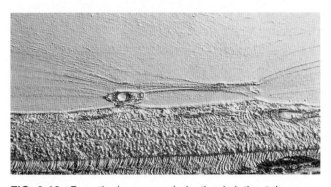

FIG. 8-12. Preretinal neovascularization is intimately associated with the cortical vitreous. From ref. 19, published courtesy of Springer-Verlag.

electrolytes, are removed by the transport mechanisms of the **retinal pigment epithelium** (RPE) and retinal vascular endothelium, but lipid remains in the retina in the form of ''hard exudates.'' The lipid is phagocytized by **microglial cells** (Fig. 8-15). Both edema and exudates are most abundant in the outer plexiform layer, but they also are present in the inner nuclear and ganglion cell layers. The exact mechanism by which edema and exudates cause diminished visual acuity is not known.

Hemorrhages

Hemorrhages in the nerve fiber layer of the retina are linear because the extravascular blood becomes aligned parallel to the axons within this layer of the retina (Fig. 8-16). Rounded **dot-and-blot** hemorrhages are in the nuclear and plexiform layers where they displace the neurons and glial cells and are limited at the periphery by undamaged neurons and Mueller cells (Fig. 8-17).

Clinically, the most important type of hemorrhage that occurs in diabetics is the **preretinal** or **vitreous hemorrhage** (Fig. 8-18). As described earlier, the neovascularization that occurs in diabetics becomes intimately associated with the cortical vitreous. When a posterior vitreous detachment occurs in a diabetic patient, the vitreous puts traction on the neovascular complex and often a vitreous hemorrhage occurs. This hemorrhage may initially be limited to the preretinal space; however, it usually also diffuses into the vitreous cavity.

Blood present within the vitreous cavity is broken down into hemoglobin globules and ghost cells (Fig. 8-19). If

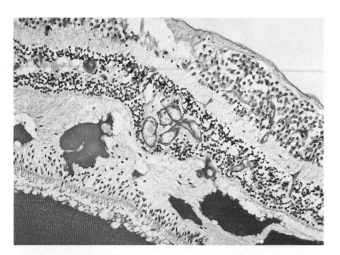

FIG. 8-14. Prominent intraretinal microvascular abnormalities and surrounding retinal edema. Edema is present in the outer plexiform layer.

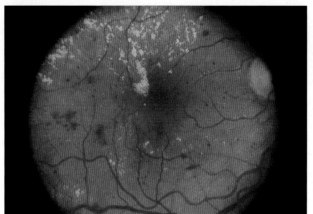

A

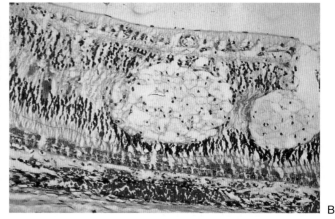

B

FIG. 8-15. (A) Hard exudates. **(B)** Lipid is phagocytized by microglial cells within the retina. From Green WR and Wilson DJ. Histopathology of diabetic retinopathy. In Franklin RM, ed. *Retina and vitreous.* New York: Kugler, 1993;63–81.

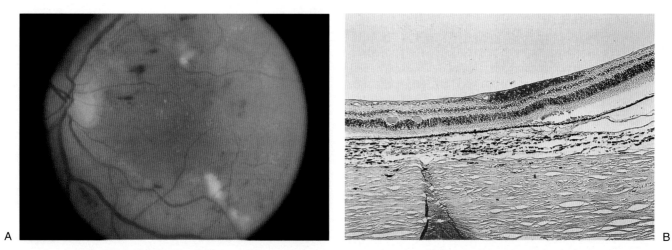

A

B

FIG. 8-16. (A) Nerve fiber-layer hemorrhage. **(B)** Hemorrhage in the nerve fiber layer spreads out parallel to the nerve fibers.

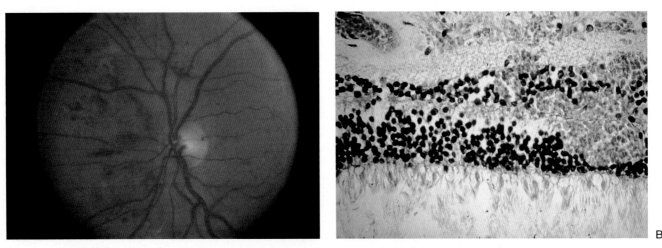

FIG. 8-17. (**A**) Rounded "dot-and-blot" hemorrhages. One nerve fiber layer hemorrhage is also present. (**B**) Dot-and-blot hemorrhages are present in the deeper retinal layers, where expansion of the hemorrhage is limited by the adjacent glial cells.

the latter gain access to the anterior chamber, ghost-cell glaucoma may ensue.

Cotton-Wool Spots

Cotton-wool spots, which are microinfarctions of the nerve fiber, have been reproduced experimentally and have been shown to represent interruptions of axoplasmic flow.[22] In flat preparations of the retina, the capillary bed beneath the cotton-wool spot is acellular and the feeding arteriole is occluded indicating these lesions are due to arteriolar occlusion. By light microscopy, the ganglion cell and nerve fiber layers are thickened by a sharply circumscribed lesion (Fig. 8-20). Within the lesion are **cytoid bodies,** which are globular structures 10 to 20 μm in diameter. By electron microscopy, the cytoid body has been shown to be degenerated axoplasmic organelles (mitochondria, neurofilaments, and endoplasmic

reticulum).[23] After resolution of the cotton-wool spot, inner retinal ischemic atrophy may be present, producing a local area of retinal thinning (described clinically as the **retinal depression sign**).[24]

Traction Retinal Detachment

Persistent traction on the retina by a partially detached vitreous or cell-mediated contraction from preretinal neovascular complexes can result in various degrees of retinal changes. Traction can produce **schisis cavities** within the retina. Avulsion of a retinal vessel (venous loop) may occur. In some instances, detachment of the retina from the underlying RPE may occur, producing a traction retinal detachment (Fig. 8-21). With prolonged detachment of the retina, the photoreceptor layers atrophy and glial cells proliferate.

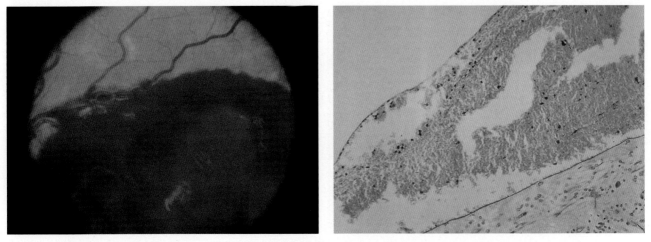

FIG. 8-18. (**A**) Preretinal hemorrhage obscures underlying retinal vessels. (**B**) Preretinal hemorrhage, sandwiched between the internal limiting membrane and the posterior hyaloid. From Green WR, Wilson DJ. Histopathology of diabetic retinopathy. In: Franklin RM, ed. *Retina and vitreous.* New York: Kugler, 1993;63–81.

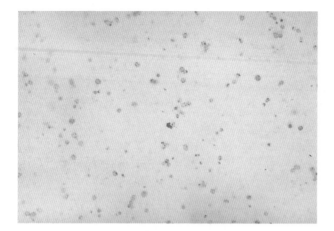

FIG. 8-19. Hemoglobin globules and ghost cells.

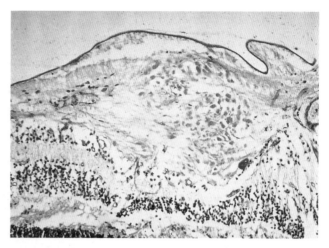

FIG. 8-20. Globular structures in the nerve fiber layer known as *cytoid bodies*.

Histopathology of Diabetic Retinopathy Treatment

Photocoagulation

Various types of photocoagulation have been used to treat diabetic retinopathy. The Diabetic Retinopathy Study was a prospective, randomized trial that demonstrated the efficacy of **panretinal photocoagulation** in treating proliferative diabetic retinopathy and preventing clinical blindness from it.[25] Similarly, the Early Treatment of Diabetic Retinopathy Study demonstrated the efficacy of **focal photocoagulation** in the treatment of diabetic macular edema.[26] All the different wavelengths of light used in the treatment of diabetic retinopathy have in common their ability to be absorbed by the intraocular tissues and to subsequently inflict thermal injury to the absorbing and adjacent tissues. The location and the extent of the injury depends on the wavelength and the intensity of the light, the duration of application, and the density of the absorbing pigment within the tissue.

The most commonly employed source of light for photocoagulation is the argon laser (Fig. 8-22). It produces blue-green light with wavelengths of 483 and 514 nanometers. As currently used in peripheral retinal photocoagulation, the argon laser results in variable destruction of the inner retina, destruction of the RPE, and occlusion of the choriocapillaries (Fig. 8-23).[27] These lesions heal by proliferation of the adjacent RPE to heal the defect (Fig. 8-24) and glial scarring. In a small number of lesions, Bruch's membrane is ruptured, but only rarely does choroidal neovascularization occur as a complication.

A blue-light absorbing pigment, called **xanthophyll pigment,** is present within the central 2 degrees of the retina. Argon blue-green laser treatment to this region of the retina prominently damages the inner retina due to

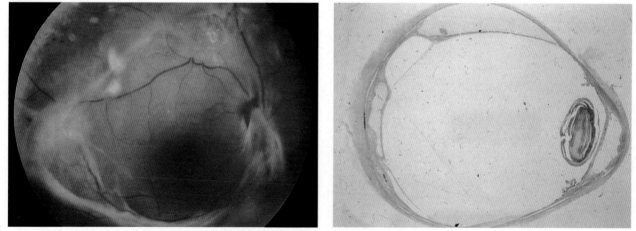

FIG. 8-21. (**A**) Traction retinal detachment superiorly due to preretinal fibrovascular tissue. (**B**) Traction retinal detachment with retina elevated from the underlying retinal pigment epithelium. From Green WR, Wilson DJ. Histopathology of diabetic retinopathy. In: Franklin RM, ed. *Retina and vitreous.* New York: Kugler, 1993;63–81.

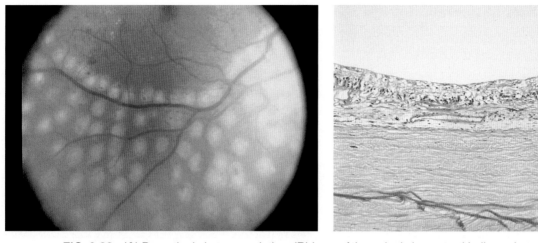

FIG. 8-22. (**A**) Panretinal photocoagulation. (**B**) Loss of the retinal pigment epithelium, photoreceptors, and a portion of the inner nuclear layer in a peripheral area of photocoagulation.

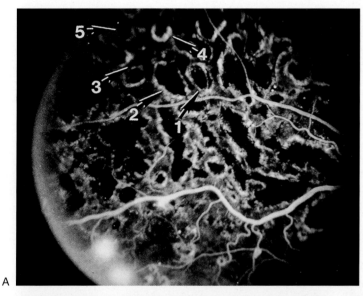

FIG. 8-23. (**A**) Fluorescein angiogram of laser photoco-agulation burns. Numbers correspond to numbers in B. (**B**) Defects in this injected plastic cast of the choriocapil-laris correspond to the photocoagulation burns. (**C**) Higher magnification of lesion #4 showing sharp demar-cation of the choriocapillaris filling defect. From Wilson DJ, Green WR. Argon laser panretinal photocoagulation for diabetic retinopathy: scanning electron microscopy of human choroid vascular casts. *Arch Ophthalmol* 125:239–242, 1987. Published courtesy of the Ameri-can Medical Association.

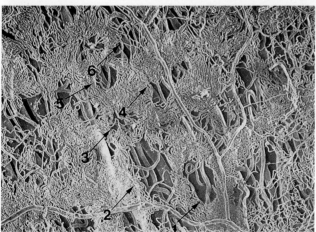

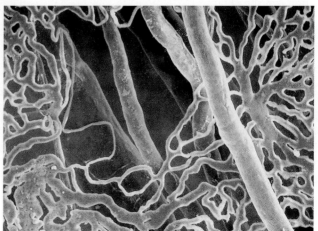

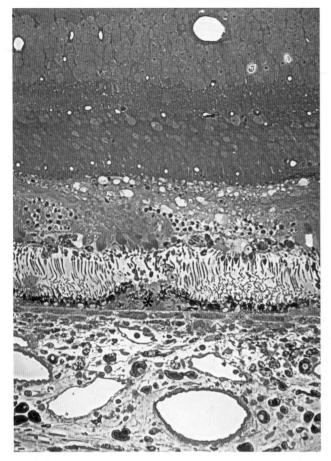

FIG. 8-24. Heaped-up retinal pigment epithelium (RPE) cells at the margin of two photocoagulation burns (*asterisk*). Cells in this area are dividing to repopulate the adjacent areas of damaged RPE.

the presence of this pigment. Consequently, when treatment is performed in this area, the blue wavelengths of the argon laser are removed by filtering. The damage produced by the argon green laser is confined to the outer retina and the choroid.[28]

Other sources of light are less commonly used in photocoagulation. Xenon photocoagulation results in full-thickness retinal injury. The Krypton laser, the diode laser, the double-frequency YAG laser, and the ruby laser produce an injury similar to the argon green laser.[29] Yellow wavelengths from the tunable dye laser are absorbed principally by hemoglobin and, therefore, are sometimes used for destroying vascular abnormalities.

The mechanism by which laser photocoagulation has a beneficial effect in proliferative diabetic retinopathy and in diabetic macular edema is not known. Several theories have been proposed to explain the regression of neovascularization that follows panretinal photocoagulation. These theories include the following: (1) destruction of ischemic retinal tissue with subsequent reduction in angiogenic factors previously produced by the ischemic tissue[30]; (2) improved oxygenation of the inner retina due to destruction

of the outer retina[31]; and (3) a decrease in the metabolic requirements of the inner retina due to loss of synaptic input to the inner retina from the outer retina.[32]

Similarly, the mechanism by which focal macular photocoagulation results in reduced macular edema is not fully understood. Wallow and associates have shown in clinicopathologic studies of human specimens that focal photocoagulation does not definitely occlude microaneurysms.[33] In an experimental study of grid macular photocoagulation, Wilson et al demonstrated that initially following grid photocoagulation, there was no apparent damage to the inner retinal capillaries. Nevertheless, between 3 days and 1 month after grid photocoagulation, there was delayed involution of the capillary bed[34] (Fig. 9-25). These studies suggest that in macular photocoagulation, the effect of laser on the retinal vessels may not be direct occlusion of the vessels, but rather a delayed indirect involution of the retinal capillaries.

Surgical Treatment

There have been few histopathologic studies of the surgical treatment of diabetic retinopathy. In most instances, surgical treatment consists of **vitrectomy** to remove vitreous hemorrhage or to repair a traction detachment of the fovea. Once the vitreous has been removed, there generally is atrophy of the neovascular complexes on the optic nerve head and in the posterior retina; however, the peripheral vitreous is never completely removed, and in some cases, there is neovascularization of the remaining anterior vitreous, so-called **anterior hyaloidal fibrovascular proliferation** (Fig. 8-26). This neovascularization can extend across the posterior lens capsule and can be the source of postvitrectomy hemorrhage and anterior traction retinal detachment.

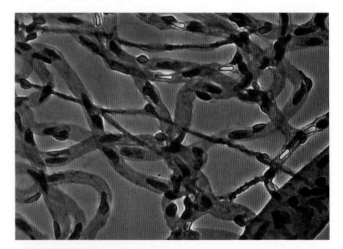

FIG. 8-25. Atrophic acellular vessels in trypsin digest preparation after grid macular photocoagulation. From ref. 34, published courtesy of the American Medical Association.

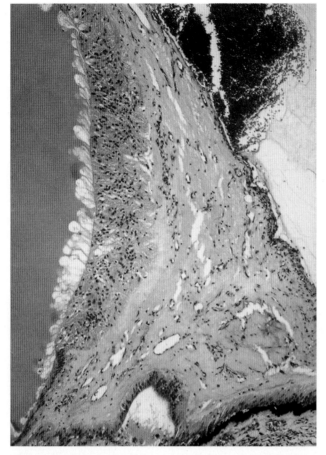

FIG. 8-26. Marked vascularization of the remaining anterior vitreous. Vascularized vitreous adherent to the ciliary epithelium and the peripheral retina produces anterior traction on the peripheral retina.

CHOROID

Previously, the choroidal vasculature was not considered to be involved with the vascular changes of diabetes. Recently, several authors have reported changes in the choroidal vasculature in patients with diabetes mellitus. These changes included **capillary dropout, beaded capillaries, arteriovenous anastomoses,** and **neovascularization.** The significance of these changes is not presently known.[35,36]

IRIS

Iris neovascularization is commonly present in patients with diabetic retinopathy. This neovascularization typically takes the form of nonprogressive neovascularization of the pupillary border with mild **ectropion uvea.** In some cases, and particularly after vitrectomy, iris neovascularization may be more severe. In these cases, **peripheral anterior synechia** formation with subsequent **neovascular glaucoma** may develop.

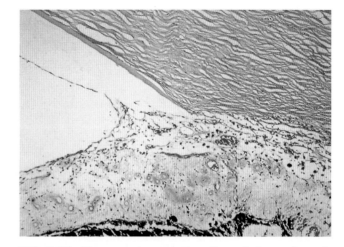

FIG. 8-27. Fine vessels present on the anterior surface of the peripheral iris and adherent to the trabecular meshwork. Corneal endothelium is artifactitiously detached.

The histologic features of iris neovascularization are the presence of fine vessels on the anterior surface of the iris and ectropion uvea (Fig. 8-27). With time, the iris surface vessels may become covered with a basement membrane structure resembling Descement's membrane. This membrane can extend across the trabecular meshwork creating a "pseudoangle."

In patients with chronic hyperglycemia, the iris pigment epithelium becomes laden with glycogen. This results in the histologic appearance of **lacy vacuolization** (Fig. 8-28).

CORNEA

The corneal epithelial basement membrane is thickened in diabetics. This also is true of the basement membrane of other intraocular epithelial cells such as the nonpig-

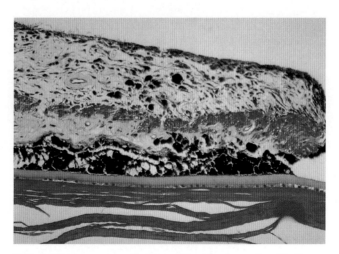

FIG. 8-28. Lacy vacuolization of the iris pigment epithelium.

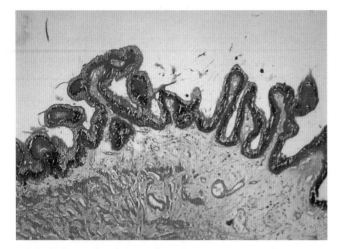

FIG. 8-29. Marked thickening of the basement membrane of the nonpigmented ciliary epithelium.

mented ciliary body epithelium (Fig. 8-29). The thickened basement membrane of the corneal epithelium is significant in that it predisposes these patients to recurrent corneal erosions and prolongs the healing of any epithelial defect. Azar and associates have produced evidence that the number of epithelial adhesion plaques are reduced in the corneal epithelial cells of diabetic patients.[37]

REFERENCES

1. The Diabetes Control and Complications Trial Research Group. The effect of intensive treatment of diabetes on the development and progression of long term complications in insulin dependent diabetes mellitus. *N Eng J Med* 1993;329:977–986.
2. Atkinson MA, Maclaren NK. The pathogenesis of insulin-dependent diabetes mellitus. *N Eng J Med* 1994;331:1428–1436.
3. Scriver CR, Beudet AL, Sly WS, Valle D, eds. *Daniel Foster: diabetes mellitus.* New York: MacGraw-Hill, 1989:chap 10.
4. Kinoshita JH. Aldose reductase in the diabetic eye. XLIII Edward Jackson Memorial Lecture. *Am J Ophthalmol* 1986;102:685–692.
5. Engerman RL, Kern TS, Garment MD. Capillary basement membrane in retina, kidney, and muscle of diabetic dogs and its response to 5 years aldose reductase inhibition. *J Diabetes Complications* 1993;7: 241–245.
6. Ashton N. Studies of the retinal capillaries in relation to diabetic and other retinopathies. *Br J Ophthalmol* 1963;47:521–538.
7. Frank RN, Keirn RJ, Kennedy A, et al. Galactose induced retinal capillary basement membrane thickening: prevention by sorbinil. *Invest Ophthalmol Vis Sci* 1983;24:1519–1524.
8. Robison WG Jr, Kador PF, Kinoshita JH. Retinal capillaries: basement membrane thickening by galactosemia prevented with aldose reductase inhibitor. *Science* 1983;221:1177–1179.
9. Sorbinil Retinopathy Trial Research Group. A randomized trial of sorbinil, an aldose reductase inhibitor, in diabetic retinopathy. *Arch Ophthalmol* 1990;108:1234–1244.
10. Cogan DG, Toussaint D, Kuwabara T. Studies of retinal vascular patterns IV. Diabetic retinopathy. *Arch Ophthalmol* 1961;66:100–112.
11. Kuwabara T, Cogan DG. Studies of retinal vascular patterns. VI. Mural cells of the retinal capillaries. *Arch Ophthalmol.* 1963;69: 492–502.
12. Orlidge A, D'Amore P. Inhibition of capillary endothelial cell growth by pericytes and smooth muscle cells. *J Cell Biol* 1987;37: 277–299.
13. de Venecia G, Davis M, Engerman R. Clinicopathologic correlations in diabetic retinopathy. I. Histology and fluorescein angiography of microaneurysms. *Arch Ophthalmol* 1976;94:1766–1773.
14. Toussaint D, Dustin P. Electron microscopy of normal and diabetic retinal capillaries. *Arch Ophthalmol* 1963;70:140–152.
15. Bloodworth JMB Jr, Molitor DL. Ultrastructural aspects of human and canine diabetic retinopathy.
16. Kuwabara T, Cogan DG. Retinal vascular patterns. VII. Acellular change. In: Bettman J, ed. *Vascular disorders of the eye.* St. Louis: Mosby, 1966;77–86.
17. The Diabetic Retinopathy Study Research Group. Preliminary report on the effects of photocoagulation therapy. *Am J Ophthalmol* 1976;81:383–396.
18. Robbins SG, Mixon RN, Wilson DJ, et al. Platelet-derived growth factor ligands and receptors immunolocalized in proliferative retinal diseases. *Invest Ophthalmol Vis Sci* 1994;35:3649–3663.
19. Faulborn S, Bowald S. Microproliferations in proliferative diabetic retinopathy and their relationship to the vitreous: corresponding light and electron microscopic studies. *Graefe's Arch Clin Exp Ophthalmol* 1985;223:130–138.
20. Wallow IHL, Geldner PS. Endothelial fenestrae in proliferative diabetic retinopathy. *Invest Ophthalmol Vis Sci* 1980;19:1176–1183.
21. Wallow IHL, Greaser ML, Stevens TS. Actin filaments in diabetic fibrovascular preretinal membrane. *Arch Ophthalmol* 1981;99: 2175–2181.
22. McLeod D, Marshall J, Kohner EM, et al. The role of axoplasmic transport in the pathogenesis of cotton-wool spots. *Br J Ophthalmol* 1977;61:177–191.
23. Shakib M, Ashton N. Focal retinal ischaemia. II. Ultrastructural changes in focal retinal ischaemia. *Br J Ophthalmol* 1966;50:325–384.
24. Goldbaum MH. Retinal depression sign indicating a small retinal infarct. *Am J Ophthalmol* 1978;86:45–55.
25. Diabetic Retinopathy Study Research Group. Photocoagulation treatment of proliferative diabetic retinopathy: clinical application of Diabetic Research Study (DRS) findings, DRS report number 8. *Ophthalmology* 1981;88:583–600.
26. Early Treatment Diabetic Retinopathy Study Research Group. Early photocoagulation for diabetic retinopathy. *Ophthalmology* 1991;98: 766–785.
27. Wallow IHL, Davis MD. Clinicopathologic correlation of xenon arc and argon laser photocoagulation: procedures in human diabetic eyes. *Arch Ophthalmol* 1979;97:2308–2315.
28. Smiddy WE, Fine SL, Green WR, et al. Clinicopathologic correlation of krypton red, argon blue-green, and argon green laser photocoagulation in the human fundus. *Retina* 1984;4:15–21.
29. McMullen WW, Garcia CA. Comparison of retinal photocoagulation using pulsed frequency-doubled neodymium-YAG and argon green laser. *Retina* 1992;12:265–269.
30. Michaelson IC. The mode of development of the vascular system of the retina, with some observations on its significance for certain retinal diseases. *Trans Ophthalmol Soc UK* 1948;68:137–180.
31. Wolbarsht ML, Landers MB III, Rand L. Modification of retinal vascularization by interaction between retinal and choroidal circulation. *Invest Ophthalmol Vis Sci* 1978;17(suppl):224.
32. Wilson DJ. Intraocular neovascularization and retinal energy metabolism. *Arch Ophthalmol* 1989;107:953.
33. Wallow IHL, Bindley C. Focal argon treatment of diabetic macular edema. *Invest Ophthalmol Vis Sci* 1988;29(suppl):36.
34. Wilson DJ, Finklestein D, Quigley HA, et al. "Grid" macular photocoagulation: a quantitative histologic study of the effect on the primate retinal capillaries. *Arch Ophthalmol* 1988;106:100–105.
35. Fryczkowski AW, Sato SE, Hodes BL. Changes in the diabetic choroidal vasculature: scanning electron microscopy findings. *Ann Ophthalmol* 1988;20:299–305.
36. McLeod DS, Lutty GA. High resolution histologic analysis of the human choroidal vasculature. *Invest Ophthalmol Vis Sci* 1994;35: 3799–3811.
37. Azar DT, Spurr-Michaud SJ, Tisdale AS, et al. Altered epithelial-basement membrane interactions in diabetic corneas. *Arch Ophthalmol* 1992;110:537–540.

Ophthalmic Pathology with Clinical Correlations,
edited by Joseph W. Sassani, M.D.
Lippincott-Raven Publishers, Philadelphia © 1997.

CHAPTER 9

Trauma and Wound Healing

J. Douglas Cameron

The eye is exposed to many types of trauma, which all may lead to visual impairment. The visual outcome is difficult to predict, however, unless the natural history of the specific trauma is known.[1-3] For example, corneal abrasions may cause immediate visual loss and extreme pain, but usually do not cause permanent vision loss. Conversely, alkali injuries may be remarkably free of signs and symptoms initially, but eventually may cause ocular destruction. Intermediate between these two extremes in outcome is **commotio retinae,** a situation in which the initial signs and symptoms are variable and often not predictive of final functional outcome.

FUNDAMENTAL PATHOLOGIC PROCESSES IN OCULAR TRAUMA

Hemorrhage

Hemorrhage frequently is associated with ocular trauma. The degree of damage is related to the specific tissues involved and the amount of blood actually extravasated. Among the most damaging of hemorrhagic events is **expulsive choroidal hemorrhage,** which is arterial hemorrhage into the potential space between the choroid and sclera.[4-6] The choroid is only loosely attached to the sclera except at the scleral spur, the scleral canal of the optic nerve, and the entry sites of arteries and exit sites of the vortex veins. Arterial hemorrhage may occur during sudden shifts of intraocular pressure, eg, during cataract surgery or following perforation of a corneal ulcer. Sudden reduction of intraocular pressure establishes shearing forces that may cause disruption of an artery as it passes from the rigid sclera into the mobile tissues of the choroid. In the case of elderly individuals with rigid arterial walls, the vessel may not be able to constrict in a hemostatic

manner. The result is anterior displacement of the choroid, retina, vitreous, and lens toward and through the region of least pressure, which is the wound (Fig. 9-1). All internal contents of the globe may be extruded with extensive hemorrhage (Fig. 9-2).

Hemorrhage into the anterior chamber may result in glaucoma from multiple mechanisms. Red blood cells or the macrophages that attempt to remove them may occlude the trabecular meshwork, leading to secondary open-angle glaucoma. Obstruction to aqueous flow between the iris and lens by blood clot can lead to pupillary block and secondary angle-closure glaucoma.

Opacification of the corneal stroma by accumulated blood breakdown products is called **corneal blood staining**[7] (Fig. 9-3). This occurs when hemoglobin released from extravasated red blood cells crosses the endothelium and Descemet's membrane as small disassembled molecules, which reaggregate within the corneal stroma. The degree of opacification depends on multiple variables, including the amount of hemorrhage, the length of time from the original hemorrhage, the degree of intraocular pressure elevation, and the integrity of the endothelial cell barrier. In most cases, Descemet's membrane remains intact. The particles can be seen in histologic sections as discrete, uniform, reddish brown, somewhat angulated fragments, usually concentrated in the central corneal stroma (Fig. 9-4). The hemoglobin fragments are cleared very slowly by phacolytic and biochemical processes within the stroma. Blood staining of the cornea in childhood can result in dense amblyopia.

Toxic damage to ocular epithelial cells by iron cations is called **hemosiderosis bulbi** when the source of iron is from degenerating blood, and **siderosis bulbi** when the source of iron is from a foreign body.[8] In either event, the iron cation damages intracellular enzyme systems, leading to cellular dysfunction and cellular death. The cells at greatest risk are those with the highest metabolic rate, such as the epithelial cells of the lens (leading to a siderotic cataract) and the endothelial cells covering the

J. D. Cameron: Hennepin County Medical Center, Minneapolis, Minnesota 55415.

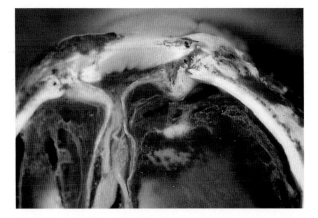

FIG. 9-1. Expulsive choroidal hemorrhage. Gross photograph of blood collecting in the suprachoroidal space, forcing the uveal tract and retina centrally. The surgical wound had been closed intraoperatively.

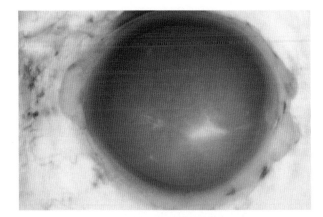

FIG. 9-3. Corneal blood staining. Gross photograph of a cornea impregnated with pigment derived from the fragmentation and displacement of red blood cells. The opaque cornea appears golden brown.

trabecular meshwork (leading to a type of secondary open-angle glaucoma). The ions also damage the cells of the retina, which are replaced by a glial reaction (Fig. 9-5).

The natural involution of extravasated red blood cells involves a stage in which they change from pliable biconcave discs to rigid spheres[9] (Fig. 9-6). Hemoglobin remaining within these **ghost cells** accumulates along the external plasma membrane as **Heinz bodies.** Usually, this stage is of no functional consequence except when the cells accumulate in the trabecular meshwork. The rigid forms cannot pass through the physical barrier of the trabecular meshwork, and they accumulate causing secondary obstruction and glaucoma. Treatment may require removing the red blood cells by irrigating the anterior chamber to reestablish normal aqueous outflow. Ghost cells are not often identified in paraffin-embedded sections because of their osmotic fragility. They are best seen by viewing an aqueous or vitreous aspirate by phase-

contrast microscopy or by standard cytology preparation techniques (cytospin) (Fig. 9-7).

The red blood cells found in various hemoglobinopathies, such as sickle cell anemia, also are rigid, and may obstruct the trabecular meshwork.[10] In states of hypoxemia, these cells may cause vascular obstruction and thrombosis, leading to markedly destructive entities such as anterior segment necrosis.

Hemorrhage in the posterior segment of the eye may cause significant visual impairment over an extended period because mechanisms for clearing blood are extremely limited in this region. Extravasated red blood cells in the vitreous often degenerate in situ instead of being processed by macrophages and eliminated through vascular channels as they usually would be in other parts of the body. Partially degenerated red cell membranes associated with partially catabolized hemoglobin may accumulate on the free surface of a detached vitreous to form an *ochre membrane* (Fig. 9-8). This membrane is important

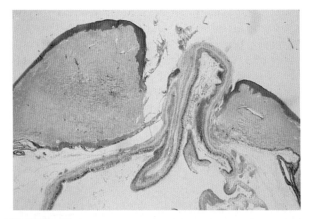

FIG. 9-2. Expulsive choroidal hemorrhage. Photomicrograph of a case in which the wound could not be closed allowing the retina to be prolapsed externally.

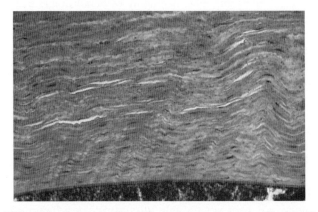

FIG. 9-4. Cross-section of a cornea stained with blood breakdown products. There is often a gradient of density from the posterior cornea, where gross hemorrhage can be seen, to the anterior cornea, where the pigment is less dense.

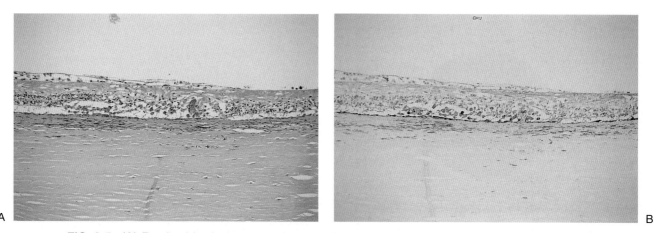

FIG. 9-5. (**A**) Routine histologic preparation and (**B**) special stain for iron of retina in siderosis bulbi.

because it may be misinterpreted ultrasonographically as a retinal detachment. The red cell membranes are degraded to cholesterol, which may be seen as red-gold to golden brown mobile particles in the dependent portion of the vitreous cavity in the liquid vitreous (synchesis scintillans) (Fig. 9-9). This latter condition must be distinguished from **asteroid hyaloid bodies,** which are fixed calcium soaps within the formed vitreous. When tissue is processed for paraffin-embedded sections, cholesterol is dissolved by organic solvents used to prepare the tissue for sectioning leaving voids in the paraffin, known as **cholesterol clefts.** Cholesterol clefts only indicate the presence of extensive amounts of cholesterol and may be seen in conditions without extravasation of red blood cells, such as Coats' disease in which incompetent retinal blood vessels leak plasm proteins.

The presence of degenerating red blood cells and extravasated plasma often stimulates the eye's repair mechanisms. The principal repair mechanism is the production of fibrovascular tissue outside of the retina and of fibro-

glial tissue within the retina.[11,12] The difference in occurrence of these two forms of repair processes is due to the fact that the intraretinal glial cells are not capable for forming extracellular collagen, but form a repair structure by producing intracellular elements.

Extraretinal fibrovascular proliferation within both the anterior chamber and the posterior segment can result in displacement of tissue by contractile forces of fibroblasts, which develop characteristics of smooth muscles (myofibroblasts). In the anterior chamber, this type of reaction may produce peripheral anterior synechiae and fibrosis. In the posterior chamber, fibrous organization of a vitreous hemorrhage may produce total tractional retinal detachment. Organization of hemorrhage on the anterior vitreous face across the posterior chamber may stimulate formation of a *cyclitic membrane,* which originates in the region of the anterior border of the vitreous base and extends parallel to the iris diaphragm but posterior to the crystalline lens. Contraction of a cyclitic membrane does not influence the retina, but pulls the ciliary body from the overlying sclera causing ciliary body dysfunction and ocular hypotony.[13]

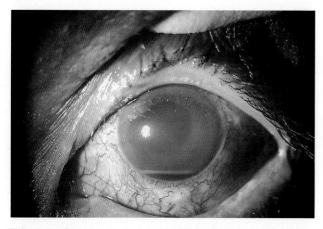

FIG. 9-6. Ghost-cell glaucoma. Clinical photograph of partially denatured red blood cells in the inferior anterior chamber angle. The distinctive khaki color is a helpful clue in distinguishing ghost-cell glaucoma from a fresh hyphema.

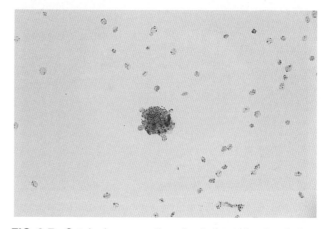

FIG. 9-7. Cytologic preparation of cells from ghost-cell glaucoma showing individual red blood cell remnants.

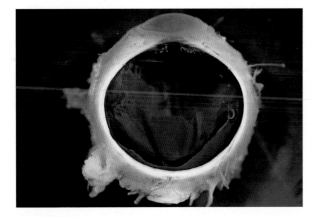

FIG. 9-8. Gross photograph of blood accumulating on the face of a detached vitreous. The retina is attached. The density of the blood may give a false impression of a detached retina by echography.

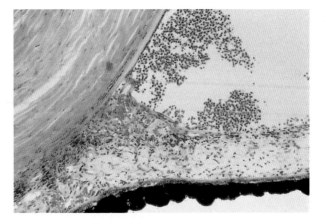

FIG. 9-10. Photomicrograph of peripheral anterior synechiae. The anterior surface of the iris has come in contact with the posterior surface of the cornea, causing total obstruction of aqueous outflow.

Inflammation

Inflammation associated with ocular trauma may be stimulated by hemorrhage, foreign material introduced at injury, tissue necrosis, and immune reaction to newly exposed antigens.

Disruption of tissue often leads to tissue necrosis. The degree of necrosis may be limited for well-defined wounds, such as those created by a knife or other sharp object, but may be extensive in crush injuries. The degree of injury also is influenced by interruption of vascular channels supplying the adjacent tissue.

The inflammatory process itself may further compromise tissue and its function. The anterior chamber angle is particularly vulnerable, either to direct injury to the trabecular meshwork or to functional compromise, like that caused by peripheral anterior synechiae formation

(Fig 9-10). Inflammation in the pupillary space may generate a membrane at the plane of the pupil (occlusio pupillae) or complete posterior synechiae (seclusio pupillae) (Fig. 9-11). The delicate microenvironment of the lens can be totally disrupted by even small amounts of inflammation, thereby leading to posterior subcapsular cataract or anterior subcapsular fibrous plaque (Fig. 9-12).

Inflammation in the vitreous also is a potential source of transvitreal membranes composed of myofibroblasts, which have the potential to contract, leading to traction retinal detachment. Inflammation in the choroid may cause serous retinal detachment and can result in subretinal neovascularization if Bruch's membrane is ruptured.

An inflammatory process that is especially important in the setting of ocular trauma is **sympathetic ophthalmia** both because it is unique to the eye, and because

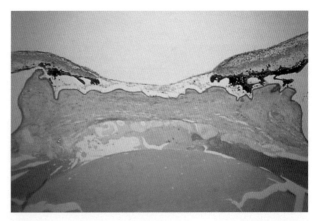

FIG. 9-11. Photomicrograph of an eye removed because of persistent inflammation. The posterior surface of the iris has become adherent to the anterior surface of the lens, obstructing aqueous outflow from the posterior chamber to the anterior chamber (seclusio pupillae). Also, delicate membrane has formed across the pupillary space (not seen in this photograph) causing occlusio pupillae.

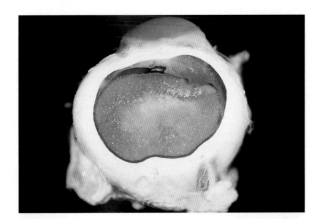

FIG. 9-9. Gross photograph of a phthisical eye with multiple cholesterol crystals in the subretinal space. The crystals are a degradation product of long-staining intraocular hemorrhage.

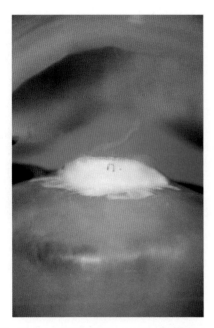

FIG. 9-12. Gross photograph of a crystalline lens with a discrete anterior subcapsular cataract. The environment due to persistent inflammation in the anterior chamber caused fibrous metaplasia of the anterior crystalline lens epithelium.

the final result may be bilateral blindness from unilateral injury.[14,15] Sympathetic ophthalmia is a diagnosis that can be established with certainty only with the combination of clinical and histologic inflammation. Precision in its diagnosis is important because the treatment may involve extremely long courses of antiinflammatory agents or cytotoxic agents.

Sympathetic ophthalmia may follow either accidental or surgical trauma. The incidence with accidental trauma is approximately 2 of every 1000 cases and is 1 in 10,000 cases with surgical trauma. The injured eye is termed the **exciting eye** and the noninjured eye is called the **sympathizing eye.** The inflammation is an autoimmune type of delayed hypersensitivity stimulated by retinal antigens most likely derived from the photoreceptor outer segments. Often, uveal tissue is incarcerated within the wound, although sympathetic ophthalmia has been reported to follow vitrectomy and cyclocryotherapy in which there apparently was no tissue prolapse.

The onset of sympathetic ophthalmia may occur between 5 days and several decades after the initial injury. Usually more than 14 days are required for the process to become clinically evident. More than 65% of cases begin between 2 weeks and 2 months after injury. The earliest clinical sign of sympathetic ophthalmia may be decreased accommodative range of the sympathizing eye followed by frank granulomatous anterior uveitis.

Histologically, there is a diffuse lymphocytic infiltrate of the uveal tract composed primarily of T lymphocytes. Epithelioid histiocytes and inflammatory giant cells, some of which contain melanin pigment, also are a prominent

feature. Eosinophils may be present early in the course of the disease, but plasma cells most often are not noted. Although there may be an extensive choroidal infiltrate, typically, the choriocapillaris is not involved. A classic feature is the presence of nodular accumulations of histiocytes between retinal pigment epithelium and Bruch's membrane called **Dalen-Fuchs nodules.** A perivascular infiltrate of chronic inflammatory cells may be prominent within preserved areas of retina. There is a 23% to 45% coassociation of sympathetic ophthalmia with phacoantigenic uveitis (previously called phacoanaphylactic endophthalmitis).

Glaucoma

Several mechanisms cause glaucoma in traumatized eyes. The glaucoma may follow the initial injury by hours or days (eg, in the case of hemorrhage obstructing the trabecular meshwork) or by decades (eg, subclinical damage combining with aging changes).[16]

Several mechanisms associated with hemorrhage have already been discussed (ghost-cell glaucoma, physical obstruction of the trabecular meshwork or pupil, siderotic damage to the trabecular meshwork, and anterior synechiae). In addition, disruption of the insertion of the longitudinal muscle bundle of the ciliary body to the scleral spur, known as *cyclodialysis,* may be followed initially by hypotony, but if the cleft closes spontaneously, there is a risk of an acute pressure elevation.

A delayed glaucoma mechanism is the migration of corneal endothelial cells over the adjacent trabecular beams in areas where the native trabecular endothelium has been damaged or lost. The migrating corneal endothelium may produce a Descemet's-like basement membrane, which may obstruct aqueous outflow.[17]

Displaced crystalline or artificial intraocular lenses, whether subluxed (partially dislocated) into the pupillary space or luxated (completely dislocated) into the anterior chamber, may result in pupillary block and secondary closed-angle glaucoma. A damaged lens also may undergo *phacolysis* in which denatured lens protein leaks through the lens capsule of a mature cataract, resulting in secondary open-angle glaucoma from obstruction of the trabecular meshwork by the proteinaceous material itself or by the macrophages that ingest it. The released protein does not appear to cause a type II hypersensitivity response as is found in phacoantigenic uveitis.

Surface epithelium, generally from the region of the limbus, may enter the eye at the time of injury or through a fistulous tract and then proliferate along the surface of Descemet's membrane or on the anterior iris.[18] In these areas, the stratified squamous epithelium may result in segmental corneal edema; however, if the squamous epithelium grows over the trabecular beams, the trabecular meshwork is altered and occluded by a fibrous tissue reaction to the overlying epithelial cells (Fig. 9-13).

DEGENERATION OF THE EYE FOLLOWING TRAUMA (PHTHISIS BULBI)

Following severe trauma or prolonged inflammation, the eye degenerates in a series of stages. *Phthisis bulbi* is the final degenerative state of the eye. In this condition, the globe shrinks to half its former diameter and becomes "squared off" by the continuing pressure of the four rectus muscles (Fig. 9-14). No intraocular structures can be identified except for an occasional calcified and degenerated lens, portions of remaining iris pigment epithelium, and various degrees of fibrous or osseous metaplasia in the plane of the retinal pigment epithelium. This condition may follow a diverse group of clinical problems such as retinopathy of prematurity or uveitis, but it is most often encountered in traumatized eyes. The common denominator is loss of intraocular pressure causing sustained hypotony and loss of nutrition to the tissues within the eye. The natural contractility of the sclera causes collapse of the eye and apparent thickening of the posterior sclera.

Two major stages of ocular degeneration precede phthisis bulbi. The first of these stages is **atrophia bulbi without shrinkage.** Initially, the size and shape of the eye are maintained. The sclera is of normal size, and the intraocular pressure is in the normal range. The structures most sensitive to loss of nutrition are the crystalline lens, which

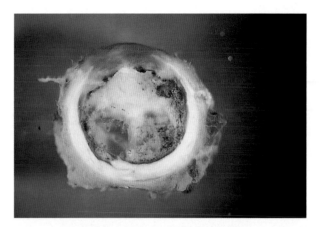

FIG. 9-14. Gross photograph of a phthisical eye. The globe is compressed by the four rectus muscles changing the overall contour of the eye from spherical to "squared." The internal contents of the eye are severely atrophic and disorganized. The posterior sclera markedly thickens. The peripheral corneal tissue often invaginates into the anterior chamber.

becomes opaque, and the neurosensory retina, which loses light-sensitive tissue while retaining more resistant glial cells. The retinal pigment epithelium becomes incompetent and allows accumulation of subretinal serous fluid. The retinal pigment epithelial cells may undergo metaplastic transformation (change from one type of differentiated cell to another), taking on the form of fibroblasts producing collagenous tissue or osteoblasts producing bone (Fig. 9-15). The endothelial cells lining the trabecular meshwork may degenerate and not allow filtration of aqueous.

The penultimate degenerative stage is **atrophia bulbi with shrinkage,** in which ciliary body dysfunction leads to progressive diminution of intraocular pressure. The

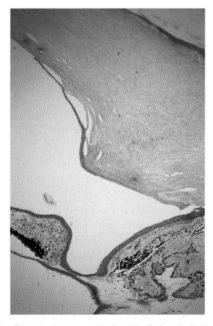

FIG. 9-13. Photomicrograph of epithelial cells lining the posterior surface of the cornea and the internal surface of the trabecular meshwork. The epithelial cells obstruct aqueous outflow and modify the structure of the collagen of the trabecular beams, causing irreversible scarring.

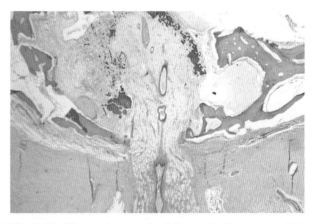

FIG. 9-15. Photomicrograph of tissue in the plane of the retinal pigment epithelium. The area has become filled with metaplastic bone, probably originating from the retinal pigment epithelium itself. The bone is clearly visible by all imaging techniques. Hematopoietic tissue may develop within the ectopic bone.

globe becomes smaller, and the scleral contour is altered both by contraction of scar tissue adjacent to the sclera and orbital tissue and by rectus muscle pressure. The anterior chamber collapses. The cornea becomes vascularized, opaque, and frequently becomes corrugated, with the most prominent folds in the region of the limbus. Internal structures of the eye are in a more advanced state of degeneration, but remain histologically identifiable. This stage progresses to phthisis bulbi.

Pathologic Anatomy and Physiology

Risk factors secondary to structure are characteristics and special features that make a tissue particularly vulnerable to injury. For example, the orbicularis oculi muscle tends to separate lid margin lacerations. This tissue characteristic actually exacerbates wounds in this region. Similarly, structures are particularly vulnerable to injury at their sites of attachment to other tissues because of the concentration of forces at these points. The attachment of the iris diaphragm to the face of the ciliary body and the attachment of the retina at the ora serrata are two examples of structural relationships that tend to exacerbate injuries in these areas. On the other hand, a tissue characteristic may tend to decrease the complexity of a wound. For example, swelling of the corneal stroma may actually self-seal small full-thickness corneal lacerations.

Certain mechanisms of injury may be much more common in one tissue than in another. For example, mechanical injuries are more common in the cornea than in the retina. Conversely, vascular-mediated injury is more common in the retina than in the cornea.

The specific reaction to injury varies considerably among tissues. This characteristic is particularly true of the ocular tissues, which tend to be highly differentiated and specialized. For example, the transparent cornea, which is composed almost exclusively of extracellular material, and the transparent retina, which has almost no extracellular space, are both vulnerable because transparency depends on the uniformity of their components, whether cellular or extracellular. In these tissues, the healing process, even in the best of circumstances, restores their structural integrity but not the regularity of structure that is the key to their transparency.

Knowledge and understanding of the projected clinical course for the specific injury are key to planning a treatment strategy aimed at minimizing potential vision loss. For example, the late scarring process of alkali injury must be anticipated so a treatment regimen to prevent it can be devised.

Eyelids

The eyelids are subject to the same mechanisms of injury as the rest of the cutaneous surface including abra-

sion, laceration, concussion, thermal injury (including electrical), chemical contact, and radiation. The eyelids and associated structures protect the eye from the environment and maintain the cornea by producing and distributing tears. Movement of the eyelids is accomplished by the neuromuscular apparatus of the orbicularis oculi, with its origin and insertion at the nasal orbit, and by the levator muscle and aponeurosis, which are relatively exposed at the superior orbital rim. The facial nerve, which innervates the orbicularis, is vulnerable because of its long course through the soft tissue of the midface to the orbicularis. The eyelid skin surface is only loosely attached to the underlying connective tissue, which provides an expandable compartment for edema fluid or extravasated blood.

An especially damaging injury is laceration of the lid margin. The orientation of the fibers of the orbicularis tend to separate the margins of the wound, causing notching of the lid margin (Fig. 9-16). The lid margin is the principal instrument of tear distribution. Any malposition of it relative to the ocular surface, such as occurs with disruption of the neuromuscular apparatus of the lid, may seriously disrupt proper nutrition to the anterior cornea.

The tears are drained from the ocular surface through the nasal lacrimal duct system. This system is vulnerable to injury because it is anchored as part of the medial canthal tissue complex and is subject to disruption by shearing forces. Laceration or avulsion of the canalicular drainage apparatus prevents exit of tears, causing the tears

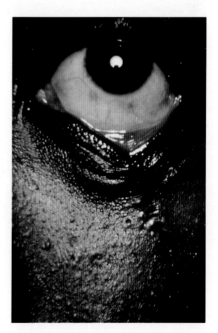

FIG. 9-16. Clinical photograph of marked distortion of the eyelid margin secondary to scarring of a full-thickness cutaneous laceration perpendicular to the eyelid margin. Reconstructive surgery is necessary to preserve the eye's function.

to spill over the cutaneous surface and resulting in maceration of the keratinized squamous epithelium.

The eyelid skin heals in the same manner as the rest of the cutaneous surface.[19,20] Initially, the wound is stabilized by hemostatic mechanisms and the extravasation of fibrin. The fibrin forms a temporary layer protecting vulnerable underlying soft tissue from drying and from contamination by microorganisms. This protein-rich material also contains the signals necessary to direct the next cellular stage of healing. The temporary fibrin surface membrane contains fibronectin, a protein capable of influencing cell movement and direction. Adjacent healthy epithelial cells migrate over the fibronectin surface until cell contiguity is established. While migrating, the epithelial cells produce protein signals that affect the activity of the fibroblasts, such as the production of collagen and of proteolytic enzymes including collagenase. When continuity is reestablished, the epithelial cell layer is much thinner than normal at only one to two cell diameters thick. Normal thickness is established by cellular division of the newly migrated cells and by differentiation of the cells, which reestablishes the capability to prevent soft-tissue dessication. As the epithelium differentiates, it stops producing stimulating peptides.

During epithelial movement, underlying undamaged fibroblasts and vascular endothelial cells migrate to reestablish structural integrity in the wounded area. This activity of the subepithelial tissues also is modulated by the influence of fibronectin and associated proteins. The newly formed tissue composed of delicate blood vessels, fibroblasts, newly synthesized collagen, and extracellular matrix is called **granulation tissue** because it has the appearance of small granules on the surface of the wound (Fig. 9-17). The production of granulation tissue is quite different in origin and clinical significance from granulomatous inflammation, which is an inflammatory process characterized by the presence of multiple histiocytes and, possibly, multinucleated giant cells (see Chapter 3).

The granulation tissue scaffolding is also temporary. Through the process of tissue resorption and replacement (soft-tissue modeling), reparative tissue that, at best, restores tissue continuity and structural support, is produced. Nevertheless, highly specialized tissue, such as the hair follicles (including eyelashes), exocrine glands, and even the tarsal plate, are not regenerated. The specialized functions offered by these tissues are lost. The eyelid skin, however, has the functional advantage of being richly supplied with blood vessels that accelerate the wound healing process relative to skin on other body areas such as the trunk.

The Conjunctiva

The conjunctiva is a mucous membrane, a thin cellular tissue with a surface that is usually covered by a mucous layer to prevent tissue drying. The conjunctiva allows full movement of the eye within the orbit and forms an anterior covering of orbital tissue. The conjunctiva also provides a conduit for the flow of tears to the cornea. *Goblet cells,* which produce mucus, are located in focal areas throughout the conjunctiva but primarily at the nasal semilunar fold. Accessory lacrimal tissue also is present but primarily in the forniceal regions. The conjunctiva is only loosely adherent to Tenon's capsule, creating a potential space for the accumulation of blood, which is readily apparent clinically even from minor hemorrhage, and for air from paraorbital sinuses through orbital wall fractures. The conjunctiva's transparency is not essential to its function. Subconjunctival blood usually is of no clinical consequence except in blunt trauma in which the hemorrhage may hide an occult scleral rupture.

Lacerations of the conjunctiva, up to 1 cm in length, generally heal quickly and completely (even without sutures) in the protective environment provided by the eyelids. The surface epithelial cells migrate and proliferate in a manner similar to the cutaneous epithelium. Unfortunately, the underlying fibrovascular tissue responds, proliferates, and undergoes remodeling to form a repair tissue, which is much less delicate and less pliable than the native tissue.

The conjunctiva is particularly vulnerable to surface injury from chemical agents, primarily alkali.[21,22] The most common alkali agents are ammonia (including fertilizer), cleaning solutions, sodium hydroxide (lye), potash (caustic soda), and lime. Lime, which is usually in particulate form, can lodge in the fornices and act as a slow-release agent of alkali solution.

High-pH substances readily dissolve cellular membranes including cellular-rich tissue, such as the nonkeratinized superficial squamous epithelial cells of the con-

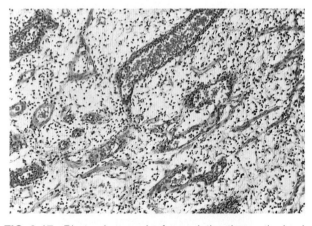

FIG. 9-17. Photomicrograph of granulation tissue, the basic building block for wound healing outside of the central nervous system. This example is from an inappropriately extensive wound healing response of the tarsal conjunctiva. The condition is often erroneously referred to as *pyogenic granuloma.*

junctiva and the vascular endothelial cells. The epithelial surface is quickly stripped away leaving the underlying fibrovascular tissue exposed. The collagenous component of the substantia propria is relatively resistant to the chemical change; however, the fibroblasts, vascular endothelial cells, and resident lymphocytes and plasma cells are quickly destroyed. The vessels at the periphery of the injured tissue become thrombosed because clotting factors are activated, thereby adding ischemic insult to partially damaged tissue. Tissue damage occurs as deep as the chemical agent can diffuse. There are no natural tissue barriers to control the inevitable pH change. In the case of high concentrations of alkali, the damage may extend well into the eye and destroy the trabecular meshwork and the lens capsular epithelium and cortex.

The major components of the wound healing process are lost when alkali injuries occur. Epithelial cells often must migrate from great distances and over a surface damaged by the original alkali injury. In many cases, the epithelium may not completely cover the defect caused by necrotic tissue. The partially healed epithelium continues secreting peptides to simulate the early fibrovascular response, producing, in effect, an excessive amount of proteolytic remodeling enzymes such as collagenase. The abnormal wound healing response, therefore, contributes to ongoing tissue destruction. Only when epithelial continuity is restored can beneficial fibrous support be formed. The specialized components of the epithelium, such as the goblet cells and accessory lacrimal tissue, are not restored leaving the conjunctival surface dysfunctional and susceptible to additional injury as from infection.

In contrast to injury caused by alkali, injury to deeply situated tissues by acidic solutions is often prevented by a permeability barrier created in the corneal epithelium and superficial stromal by proteins coagulated after being exposed to acid.[23] The most common agents causing this type of injury are sulfuric acid (battery acid), sulfurous acid (refrigerant), and hydrochloric acid. Hydrofluoric acid is an exception to the general rule in that it destroys cell membranes and can penetrate deeply into the corneal stroma where it shortens collagen fibrils. Nevertheless, the damage tends to be less severe than that seen with alkali injuries.

The aim of initial therapy in chemical injuries is to restore normal tissue pH and to minimize tissue damage. The goal of subsequent therapy is to assist reepithelialization by minimizing inflammation, preventing infection, and controlling production of indigenous proteolytic enzymes. Even with aggressive therapy, severe vision loss may result from chemical agents, especially alkali.

The conjunctiva in the interpalpebral space is exposed to ultraviolet light, which may cause degeneration of the collagen of the conjunctival substantia propria. This damage is evidenced histologically by a bluish coloration in hematoxylin-eosin stained tissue (elastoid degeneration).[23] This altered collagen appears clinically as a yel-low, moderately well-outlined subepithelial mass at the temporal or nasal conjunctiva (pinguecula). The altered collagen induces a fibrous tissue response, which may extend onto the cornea as a **pterygium.** As the collagen degenerates further, a granulomatous inflammatory response may develop simulating neoplastic growth. In advanced cases, the altered collagen may undergo dystrophic calcification. Surgical excision usually is indicated only when there is a clinical suspicion of neoplasia or if the corneal process threatens visual function.

The Cornea

Transparency is both the cornea's asset and its Achilles heel. The cornea's ability to transmit light is the result of tissue homogeneity and the strict spatial relationships of the corneal collagenous fibers provided by intracollagenous proteoglycans and small caliber collagen subtypes. The squamous corneal epithelium, like that of most surface membranes, has a high rate of turnover, constantly renewing those cells lost through normal age-related attrition and minor trauma. The water content of the corneal stroma is strictly controlled both by biochemical attributes of proteoglycans, which comprise the mucopolysaccharide spacing collagenous bundles, and by the pumping activity of both the corneal epithelium and endothelium. Through these mechanisms, the corneal stroma is maintained in a state of relative dehydration. Damage to these control mechanisms increases hydration, seen clinically as corneal edema.

Bowman's membrane is composed of randomly arranged type I collagen fibers, which are not renewable if destroyed by injury (Table 1). There is no mechanism of regeneration. The corneal stromal collagen is grouped into lamellae extending across the diameter of the cornea from limbus to limbus. There is a suborganization of the collagen bundles to counter the forces of the longitudinal muscle of the ciliary body on the scleral spur, the dynamic actions of the rectus muscles, and the weight and motion of the upper lid. Lacerations extending to various depths of the stroma cause different resultant forces initially and throughout the healing process.

Descemet's membrane, like most basement membranes, is composed of fibronectin, laminin, and type IV

TABLE 1. *Types of collagen commonly found in the eye*

Type*	Location
Type I	Sclera, cornea
Type II	Vitreous
Type III	Repair and paravascular tissue
Type IV	Basement membranes (Descemet's membrane)

* Multiple other types of collagen have been identified. Many are associated with the anchoring complexes of epithelial cells to substratum.

collagen. It is produced by the corneal endothelial cells and tends to thicken throughout life. No structural connections exist between the anterior surface of Descemet's membrane and the posterior surface of the corneal stroma. Shearing forces exerted on Descemet's membrane, as sometimes occurs during the formation of limbal wounds, may detach Descemet's membrane into the anterior chamber. Because the normally dehydrated corneal stroma is exposed to the aqueous by the detachment, the hydrophilic corneal stromal proteoglycans cause the corneal stroma to swell and become relatively opaque.

The **endothelium** is only a single cell layer thick, not readily renewable, and only loosely adherent to Descemet's membrane. Mechanical trauma during anterior segment surgery may seriously compromise the dehydration role of endothelial tissue, leading initially to corneal edema and possibly to bullous keratopathy. The cornea receives its nutrition from the tears, the aqueous, and limbal vessels. The limbal circulation is composed of terminal branches of both the conjunctival network and, through intrascleral collaterals, the anterior ciliary circulation. Of the three sources of nutrition, only the vascular system is able to respond to relative corneal malnutrition or ischemia. The presence of blood vessels in the cornea as a response to injury compromises transparency by altering collagen fiber spatial relationships, altering the chemical makeup of proteoglycans, and imposing opaque hemoglobin-containing red blood cells.

Corneal reaction to injury depends on the extent of damage to corneal cell types. Generally, the epithelium responds initially by migration of uninjured cells at the border of the lesion followed by mitosis once cell continuity is reestablished. The keratocytes of the corneal stroma are modified fibrocytes, which serve mainly to maintain structural collagen and proteoglycans. When stimulated by injury, the keratocytes are capable of migrating to the injured site and producing both collagen and proteoglycans; however, both the collagen and the proteoglycans are not identical to the native substances formed embryologically. The reparative tissue cannot reestablish the homogeneity necessary to allow normal transmission of light. Corneal endothelial cells are capable of only limited regeneration. Endothelial defects are healed principally by migration of surrounding uninjured cells; however, once cell continuity is reestablished, mitosis does not follow as is seen in the epithelium. The remaining endothelial cells are spread over a much larger surface area than they were before the injury and may be too overextended to maintain the normal relative dehydrated state of the overlying stroma.

Corneal abrasion is the clinical term indicating mechanical, radiant (ultraviolet light), or chemical damage to the cornea. This results in localized loss of corneal epithelial cells, sparing the underlying supportive structures including Bowman's membrane, corneal stroma, and, often, the corneal epithelial basement membrane.

When there is a defect in the corneal epithelium, the tissue barrier to microbes is lost. Other steady-state functions of the corneal epithelium also are lost including cytokine production to limit collagenase production by fibroblasts and superoxide dismutase production to neutralize free radicals. Generally, the cornea is rapidly resurfaced by cells generated from stem cells located permanently at the limbus, and there is no significant disturbance of the epithelium–stroma steady state[24] (Fig. 9-18). Occasionally, following injury by tree branches, fingernails, and other organic materials, regenerating epithelial cells do not form tight adhesions to the basement membrane. Additionally, the basement membrane itself may have been damaged or absent as a result of the injury. As a result of the inadequate epithelial adhesion, the epithelium may be lost following subsequent minor trauma or even the wiping action of the eyelids (recurrent erosion).

Corneal foreign bodies and superficial lacerations result in injury to Bowman's membrane and to variable amounts of anterior corneal stroma. Generally, epithelial wound healing follows the pattern outlined for corneal abrasion; however, Bowman's membrane is not repaired by fibrous tissue. The anterior stromal defect is filled in by proliferating epithelial cells (epithelial acanthosis) resulting in the formation of an epithelial facet (Fig. 9-19). On slit-lamp examination, the facet is seen as a translucent area of the anterior cornea. The epithelial facet generally does not interfere with visual function.

Full-thickness lacerations of the cornea cause immediate tissue reaction at all levels. The corneal stroma, which normally is relatively dehydrated, swells when exposed to tears and aqueous. The degree of swelling may be sufficient to close a small linear or shelved laceration creating a water-tight wound. These self-sealing lacerations may not need additional suturing. Larger anterior corneal wounds are prevented from self-sealing by retrac-

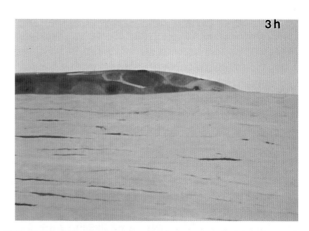

FIG. 9-18. Photomicrograph of the rounded leading edge of healing corneal epithelial cells. The cells migrate centrally by a complex interaction of alterations of the cell cytoskeleton and differential adhesion of the cell surface with the underling extracellular matrix.

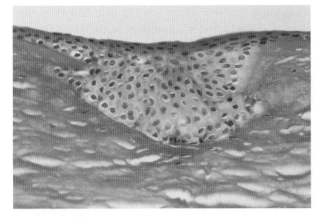

FIG. 9-19. Photomicrograph of a superficial injury to the cornea involving Bowman's membrane. Bowman's membrane itself does not regenerate, and there is limited fibrous reaction in the anterior corneal stroma. Surface epithelial cells fill the defect to restore the overlying corneal contour, the primary refractive surface of the eye.

tion or gaping of Bowman's membrane. Similarly, wounds involving the posterior cornea are held open by both retraction and inward curling of Descemet's membrane toward the corneal stroma. The net result in extensive untreated wounds may be incomplete wound closure and the formation of a fistulous tract, which allows loss of aqueous, leading to a collapsed anterior chamber and invasion of microbes into the eye. In time, the surface epithelium also may use a fistulous tract to enter the anterior chamber and cover the anterior chamber angle structures (epithelial downgrowth) causing secondary glaucoma (see Chapter 7).

As was noted previously, corneal endothelial cells are capable of only limited mitotic division and generally reestablish continuity by the spreading of adjacent surviving cells to cover the defect. Unlike Bowman's membrane, Descemet's membrane is reproduced by endothelial cells, although the new basement membrane always is thinner. Whether the corneal cells reestablish relative stroma dehydration and clarity depends on many factors, the most important of which is the extent of cell loss.[24] Occasionally, corneal endothelial cells respond to injury by *fibrous metaplasia,* differentiation of one mature cell type to another mature cell type. The result is an opaque retrocorneal fibrous plaque.

Alkali injury often involves the corneal stroma (Fig. 9-20). Initial penetration of the alkali causes cation binding to collagen and glycosaminoglycans. This chemical change causes hydration of the proteoglycans and shortening and thickening of the collagen fibrils. The alkali also destroys keratocyte membranes. Destruction of corneal nerves causes corneal anesthesia, which minimizes initial symptoms. The early stages of repair may be limited by destruction of epithelial stem cells at the limbus. If the stem cells are totally destroyed, epithelial regeneration may be permanently deficient. In the later stages, much

of the corneal damage is due to leukocytes producing proteases, including collagenase, which delays reepithelialization. Keratocytes remodel corneal stroma by removing damaged collagen with collagenase, and by producing both collagen and proteoglycans. Occasionally keratocytes produce excessive amounts of collagenase, leading to the formation of a sterile corneal ulcer. There is little or no contribution of collagenase from the epithelium. Definitive healing of the cornea, however, can be accomplished only after the epithelial cover is fully reestablished. Treatment strategies include limiting the amount of alkali by flushing with neutral pH solutions, promoting epithelial healing, limiting the inflammatory response with citrate (decreased polymorphonuclear leukocyte activity) and steroids, supplying compounds such as ascorbate, which are necessary for collagen production, and preventing bacterial and fungal secondary infection.

As is true of the conjunctiva, injury to the cornea by acids tends to be superficial. The acid denatures the surface proteins causing sterile ulceration of the superficial corneal stroma. Nerve endings in the corneal epithelium and anterior stroma may be destroyed, which may limit the degree of pain associated with the injury. The cornea often heals with anterior stromal scarring and vascularization.

Blunt injury to the cornea causes deformation of tissues. The least elastic, such as Descemet's membrane, may rupture causing transient corneal edema (acute hydrops) because of exposure of the stroma to aqueous. As with corneal wound healing from other causes, Descemet's membrane may regenerate allowing the cornea to clear. Scrolls of Descemet's membrane at the margin of

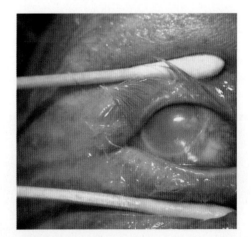

FIG. 9-20. Clinical photograph of a corneal alkali injury. The cornea is translucent generally and opaque centrally in an area of extensive corneal stromal degeneration. The normal healing mechanisms are limited because of necrosis of limbal stem cells and of keratocytes. The proteoglycans are dentured by high-pH fluids. Intravascular coagulation is caused by alkali penetrating into the vessel lumen and initiating the coagulation cascade. Downstream ischemia adds to the damage from direct alkali injury.

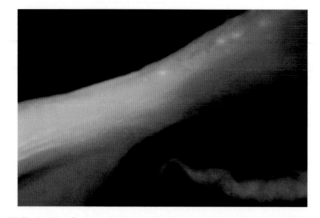

FIG. 9-21. Gross photograph of a meridional section of human limbal tissue. Note the relative thinness of the limbal tissue at the junction of the more opaque scleral tissue and the blue-tinged corneal tissue.

the initial rupture do not generally interfere with vision. Less severe, focal blunt trauma may cause temporary dysfunction of corneal endothelium leading to focal areas of corneal edema due to endothelial pump dysfunction.

The Sclera

The sclera has multiple points of structural weakness. Anteriorly, in the region of the limbus, the external scleral sulcus, containing the insertion of Tenon's capsule and the conjunctiva, lies directly over the internal scleral sulcus containing the trabecular meshwork. This spatial arrangement effectively reduces the thickness of the sclera in that region from approximately 1 mm to approximately 0.5 mm (Fig. 9-21). Sudden increased intraocular pressure, like that which occurs with blunt trauma, may rupture the globe at the limbus through this area[25,26] (Fig 9-22). The rupture also may extend posteriorly in the meridian of a rectus muscle because the sclera is also reduced to approximately 0.5-mm thickness immediately

posterior to the site of the muscle insertion (Fig. 9-23). Similarly, the sclera in the region of the insertion of the superior oblique tendon is thin and vulnerable. The muscular insertion of the inferior oblique, however, is not associated with an increased risk of scleral perforation.

The dura of the optic nerve inserts directly into the sclera in the region of a rich arterial pressure. Acceleration–deceleration injuries sometimes associated with child abuse may cause hemorrhage both within the subdural and subarachnoid space and within the sclera itself.

The Anterior Chamber Angle

The anterior chamber angle is the anchoring site of the ciliary musculature and (indirectly through the tissues of the face of the ciliary body) of the iris diaphragm to the scleral spur or roll. A peripheral drainage system, including the trabecular meshwork and Schlemm's canal, is present in a recess of the sclera (the internal scleral sulcus). This drainage route allows egress of aqueous by means of multiple collector channels to the episcleral vascular plexus. Anteriorly, the trabecular beams, which are composed of endothelium-covered collagenous columns, extend from the termination of Descemet's membrane to the scleral spur. Posteriorly, the longitudinal muscle of the ciliary body inserts into the scleral spur and is contiguous with the most internal trabecular beams. The iris root does not insert directly onto the scleral spur but is indirectly connected via the delicate collagenous tissue of the ciliary body face. The principal arterial trunk of the

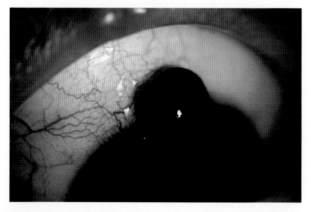

FIG. 9-22. Clinical photograph of ruptured limbus allowing the iris to become externalized and appear as a pigmented limbal mass.

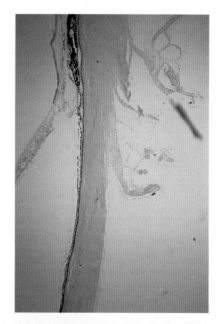

FIG. 9-23. Photomicrograph of the sclera at the site of insertion of a rectus muscle. Here, too, the sclera thins to approximately half the thickness of the surrounding tissue, making this site at high risk for perforation.

vascular system of the ciliary body lies near the surface of the ciliary body face.

The anterior chamber angle is vulnerable, particularly to blunt injury, because a confluence of forces is often directed to this area, primarily at the scleral spur. All of the anterior chamber angle structures are relatively inelastic. Any change of tension, such as that due to altered hydrostatic forces associated with deforming blunt injury, is transmitted by the fluid within the eye as a shock wave, which impacts throughout the eye and may cause tissues to rupture. Disinsertion of the ciliary body's longitudinal muscle attachment to the scleral spur (cyclodialysis) permits aqueous access to the suprachoroidal space and may result in ocular hypotony. Tearing of the iris insertion at the ciliary face causes **iridodialysis,** which is expressed clinically as a displaced and distorted pupil, and a hiatus of the peripheral iris diaphragm (Fig. 9-24). Rupture of the ciliary body face, in the plane between the longitudinal muscle of the ciliary body and the more internally situated circular and oblique muscles, is reflected clinically as a sectorial area of anterior chamber deepening due to posterior displacement of the iris diaphragm (recession of the anterior chamber angle)[27,28] (Fig. 9-25). Injury to the trabecular beams cannot often be identified clinically, but may result in increased intraocular pressure, which may develop months or years after the initial injury.

The most common source of injury to the anterior chamber angle is blunt ocular trauma, which often produces hemorrhage into the anterior chamber (hyphema)[29] (Fig. 9-26). The hemorrhage usually is caused by stretching of limbal tissue associated with equatorial scleral expansion and posterior displacement of the lens–iris diaphragm during blunt trauma. Increased hydrostatic pressure tears the major arterial circle of the ciliary body located in the anterior ciliary musculature or tears one of the meridional vessels supplying the iris via the insertion

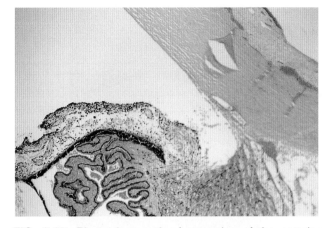

FIG. 9-25. Photomicrograph of recession of the anterior chamber angle, illustrating laceration into the anterior face of the ciliary body. In time, the ciliary body assumes a more fusiform configuration.

of the iris diaphragm into the face of the ciliary body. The blood within the anterior chamber initially may obscure the injuries to its structures. After the hemorrhage clears, the clinical signs may be limited to gonioscopic findings of recessed anterior chamber angle or small areas of iridodialysis.

Associated ocular findings include traumatic mydriasis (damage to sphincter muscle or sympathetic nerves), traumatic miosis (inflammation and dysfunction of dilator muscles), corneal blood staining (accumulation of hemoglobin breakdown products in the corneal stroma), and "eight-ball" hyphema (extensive hemorrhage into the anterior chamber with disruption of aqueous outflow and deoxygenation of hemoglobin in the extravasated blood, giving the blood a characteristic dark color)[30,31] (Fig. 9-27).

The Iris

The iris diaphragm regulates the amount of light entering the eye. The sphincter muscle makes up the central

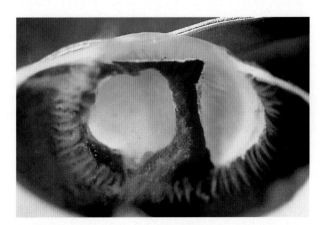

FIG. 9-24. Gross photograph of dialysis of the iris from its insertion into the face of the ciliary body. There is a high likelihood of concurrent damage to the adjacent trabecular meshwork.

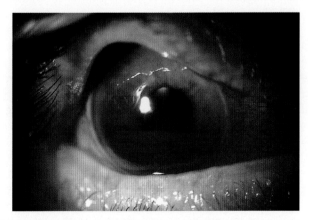

FIG. 9-26. Clinical photograph of blood layered out in the dependent portion of the anterior chamber angle. The blood, eventually, filters through the trabecular meshwork.

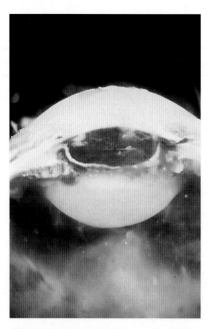

FIG. 9-27. Gross photograph of extensive hemorrhage into the anterior chamber, known as "eight-ball" hemorrhage. The blood is immobile and quickly becomes deoxygenated. The darkening color is an omnious prognostic sign for salvaging the eye.

border of the pupil. This muscle is not elastic and is easily ruptured. The blood supply is via meridional end arteries, which traverse the iris root from the major arterial circle of the ciliary body. The iris root inserts into the anterior face of the ciliary body via a small number of delicate collagenous columns containing blood vessels. The muscular components of the iris do not extend into the face of the ciliary body. The iris is supported primarily by resting on the anterior surface of the lens. Weakening of the lens zonular attachments to the ciliary body may causes the iris to "flutter" (iridodonesis), or may permit anterior–posterior movements of the lens (phacodonesis). These relative movements of the iris and lens may change aqueous dynamics and can result in a form of pupillary block closed-angle glaucoma.

The iris is most often injured by blunt trauma. The iris may be torn at its root (iridodialysis) or the sphincter muscle may tear creating single or multiple notches along the pupillary margin. Both injuries can interfere with the ability of the iris to control the amount of light entering the eye. In addition, melanin pigment from the iris pigment epithelium may be released at the time of the initial injury, giving the false impression of white blood cells (anterior iritis) in the anterior chamber.

Abnormal placement of the iris often is a complicating factor in penetrating wounds of the anterior segment. Because the iris has the consistency of wet tissue paper, it is often swept into the wound along with the egress of aqueous through the wound. At times, the iris tissue may occlude the wound and temporarily reestablish a relative water-tight seal for the eye; however, with time, this iris tissue may act as a conduit for microorganisms or surface epithelial cells to gain access to the eye. Whether to reposition the iris through a penetrating wound is often a difficult decision that requires the clinician to weigh the advantage of reestablishing the ocular light control mechanisms with the risk of promoting endophthalmitis or epithelial downgrowth.

The Crystalline Lens

The crystalline lens is a biconvex transparent structure composed of fibers maintained by cell bodies located only along its anterior hemisphere. The lens is suspended by delicate acellular structures (zonules) extending though the posterior chamber to the region of the vitreous base.

Lens transparency depends on its relative dehydration and on the homogeneity of the lens fiber arrangement. Ingress of fluid though a hiatus in the lens capsule disrupts the strict arrangement of fibers leading to opacification. Alterations of aqueous fluid dynamics in the posterior chamber, such as that associated with hemorrhage or acute elevations of intraocular pressure, may interrupt the nutrition of the lens epithelial cells leading to a type of ischemia.

Lens epithelial cells are capable of responding to stress from any cause only by undergoing fibrous metaplasia.[32] An anterior subcapsular cataract is a collagenous plaque that forms as a result of fibrous metaplasia of anterior lens epithelium following trauma to this area. The cataract often is densely opaque and may be nonprogressive if the trauma is limited to a single event.

Overwhelming injury to the lens cells disrupts the homogeneity of the tissue, leading to lens opacification. Capsular rupture allows aqueous to enter and disrupt cortical tissue both by mechanical separation and by increased hydration. This type of injury often leads to total opacification of the lens. Additionally, exposure of nondenatured lens protein to the immunologic system may result in an autoimmune delayed hypersensitivity response known as **phacoantigenic uveitis** (formerly called phacoanaphylactic endophthalmitis), which is characterized by zonal granulomatous inflammation.[33] In contrast, leakage of denatured lens protein into the anterior chamber, as is seen in a mature cataract, is characterized by phagocytosis of the proteinaceous material by macrophages (phacolytic glaucoma).

A **Vossius ring** is the result of forceful compression of the iris pigment epithelium against the anterior surface of the lens (Fig. 9-28). The intracellular pigment is dislodged from the iris pigment epithelial cells and adheres to the anterior lens capsule in a meridional pattern reflecting the meridional corrugations of the posterior iris surface. There may be an associated anterior subcapsular or anterior cortical cataract.

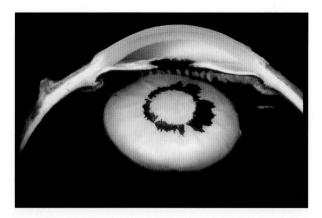

FIG. 9-28. Gross photograph of a Vossius ring, which is iris pigment displaced onto the anterior surface of the lens by forces compressing the iris against the lens.

The zonular support of the lens may be disrupted, particularly by blunt trauma causing partial (subluxation) or total (luxation) displacement of the lens (Fig. 9-29). The lens may be displaced anteriorly to cause a type of obstructive glaucoma or may be lost into the vitreous cavity. Totally dislodged lenses may be extruded from the eye through a penetrating wound as small as 3 to 4 mm. Subluxed lenses are often recognized clinically by movements of an unsupported iris (iridodonesis) or by herniation of formed vitreous into the anterior chamber. The displaced vitreous also may interrupt aqueous outflow causing a type of pupillary obstructive (block) glaucoma.

The Vitreous

The vitreous is a gelatinous structure composed of hyaluronic acid and type II collagen. It is important in embryologic development of the eye, but undergoes degeneration beginning in the first decade of life. The clinical importance of the vitreous lies mainly in its strong attachment to the region of the ora serrata anteriorly (the vitreous

base) and to areas of relative attachment over the retinal blood vessels, the paramacular region, the region of the optic disc, and regions of pathologic adherence such as at the border of lattice degeneration.

The vitreous is a prolonged repository of extravasated blood. Without direct access to either the venous circulation or to lymphatics, the blood components tend to involute in situ.

The inertia of the vitreous is important in the mechanism of retinal hole formation secondary to blunt injury. Displacement of the vitreous relative to the retina, particularly near the ora serrata, frequently creates retinal holes or tears at the areas of attachment; nevertheless, avulsion of the retina from its insertion at the vitreous base (retinal dialysis) is uncommon[34] (Fig. 9-30). The presence of preexisting retinal pathology, such as lattice degeneration, may predispose to retinal hole formation and subsequent retinal detachment from blunt trauma.

The Retina

The retina is a tract of the brain composed of tissues with vulnerabilities and reaction patterns similar to those found in the central nervous system. The retinal tissue is segregated from the general circulation by a blood–retinal barrier similar to the brain, which is protected by a blood–brain barrier. The barrier actually is composed of specialized attachments of the retinal vascular endothelium and of the retinal pigment epithelium. Any breach of these junctions markedly compromises the microenvironment of the retinal tissue, both mechanically and biochemically.

The correlate for the fibroblast in the central nervous system and retina is the glial cell. The fibroblast functions, in part, by producing extracellular collagen (fibrosis) in the repair process. The glial cell, however, is not capable of producing extracellular materials and can function in repair only by changing its cellular configuration to breach a defect (gliosis). Fibrous tissue can be maintained

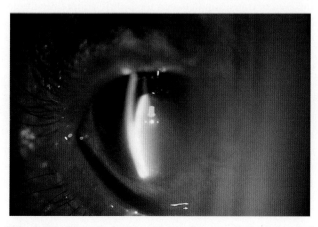

FIG. 9-29. Clinical photograph of a lens partially dislocated inferiorly into the vitreous.

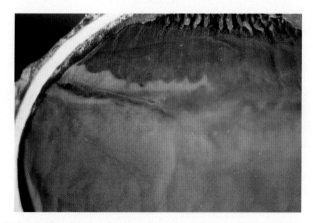

FIG. 9-30. Gross photograph of avulsion of the vitreous base from the pars plana. In this case, the peripheral retina remained intact.

in a much more hypoxic environment than can reactive glial cells; however, reactive glial cells can be maintained in a more hypoxic environment than can intact photosensitive or photoprocessing cells. There is no mechanism to replace highly differentiated retinal cells lost due to injury.

Retinal transparency depends on its relative thinness, lack of blood vessels, and near-perfect homogeneity of cells (maintained in part by lack of extracellular fluid). The retina is attached only at the ora serrata and the parapapillary regions. It is highly dependent on a continuous and abundant supply of oxygen and nutrients delivered mainly via the choriocapillaris of the choroidal circulation. The indigenous retinal circulation is secondary and supplies mainly the transmission portions of the retina, the ganglion cell and nerve fiber layers. Disruption of the retinal vascular supply leaves the posterior layers of the retina intact.

The architecture of the retina is modified in the region of the macula and at the retinal periphery. The microanatomy of the macular portion of the retina permits maximum direct access of light to the photoreceptors. The photoreceptor density is greatest in the area of the foveola centralis where each photoreceptor is served by a higher ratio of ganglion cells. The structural modification in the foveola includes an avascular zone of approximately 0.40 mm. To be adequately supplied with nutrients, the retinal tissue is thinned to fall within the diffusion capacity of oxygen and nutrients from choriocapillaris. The macular area is particularly vulnerable to vascular insult and to forces transmitted through attached cortical vitreous.

Blunt injury to the retina (commotio retinae) disrupts the photoreceptor layer seen clinically as a relatively well-demarcated region of deep retinal opacity.[35,36] Although the condition has been called **Berlin's edema,** the retinal tissues are not edematous. Usually, the architecture of the retina is restored within several days.

Rupture of Bruch's membrane and choroid, however, often causes permanent vision loss if the macular area is involved (Fig. 9-31). The cause of this type of injury usually is severe compression of the globe. Bruch's membrane, which is relatively inelastic, tends to rupture in a curvilinear pattern concentric to the optic disc that tends to extend into the area of the macula. The main reason for vision loss is damage to the overlying retina, which may not be visible clinically.[37,38] The rupture site, in later years, may allow new blood vessels from the choriocapillaris to access the subretinal space resulting in subretinal neovascular membrane formation. Histologically, there is a rupture of Bruch's membrane with separation of the retinal pigment epithelium. The overlying retina often is atrophic.

Purtscher's retinopathy is not caused by direct trauma to the globe but is the result of arteriolar occlusion from microembolization. The emboli may consist of aggregations of white blood cells made cohesive by compliment

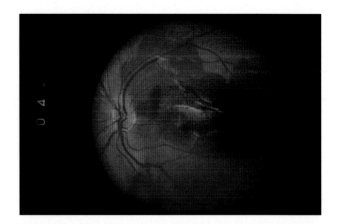

FIG. 9-31. Clinical photograph of choroidal rupture. The hiatus in the uveal tract can be seen as a curvilinear area concentric to the disc where internal sclera is exposed and reflects light.

activation or may be due to fat or to air embolism generated at a site of nonocular injury, often involving the chest or long bones.[39,40] In mild cases, the condition may be seen only as nerve fiber layer infarcts in the peripapillary region, or with more extensive injury, larger areas of retinal necrosis and retinal hemorrhage may be observed. The prognosis for return of visual function is guarded and most patients lose some vision.

Holes in the macula following trauma often are due to postconcussion necrosis of the foveola with or without surrounding cystoid macular edema. A hole may form following rupture of an intraretinal cyst many weeks or months after the episode of trauma.

The peripheral retina is much thinner than the posterior retina. The most peripheral retina often is thin enough to be supplied totally by the choriocapillaris, permitting the peripheral intraretinal vascular system to be inconspicuous or nonexistent. The vitreous base in tightly adherent to the surface of the retina for several millimeters posterior to the ora serrata. The thin peripheral retina in this region is particularly vulnerable to traumatic disruption at the area of transition between the tightly adherent vitreous base and the more loosely attached preequatorial retina (Fig. 9-32). Sudden changes in the inertial forces applied to the vitreous may be transmitted to the posterior vitreous base resulting in retinal hole formation.[41]

Traumatic tears leading to retinal detachment tend to occur in an area of preexisting weakness, such as in lattice degeneration, or unusual anchoring, such as a chorioretinal scar. Even if a hole in the retina is formed at the time of injury, the retina may not become detached until weeks or months later when the overlying vitreous degenerates and allows separation of the retina by liquid vitreous dissecting between it and the underlying pigment epithelium. The retinal injury may be extensive and cause giant tears (greater than 90 degrees of the circumference) of the peripheral retina. The vitreous base itself may become

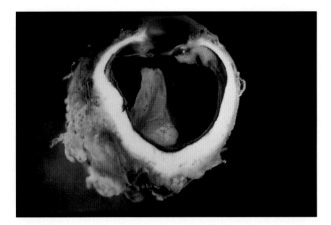

FIG. 9-32. Gross photograph of an eye with total retinal dialysis and total retinal detachment.

avulsed from the peripheral retina and the posterior pars plana.

Both the peripheral retina and the posterior retina are subject to deformation and detachment due to contractile myofibroblastic membranes formed as a repair response to injury. The source of the fibroblasts may be circulating monocytes, transformed retinal pigment epithelial cells, or fibroblasts from the choroid. The last two sources require a break in the retina to cause epiretinal membranes. The contractile activity of the myofibroblasts is beneficial in wound closure and in the restoration of anatomic integrity to injured tissue. On the surface of the retina, however, this contractile activity leads to deformation of the internal smooth surface of the retina, causing visual distortion, or to traction on the retinal surface, leading to retinal detachment. This same mechanism leads to pathologic changes along the anterior vitreous border, posterior to the lens, and internal to the pars plana of the ciliary body. In this latter case, the fibrous contractile membrane (cyclitic membrane) uses the anterior vitreous face to form a membrane anchored circumferentially at the pars plana. With contraction of this membrane, the entire ciliary body becomes detached causing ocular hypotony.

The Optic Nerve

The functional component of the optic nerve has the consistency of butter. This neural axonal tissue is supported by the relatively inelastic tissues of the dura externally and the pia infiltrating throughout the nerve. The axons pass through a relatively weak area of the scleral coat, which is surrounded by an area of relative strength where the dura of the optic nerve inserts into the posterior sclera. The entire optic nerve/scleral complex is supplied by an intricate network of vessels within the sclera (circle of Zinn-Haller) and within the nerve itself from branches of the ophthalmic artery and central retinal artery.

During severe facial or other anterior head trauma, the globe may be displaced relative to the optic nerve. The shearing forces created may first disrupt the delicate axonal material, then the vascular components of the optic nerve, and finally its collagenous coverings. Therefore, even with moderate globe displacement, the axonal component of the optic nerve may be functionally transected leaving the central vascular compartment intact (Fig. 9-33). Transection of the dural component of the optic nerve at its attachment to the sclera is rare.[42]

INTRAOCULAR FOREIGN BODIES

The reaction of ocular tissues to intraocular foreign bodies is determined by the site of entry, the trajectory through the globe, the exit site, and the size, shape, and makeup of the foreign material.[43,44]

The cornea is the most common entry site for intraocular foreign bodies. Its trajectory through the eye, and the types of tissue it penetrates are determined by its speed and other energy-related forces. Those objects with sufficient energy penetrate the posterior ocular wall to involve orbital tissue (a double perforating injury).[54] Additional injury may be generated by hemorrhage if the foreign body encounters vascularized tissue such as the uveal tract and the retina. Hemorrhage within such a tract, particularly if it traverses the vitreous, may organize with myofibroblasts, causing tractional retinal detachment.

Several foreign-body characteristics are important in determining the extent of the initial injury and the tissue response to the presence of the foreign material. Large blunt objects are not as likely to penetrate the globe as are small sharp ones. Once inside the eye, small sharp objects are more likely to migrate through adjacent tissue and possibly to the surface of the eye. The object may be propelled by micromovements within the eye generated by the action of extraocular muscles, aqueous convection currents, or movements of the eyelids. Organic materials, such as vegetable matter (wood), or cilia are

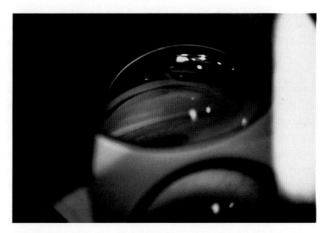

FIG. 9-33. Goniophotograph of a Kayser-Fleischer ring from copper deposition in Descemet's membrane.

most likely to generate a foreign-body granulomatous inflammatory reaction. These materials also are the most likely to act as a vehicle for intraocular implantation of microbial organisms because of surface contamination of the material. Small metallic foreign bodies (including bullet fragments) tend to be heated when they are generated and are more likely to be sterile when they penetrate the globe. BB pellets, although not projected at a high enough velocity to become heated, do transmit sufficient force to the eye to cause extensive damage.[45,46]

Copper and iron are commonly encountered foreign-body materials that are likely to provoke tissue damage beyond initial mechanical injury. Pure copper induces a massive suppurative inflammatory reaction potentially causing panophthalmitis and loss of the eye.[47,48] Alloys of copper are proportionally less toxic to a level of approximately 60% copper. Materials with less copper may be encased in fibrous tissue following a more localized suppurative inflammatory response. Copper ions may be released from copper alloy foreign bodies and be deposited in basement membranes of the eye (chalcosis). Deposition of copper in Descemet's membrane and posterior corneal stroma produces a **Kayser-Fleischer ring** (Fig. 9-33). Copper deposition in the lens capsule causes a **sunflower cataract.** Copper also may be deposited in the lens zonules and in the retina.

Siderosis is toxic damage from iron ions originating in ferrous foreign materials. Toxic iron damage from ions originating in hemoglobin is called **hemosiderosis.** The divalent ferrous ion is more toxic to cell enzyme systems than is trivalent ferric ions. The ions interfere with vital intracellular enzymes particularly in the photoreceptor cells of the retina. Initially, the cellular damage is limited to edema, which is reversible. In a short period, the outer retina becomes necrotic, an irreversible change. The Mueller cells are relatively resistant and remain to maintain the overall cellular architecture of the retina. All ocular epithelial cells and the endothelial cells of the trabecular beams are subject to damage by siderosis. Loss of endothelial cell maintenance of the trabecular beams results in trabecular fibrosis and secondary open-angle glaucoma. Toxic damage to lens epithelial cells causes a rusty-appearing **siderotic cataract.** The iris sphincter and dilator muscles may become dysfunctional because of iron ion toxicity. Some iron foreign bodies may become encapsulated by fibrous tissue, which in turn, becomes stained by iron ions resulting in a pigmented mass that may resemble a malignant melanoma.

Lead, zinc, nickel, aluminum, and mercury also are toxic to tissues by various mechanisms but are less frequently encountered. Stone, rock, clay, carbon, glass, and some plastics are relatively inert and are more likely to cause damage from mechanical factors. Precious metals (gold and silver) are essentially inert. Platinum may undergo slow biodegradation by hydrolysis.

Retained vegetable matter in the eye may cause a marked inflammatory reaction (Fig. 9-34).

TISSUE-SPECIFIC SURGICAL TRAUMA

Surgical procedures are designed to accomplish a mechanical change in tissue with minimal damage to surrounding tissues. The main difference between accidental and surgical trauma is that the natural history of surgical procedures is more predictable than the natural history of accidental injuries. Nonetheless, there are individual circumstances in which the tissue reaction to surgical procedures deviates from the usual natural history and either negates the intended surgical goal or causes undesirable tissue changes. It is important to understand the tissue changes that occur during surgical trauma in order to recognize deviations from the expected course of healing and to intervene, when possible, in a timely manner to prevent further complications.

The most common reason for ocular function loss following intraocular surgery is the development of glaucoma, ultimately leading to phthisis. The glaucoma may be caused by several mechanisms including both closed- and open-angle varieties. All types of intraocular procedures have the potential for a complicated course; however, procedures involving more serious primary ocular disease (eg, diabetes mellitus) or following multiple prior surgical procedures are more likely to follow a complicated postoperative course.[49–51]

Surgical Procedures of the Eyelids

Surgical procedures of the eyelid skin are intended to maintain function of the orbicularis oculi, the lid margin, and the tear drainage system. Incisions are placed in pre-existing lid creases in an orientation that does not alter the lid margin contour and that minimizes the effects of

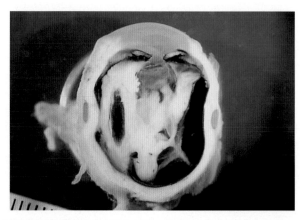

FIG. 9-34. Gross photograph of an eye removed because of an intense inflammatory reaction to retained vegetable matter (cattail).

fibrovascular tissue contraction. Complications include lid notch formation and eyelid malposition.

The gray line is an important surgical landmark for dividing the anterior compartment of the eyelid, containing the orbicularis and ciliary follicles, from the posterior compartment, containing the tarsal plate and the meibomian glands. It is an area of relative avascularity created by the muscle of Riolan and is located anterior to the orifices of the meibomian glands and posterior to the line of cilia.

Wound healing of the skin is an orchestrated series of events controlled by a complicated series of positive and negative controls operating through a system of regulatory proteins. These substances consist of cytokines, growth factors, and enzyme systems (most of which are proteases) effected primarily through a monocyte macrophage cell population. Following injury to full-thickness dermis, coagulation systems reestablish hemostasis. The surface epithelial cells are the first to act by migrating in a plane between healthy and necrotic tissue to cover and protect the underlying dermis and, ultimately, to expel necrotic debris. Once the surface is covered, fibroblasts, derived from native fibrocytes and converted monocytes, begin dermal repair, first by migrating into the area of injury and ultimately by producing extracellular materials such as collagen and proteoglycans to recreate architectural integrity. Highly differentiated structures such as hair follicles, eccrine glands, apocrine glands, and sebaceous glands are not regenerated. With time, remodeling of the dermal component reacts to prevailing or changing tissue tensions. To expedite healing of skin wounds, all accessible debris should be removed to minimize inflammation and to decrease the possibility of infection. In addition, wound edges are reapposed with the smallest number of finest appropriate sutures to minimize the dermal reaction.[52]

Surgical Procedures on the Episclera

Several surgical procedures, including extraocular muscle surgery, retinal reattachment surgery, and glaucoma filtering procedures involving setons, primarily involve the surface of the sclera in the orbit. The episcleral tissue is highly reactive and is capable of producing extensive amounts of dense fibrovascular tissue in a relatively short period. In the setting of retinal reattachment surgery, this property is a definite advantage in securing retinal buckling elements to the surface of the globe; however, it is a definite disadvantage in glaucoma filtering surgery. Therefore, antimetabolites often are used to blunt the formation of fibrous tissue in the region of intended filtration in glaucoma procedures.

Complications related to strabismus surgery include improper position of muscle reattachment and the formation of epithelial inclusion cysts by surface epithelial cells trapped within and beneath the conjunctival incision closure.[53,54]

Complications of retinal reattachment surgery include damage to vortex veins potentially causing choroidal effusion or delayed resorption of subretinal fluid. Removal of too many muscles, especially in the setting of hyperviscosity syndromes or sickle cell disease, may cause anterior segment necrosis. Acute elevations of intraocular pressure may be seen with tight scleral buckles and from excessive expansion of intraocular therapeutic gasses. The synthetic material used for scleral buckles (eg, encircling elements, bands, sponges) may migrate through the conjunctiva creating a risk of infection or, rarely, may migrate into the eye itself.

Surgical Procedures at the Limbus

Most ocular surgical procedures are performed at the limbus, even though the term *limbus* is variably defined. For the anatomist, the area is defined by a change in the nature and orientation of lamellae of the collagen from the cornea to the sclera. For the pathologist, the termination of Bowman's membrane and Descemet's membrane is a convenient landmark. The surgeon, however, identifies the limbus by the change in density of the collagen from the region of the scleral spur peripherally to the area of the internal scleral sulcus, which houses the trabecular meshwork and the canal of Schlemm. Clinically, this change is recognized as a blue translucent region, which when used as an incision point, guides the surgeon into the anterior chamber that is anterior to Schwalbe's line and well central to the trabecular meshwork structures.

Healing of the tissues at the limbus involves characteristics of both dermis wound healing (described earlier) and corneal wound healing (described later in this chapter). The initial event in the healing of most limbal wounds is the production of a fibrin coagulum in the subepithelial space of the conjunctiva in a defect of the episcleral tissue. The coagulum acts both as an adhesive that holds the wound edges together, and as a scaffolding for ingrowth of fibrovascular tissue from surrounding uninjured episcleral tissue. The wound is quickly resurfaced migration and mitosis of conjunctival epithelial cells. Healing of the remainder of the external surface of the wound is similar to that of the dermis; however, the healing process at the limbus appears to be slower and less complete than that found in cutaneous tissues. The posterior extent of limbal wounds in the region of Descemet's membrane heals as does other areas of the posterior cornea. Endothelial cells participate in sliding but undergo limited mitotic divisions of endothelial cells. There is limited fibrous proliferation of the keratocytes of the paucicellular stroma. Finally, there is proliferation of scleral fibroblasts. The limbal wound, even under ideal conditions, does not reestablish the full tensile strength of the native limbal tissues.[55,56]

The incision for cataract extraction is the most commonly used limbal wound. The circumferential extent of the wound has become smaller with the development of phacoemulsification and foldable intraocular lenses. Decreasing wound size reduces but does not eliminate complications related to limbal wound healing, primarily postoperative astigmatic error. Improper placement of the wound or suturing techniques may lead to unacceptable degrees of postoperative astigmatism.

There is no physical adhesion between the posterior surface of the corneal stroma and the anterior surface of Descemet's membrane. Descemet's membrane may be stripped away during creation of an incision, thereby exposing the posterior corneal surface to aqueous. Sudden corneal edema and opacification, usually limited to the area of stripped Descemet's membrane, is the characteristic clinical sign of this problem.[57] In addition, undue tension on the iris root may cause either **iridodialysis,** separation of the iris root from the face of the ciliary body, or **cyclodialysis,** separation of the insertion of the longitudinal muscle of the ciliary body from the scleral spur. Iridodialysis may induce intolerable glare postoperatively, and cyclodialysis seriously disrupts aqueous fluid dynamics, most often causing profound hypotony. Excessive traction also may be transmitted to the peripheral retina, creating a risk of retinal hole formation leading to retinal detachment.

The limbal wound may act as a fistulous tract allowing downgrowth of epithelial cells or ingrowth of fibrous tissue into the anterior chamber. Epithelial downgrowth, in most cases, gains access though an inconspicuous hiatus in the limbal wound. The epithelial cells grow over any available surface and modify that substratum to suit the epithelial cells' particular requirements. The region in which epithelial cells replace corneal endothelial cells is recognized clinically as a translucent region of the posterior cornea (usually contiguous with the limbal wound) and demarcated from the surrounding normal transparent cornea by a sharply defined line. Epithelial cells on the anterior iris surface are nearly invisible, but may, on occasion, efface iris crypts. Epithelial cells on the posterior cornea and anterior iris are of limited clinical significance; however, when they grow over the trabecular meshwork they mechanically obstruct aqueous outflow, both because of the physical presence of the epithelial cells and because of fibrous modification and functional destruction of the trabecular beams. The fibrous modification of the trabecular beams is irreversible even if the overlying epithelial cells are removed or destroyed. Prevention through careful attention to wound construction is the best way to treat this intractable form of glaucoma.

Fibrous ingrowth is an abnormal proliferation of fibrous tissue, most often originating from episcleral tissue, into the anterior chamber and sometimes onto the trabecular meshwork.[58] Fibrous ingrowth is much more likely to be found in the setting of accidental trauma involving tissue incarceration than in surgical trauma.

Wound healing aberrations of limbal wounds may be clinically significant. A fibrovascular strand may extend from the internal aspect of the wound into the anterior chamber. Occasionally, this delicate tuft of vessels bleeds, resulting in recurrent episodes of microhyphema (sputtering hyphema syndrome of Swann) recognized clinically between episodes by the presence of multiple "high water marks" of red blood cells adherent to corneal endothelium in dependent areas of the anterior chamber.[59] Laser treatment of the exposed vessels at the posterior wound edge within the anterior chamber usually corrects the problem.

The natural history of a limbal wound consists of continuous remodeling to accommodate changing wound stresses. Generally, the amount of tissue resorption equals the amount of tissue production. In elderly individuals, however, the resorption may exceed production because of dietary or other tissue factors related to aging. In such cases, the limbal wound becomes weak and ectatic even in the presence of normal intraocular pressure. The ectatic area often is lined by anterior uveal tissue (anterior staphyloma) and may be misinterpreted as extraocular extension of an intraocular malignant melanoma. The ectatic area transmits light on transillumination thereby excluding the possibility of a solid neoplasm, which would not transmit light. On occasion, mild blunt trauma may rupture a staphylomatous region.

The limbal wound also may allow implantation of microbes, most often during the intraoperative period. Bacterial infections usually cause symptoms within the first several postoperative days; however, infections by fungi and low virulence bacteria may not be manifest for several weeks or months.[60] A peculiar infectious process involving the crystalline lens capsular remnants of extracapsular cataract surgery is caused by such bacteria. Organisms (usually *Propionibacterium acne*) are protected within the lens capsule and proliferate to the point where colonies of bacteria are visible as opaque spherules.[61,62] The infection often causes signs of low-grade anterior uveitis, which may be transiently responsive to antiinflammatory agents. The definitive treatment requires either appropriate antimicrobial agents or surgical removal of the remaining lens capsular remnants. Other organisms, such as *Staphylococcus epidermidis* and *Candida parapsilosis,* have also been reported to cause this syndrome.

The lens epithelial cells remaining after extracapsular cataract extraction may migrate or proliferate over the scaffold afforded by the posterior capsule, causing significant opacification within the visual axis. This condition usually is corrected by a Nd-YAG laser capsulotomy. Proliferation of lens cells to form small translucent to opaque spheroids known as **Elschnig's pearls** are usually of no clinical significance.

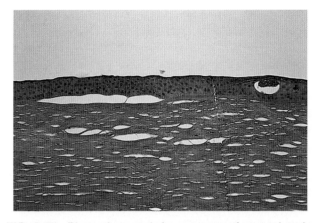

FIG. 9-35. Photomicrograph from a case of corneal endothelial decompensation syndrome. The stroma is somewhat swollen. Multiple subepithelial bullae and intraepithelial cysts are present.

Intraocular Lens Surgery

Intraocular lens implantation has been a successful procedure because the material that most intraocular lenses are made of, known as **polymethylmethacrylate** (PMMA), is biologically inert, even though the monomer of this compound, monomethylmethacrylate, is highly toxic to corneal endothelial cells.[63]

Iris-supported lenses were among the first types to be used in large quantities in the era of intracapsular cataract surgery. The PMMA **optic** was supported in the pupillary space by loops called **haptics** constructed of several different types of material including nylon, Supramid, and platinum. The lenses were technically difficult to insert, and the lens loops often abraded the pupillary margin or lacerated the sphincter muscle. The lens often was secured to the iris with transiridial nylon sutures which can undergo hydrolysis in the posterior chamber, leading to dislocation of the intraocular lens either anteriorly into the anterior chamber or posteriorly into the vitreous. The relatively heavy weight of iris-supported lenses, and the increased mobility of the pseudophakos–iris–diaphragm in the absence of support from the crystalline lens or the posterior capsule could set up inertial forces within the eye as a result of normal ocular movements. These forces could be transmitted to the delicate structures of the macula via the vitreous. These forces or ill-defined inflammatory mechanisms were believed to result in cystoid macular edema (Irvine-Gass-Norton syndrome), which may be only partially responsive to antiinflammatory agents.[64,65]

Anterior chamber intraocular lenses spanned the transition from intracapsular cataract surgery to extracapsular cataract surgery. The anterior chamber lenses were quickly associated with the **UGH syndrome,** characterized by uveitis, glaucoma, and hyphema. Initially, the condition was thought to be caused by a specific type of intraocular lens; however, it was later recognized that the syndrome was due to mechanical abrasion of the delicate tissues of the anterior chamber angle by haptics.[66]

Posterior chamber lenses became practical with the widespread use of extracapsular cataract surgery, particularly with phacoemulsification. Most tissue-related problems involving the use of these lenses relates to dislocation of the lens in the setting of weakened zonular support often in the presence of pseudoexfoliation. The surgical goal is to implant the optic and both haptics within the residual lens capsule thereby placing the lens in the most "physiologic" location possible.

The most common clinical problem associated with all lens types, but less so with posterior chamber intraocular lenses, has been corneal endothelial decompensation syndrome. The endothelial decompensation may be secondary to an intrinsic endothelial abnormality, such as Fuchs' dystrophy, may be related to intraoperative mechanical trauma to the endothelium or may be secondary to postoperative anterior uveitis or physical displacement of the intraocular lens. With loss of endothelial cell function, the corneal stroma becomes progressively more edematous, leading to secondary changes of the corneal epithelium including subepithelial bullae and fibrous pannus, aberrant intraepithelial basement membrane deposition, and even infectious anterior corneal stromal ulceration associated with ruptured bullae (Fig. 9-35).

Manufacturing defects of intraocular lenses have occasionally caused significant intraocular complications. For example, polishing compound retained on the surface of the intraocular lenses has caused anterior uveitis (Fig. 9-36).

Surgical Procedures on the Cornea

Until recently, the most common surgical procedure on the cornea was **penetrating keratoplasty** (corneal transplantation) for keratoconus or for complications of the corneal endothelial decompensation syndrome.

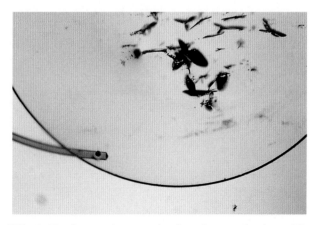

FIG. 9-36. Gross photograph of an intraocular lens. The central lens defects are due to improper focusing of a YAG laser.

Full-thickness wounds of the cornea heal in their anterior region in a manner similar to skin and episclera; however, because of the relative elasticity of Bowman's membrane, the anterior aspect of a corneal wound tends to gape (Fig. 9-37). The underlying corneal stroma swells from exposure to aqueous and tears. Occasionally, the swelling is of sufficient magnitude to appose well-aligned wounds. The corneal epithelium migrates into the anterior wound gape to the depth of stromal apposition and then proliferates to fill the anterior wound gape forming an epithelial facet. Eventually, keratocytes migrate into the area of injury to produce reparative extracellular materials. The new extracellular matrix tissue is biochemically dissimilar to the native tissue and is not transparent. As the anterior corneal contour is reestablished, the epithelial cell facet regresses to leave a surface epithelium of near-normal thickness. The posterior portion of the wound may be partially filled with fibrin-like material generated in the anterior chamber. The posterior keratocyte density is much less than the anterior keratocyte density making the posterior keratocytic response slower than that observed anteriorly.

Endothelial cells do not have the capacity to undergo significant degrees of mitosis. Adjacent uninjured endothelial cells migrate over the posterior surface of the wound. Individual endothelial cells become thinner and spread over a larger area than those cells in uninjured areas of the cornea. Eventually, the displaced endothelial cells produce a new thinner Descemet's membrane in the interface between the healed stroma and the reparative endothelial cells. Endothelial cells are capable of undergoing fibrous metaplasia to produce extracellular collagen and a retrocorneal fibrous plaque. These plaques are commonly found at the posterior aspect of keratoplasty wounds (stromal ingrowth) and are found in cases of severe corneal trauma or severe anterior segment inflammation.

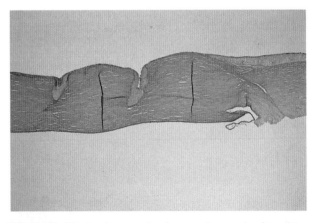

FIG. 9-37. Photomicrograph of corneal wounds placed two years prior to penetrating keratoplasty. The wound separate easily through nearly their entire length during routine paraffin processing, indicating incomplete wound healing.

Penetrating keratoplasty wounds rarely are the site of ingress for squamous epithelial cells (epithelial downgrowth syndrome). Keratoplasty wounds remodel as do most wounds, which accounts for some variability of astigmatism in the postoperative period. Graft failure usually is due to a variation of the corneal endothelial decompensation syndrome. Endothelial rejection may be a source of endothelial injury in this setting. Full-thickness graft rejection has been greatly reduced by the use of antiinflammatory and cytotoxic agents. Surgical complications occasionally involve incomplete removal of host tissues, usually limited to retention of the host Descemet's membrane. Donor tissue may harbor microorganism and cause endophthalmitis.[60]

Lamellar keratoplasty and epikeratophakia create a large graft– host interface in a plane parallel to the surface of the cornea. There are few mechanisms by which architectural support can be established in this surgical plane and the junction remains weak. An intrastromal cystic cavity may be formed. The junction of graft and host also may harbor ingrowth of epithelium, creating a nutritional barrier to the graft and often graft loss.

Radial keratotomy involves a series of penetrating wounds of the anterior corneal surface, but not perforation of full-thickness cornea. The wound healing process is limited to that characteristic of the anterior corneal stroma. It has often been observed, however, that although the epithelial facet forms in a timely manner, there is limited or no response from the surrounding stromal tissue. The epithelial facet may remain for months to years after the procedure. The lack of a meaningful stromal healing response creates a cornea that is susceptible to rupture from forces weaker than those required to disrupt native corneal tissue. Inadvertent perforations of the cornea at the time of radial keratotomy increase the risk of microbial and epithelial invasion of the anterior chamber.[67]

Implantation of synthetic materials in the corneal stroma, either to alter the anterior contour of the cornea or to alter the index of refraction of the cornea, has the common problem of creating a barrier to diffusion of nutrients across the stroma. Anterior and posterior ulceration of the cornea associated with extrusion of the synthetic implant are common occurrences.[68] Use of a ring of material not involving the visual axis of the cornea is currently being investigated.

The excimer laser removes tissue by delivering sufficient energy via a specific wavelength of light (193 nm) to disrupt intermolecular bonds of tissue in a short enough period to minimize damage to surrounding tissue.[69] Removal of large amounts of tissue stimulates a wound healing response in the corneal tissue. This response may reverse the desired refractive effect. Removal of lesser amounts of tissue gives less refractive effect, but stimulates less of a negating tissue response. Unless deep corneal penetrations are used, the endothelial cell layer appears to be uninfluenced by the application of the laser energy.

Surgical Procedures at the Pars Plana

Precise intraocular entry via the pars plana is the least risky route into the posterior chamber and the vitreous compartment. At the pars plana, the two layers of neuro-epithelium—the natural anterior extensions of the plane of the retina and the retinal pigment epithelium—are tightly adherent and unlikely to separate with mechanical penetration. Thus, there is less chances of ciliochoroidal or retinal detachment. Potential complications include inaccurate placement of the wound to involve the vascular structures of the pars plicata or posterior placement through the peripheral retina. The wound tract also is a possible access route for episcleral tissue to enter the eye, create a fibrous ingrowth, and cause traction retinal detachment or displacement of the crystalline lens.[70] Vitrectomy procedures also may adversely affect the biochemical microenvironment of the lens leading to cataract formation. Undue traction on the vitreous base may cause holes to form in the peripheral retina and result in a retinal detachment.

Surgical Procedures on the Retina

Most retinal surgical procedures involve laser surgery or retinal reattachment procedures, which usually are accomplished by external means such as the application of a scleral buckle. Only infrequently is the retina directly manipulated. The most common direct retinal surgical procedure involves removing delicate epiretinal membranes, which distorts the internal contour of the retina by creating traction on the internal limiting membrane. Complications of this procedure include inadvertent penetration of the retina itself and intraoperative hemorrhage.

Healing of mechanical wounds of the retina is rarely observed, although Mueller cells, theoretically, are capable of repairing small rents. The most common healing response of the retina is to thermal injury, most often following cryotherapy or photocoagulation. Application of either extreme heat or cold causes necrosis of both the retinal pigment epithelium and most of the cells of the overlying neurosensory retina. Under ideal conditions, extracellular materials of the retina such as the internal limiting membrane, basement membrane of vascular channels, and the basement membrane of the retinal pigment epithelium (a portion of Bruch's membrane) remain intact to provide a reparative scaffold for regenerating cells. Adjacent uninjured retinal pigment epithelial cells become depigmented and fusiform and migrate into the area of necrosis following removal of necrotic debris by macrophages. Likewise, adjacent surviving Mueller cells migrate into the defect of the neurosensory retina. When these two cell masses come in contact, they form strong intercellular attachments (desmosomes) and effectively seal the two layers of the retina creating a "chorioretinal scar" although the choroid is not directly involved.

Complications of retinal laser or cryosurgery are most commonly seen when one of the extracellular boundaries is breached by the application of excessive amounts of energy. If Bruch's membrane is interrupted, fibrovascular tissue from the choroid may migrate into the adjacent subretinal space leading to photoreceptor dysfunction and possible subretinal hemorrhage and the formation of a disciform scar. Breaching of the internal limiting membrane may lead to the creation of epiretinal membranes that may distort the internal contour of the retina. Rupture of vascular basement membranes can lead to immediate intraoperative hemorrhage or delayed hemorrhage as thrombosed vessels are recanalized in the postoperative period.

REFERENCES

1. Schein OD, Hibberd PL, Singleton BJ, et al. The spectrum and burden of ocular injury. *Ophthalmology* 1988;95:300.
2. Fuller DG, Hutton WL. Prediction of postoperative vision in eyes with severe trauma. *Retina* 1990;10:20.
3. Barr CC. Prognostic factors in corneoscleral lacerations. *Ophthalmology* 1983;101:919.
4. Manshot WA. The pathology of expulsive choroidal hemorrhage. *Am J Ophthalmol* 1955;40:25.
5. Purcell JJ, Krachmer JH, Doughman DJ, Bourne WM. Expulsive choroidal hemorrhage in penetrating keratoplasty. *Ophthalmology* 1982;89:41–43.
6. Speaker MG, Guerriero PN, Met JA, et al. A case-control study of risk factors for intraoperative suprachoroidal expulsive hemorrhage. *Ophthalmology* 1991;98:837–842.
7. McDonnell PJ, Green WR, Stevens RE, et al. Blood staining of the cornea: light microscopic and ultrastructural features. *Ophthalmology* 1985;92:1668.
8. Gerkowicz K, Prost M, Wawrzyniak M. Experimental ocular siderosis after extrabulbar administration of iron. *Br J Ophthalmol* 1985;69:149.
9. Campbell DG, Simmons RJ, Grant WM. Ghost cells as a cause of glaucoma. *Am J Ophthalmol* 1976;81:441–450.
10. Goldberg MF. Sickled erythrocytes, hyphema and secondary glaucoma. *Ophthalmic Surg* 1979;10:17.
11. Gregor Z, Ryan SJ. Combined posterior contusion and penetrating injury in the pig eye. II. Histologic features. *Br J Ophthalmol* 1982;66:799.
12. Vergara O, Ogden T, Ryan S. Posterior penetrating injury in the rabbit eye: effect of blood and ferrous ions. *Exp Eye Res* 1989;49:1115.
13. Cleary PE, Ryan SJ. Experimental posterior penetrating eye injury in the rabbit. II. Histology of the wound, vitreous, and retina. *Br J Ophthalmol* 1979;63:321.
14. Lubin JR, Albert DM, Weinstein M. Sixty-five years of sympathetic ophthalmia: a clinicopathologic review of 105 cases. *Am J Ophthalmol* 1980;87:109–121.
15. Lewis ML, Gass JDM, Spencer WH. Sympathetic uveitis after trauma and vitrectomy. *Arch Ophthalmol* 1978;96:263–267.
16. Herschler J. Trabecular damage due to blunt anterior segment injury and its relationship to traumatic glaucoma. *Trans Am Acad Ophthalmol Otolaryngol* 1977;83:239.
17. Colosi NJ, Yanoff M. Reactive corneal endothelialization. *Am J Ophthalmol* 1977;83:219–224.
18. Jensen P, Minckler DS, Chandler JW. Epithelial ingrowth. *Arch Ophthalmol* 1977;95:837–842.

19. Croft CB, Tarin D. Ultrastructural studies of wound healing in mouse skin. I. Epithelial behavior. *J Anat* 1970;106:63–77.

20. Croft CB, Tarin D. Ultrastructural studies of wound healing in mouse skin: II. Dermal-epidermal relationships. *J Anat* 1970;106: 79–91.

21. Paterson CA, Pfister RR, Levinson RA. Aqueous humor pH changes after experimental alkali burns. *Am J Ophthalmol* 1975;79:414.

22. Pfister RR. The alkali-burned cornea. I. Epithelial and stromal repair. *Exp Eye Res* 1976;23:1217–1222.

23. Austin P, Jakobiec FA, Iwamoto T. Elastodysplasia and elastodystrophy as pathologic basis of ocular pterygium and pinguecula. *Ophthalmology* 1984;90:96.

24. Ebato B, Friend J, Thoft R. Comparison of limbal and peripheral human corneal epithelium in tissue culture. *Invest Ophthalmol Vis Sci* 1988;29:1533–1537.

25. Russell SR, Olsen KR, Folk JC. Predictors of scleral rupture and the role of vitrectomy in severe blunt ocular trauma. *Am J Ophthalmol* 1988;105:253.

26. Cherry PMH. Rupture of the globe. *Arch Ophthalmol* 1972;88:498.

27. Wolff SM, Zimmerman LE. Chronic secondary glaucoma associated with retrodisplacement or iris root and deepening of the anterior chamber angle secondary to contusion. *Am J Ophthalmol* 1962;54: 547.

28. Kaufman JH, Toplin DW. Glaucoma after traumatic angle recession: a ten-year prospective study. *Am J Ophthalmol* 1974;78:648.

29. Wittenmann GJ, Brubaker SJ, Johnson M, et al. Traumatic hyphema in a defined population. *Am J Ophthalmol* 1988;106:123.

30. Caprioli J, Sears ML. The histopathology of blackball hyphema: a report of two cases. *Ophthalmic Surg* 1985;15:491.

31. Wolter JR, Henderson JW, Talley TR. Histopathology of blackball clot around four days after total hyphema. *J Pediatr Ophthalmol Strabismus* 1971;8:15.

32. Font FL, Brownstein S. A light and electron microscopic study of anterior subcapsular cataracts. *Am J Ophthalmol* 1974;78:972–984.

33. Marak GE, Font RL, Czawlytko LN, Alepa FP. Experimental lens-induced granulomatous endophthalmitis: preliminary histopathologic observations. *Exp Eye Res* 1974;19:311.

34. Ross WH. Traumatic retinal dialyses. *Arch Ophthalmol* 1981;99: 1371.

35. Blight R, Hart JCD. Structural changes in the outer retinal layers following blunt mechanical trauma to the globe: an experimental study. *Br J Ophthalmol* 1977;61:573–587.

36. Sipperley JO, Quigley HA, Gass JDM. Traumatic retinopathy in primates: the explanation of commotio retinae. *Arch Ophthalmol* 1978;96:2278.

37. Aguilar JP, Green WR. Choroidal rupture: a histopathologic study of 47 cases. *Retina* 1984;4:269.

38. Wyszynski RE, Grossniklaus HE, Frank KE. Indirect choroidal rupture secondary to blunt ocular trauma. *Retina* 1988;8:267.

39. Shapiro I, Jacob HS. Leukoembolization in ocular vascular occlusion. *Ann Ophthalmol* 1982;14:60–62.

40. Kincaid MC, Green WR, Knox DL, Mohler C. A clinicopathological case report of retinopathy of pancreatitis. *Br J Ophthalmol* 1982; 66:219–226.

41. Benson WE. The effects of blunt trauma on the posterior segment of the eye. *Trans Pa Acad Ophthalmol Otolaryngol* 1984;37:26.

42. Williams DF, Williams GA, Abrams GW, et al. Evulsion of the retina associated with optic nerve evulsion. *Am J Ophthalmol* 1987; 104:5.

43. Honda Y, Asayama K. Intraocular graphite pencil lead without reaction. *Am J Ophthalmol* 1985;99:494.

44. Potts AM, Distlet JA. Shape factor in penetration of intraocular foreign bodies. *Am J Ophthalmol* 1985;100:183.

45. Sternberg P, deJuan E, Green WR, et al. Ocular BB injuries. *Ophthalmology* 1984;91:1269.

46. Brown GC, Tasman WS, Benson WE. BB-gun injuries to the eye. *Ophthalmic Surg* 1985;16:505.

47. Schmidt JGH. Intravitreal cupruferous foreign bodies: electroretinograms and inflammatory processes. *Doc Ophthalmol* 1988;67:253.

48. Rao NA, Tso MOM, Rosenthal AR. Chalcosis in the human eye. *Arch Ophthalmol* 1976;94:1379.

49. Bettman JWJ. Pathology of complications of intraocular surgery. *Am J Ophthalmol* 1969;81:1037.

50. Kimble JA, Morris RE, Witherspoon CD. Globe perforation from peribulbar injection. *Arch Ophthalmol* 1987;105:749.

51. Borges J, Zony-Yi L, Tso MOM. Effects of repeated photic exposures on the monkey macula. *Arch Ophthalmol* 1990;108:727–733.

52. Anderson RL. Visual loss after blepharoplasty. *Arch Ophthalmol* 1981;99:2205.

53. Greenberg DR, Ellenhorn NL, Chapman LT, et al. Posterior chamber hemorrhage during strabismus surgery. *Am J Ophthalmol* 1988; 106:634.

54. Gottlieb F, Castro JL. Perforation of the globe during strabismus surgery. *Arch Ophthalmol* 1970;84:151–156.

55. Flaxel JT, Swan KC. Limbal wound healing after cataract extraction. *Arch Ophthalmol* 1969;81:653–659.

56. Flaxel JT. Histology of cataract extraction. *Arch Ophthalmol* 1970; 83:436–444.

57. Kozart DM, Eagle RCJ. Stripping of Descemet's membrane after glaucoma surgery. *Ophthalmic Surg* 1981;12:420–423.

58. Swan KC. Fibroblastic ingrowth following cataract extraction. *Arch Ophthalmol* 1973;89:445–449.

59. Swan KC. Late hyphema due to wound vascularization. *Trans Am Acad Ophthalmol Otolaryngol* 1996;81:138–144.

60. Pfugfelder SC, Flynn TW, Zwickey TA, et al. Exogenous fungal endophthalmitis. *Ophthalmology* 1988;95:19.

61. Meisler DM, Palestine AG, Vastine DW, Demartini DR, et al. Chronic propionibacterium acne endophthalmitis after extracapsular cataract extraction and intraocular lens implantation. *Am J Ophthalmol* 1986;102:733–739.

62. Beatty RF, Robin JB, Trousdale MD. Anaerobic endophthalmitis caused by propionibacterium acnes. *Am J Ophthalmol* 1986;101: 114.

63. Turkish L, Galin MA. Methylmethacrylate monomer in intraocular lenses of polymethylmethacrylate. Cellullar toxicity. *Arch Ophthalmol* 1980;98:120–121.

64. McDonnell PJ, de la Cruz ZC, Green WR. Location and composition of haptics of posterior chamber lenses. *Ophthalmology* 1987; 94:136–142.

65. Champion R, McDonnell PJ, Green WR. Histopathologic characteristics of a large series of autopsy eyes. *Surv Ophthalmol* 1985;30: 1–32.

66. Ellingson FT. Complications with the Choyce Mark VIII anterior chamber lens implant. *AIOIS Journal* 1977;3:199–200.

67. Binder PS, Nayak SK, Deg JJK, Zavala E, Sugar J. An ultrastructural and histochemical study of long-term wound healing after radial keratotomy. *Am J Ophthalmol* 1987;213:432–440.

68. Samples JR, Binder PS, Zavala EY, Baumgartner SD, Deg JJK. Morphology of hydrogel implants used for refractive keratoplasty. *Invest Ophthalmol Vis Sci* 1984;25:843–850.

69. Taylor DM, L'Esperance FAJ, Del Pero RA, et al. Human excimer laser lamellar keratectomy: a clinical study. *Ophthalmology* 1989; 96:654–664.

70. Fauborn J, Conway BP, Machimer R. Surgical complications of pars plana vitreous surgery. *Ophthalmology* 1978;96:116–125.

Ophthalmic Pathology with Clinical Correlations,
edited by Joseph W. Sassani, M.D.
Lippincott-Raven Publishers, Philadelphia © 1997.

CHAPTER 10

Uvea (Including Melanoma)

Kerry E. Hunt and Ben J. Glasgow

The **uvea** consists of the iris, ciliary body, and choroid. Conditions affecting the uvea include neoplastic, infectious, inflammatory, and degenerative diseases, trauma, and congenital abnormalities. This chapter describes the normal anatomy and presents the common pathologic disorders of the uveal tract. Trauma, uveitis, glaucoma, and conditions of the uveal tract unique to the pediatric age are discussed elsewhere.

ANATOMY AND HISTOLOGY

The uvea is one contiguous structure with distinct anatomic and physiologic regional differences. The three uveal structures share a rich interconnected vascular system. The posterior choroid is supplied by multiple **short posterior ciliary arteries** that penetrate the sclera and enter the choroid close to the optic nerve. The anterior choroid, ciliary body, and iris are supplied by two long posterior ciliary arteries and seven **anterior ciliary arteries**. The posterior ciliary arteries pass through the sclera and enter the choroid posteriorly. They pass through the choroid, anastomosing with the anterior ciliary arteries that penetrate the sclera after traveling with and supplying the rectus muscles. Venous drainage occurs from several large vortex veins located just posterior to the equator in each quadrant. Individual variation does occur. The **blood–ocular barriers** associated with the uveal circulation include the endothelium of the iris vessels, the nonpigmented ciliary epithelium, and the retinal pigment epithelium.

Numerous dendritic melanocytes throughout the uvea absorb light. The rich vascularity and abundant melanin give the uvea its dark color. Fibroblasts, nerves, and connective tissue are integral parts of the uvea.

K. E. Hunt and B. J. Glasgow: Jules Stein Eye Institute, UCLA School of Medicine, Los Angeles, California 90024.

Iris

The **iris** divides the anterior and posterior chambers, forms the pupillary aperture that controls the amount of light entering the eye, and contributes to depth of focus. The irregularity of the surface of the iris is caused by blood vessels, fibrous stromal bands, intervening crypts, and contraction furrows. Iris color is determined by the number and pigment content of stromal melanocytes.

The iris contains four important layers: the **anterior border layer**, the **stroma**, the **dilator muscle**, and the **iris pigment epithelium**. The anterior border layer is a condensation of stromal cells and melanocytes. In some areas the border layer is absent. The stroma is made of collagen fibers, dendritic melanocytes, **clump cells**, blood vessels, nerves, and the sphincter muscle. Clump cells are heavily pigmented cells that are most numerous near the sphincter muscle and iris root. Most clump cells are pigment-containing macrophages. Some have a surrounding basement membrane and are neuroepithelial in origin.[1] The **sphincter** and **dilator muscles** are smooth muscle. They are derived from the outer layer of the optic cup and are therefore neuroectoderm. The nuclei of the dilator muscle cells lie within the pigmented cytoplasm posterior to the muscle fibers. The **iris pigment epithelium**, the most posterior layer, consists of irregular cuboidal cells with densely packed round uniform pigment granules. It is derived from the inner layer of the optic cup.

Ciliary Body

The **ciliary body** is composed of two parts, the **pars plicata** and the **pars plana**. The pars plicata, a series of about 70 radially oriented projections called the ciliary processes, makes up the anterior 2 mm of the ciliary body. The pars plana is contiguous with the pars plicata anteriorly and the choroid posteriorly. It is flat and makes up the posterior 4 to 4.5 mm.

The **ciliary body** is composed of six layers. From internal to external, they are the **internal basement membrane** or **basement membrane of the nonpigmented ciliary epithelium**, the **nonpigmented ciliary epithelium**, the **pigmented ciliary epithelium**, the **basement membrane of the pigmented ciliary epithelium**, the **vessel layer**, and the **ciliary muscle**. The nonpigmented ciliary epithelium is contiguous with the pigmented iris epithelium in the ciliary sulcus and with the neurosensory retina at the ora serrata. The cells are cuboidal anteriorly and become more columnar near the ora serrata. Tight junctions between nonpigmented epithelial cells form the blood–ocular barrier in this area. The nonpigmented ciliary epithelium is the site of aqueous production. The pigmented ciliary epithelium is contiguous with the iris dilator muscle at the iris root and with the retinal pigment epithelium at the ora serrata. The cells are cuboidal and densely packed with round melanin granules. The vessel layer is a continuation of the choroidal vasculature in the pars plana. Large capillary tufts from the long posterior ciliary vessels are present in the ciliary processes. Capillaries in the ciliary body are permeable to plasma proteins because of large pores in their walls.[2] The **major vascular circle of the iris**, which is not part of the vascular layer, is located in the most anterior portion of the ciliary body near the iris root. The ciliary muscle is divided into three groups of fibers. The innermost circular fibers and the central radial fibers contribute to zonular tension on the lens and accommodation. The outermost longitudinal fibers insert into the scleral spur and help modulate aqueous outflow. The suprachoroidal tissue plane is a potential space between the ciliary muscle and the sclera.

Choroid

The **choroid** is a delicate vascular structure that begins at the ora serrata, where it merges imperceptibly with the ciliary body, and ends at the optic nerve. It is attached to the sclera by fine connective tissue strands and by the numerous nerves and vessels that enter the eye posteriorly.

There are four layers of the choroid. From internal to external, they are **Bruch's membrane**, the **choriocapillaris**, the **stroma**, and the **lamina fusca**. Bruch's membrane is composed of five structures. Innermost is the basement membrane of the retinal pigment epithelium. An elastic layer is centrally located between collagenous layers. The outermost layer is the basement membrane of the choriocapillaris. The choriocapillaris is a single layer of fenestrated capillaries adjacent to Bruch's membrane. It supplies substrates of metabolism to the retinal pigment epithelium and the outer retinal layers. The stroma is composed mostly of medium to large choroidal vessels, the largest of which lie in the outermost portions. Ciliary nerves are numerous. The long ciliary nerves are large

nerves that enter the eye posteriorly and extend to the ciliary body within the choroid near the horizontal plane. Scattered dendritic melanocytes and loose fibrous tissue are present between vessels. The lamina fusca contains densely packed melanocytes, collagen, and elastic fibers. These elements extend through the sclera around blood vessels and nerves in emissarial canals.

IRIS CYSTS

Iris cysts may be congenital or acquired and are lined by surface epithelium or neuroepithelium.[3] The origin of **primary stromal cysts** is unknown; secondary cysts arise from implanted surface epithelium from surgical or nonsurgical trauma. Stromal cysts may grow to a large size and obstruct the pupil or cause secondary angle-closure glaucoma. They lie within the iris stroma and have an epithelial lining that resembles corneal epithelium or conjunctival epithelium if goblet cells are present.

Primary iris epithelial cysts are lined by the inner layer of neuroepithelium and are much more common than stromal cysts. Cysts arising from the nonpigmented ciliary epithelium of the ciliary processes have traditionally been grouped with iris cysts and together are sometimes referred to as **sulcus cysts**. The majority (85%) of epithelial cysts, in which the site of origin can be established, arise from the peripheral iris or ciliary processes.[3] Cysts arising in or near the pupillary aperture can be seen directly or after pupillary dilation. Peripherally located cysts commonly cause anterior bulging of the iris visible with slit-lamp biomicroscopy and require wide dilation and gonioscopy to be seen directly. Rarely, iris epithelial cysts separate from the iris and float free in the anterior chamber or vitreous. Secondary iris epithelial cysts are associated with miotic drug therapy and regress with discontinuance of drug use. Therapy for iris cysts is not required unless visual disturbance or pupillary block occurs.

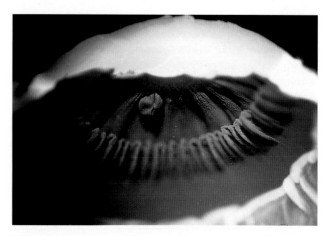

FIG. 10-1. Gross appearance of a pigment epithelial cyst of the mid iris.

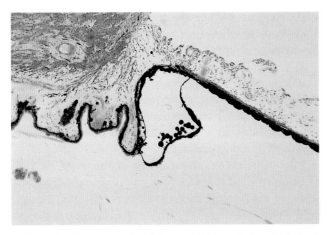

FIG. 10-2. Pigment epithelial cyst of the peripheral iris (sulcus cyst). The cyst is located at the junction of the iris and the ciliary processes and is lined by pigmented epithelium.

Iris epithelial cysts are lined by pigmented epithelium if they arise strictly from the posterior surface of the iris (Fig. 10-1). These cysts are formed by a separation of the two layers of iris pigment epithelium. Cysts arising near the ciliary sulcus may be lined by pigmented or nonpigmented epithelium or both (Fig. 10-2). The bases of these cysts are lined by both inner and outer epithelial layers, indicating that they arise from a proliferation of inner neuroepithelial cells rather than a separation of the inner and outer layers.[4]

PARS PLANA CYSTS

Pars plana cysts are not true cysts; rather, they represent a separation of the pigmented and nonpigmented ciliary epithelium filled with hyaluronic acid (Fig. 10-3). They increase with age and are found in a third of persons over age 70.[5] Pars plana cysts vary from small lesions (less

than 0.5 mm in diameter) near the ora serrata to large bullous lesions (2 to 3 mm wide), spanning the whole pars plana anterior to posterior. They can become confluent, forming ever-larger bullous lesions. Occasionally, larger cysts develop a white fibrous base called a **Snell plaque** (Fig. 10-4). Opaque cysts filled with proteinaceous material occur in hyperproteinemic states and in persons with liver disease (Fig. 10-5).

IRIDOSCHISIS

Iridoschisis is an atrophic condition characterized by splitting and separation of iris stromal fibers. Extensive atrophy may lead to total baring of the muscular and epithelial layers. This rare condition is causally associated with iritis, trauma, angle-closure glaucoma, and the use of miotics.[6]

IRIS HETEROCHROMIA

Differences in color between a person's eyes are caused by various conditions (Table 1). Increased melanin and deposition of iron pigment make the involved iris appear darker. Increased vascularity may impart a red or orange color. In general, stromal atrophy makes the iris lighter in color; however, atrophy in lightly pigmented eyes can uncover the pigment epithelium and make the involved eye appear darker.

UVEAL EDEMA/UVEAL EFFUSION SYNDROME

Uveal edema is characterized by the accumulation of fluid within the choroid and ciliary body. Enough exudation can occur to cause choroidal or ciliary body detach-

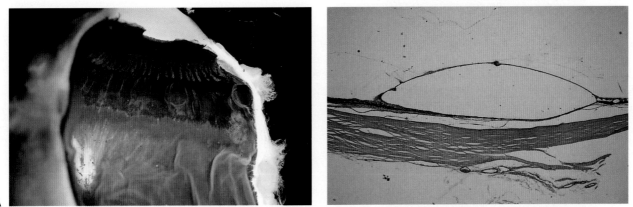

A   B

FIG. 10-3. (A) Gross appearance of several pars plana cysts. The pars plana clear cyst on the right is divided so that the cavity is visible. **(B)** Section shows bullous separation of the pigmented and nonpigmented ciliary epithelium extending to the ora serrata where there is typical cystoid degeneration of the peripheral retina.

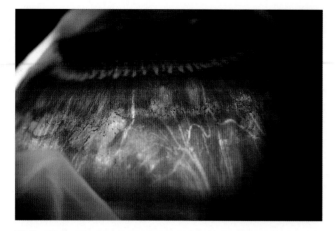

FIG. 10-4. Gross appearance of a large pars plana cyst with a white fibrous base (Snell plaque).

ment from the sclera. Fluid preferentially accumulates beneath the ciliary body and anterior choroid due to regional differences in uveoscleral attachment fibers.[7] Strong uveal anchoring sites at the scleral spur, optic nerve, vortex veins, and ciliary vessels explain the lobular clinical appearance of large uveal detachments. Chronic effusion may cause disruption of the retinal pigment epithelium and breakdown of the blood–ocular barrier. Exudate then can enter the subretinal space, causing retinal detachment.

Uveal detachment can lead to acute angle-closure glaucoma due to anterior rotation of the ciliary body and pupillary block from anterior displacement of the lens. Conversely, hypotony may result from chronic uveal effu-

sion. Mechanisms causing hypertony include decreased aqueous production from detachment of the ciliary body, increased uveoscleral outflow, or both.

The most common cause of choroidal detachment is hypotony from surgical or nonsurgical trauma, which leads to choroidal vascular dilatation and fluid exudation. Extreme systemic hypertension, uveal inflammation, nanophthalmos, and sources of uveal traction are other causes of choroidal edema.

Idiopathic serous detachment of the uvea, or uveal effusion syndrome, is a chronic progressive condition that leads to exudative retinal detachment.[8] Retinal pigment epithelium abnormalities with streaks of hyper- and hypopigmented areas (''leopard spots'') are seen clinically. Gross examination of the eyes usually shows exudative retinal detachment, pigment epithelium changes, detached and edematous ciliary body and anterior choroid, and a thickened sclera. Histologically, hypertrophy and hyperplasia of the retinal pigment epithelium and edema and mild chronic inflammation of the uvea are seen. Thickened scleral fibers and vortex vein abnormalities have been found in many cases. Increased amounts of glycosaminoglycans have been demonstrated within the sclera. Electron microscopy shows an increased diameter of scleral collagen fibrils and deposition of glycosaminoglycans.[9] The pathophysiology of this condition is believed to be reduced transscleral flow of uveal proteins and fluids due to the accumulation of glycosaminoglycans and scleral swelling. This appears to have been the same mechanism of chronic choroidal effusion in a patient with **Hunter syndrome.**[10] Treatment has been directed at in-

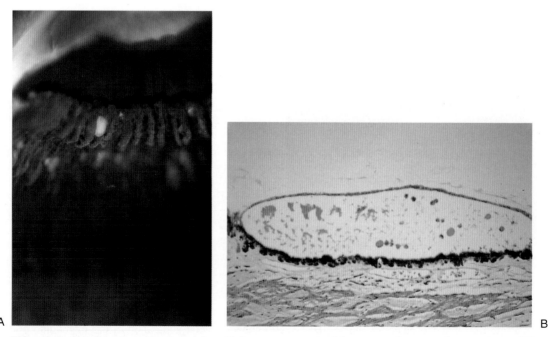

FIG. 10-5. (A) Gross appearance of multiple opaque cyst of the pars plicata and pars plana. **(B)** Proteinaceous fluid fills the cyst.

TABLE 1. *Iris heterochromia:
conditions and mechanisms*

Increased stromal melanin
  Diffuse nevus
  Diffuse melanoma
  Ocular melanocytosis
  Oculodermal melanocytosis
  Iris nevus syndrome
Decreased stromal melanin
  Congenital Horner syndrome
  Iris atrophy
  Fuchs heterochromic iridocyclitis
  Chronic iritis
  Acute angle-closure glaucoma
  Essential iris atrophy
  Waardenburg syndrome
  Bicolored irides of Hirschsprung disease
Increased vascularity
  Rubeosis iridis
  Juvenile xanthogranuloma
Deposition of material
  Siderosis
  Hemosiderosis
Others
  Leukemic infiltration

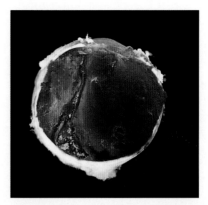

FIG. 10-6. Choroidal hemorrhage following penetrating trauma. The anterior segment structures were expulsed by choroidal hemorrhage.

creasing scleral or venous flow by lamellar scleral resection or decompression of vortex veins.[11]

UVEAL HEMORRHAGE

Expulsive choroidal hemorrhage can occur in the setting of rapid reduction of intraocular pressure. Exudation with or without mild hemorrhage from small choroidal vessels causes expansion of the choroid and tension on penetrating posterior ciliary vessels. Rupture of these vessels leads to massive hemorrhage within the suprachoroidal space (Fig. 10-6). Ocular structures are expulsed by the rapidly expanding choroidal hemorrhage. Blood can extend into the subretinal space and vitreous. Histopathologic examination has demonstrated ruptured penetrating posterior ciliary arteries in a few cases. Arteriolar fragility has been implicated as contributing to the development of expulsive choroidal hemorrhage because patients with hypertension and advanced age are at greatest risk for developing expulsive hemorrhage during intraocular surgery. Causes of expulsive choroidal hemorrhage are listed in Table 2.

Subacute hemorrhages can lead to hemorrhagic uveal detachment. The clinical presentation is similar to that of serous uveal detachment. Localized choroidal hemorrhages may accompany choroidal ruptures from blunt ocular trauma.

Organization of choroidal hemorrhage is followed by fibrovascular proliferation. Dense collagenous membranes form, and with time osseous or fatty metaplasia may occur.

ACQUIRED NEUROECTODERMAL TUMORS OF THE CILIARY BODY

Fuchs Adenoma/Hyperplasia

Fuchs adenoma (also known as coronal adenoma or **pseudoadenomatous hyperplasia**) is an acquired benign lesion of the nonpigmented ciliary epithelium. Fuchs adenomas are the most common tumors of the eye: they occur in up to 31% of patients in autopsy series and increase in prevalence with age.[12] It is unknown whether these tumors represent true neoplasms or hyperplasias. Generally, they cause no ocular symptoms and are discovered at autopsy. They may cause sectoral cataracts or simulate iris or ciliary body neoplasms.[13,14]

Fuchs adenomas are small (less than 1.4 mm) white nodules on or within ciliary processes (Fig. 10-7). Rarely, they are pigmented due to overlying pigmented ciliary epithelium. Histologically, these tumors are composed of sheets and chords of hyperplastic nonpigmented ciliary epithelium with thick deposits of eosinophilic, periodic acid–Schiff (PAS)-positive basement membrane-like material. Immunohistochemical and electron microscopic studies indicate that the cells closely resemble the nonpigmented epithelium of the ciliary processes and that the extracellular material is

TABLE 2. *Causes of expulsive
choroidal hemorrhage*

Intraocular surgery
Penetrating trauma
Perforating corneal ulcer
Malignant melanoma
Spontaneous hypotony
Thrombocytopenia
Choroidal vascular aneurysm

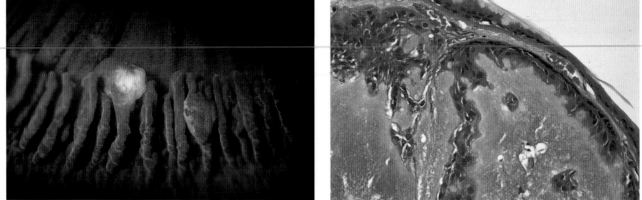

FIG. 10-7. Fuchs adenoma. (**A**) A typical adenoma covered by nonpigmented epithelium is shown on the left. An adenoma covered by pigmented epithelium is on the right. (**B**) Fuchs' adenoma showing cords of nonpigmented ciliary epithelium and thick hyalinized basement membrane material.

most likely dense deposits of epithelial basement membrane material.[15]

If necessary, fine-needle aspiration biopsy can be performed to rule out a malignant melanoma of the ciliary body. Aspiration biopsy reveals cohesive groups of nonpigmented epithelial cells around pink extracellular matrix material with hematoxylin and eosin (H&E) stain. The nuclei are round to oval with homogeneous chromatin and small nucleoli.[16]

Adenoma/Adenocarcinoma of the Nonpigmented Ciliary Epithelium

Neoplasms of the nonpigmented epithelium of the ciliary body are rare tumors that are frequently mistaken for other lesions. Simulating lesions include amelanotic melanoma, metastatic tumors, and leiomyomas of the ciliary body. Clinically, these tumors present as yellow to tan endophytic lesions that do not block transillumination. Ultrasound demonstrates high internal reflectivity compared to melanomas. The correct diagnosis usually becomes evident on histologic analysis after tumor removal.

Adenomas and carcinomas are differentiated by evidence of tissue invasion and the amount of cellular atypia; however, precise categorization is often not realized for nonpigmented epithelial tumors. Adenomas may be classified as solid, papillary, or **pleomorphic**.[17] Cells may form sheets, tubuloacinar structures, or solid masses. Occasionally, cells are embedded in a mucoid stroma (Fig. 10-8). Mitotic figures are rare, and there is minimal nuclear pleomorphism.

Carcinomas of the nonpigmented ciliary epithelium are rare and display a broad spectrum of differentiation. A proposed classification of these tumors includes glandular or papillary, pleomorphic of low grade, pleomorphic with hyaline stroma, and anaplastic types.[18] There seems to be

a propensity for poorly differentiated tumors in phthisical eyes associated with trauma or longstanding inflammation, leading some to believe they arise from neoplastic transformation of reactive hyperplasia of the ciliary epithelium.[18,19] Some cells may contain pigment. Intraluminal hyaluronidase-sensitive mucopolysaccharides are found within the tumor.[20] This may be a helpful distinguishing feature from metastatic adenocarcinomas that possess intracellular mucopolysaccharides.[21]

Immunohistochemistry and electron microscopy can be used to differentiate nonpigmented ciliary epithelium adenomas and adenocarcinomas from other intraocular lesions. Ciliary body adenomas and adenocarcinomas react with antibodies to intermediate filaments, vimentin, and S-100. Reactions to cytokeratin and HMB-45 are negative.[22] Ultrastructural features include desmosomes between tumor cells, areas of thick multilaminated basement membrane, intracytoplasmic filaments, and intercellular lumens with microvillous processes.

Adenoma/Carcinoma of the Pigmented Ciliary Epithelium

Acquired tumors of the pigmented ciliary epithelium are rare and are usually mistaken for malignant melanoma of the ciliary body. Diagnosis is made at the time of enucleation or local resection. Both adenomas and adenocarcinomas of the pigmented ciliary epithelium have been described. The distinction is based on subjective criteria such as invasion or cellular pleomorphism, although several locally invasive tumors have been labeled adenomas.[23]

Solid, papillary, and vacuolated patterns have been described; the vacuolated or cystic variety appears to be the most characteristic (Fig. 10-9). The tumors are composed of large pigmented cells arranged in sheets, chords, and nodules. Vacuoles containing hyaluronidase-resistant mu-

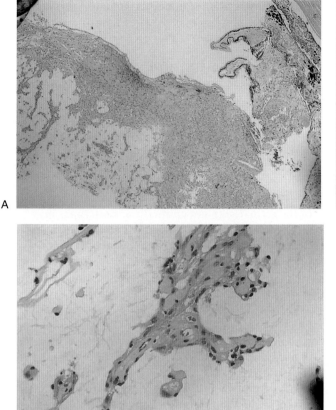

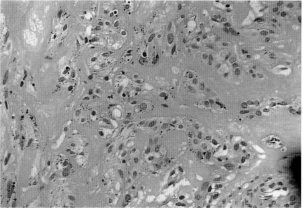

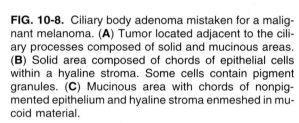

FIG. 10-8. Ciliary body adenoma mistaken for a malignant melanoma. (**A**) Tumor located adjacent to the ciliary processes composed of solid and mucinous areas. (**B**) Solid area composed of chords of epithelial cells within a hyaline stroma. Some cells contain pigment granules. (**C**) Mucinous area with chords of nonpigmented epithelium and hyaline stroma enmeshed in mucoid material.

copolysaccharides are present throughout the tumor. Large melanin granules and macromelanosomes are present in the cells containing pigment.

Electron microscopy demonstrates tight cell junctions, well-developed basement membrane, and intracytoplasmic and intercellular spaces lined with microvilli. Immunohistochemistry in one case showed positive staining to cytokeratin and S-100 but negative staining to vimentin, HMB-45, neurofilaments, and epithelial membrane antigen.[24]

BENIGN REACTIVE LYMPHOID HYPERPLASIA (INFLAMMATORY PSEUDOTUMOR) OF THE UVEA

Benign reactive lymphoid hyperplasia, or **idiopathic inflammation of the uveal tract**, is a rare condition that masquerades as a primary uveal or metastatic tumor, lymphoma, leukemia, or infectious uveitis. Clinical diagnosis is extremely difficult and is considered after exclusion of the conditions mentioned.[25] The diagnosis is usually made at the time of enucleation.[26]

Isolated iris involvement is rare. **Inflammatory pseudotumor of the ciliary body** is frequently part of diffuse uveal involvement. Associated signs of uveal pseudotu-

mor include decreased vision, retinal detachment, elevated intraocular pressure, iridocyclitis, and signs of orbital inflammation.

Histologic diagnosis of the enucleation specimen is made by identifying features of benign lymphoid hyperplasia: a mixed cellular response, predominance of mature lymphocytes, and lymphoid follicles with reactive cen-

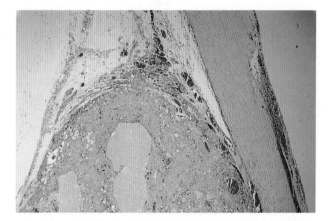

FIG. 10-9. Cystic variety of an adenoma of the pigmented ciliary epithelium. The tumor is composed of variably pigmented epithelial cells forming sheets and tubules.

ters. Helpful but nonspecific immunohistochemical findings include mixed B- and T-lymphocyte and polyclonal light chain surface markers. Degeneration, hyperplasia, and fibrous metaplasia of the retinal pigment epithelium, drusen, and extension of inflammation into the optic nerve have been observed.

The correct diagnosis is suggested by benign cellular characteristics in biopsy specimens, or mixed inflammatory cells lacking atypical features in cytologic specimens. Granulomatous inflammation raises other possibilities such as infection, sympathetic uveitis, or Harada disease.

PRIMARY TUMORS OF THE UVEA

Choroidal Osteoma

Choroidal osteoma, or **choroidal osseous choristoma**, is characterized by the formation of compact bone within the posterior choroid.[27] Young women seem to be the most frequently affected. The etiology of osseous choroidal tumors is unknown. Some cases of secondary choroidal ossification have followed inflammatory diseases of the orbit or choroid, systemic malignancy, and hypoparathyroidism.[28-30] Primary lesions, not associated with other conditions, are believed to represent choristomatous tumors. Choroidal osteomas have been reported in at least three families, implicating an inherited basis similar to most choristomas.[31-33]

Bone formation occurs adjacent to the optic nerve and with ophthalmoscopy has a white to orange color with irregular scalloped borders (Fig. 10-10). Retinal pigment epithelium changes are sometimes seen. Radial growth and decalcification of bone have been observed.[34] Ultrasonography shows a highly reflective area in the involved choroid even at very low decibel settings. Computed topography (CT) scans demonstrate radiopaque choroidal plaques of bone density as well. Magnetic resonance imaging (MRI) did not demonstrate the typical negative image of bone in 1 patient,[35] and the role of MRI in the diagnosis of choroidal osteoma has yet to be determined. Some patients have developed choroidal neovascular membranes associated with these tumors.

Histopathologic studies show dense cancellous bone, vascularized fatty marrow spaces, and all the normal cellular constituents of bone.[36,37] In some areas, Bruch's membrane is intact but compressed, and the retinal pigment epithelium and outer retina show focal atrophic changes.

Hemangioma

Hemangiomas are **vascular hamartomas**. Hemangiomas of the iris and ciliary body are rare, and the validity of many clinically reported cases is questionable. Many represent tumors of juvenile xanthogranuloma or highly vascular areas of other tumors.

Choroidal hemangiomas present with two growth patterns: diffuse and localized.[38] The **diffuse type** is associated with **Sturge-Weber syndrome**. Clinically, involved areas cannot be distinguished from uninvolved areas; however, the involved fundus has a deep-red hue compared to the fellow eye. Localized tumors have no associated systemic abnormalities and present as well-demarcated lesions (Fig. 10-11). Progressive growth of localized lesions is unusual.[39] Pigmentary changes are seen due to compressive effects on the adjacent choroid and atrophy and hyperplasia of the retinal pigment epithelium. Both types may have an associated retinal detachment or neovascular glaucoma. Elevated episcleral venous pressure and incomplete development of the aqueous drainage pathways are other mechanisms leading to glaucoma in patients with diffuse hemangiomas of the choroid.

Diffuse hemangiomas often are composed of a mixture of **capillary** and **cavernous** components. Localized hemangiomas are usually composed of cavernous or mixed vascular areas and rarely show only capillary formation (Fig. 10-12). Classification as capillary versus cavernous hemangioma depends on the size of the vascular channels. **Capillary hemangiomas** consist of small vessels lined by flat, inconspicuous endothelial cells. Blood elements are found within the vessels, and the vascular channels are surrounded by loose edematous connective tissue. **Cavernous hemangiomas** also contain thin-walled blood vessels lined by a flat endothelium; however, their vascular spaces are much larger and are separated by fibrous septa. Smooth muscle is absent in both cavernous and capillary hemangiomas. There is a complete lack of cellular proliferation, indicating that these lesions may represent vascular anomalies rather than neoplastic lesions. Seventy-five percent of localized hemangiomas have well-demarcated histologic borders; the other 25%, and all diffuse hemangiomas, have poorly defined borders. Diffuse hemangiomas also demonstrate engorgement of the normal choroidal vessels. The overlying retinal pigment epithelium frequently shows atrophy, hyperplasia, fibrous membrane formation, and ossification. Loss of the blood−retinal barrier can lead to cystic retinal changes, atrophy, and detachment.

Leiomyoma/Mesenchymal Leiomyoma

Leiomyomas are rare benign tumors displaying smooth muscle differentiation. In the uveal tract, they are thought to arise from sites of normal smooth muscle, such as the iris sphincter and dilator muscles, ciliary body smooth muscle, vascular smooth muscle, or from undifferentiated mesenchymal cells. Most cases have occurred in the iris

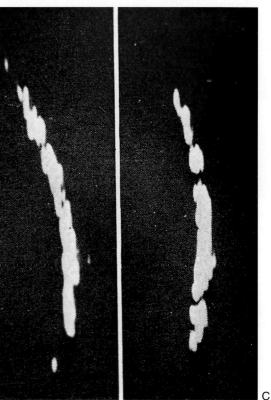

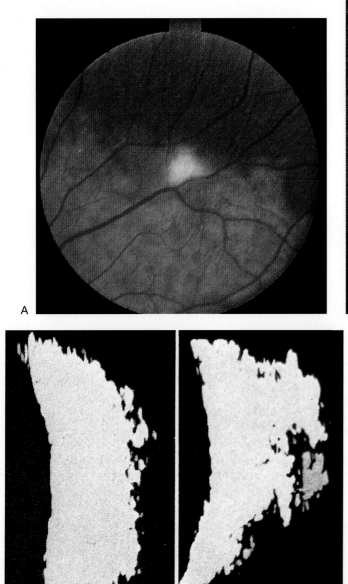

FIG. 10-10. (A) Clinical photo of a choroidal osteoma showing irregular borders and disturbance of the retinal pigment epithelium. (B) B-mode ultrasound shows a highly reflective choroidal mass at 80 dB setting. (C) High reflectivity remains at a setting of 50 dB. (Cunha SL. Osseous choristoma of the choroid: a familial disease. *Arch Ophthalmol* 1984;102:1052.)

and ciliary body and were mistaken clinically for a nodular amelanotic melanoma. There are no clinical features that reliably distinguish these from other uveal tumors; however, there are features that should lead one to consider the diagnosis of leiomyoma. Leiomyomas of the eye are usually found in females less than age 45. They usually arise in the ciliary body and lack a transillumination shadow.[40] Leiomyomas account for 0% to 14.5% of iris tumors in reported surgical series.[41,42] Only two cases have been reported in the choroid.[43]

Ultrasound and fluorescein angiography are frequently not helpful in the diagnosis due to the location of these tumors. Normal uvea over the tumor may suggest a leiomyoma rather than a melanoma. MRI performed on one large ciliochoroidal leiomyoma showed hyperintense T1-weighted images, hypointense T2-weighted images, and

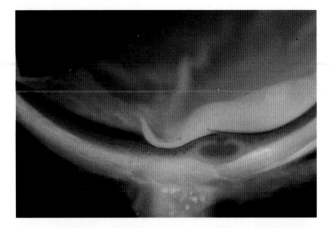

FIG. 10-11. Localized choroidal hemangioma. Well circumscribed hemangioma in an autopsy specimen of a newborn child.

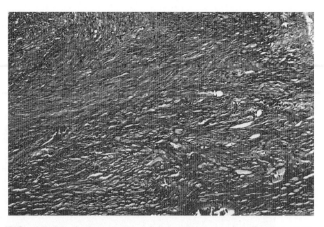

FIG. 10-13. Leiomyoma of the ciliary body. Tumor composed of tightly packed spindle-shaped cells with eosinophilic cytoplasm and long blunt-ended nuclei.

marked enhancement with gadolinium.[40] The ability of MRI to distinguish leiomyoma and amelanotic melanoma has not been fully delineated.

Light microscopic features of leiomyoma include tightly packed spindle-shaped cells with a moderate amount of eosinophilic cytoplasm and little or no intercellular stroma (Fig. 10-13). Nuclei are oval with blunted ends and may demonstrate palisading. Light microscopy has limited value because other tumors such as amelanotic spindle-cell melanomas, nevi, neurofibromas, and neurilemmomas have similar features. It is often necessary to use immunohistochemistry or electron microscopy to differentiate leiomyomas from other spindle-cell tumors.

Ultrastructural features of leiomyomas include numerous parallel intracytoplasmic filaments with associated oval to fusiform densities, numerous dense bodies and

pinocytotic vesicles associated with the plasma membrane, and a surrounding basement membrane.[44] The absence of melanosomes helps distinguish leiomyoma from amelanotic spindle-cell melanoma. Mesenchymal leiomyoma of the ciliary body has light and electron microscopic features of both smooth muscle and neural tissue.[45]

Immunohistochemistry may be helpful in the diagnosis of uveal leiomyomas. Smooth muscle cells normally stain positively with smooth muscle actin and the intermediate filaments desmin and vimentin. They do not react with HMB-45 or S-100, both of which are frequently used to detect melanocytic cell lines. In one series, cases previously diagnosed as intraocular leiomyoma were examined with immunohistochemical markers.[46] All of 20 iris leiomyomas and four leiomyosarcomas, as well as one of three ciliary body leiomyomas, were reclassified as melanocytic lesions based on immunohistochemistry. Immunohistochemical and ultrastructural findings were confirmatory in one case.[40]

Fine-needle aspiration biopsy smears show spindled cells with blunt-ended oval nuclei and an absence of melanin granules. Electron microscopy and immunohistochemistry can be performed on aspirated material.

Neurofibroma/Neurilemmoma

Schwann cell tumors (neurofibromas and neurilemmomas) of the uveal tract are rare. The choroid is the most commonly reported site.[47] Some cases have been associated with neurofibromatosis.

Neurilemmomas are encapsulated proliferations of Schwann cells (Fig. 10-14). Classically, they display **Antoni A** and **B** areas. The former are areas of tightly packed bundles of spindle-shaped cells with nuclear palisading and cytoplasmic process fibrillary formations. The latter are areas with a more haphazard arrangement of round

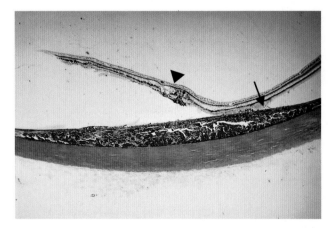

FIG. 10-12. Localized cavernous hemangioma of the choroid. There is a plaque-like proliferation of large vascular channels. There is subretinal fluid (*arrow*) and cystoid degeneration of the retina (*arrowhead*).

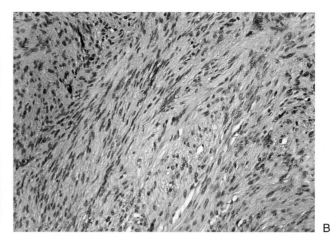

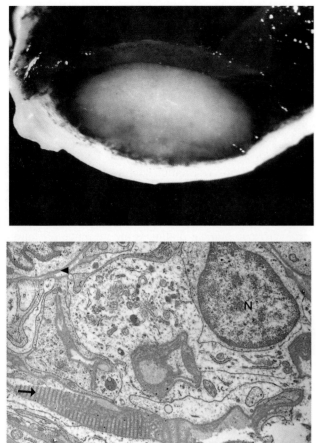

FIG. 10-14. Neurilemmoma (schwannoma) of the choroid. (**A**) Gross appearance of the tumor. (**B**) Histology shows interlacing bipolar spindle cells with vacuolated nuclei. (**C**) Ultrastructural features include extracellular long-spaced collagen with cross-banding (Luse bodies) (*arrow*) and surrounding basal lamina (*arrowhead*). N, nucleus. (Fan JT, Campbell RJ, Robertson DM. A survey of intraocular schwannoma with a case report. *Can J Ophthalmol* 1995;30:37. Reprinted with permission of the *Canadian Journal of Ophthalmology,* courtesy of Dr. Jean Campbell).

and spindle-shaped cells in a background of abundant mucoid material. One case of a **melanotic schwannoma** arising from the choroid, a tumor usually arising in soft tissues or peripheral nerves, has been reported.[48]

Neurofibromas are nonencapsulated tumors composed of Schwann cells, endoneural fibroblasts, axons, and fibrous connective tissue. Plexiform neurofibromas are Schwann cell proliferations of peripheral nerves confined within the nerve sheath. Both are composed of wavy bundles of cells with indistinct cell borders, bent nuclei, and a variable amount of stromal collagen. Axons are sometimes evident in H&E-stained sections but are better demonstrated with Bodian stain.

Electron microscopy of neurilemmomas shows features of Schwann cells: sparse intracytoplasmic organelles, long cytoplasmic processes, filaments and microtubules, and a surrounding basement membrane that may be banded in areas (Luse bodies). Neurofibromas' ultrastructural features are more like neural fibroblasts than Schwann cells. Cytoplasmic filaments and pinocytotic vesicles are present, but basement membrane formation is less complete than with neurilemmomas. Immunohistochemical stains for S-100 are usually positive in these and other tumors of neural crest origin.[49]

SECONDARY TUMORS OF THE UVEA

Leukemia

The eyes are involved in up to 90% of patients with **leukemia**; the uvea is involved in up to 85% of these eyes.[50–52] This high rate of ocular involvement may be due in part to high peripheral blood leukocyte counts at the time of death.[53] Clinical ocular involvement may be the presenting sign of acute leukemia or leukemic relapse.[54,55]

Involvement of the anterior segment is detected clinically and pathologically in about 1.5% of patients with leukemia, and it is seen most commonly with acute lymphocytic leukemia.[52,56,57] Manifestations include decreased vision, iris heterochromia, aqueous cells, hypopyon, glaucoma, and spontaneous hyphema. Leukemia in the posterior segment presents with retinal hemorrhages, cotton-wool patches, retinal infiltrates, retinal detachment, optic nerve infiltration, and pigmentary changes. Fluorescein angiography shows nonspecific diffuse leakage at the level of the retinal pigment epithelium.

Histologically, mild diffuse infiltration of the uvea by

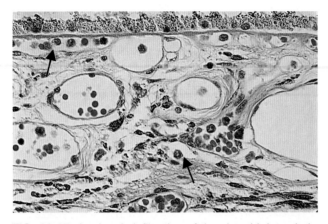

FIG. 10-15. Leukemic infiltration of the choroid. Lymphoblastic cells are present in the choroidal vessels and stroma (*arrows*).

leukemic cells is often evident (Fig. 10-15). Iris involvement, when present, is denser at the iris root and near the sphincter.[51] The choroid is thickened by leukemic cells, and there may be atrophy, hyperplasia, and hypertrophy of the retinal pigment epithelium. Serous retinal detachment, cystoid retinal edema, loss of photoreceptors, and drusen are also seen.

Unilateral involvement in a patient with leukemia may raise the question of an infectious endophthalmitis, because these patients frequently are immunosuppressed. Cytologic examination of ocular fluids, or of fine-needle aspiration biopsy material, may demonstrate malignant cells and confirm leukemic eye involvement.

Lymphoma

Systemic lymphoma affects the eye less often than does leukemia: about 7% of patients dying of lymphoma have ocular involvement histologically.[58] Large cell lymphoma is the most common form of intraocular lymphoma. Antiquated misnomers such as **reticulum cell sarcoma** or **histiocytic lymphoma** should not be used to describe these neoplasms. There is a sarcoma putatively arising from reticulum cells of the skin that is more deserving of the name "reticulum cell sarcoma." The cause of intraocular lymphoma is unknown, but recent studies have implicated viruses in some patients.[59,60]

In general, uveal infiltration by large cell lymphoma occurs in association with systemic involvement. Conversely, the vitreous, retina, subpigment epithelial space, and optic nerve are involved when the lymphoma is localized to the central nervous system. Summaries of previously reported cases are presented elsewhere.[61,62] One characteristic clinical finding is the presence of multiple retinal pigment epithelial detachments.

Histologically, uveal involvement is characterized by diffuse infiltration of the uvea and adjacent structures by atypical lymphocytes (Fig. 10-16). Other findings include retinal pigment epithelium atrophy and hyperplasia, retinal detachment, and outer retinal atrophy.

Metastatic Solid Tumors

Metastatic tumors are the most common intraocular malignancy. Clinically, less than 2.5% of patients with malignant solid tumors have ocular metastases.[63] The incidence in autopsy series is as high as 12%.[64] The eye is about seven times more likely to be involved by metastatic tumor than the orbit. The choroid is the most common site (57% to 95%) of ocular metastasis.[65-67] The iris is involved in up to 8% of eyes with metastatic tumor.[68] Multiple foci of tumor in one or both eyes are present in up to 21% of patients with ocular metastasis.[67]

The most common sites of **primary tumors** are the breast in women and the lung in men.[65-68] Sarcomas are less common tumors and rarely cause ocular metastasis.

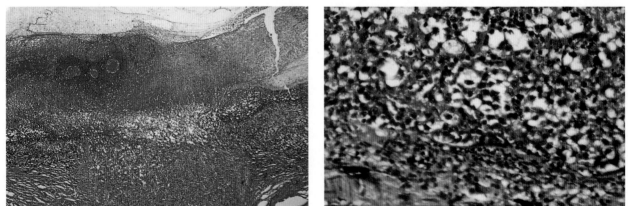

FIG. 10-16. Intraocular lymphoma of the choroid. (**A**) Diffuse infiltration of the retina, choroid, and sclera. (**B**) Dense collections of atypical lymphocytes in the choroid.

In up to 46% of ocular metastatic tumors, particularly lung carcinomas, detection of tumor in the eye precedes discovery of the primary tumor site.[65] Moreover, the primary site is not identified in about 10% of cases.[68] Other nonocular sites of metastasis are found in up to 82% of patients with uveal metastasis.[69]

Common clinical presentations for tumors metastatic to the eye include pain, red eye, inflammation, and elevated intraocular pressure in iris lesions, and a painless loss of vision and exudative retinal detachment in ciliochoroidal lesions. Iris lesions are usually white, pink, yellow, or flesh-colored, lack intrinsic vessels, and may have an associated pseudohypopyon. Choroidal lesions may be diffuse or nodular; rupture through Bruch's membrane, resulting in a mushroom or collar-button configuration, is rare in these lesions.

Most metastatic lesions are easily diagnosed because of a prior history of cancer or because of detection of a primary tumor at the time of initial evaluation of the intraocular mass. In the absence of a known primary, clinical features may prove useful to distinguish them from other choroidal tumors.[68,70] The differential diagnosis of metastatic tumors to the iris and choroid includes amelanotic melanoma, leiomyoma, lymphoid lesions, and infectious nodules. Hemangiomas also must be considered in the differential diagnosis of choroidal lesions.

Ancillary studies can be helpful, although individual tumors do not always conform to reported norms. Metastatic tumors usually lack the low internal reflectivity, choroidal excavation, and mushroom shape typical of choroidal melanoma with ultrasonography. Ultrasound is very useful for detecting a mass lesion obscured by retinal detachment. Fluorescein angiography of metastatic lesions frequently shows later hyperfluorescence than that seen with melanomas and hemangiomas. CT has not been helpful for determining the type of malignancy. Melanotic tumors have unique MRI properties, but the ability of MRI to distinguish amelanotic melanomas from metastatic tumors has not been established.

Fine-needle aspiration biopsy is especially useful for establishing a diagnosis of a primary or metastatic intraocular tumor.[71] The diagnostic technique cannot always establish the primary site of a metastatic tumor; however, the cytologic features of the lesion correspond to those of the primary tumor and, therefore, may provide important clues.

Metastatic tumors often recapitulate the differentiation of the primary tumor. Many adenocarcinomas form tubuloacinar structures and demonstrate mucin production with mucicarmine, alcian blue, or colloidal iron stains (Fig. 10-17). Breast, lung, gastrointestinal, and prostate adenocarcinomas are the most common primary sites. Small round undifferentiated cells may be found with carcinoid and small cell lung tumors. Spindle-shaped cells are indicative of sarcomas or metastatic melanoma. Metastatic tumors may be amenable to studies that identify the site of origin. For example, prostate carcinomas can be identified with immunoreactivity for prostate-specific antigen. Electron microscopy and immunohistochemistry can be useful for characterizing undifferentiated tumors.

Differentiating metastatic cutaneous melanomas and uveal melanoma can be difficult. Clues that suggest a metastatic tumor include multifocality, flat growth, ana-

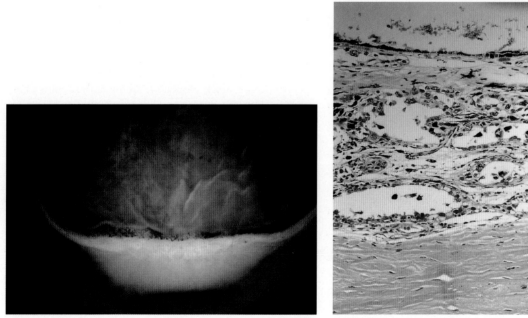

FIG. 10-17. Metastatic adenocarcinoma of the lung. (**A**) Diffuse thickening of the choroid by tumor forming tubular structures. (**B**) Atypical epithelial cells lining a large lumen.

plastic cell type, and absence of adjacent nevus cells. Monoclonal antibodies to different S-100 subtypes may be useful in differentiating cutaneous from uveal melanomas.[72] Seventeen percent of choroidal melanomas (compared to 85% of cutaneous melanomas) stain with a monoclonal antibody (MAB-079) that reacts with S-100α and S-100β polypeptides.

MELANOCYTIC TUMORS OF THE UVEA

Iris

Primary melanocytic tumors of the iris comprise a spectrum of benign and malignant neoplasms. Tumors are designated as iris lesions if more than 50% of the tumor mass lies within the iris or anterior chamber.[41] Many lesions grow slowly and have intermediate histologic characteristics that make them difficult to classify with certainty.

Freckles

Iris freckles (ephelis) are composed of small groups of hyperpigmented melanocytes in the anterior border area that form a pigmented macule clinically (Fig. 10-18). No tumor nodule is present.

Nevi

Iris nevi are melanocytic lesions that are histologically benign. They are more common in lightly pigmented persons, but their true prevalence is unknown. Systemic syndromes that have iris nevi as part of their phenotype include **neurofibromatosis type I**, **dysplastic nevus syndrome**, and **oculodermal melanocytosis (nevus of Ota)**. Ocular syndromes include **ocular melanocytosis**

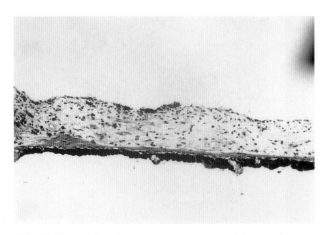

FIG. 10-18. Iris freckle composed of a small group of round, hyperpigmented melanocytes.

(**melanosis oculi**) and **iridocorneal endothelial (ICE)** syndrome.

Ninety-two percent of persons with neurofibromatosis have multiple small iris nevi (**Lisch nodules**) by age 6.[73] Typically, Lisch nodules are not present at birth but arise within the first decade of life. The absence of Lisch nodules has been used to exclude neurofibromatosis in patients with a family history of neurofibromatosis but insufficient systemic criteria for the diagnosis. Lisch nodules are not specific for neurofibromatosis. Chromosomal analysis can identify abnormalities in chromosomes 17 and 22 that are associated with **neurofibromatosis types I and II**, respectively.[74,75]

Patients with ICE syndrome may display superficial iris melanocytic aggregates in addition to endothelialization. When iris nodule formation is a prominent feature, it has been designated **Cogan-Reese** or **iris nevus syndrome**.

The **dysplastic nevus syndrome** (also labeled **BK mole syndrome** and **familial atypical multiple mole/melanoma syndrome**) is characterized by the presence of increased numbers of typical and atypical cutaneous nevi that appear early in life and increase with age. It may be sporadic or familial. Affected persons are two to three times more likely to have iris nevi and demonstrate more nevi per eye than those without the condition.[76]

Oculodermal melanocytosis and **ocular melanocytosis** present with diffuse or sectoral proliferations of benign melanocytic cells in the sclera, iris, or choroid.

Benign melanocytic cells (**nevocytes**) grow as surface plaques, infiltrate the iris stroma, or both (Fig. 10-19). Individual cells display a wide variety of shapes—in order of decreasing frequency: spindle, epithelioid, and dendritic.[41] They typically have a large cytoplasmic:nuclear ratio; small nuclei with dark, homogeneous or finely stippled nuclear chromatin; a small or absent nucleolus; and occasional nuclear vacuoles. Spindle and epithelioid lesions show variable pigmentation, whereas dendritic cells are heavily pigmented. About 3% of nevi are melanocytomas that have densely packed macromelanosomes and are black clinically. Abundant reticulin fibers are present in the intrastromal areas of nevi.

Melanoma

The median age of patients identified with iris melanoma is 40 to 50 years. Although rare in children, the tumors represent slightly less than half of uveal melanomas in persons under age 20. In contrast, there is a 1:15 ratio of iris melanomas to posterior melanomas in adults.[77] Persons with blue or gray irides have a risk of developing iris melanoma more than 10 times higher than that of those with brown irides.[78,79] Iris melanomas may be more common in patients with **neurofibromatosis**, although epidemiologic conclusions are difficult due to the rarity of reported cases.[80] For unknown reasons, iris melanomas

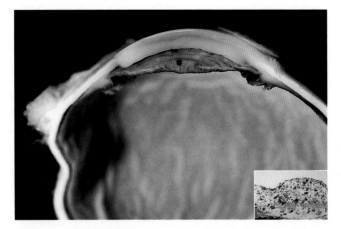

FIG. 10-19. A small iris nevus. (*Inset*) The nevus is composed of variably pigmented cells. Small spindle-shaped cells are located near the anterior border layer and epithelioid cells are present in the deep stroma.

are most common in the inferotemporal quadrant. Pigmentation is variable.

Iris melanomas diffusely infiltrate the stroma and may form surface plaques. They are composed of cytologically atypical cells that have larger nuclei, a coarser chromatin pattern, and more prominent nucleoli than nevus cells. About half of these tumors are composed purely of spindle-shaped cells. **Epithelioid cells** make up about 20% of tumors; the remaining tumors show **mixed cellular morphology**. Mitotic figures are present in essentially all melanomas. Exfoliated tumor cells and pigment-containing macrophages are sometimes found free in the chamber angle. Iris melanomas lack the abundant reticulin fiber deposition in the stroma characteristic of nevi. Nearly half of iris melanomas are found to have adjacent populations of nevocytes, suggesting that many may arise from preexisting nevi.[41]

Pigmented iris tumors that enlarge are not necessarily malignant. Tumor characteristics such as color, size, location, vascularity, and growth into the anterior chamber or on the corneal endothelium are unreliable indicators of benign or malignant behavior.[41] Clinical signs shared by benign and malignant tumors include glaucoma (secondary to peripheral anterior synechiae or blockage of the drainage pathways by pigment, melanophages, or tumor cells),[81] cataract, pupillary changes, episcleral vascular dilation, and localized corneal edema from tumor–corneal touch.

Two clinical presentations of enlarging iris tumors indicate a greater likelihood of a malignant lesion. **Ring lesions** demonstrate circumferential growth of melanocytic cells on the face of the ciliary body or chamber angle. The likelihood of malignancy is especially high when they are associated with elevated intraocular pressure. "**Tapioca melanoma**" displays a diffuse melanocytic proliferation with multifocal, translucent thickenings and elevations that resemble tapioca seeds.

The ultimate differentiation of iris nevi from melanoma rests on histopathologic analysis. Recently described diagnostic modalities that may help differentiate benign from malignant tumors include nucleolar morphometry and **quantitation of nucleolar organizer regions**.[79,82]

Metastases from iris melanomas reportedly occur in less than 4% of cases, and deaths result from metastatic disease in less than 3% of patients.[62,83] The relatively benign nature of these lesions is thought to be due to early detection and small tumor size. Survival has not been correlated with histologic cell type, as in choroidal melanoma. It is essential to determine if an iris lesion represents the most anterior portion of a ciliary body tumor, because ciliary body tumors carry a mortality rate of nearly 60%.[84,85]

Most pigmented iris tumors have a good prognosis and usually can be observed. The need for biopsy or treatment is dictated by the rate of growth, symptomatology, visual potential, resectability, and availability for continued follow-up. If necessary, biopsy may be performed by complete excisional biopsy or fine-needle aspiration biopsy, depending on the difficulty of tumor resection. Incomplete excisional biopsy is discouraged because many reports have implicated this as a causative factor in fatal outcomes. Diffuse lesions require multiple biopsy sites. Open biopsy may be indicated in this circumstance if clinicians experienced with fine-needle aspiration biopsy are unavailable.

Treatment options for iris melanomas include enucleation or complete local resection. Clinical judgment dictates the need for further treatment of incompletely excised malignant tumors because only a small percentage of tumors demonstrate recurrent growth.[41] To rule out emergence of a malignant tumor clone or inadequate sampling of the original tumor, consideration should be given to repeat biopsy of recurrent histologically benign but

TABLE 3. *Lesions simulating iris melanocytic tumors*

Primary iris cyst
  Epithelial
  Stromal
Iris foreign body
Iris atrophy
  Essential
  Secondary to other causes
Iris metastasis
Leiomyoma
Reactive lymphoid hyperplasia
Iridoschisis
Pigment epithelial hyperplasia
Epithelial downgrowth cyst

Shields JA, Sanborn GE, Augsburger JJ. The differential diagnosis of melanoma of the iris: a clinical study of 200 patients. *Ophthalmology* 1983;90:716.

clinically aggressive lesions. Iris lesions that masquerade as melanotic neoplasms are listed in Table 3.[86]

Choroid/Ciliary Body

Nevi

Choroidal nevi are proliferations of benign melanocytes (nevocytes). The reported incidence is less than 1% in children and up to 30% in adults.[87] Autopsy studies have reported an incidence of up to 20% in adults.[88] The incidence appears to increase during the second, third, and fourth decades before plateauing. Bilateral nevi are present in 3.5% of persons; multiple nevi in one eye are found in about 7% of patients.[87] Choroidal nevi far outnumber ciliary body nevi.[88,89] The incidence of choroidal nevi is two to three times greater in patients with the dysplastic nevus syndrome than in controls.[76]

Nevi appear as flat or dome-shaped, light-tan to dark-brown lesions. A rare variant, the **magnocellular nevus (melanocytoma)**, is black (see the section below on optic nerve tumors). Nevi vary in size from barely perceptible to 11 mm in diameter; 87% are less than 5.5 mm in diameter and 95% are 2 mm thick or less.[89] Enlargement is not uncommon in children and young adults but is rare in older persons and should raise the suspicion of a malignant lesion.

Clinically, about 33% of nevi develop surface drusen.[90] **Orange pigment**, which represents accumulation of **lipofuscin**, is sometimes seen but is much less common than in melanomas.[91] Other less common clinical findings associated with nevi include choroidal neovascular membranes, serous retinal detachments, and visual field defects.[92–94]

Fluorescein angiography of nevi usually demonstrates partial blockage of choroidal fluorescence during the early phase; it may remain or disappear in the late phase. Some-

times the blocked fluorescence covers an area larger than the clinically apparent lesion. Uniform background fluorescence and lack of pinpoint leakage support a benign diagnosis. Nevi with overlying pigment epithelium changes may demonstrate angiographic features common to melanomas; therefore, such findings may not be helpful in distinguishing these entities.[90]

Histologically, nevocytes may occupy the full thickness of the choroid or even expand the choroid (Fig. 10-20). If the tumor does not span the full thickness, nevocytes occupy the outermost portions of the choroid. Nevi have no mitotic activity or necrosis within the lesion. They rarely, if ever, break through Bruch's membrane or invade the sclera, although extension into emissarial canals is seen.[95] Most nevi are composed of **polyhedral cells** with abundant cytoplasm and are packed with pigment granules. Nuclei are small, with uniformly basophilic chromatin and small or absent nucleoli. These cells are similar to **magnocellular nevi** of the optic nerve. The second most common cells seen are thin **spindle-shaped cells** with slender dark nuclei. These cells usually have sparse pigment granules. Some nevi contain dendritic cells or, rarely, lipid-laden **balloon cells**. Mixtures of cell types are common. Attenuation of the choriocapillaris (31%), drusen (27%), and alterations of the pigment epithelium (25%) are common histologic findings. Exudative fluid beneath the retina and minor changes in the outer retinal layers also may be found.[87,89]

Malignant Melanoma

Epidemiology

Choroidal and ciliary body melanomas are the most common primary human intraocular malignancies. The mean age at diagnosis is 55 to 60 years; less than 2% of

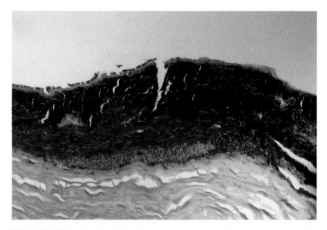

FIG. 10-20. Choroidal nevus composed of heavily pigmented round and spindle cells with homogeneous dark nuclei.

all uveal melanomas occur in patients less than age 21. One congenital ciliochoroidal melanoma has been reported.[96]

Choroidal melanoma occurs predominantly in Caucasians, whose risk is estimated to be eight to 15 times higher than blacks. Races with intermediate pigmentation appear to be at low risk as well.[97] Among Caucasians, people of northern European heritage have about a sixfold risk and persons of British heritage have a twofold risk for developing melanoma compared to persons of southern European or Mediterranean descent. Some Asians and Hispanics develop these tumors at an earlier average age than Caucasians.[98] Blacks have more severe clinical disease before enucleation and a higher rate of unsuspected melanomas in enucleated eyes.[99] Persons with light skin color and multiple (10 or more) cutaneous nevi are at greater risk.[100]

Origin

There is circumstantial evidence that melanomas arise from preexisting choroidal nevi. Occasionally, nevocytes are found adjacent to a melanoma, although this is less common than with iris melanomas (Fig. 10-21). Malignant tumors have occurred in the same location as nevi observed for many years without growth. In addition, the continuous spectrum of melanocytic tumor cells—from benign **nevus cells** to intermediate **spindle cell** A and

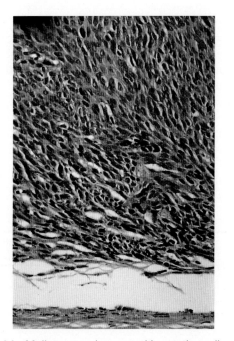

FIG. 10-21. Malignant melanoma with putative adjacent nevus cells. The tumor is composed of large spindle-shaped cells with oval nuclei and prominent nucleoli. There are numerous small round cells with bland nuclei at the base of the tumor. The tumor is artifactually separated from the sclera.

more malignant cell types—also lends support the concept of transformation from nevus to melanoma.[101]

Genetic predisposition may play a role in the development of melanoma. A few cases of melanoma in close relatives have been reported. Although the occurrence of such lesions has a low statistical probability,[102] not enough cases with possible familial inheritance have been studied to determine the mode of inheritance.[103] Uveal melanomas occurring in husband and wife suggest that a shared environmental exposure among close family members may be an alternative explanation.[97,104] Abnormalities of **chromosome 9** have been identified in **familial cutaneous melanoma** and in one case of choroidal melanoma.[105,106] Lack of a normal tumor-suppressor gene that encodes an inhibitor of cyclin-dependent kinase and is located at **9p16** may be a predisposing factor for the development of melanoma.[107]

The occurrence of simultaneous cutaneous and choroidal melanoma is rare. Of seven reported cases, at least three had **dysplastic nevus syndrome**, a condition believed to be dominantly inherited. One family had cutaneous melanoma, ocular melanoma, or dysplastic nevi in three generations.[108]

There is evidence that ultraviolet light exposure from natural sources and sun lamps is associated with an increased risk of developing choroidal melanoma.[100] However, northern Europeans, who have a relatively low level of exposure, are at greatest risk.

Ocular melanocytosis (melanocytosis oculi) and **oculodermal melanocytosis (nevus of Ota)** have been associated with an increased risk of developing melanoma.[109] Multifocal tumors have been reported in 2 patients with congenital melanocytosis.[80,110] Cases have been reported in patients with **neurofibromatosis**, although the relative risk of developing uveal melanoma is unknown.[80,111] Viruses, chemical exposure, and trauma also have been implicated as tumor-causing factors.[112–114] Several cases have occurred during pregnancy in women with prior clinically stable choroidal nevi.[115] No cases of fetal transmission of the tumor have occurred. There is evidence that pregnancy also causes accelerated growth of cutaneous melanocytic cells.

Several reports have shown an increased prevalence (up to 10%) of previously occurring, nonocular, primary malignancies in patients who subsequently develop choroidal melanoma. These data raise the possibility of an immunologic defect of tumor suppression or possibly the loss of a normal tumor-suppressor gene, like that associated with retinoblastoma, in these patients. A case-control study designed to answer that question failed to find a significant association between melanoma and systemic malignancy.[116] A **paraneoplastic syndrome** of bilateral diffuse melanocytic lesions of the uveal tract associated with systemic malignancies has been reported in 7 patients.[117] Benign cell types predominated in that study; however, some malignant-appearing cells also were seen.

Clinical Features

Forty-one percent of patients with melanoma report no symptoms.[118] The most common clinical manifestation is a change in visual acuity or visual field (40%). Pain is rare (3%) but is more common in ciliary body tumors. **Diffuse uveal melanomas** more commonly present with symptoms due to their larger size and more anterior location. A comparison of symptoms reported with all melanomas versus diffuse melanomas is shown in Table 4. Rarely, the patient's presenting symptoms may be from metastatic disease.

Elevated intraocular pressure occurs in up to 36% of eyes with posterior uveal melanoma.[119] It is more common with large tumors, those located in the ciliary body, and those associated with retinal detachment. Angle-closure mechanisms are far more common than direct invasion of the angle from the ciliary body.[81]

Exudative retinal detachment is common and varies in size from small and localized to total detachment (Fig. 10-22). The occurrence and extent of retinal detachment increase with the size of the melanoma. Retinal detachments can occur with nevi; however, lesions associated with localized serous retinal detachments of the macula are likely to be or to become melanomas.[120]

Mild aqueous iridocyclitis is, but rarely is uveitis a source of ocular discomfort. Diffuse uveal melanomas more commonly have ocular signs than do nodular tumors. Common ocular signs found in eyes with diffuse uveal melanomas are shown in Table 5. Unusual presentations of melanoma include vitreous hemorrhage,[121] panophthalmitis,[122] scleritis,[123] and orbital inflammation.[124]

Small ciliary body tumors may present with decreased vision due to cataract or astigmatic change induced by tumor contact with the lens. Localized changes in the angle architecture observable with slit-lamp biomicroscopy may be another clue to the presence of a ciliary body tumor.[125]

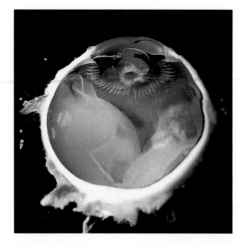

FIG. 10-22. Retinal detachment secondary to choroidal malignant melanoma. There is a total exudative detachment of the retina in this pseudophakic eye. A nodular tumor arising in the choroid and pars plana is seen in the right side of the photo.

Occasionally, posterior melanoma is discovered in enucleated eyes with **opaque media.** About 77% of these eyes are enucleated for uncontrolled glaucoma, typically with intraocular pressures of 40 to 80 mm Hg. Ultrasound is indispensable for the detection of an intraocular mass and should be performed on all eyes with opaque media.

Ophthalmoscopy

Most posterior uveal melanomas present as a discrete dome-shaped mass lesion with well-circumscribed borders (Fig. 10-23). Once a tumor breaks through Bruch's membrane, a **collar-button** or **mushroom-shaped** tumor may form. About 5% of tumors demonstrate a **diffuse pattern** of growth that is relatively flat and has irregular, ill-defined borders.[126] Color varies between and within tumors from creamy white to black. Up to 90% of choroidal melanomas contain orange pigment on their surface;

TABLE 4. *Presenting symptoms of 193 ciliary body/choroidal malignant melanomas*

Symptom	% of malignant melanomas	% of diffuse malignant melanomas
Change in vision	40	70
Pain	3	43
Red eye	30	9
Iris color change	30	4
Flashes/floaters	16	4
Others	0.5	13

Data from Servodidio CA, Abramson DH. Presenting signs and symptoms of choroidal melanoma: what do they mean? *Ann Ophthalmol* 1992;24:190, and Font RL, Spaulding AG, Zimmerman LE. Diffuse malignant melanoma of the uveal tract: a clincopathologic report of 54 cases. *Trans Am Acad Ophthalmol Otolaryngol* 1968;72:877.

TABLE 5. *Presenting signs of diffuse choroidal melanomas*

Presenting signs	% of diffuse malignant melanomas
Mass	61
Secondary glaucoma	61
Decreased vision	41
Retinal detachment	37
Cataract	24
Inflammation	15
Others	13

Font RL, Spaulding AG, Zimmerman LE. Diffuse malignant melanoma of the uveal tract: a clinicopathologic report of 54 cases. *Trans Am Acad Ophthalmol Otolaryngol* 1968;72:877.

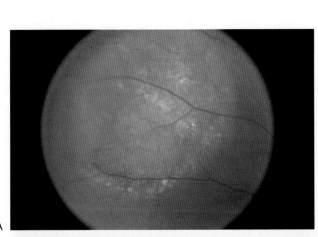

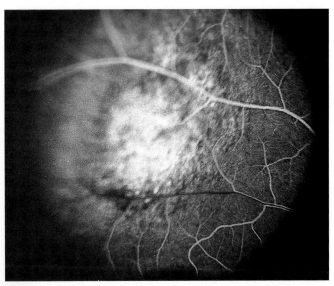

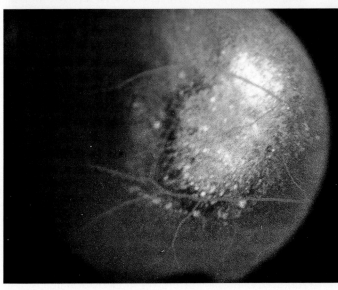

FIG. 10-23. Small choroidal melanoma. (**A**) Fundus photo showing an amelanotic dome-shaped mass with adjacent retinal detachment, overlying drusen, and pigmentary changes. (**B**) Early phase fluorescein angiogram showing patchy hyperfluorescence with blocking at the margins of the tumor. Retinal detachment causes the left side of the photograph to be out of focus. (**C**) Late phase showing persistent late hyperfluorescence over the tumor and staining of adjacent drusen.

this represents lipofuscin within retinal pigment epithelial cells and macrophages in the subretinal space.[127] These deposits are not specific, as other benign and malignant tumors accumulate lipofuscin on their surface; however, lipofuscin usually appears brown or red-brown in other lesions.[128]

Drusen are found over melanomas, although their frequency and relation to tumor growth rate are unknown. Hemorrhage may be present on the tumor surface, potentially obscuring the melanotic nature of a tumor.

Measurements of tumor diameter using indirect ophthalmoscopy are accurate in lesions less than 12 mm in diameter. Indirect ophthalmoscopy of larger lesions, however, results in considerable intraobserver differences in elevation estimates and similar large differences in estimates of tumor elevation compared to gross pathologic measurements.[129]

Diagnostic Studies

The **fluorescein angiographic** findings of choroidal melanomas are nonspecific (see Fig. 10-23). Typically, patchy early hyperfluorescence of the tumor appears in the late arterial phase and subsequently leaks. Patchy late hyperfluorescence of the whole lesion is typical and may represent staining or leakage. These characteristics are due to the loss of overlying retinal pigment epithelium, variable tumor pigmentation, and prominent vascularity composed of leaky choroidal vessels within the tumor.[90] Occasionally a discrete pattern of circulation within a tumor can be identified.

Ultrasound is the most useful tool for imaging choroidal tumors. The use of **standardized A-mode ultrasonography**, supplemented by **B-mode imaging**, demonstrates distinctive features of choroidal melanomas. Its utility is enhanced by excellent reproducibility, low cost, and lack of ionizing radiation. Findings on ultrasound suggestive of melanoma include a collar-button configuration, **low internal reflectivity**, attenuation of signal intensity, orbital shadowing, and choroidal excavation (Fig. 10-24). Low internal reflectivity is due to the tissue homogeneity characteristic of most tumors. Internal reflections caused by necrotic areas and blood lakes are seen more frequently in large tumors, which seldom present a diagnostic dilemma. **Choroidal excavation** is due to impedance of the beam and delay of reflected waves, which causes the image of the scleral interface to appear further away than it actually is. High blood flow may manifest as spontaneous pulsations. About 88% of ultrasound studies (compared with 70% of fluorescein angiograms) have findings suggestive of melanoma.[129]

Measurement of tumor height using ultrasound is highly reproducible and correlates well with height measured by gross examination and histologic section; however, it is unreliable for measuring tumor diameter.[130] The optimal method of estimating tumor size before treatment is a combination of indirect ophthalmoscopy for tumor diameter and sonography for tumor height. The reproducibility of sonographic tumor height measurements decreases in anteriorly located lesions due to difficulty in positioning the probe for measurement of the same tumor area.[129] The ability of ultrasound to detect extrascleral extension is unknown; however, one study reported 85% sensitivity in 13 cases and that some lesions less than 1 mm in diameter were detected.[131] Sonography can be useful in determining proper plaque placement and the response to radiation therapy.[132]

CT of posterior uveal melanomas is very reliable for detecting tumors greater than 2 mm in height. Contrast enhancement improves resolution. CT correlates well with histologic tumor height but is less accurate for determining greatest tumor diameter, even with reformatting. The differentiation of overlying exudative detachment from tumor is difficult, and size may be overestimated in some cases.[133] CT sometimes can detect extrascleral extension and may be better than ultrasound in this capacity.[134] CT has limited use in the evaluation of uveal melanomas because it offers little diagnostic advantage over ultrasonography, is more expensive, and carries an inherent risk of ionizing radiation exposure.

MRI is superior to CT for imaging intraocular tumors. Soft-tissue resolution is better (especially between tumor and subretinal exudate), visualization of the tumor is possible in three dimensions, and ionizing radiation is not used. Minimum tumor height for detection is 1.5 to 2.0 mm.[133,135] Melanin has a paramagnetic property, thus reducing T1 and T2 relaxation times and producing images with a high signal intensity on T1-weighted images and low signal intensity on T2-weighted images. T1-weighted images are more sensitive and show better resolution than T2-weighted images.[136] **Gadolinium enhancement** can demonstrate smaller lesions invisible on noncontrasted images. Amelanotic tumors are less well visualized than melanotic lesions, and gadolinium enhancement may be especially useful in this situation. Correlation with histopathologic tumor size and the ability to detect extrascleral extension have not been studied.

The **radioactive phosphorus** (^{32}P) test was commonly used as a diagnostic tool for detecting uveal melanoma in the past. It has lost favor because of occasional false-positive results. In addition, it requires a surgical procedure in some cases, is technically difficult to perform in posteriorly located tumors, exposes the patient to radioactivity, and requires ocular manipulation, which may significantly raise intraocular pressure. It is most useful in eyes with opaque media and a mass lacking classic melanoma features by sonography.[137] Visible lesions can be followed clinically for growth in cases of diagnostic uncertainty. The ^{32}P uptake test measures tumor mass rather

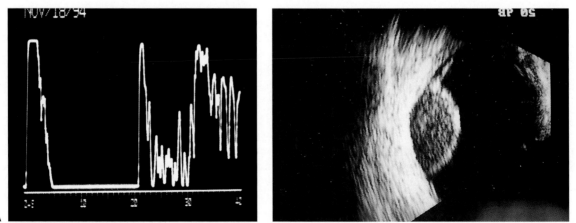

FIG. 10-24. Ultrasound of a choroidal melanoma in the same patient as Fig. 10-23. (**A**) A-scan showing a high initial tumor spike and low internal reflectivity. (**B**) B-scan showing a dome-shaped tumor in the choroid with adjacent retinal detachment. There is a high surface signal, low internal signal, mild choroidal excavation, and no evidence of extrascleral extension.

than biologic activity, which is why some benign lesions show positive results.[138]

Fine-needle aspiration biopsy can be a useful tool in the diagnosis of intraocular tumors. Cytologic diagnosis has been concordant with histology produced by fine-needle biopsy in almost 90% of cases. The criteria for cytologic diagnosis include pigmented cells with enlarged nuclei and prominent nucleoli (Fig. 10-25).[139] Spindle-shaped, epithelioid, and dendritic cells are seen, although there is variable correlation with histologic cell type, probably due to sampling error.[140] Other benign pigmented lesions (melanocytoma and retinal pigment epithelial adenoma) can be distinguished by their large melanin granules and benign cellular morphology.[141] Indications for fine-needle biopsy include diagnostic uncertainty after less invasive techniques, a patient's request for a specific diagnosis before treatment, and the desire to avoid enucleation when a metastatic tumor is suspected. Fine-needle biopsy has not been found to be reliable in identifying a primary source of metastatic intraocular lesions. Complications include intraocular hemorrhage and damage to ocular structures.[140] Several modifications of the technique have been developed to reduce the amount of vitreous hemorrhage.[142] Tumor cells have been found in needle tracts; however, transvitreal (indirect) biopsy results in significantly fewer numbers of cells within needle tracts than does direct transscleral biopsy.[143] Furthermore, the number of cells in the tracts is less than that required to produce implantation of tumor in experimental models.[144] Cells obtained from fine-needle biopsy can be used for cytomorphometry, DNA content, cell cycling analysis, immunohistochemistry, electron microscopy, in situ hybridization, and tissue culture studies.[141]

Electrooculography has been used to differentiate malignant melanoma from benign lesions. Combined use of the light peak/dark trough ratio (L/D) and interocular L/D difference (L/Dd) is 98% accurate for predicting final clinicopathologic diagnosis. The effect of melanoma on the electrooculogram appears to be independent of retinal detachment and tumor size, suggesting a diffuse influence on retinal pigment epithelial function.[145]

Recent work using **immunoscintigraphy** with monoclonal antibodies to high-molecular-weight melanoma-associated antigen showed a sensitivity of 78% and a specificity of 94% for detecting melanoma.[146] Future improvements and continued study will help define specific applications for this technology.

There are no specific **serologic tests** for uveal melanoma. Serum **carcinoma embryonic antigen (CEA)** measurements may be useful in amelanotic tumors of the choroid when metastatic lesions are in the differential diagnosis. Elevated CEA levels are more common in metastatic carcinoma to the eye (83%) than in primary choroidal melanoma (36%). Levels greater than 10 ng/mL have not been observed in uveal melanoma but are found in 58% of metastatic tumors.[147] In uveal melanomas with an elevated CEA level, monitoring of levels may be useful in detecting tumor recurrence after treatment.

The incidence of **metastatic disease** at the time of diagnosis of uveal melanoma varies from 0.5% to 6.5%. The liver is the most common site, found in nearly all patients with metastasis. Therefore, preoperative evaluation should be directed to the liver. Hepatomegaly is rare. **Lactic acid dehydrogenase** is the most sensitive serologic test (2% false-negative results) but is nonspecific (46% false-positive results). Of the imaging studies, abdominal CT is more sensitive and specific than scintigraphy and sonography. The use of MRI for detecting liver metastasis of uveal melanoma has not been studied. Given melanin's paramagnetic properties, metastatic liver lesions may be detectable when very small. Lesions as small as 10 mm have been detected by CT.[148] There seems to be no benefit to routine bone scan and brain or liver CT scan in the absence of clinical indications.[149]

Polymerase chain reaction studies have identified uveal and cutaneous melanoma cells in the peripheral blood.[150] Further evaluation of this technique is needed to establish its utility as a routine method of detecting metastatic disease.

Differential Diagnosis

One clinical study found that 52% of patients referred to an ocular oncology center with the diagnosis of posterior uveal melanoma had a **simulating lesion**.[151] The most common referral diagnoses are listed in Table 6. The rate of misdiagnoses in enucleated eyes range from 20% to 0.5%.[152–154] Lesions simulating choroidal melanoma in enucleated eyes with clear media from several large series are presented in Table 7. The improved diagnostic accuracy over the past three decades has been attributed to the use of better diagnostic modalities (indirect ophthal-

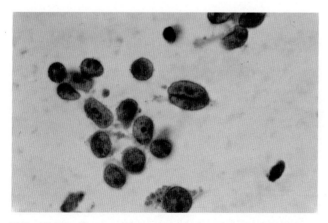

FIG. 10-25. Fine-needle aspirate of a choroidal malignant melanoma. There are round and oval pleomorphic nuclei with nuclear grooves and prominent nucleoli. Some cells contain brown pigment granules within the cytoplasm. Hematoxylin and eosin.

TABLE 6. *Clinical diagnosis of lesions referred for choroidal melanoma in eyes with clear media*

Diagnosis	% of eyes with pseudomelanoma
Nevus	28
Disciform scar	24
Congenital RPE hypertrophy	9
Hemangioma	8
Reactive RPE hyperplasia	6
Choroidal detachment	3
Hemorrhage	3
Melanocytoma	3
Retinal detachment	3
Metastatic carcinoma	1
Chorioretinitis	<1

RPE, retinal pigment epithelium.

Shields JA, Augsburger JJ, Brown GC, Stephens RF. The differential diagnosis of posterior uveal melanoma. *Ophthalmology* 1980;87:518.

moscopy, ultrasound, fluorescein angiography, and ^{32}P-uptake tests), recognition of simulating lesions, improved training of general ophthalmologists, and access to experienced consultants.

About 9% of enucleated eyes contain an **unsuspected melanoma**. The most common reasons for enucleation are severe glaucoma and blind/painful eyes.[155] Diffuse uveal melanomas present a particularly difficult problem in diagnosis. About 40% of these lesions detected histologically are unsuspected clinically.[126]

Gross Pathology

Gross descriptions of uveal melanomas should include caliper measurements of the basal and overall dimensions, tumor height, and location with regard to the ciliary body, equator, and optic nerve. The external ocular surfaces must be examined closely for evidence of extrascleral extension, especially in the areas of vortex veins and ciliary nerves and vessels. The cut end of the optic nerve should be examined closely in eyes with tumors located near the optic nerve head.

Ciliary body and choroidal melanomas present as a **nodular** or **diffuse tumor** occupying the choroidal space. Nodular tumors are usually dome-shaped (Fig. 10-26). Less common are the "classic" mushroom-shaped tumors (Fig. 10-27). This pattern represents tumor growth through Bruch's membrane. Venous stasis and intercellular edema caused by the restrictive effect of Bruch's membrane and pressure in the crowded choroidal space may also contribute to extrusion of tumor through Bruch's membrane.

Cut sections of melanoma may reveal homogeneous or variable pigmentation. Occasionally, areas with well-demarcated borders and uniform pigmentation are found within a larger tumor, suggesting proliferation of a distinct cellular clone. Necrotic areas and blood lakes can be seen within tumors.

Pathologic Findings With Prognostic Implications

Factors found to influence the prognosis of uveal melanomas include tumor size, histologic cell type, location, and pigmentation. The results of three studies from different centers that looked at these factors are shown in Table 8. No two studies agree completely on which factors are the most important, and most studies

TABLE 7. *Pathologic diagnosis in eyes with clear media enucleated for malignant melanoma*

Diagnosis	No. of eyes with diagnosis other than malignant melanoma				
	Davidorf	Chang	Ferry	Shields	Total
Retinal detachment	6	12	35	19	72 (36%)
Disciform scar	1	7	9	4	21 (10%)
Choroidal detach./hem.		5	8	4	17 (8%)
Metastatic carcinoma	2		5	3	10 (5%)
Hemangioma	1		5	4	10 (5%)
Chorioretinitis		1	8		9 (4%)
Vitreous hemorrhage		3	5	1	9 (4%)
Melanocytoma		1	4	1	6 (3%)
Reactive RPE hyperplasia		5			5 (2%)
Nevus			4		4 (2%)
Lymphoid hyperplasia		1	1		2 (1%)
Others	3	17	18	9	47 (23%)
Total eyes with pseudomelanoma*/ total eyes in study	13/369 (3.5%)	48/744 (6.4%)	100/529 (19%)	41/208 (20%)	202/1850 (10.9%)

* Some eyes contain more than one simulating lesion.

Data from Davidorf FH, Letson AD, Weiss ET, Levine E. Incidence of misdiagnosis and unsuspected choroidal melanomas. *Arch Ophthalmol* 1983;101:410; Chang M, Zimmerman LE, McLean IW. The persisting pseudomelanoma problem. *Arch Ophthalmol* 1984;102:726; Ferry AP. Lesions mistaken for malignant melanomas of the posterior uvea: a clinicopathologic analysis of 100 cases with ophthalmoscopically visible lesions. *Arch Ophthalmol* 1964;72:463; Shields JA, Zimmerman LE. Lesions simulating malignant melanoma of the posterior uvea. *Arch Ophthalmol* 1973;89:466.

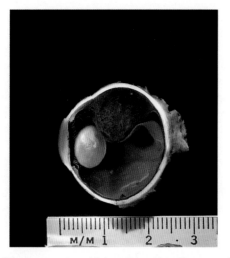

FIG. 10-26. Large choroidal malignant melanoma. Enucleation specimen showing a dome-shaped darkly pigmented choroidal tumor with adjacent retinal detachment. The tumor is displacing the lens toward the opposite ciliary body.

TABLE 8. *Prognostic factors and the relative importance of each factor in that study*

Factor	Influence on prognosis (rank)		
	Seddon	Shammas	McLean*
Cell type	+ (1)	+	+ (1)
Largest dimension	+ (2)	+ (1)	+ (3)
Location	+ (3)	+	+ (7)
Invasion to line of transection	+ (4)	–	–
Pigmentation	+ (5)	+	+ (2)
Rupture of Bruch's membrane	–	+	–
Mitotic activity	–	–	+ (5)
Scleral invasion	–	+	+ (4)

* Study on small choroidal melanomas (volume less than 1400/mm³).

+, positive (factor influences prognosis)

–, negative (no influence on prognosis)

Data from Seddon JM, Albert DM, Lavin PT, Robinson N. A prognostic factor study of disease-free interval and survival following enucleation for uveal melanoma. *Arch Ophthalmol* 1983;101:1894; Shammas HF, Blodi FC. Prognostic factors in choroidal and ciliary body melanomas. *Arch Ophthalmol* 1977;95:63; McLean IW, Foster WD, Zimmerman LE. Prognostic factors in small malignant melanomas of choroid and ciliary body. *Arch Ophthalmol* 1977;95:48.

cannot be compared with each other due to lack of inclusion of one or more important factors. Cause of death and rates of metastatic disease are not always accurate due to lack of metastatic workups, biopsy confirmation, or complete autopsy. Many studies rely on death certificates for important data on patient outcomes. Problems associated with the classification of histologic cell type are described below. Some factors tend to be codependent—for instance, larger tumors and more anteriorly placed tumors tend to have more epithelioid cells. Large numbers of patients and multivariate analytic techniques have shown that all these factors are independent predictors of outcome. Prognostic factors for melanoma have been derived from enucleation pathology specimens. Treatment modal-

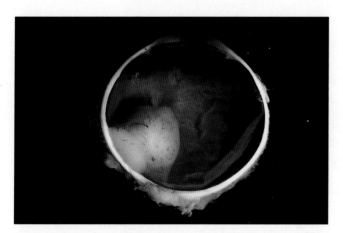

FIG. 10-27. Choroidal malignant melanoma. This amelanotic tumor has a mushroom or collarbutton shape cause by constriction from Bruch's membrane. There is exudative retinal detachment of the adjacent retina posteriorly.

ities other than enucleation necessitate the direct measurement of the available prognostic factors.

Callender was the first to show that histologic cell type provided prognostic information.[156] He described six categories based on cell type: spindle cell, which he divided into **A and B types**, **fascicular type**, **epithelioid type**, **mixed cell type**, and **necrotic**. Since that time, modifications of this system have been suggested.[157] Most pathologists now use a scheme that includes **spindle-cell type**, a combination of Callender's spindle A and B and most of the fascicular tumors; **epithelioid**; **mixed**; and **necrotic**.

The **Callender classification** can be considered a tumor-grading system, with spindle-cell tumors on the benign end of the spectrum and epithelioid cell tumors on the more malignant or less differentiated end of the spectrum. Mixed and necrotic tumors represent an intermediate grade. Shammas and Blodi found actuarial death rates at 15 years to be spindle A, 6%; spindle B, 31%; mixed, 43%; and epithelioid, 63%.[84] McLean and associates reported percent fatalities for small tumors (volume less than 1400 mm³) as spindle A, 9.1%; spindle B, 15.9%; mixed, 60.4%; and epithelioid, 100%.[85] Seddon and colleagues found that mortality increased with a greater number of epithelioid cells per high-power field.[158,159]

The rare, pure spindle A tumor is classified as a nevus by some pathologists. The rationale is the excellent prognosis these tumors have and the histologic similarity of some nevocytes and spindle A cells. Evidence to refute this concept includes liver metastases and orbital recur-

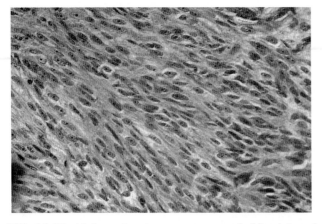

FIG. 10-28. Malignant melanoma composed of fascicles of spindle B cells.

rences with spindle cell A morphology and recurrence of spindle A tumors with mixed cell morphology.[87,160]

Morphologically, spindle cells have an elongated shape, sometimes ending in a sharp point, with oval nuclei (Fig. 10-28). Spindle A cells lack a well-defined nucleolus and often have a linear fold along the long axis of the nucleus. Spindle B cells have small, round, usually centrally located nucleoli. Spindle cells sometimes display arrangement in columns or fasciculi with nuclear palisading. Epithelioid cells are round or polygonal, with large round or oval nuclei (Fig. 10-29). Although originally described as large cells, smaller epithelioid cells are now recognized. The nuclei have distinct round nucleoli, possibly multiple. Multinucleated cells may be present.

The Callender classification scheme has many shortcomings. First, it is a subjective grading system that lacks a clear distinction between cell types because these cells fall on a continuous cytologic spectrum from "benign" spindle A cells to large epithelioid cells. One study found that four out of six ophthalmic pathologists could agree on cell type only 86% of the time.[161] Another problem is that the percentages of each cell needed to assign a tumor type have never been clearly defined or universally accepted. For example, are tumors mixed when 5%, 10%, or 20% of the cells are epithelioid?

Tumor sampling also can cause variation in grading of these tumors. Distant areas of the tumor may contain different cell types; this can lead to erroneous determination of the predominant cell type. Other features such as extrascleral extension, necrosis, pigmentation, and other prognostic factors discussed below may be missed if the tumor is not examined thoroughly.

Pigmentation can vary with all cell types. Increased pigmentation worsens the prognosis, although it is less significant than other factors. Silver stains or electron microscopy may be useful in identifying melanosomes in amelanotic tumors if necessary. Heavy pigmentation may require bleaching of the microslide to visualize nuclear detail (see Fig. 10-29).

Balloon cells have been identified within melanomas 10% to 14% of the time. Balloon cells appear as large, vacuolated cells with scant amounts of dispersed pigment granules and a single nucleus (Fig. 10-30). Balloon cells frequently are arranged in an alveolar pattern separated by multiple capillaries. These cells stain positively with oil red-O, indicating that lipids are responsible for the vacuolated appearance. Ultrastructurally, nonmembrane-bound vacuoles are present among interspersed melanosomes and premelanosomes. Occasionally, a tumor is

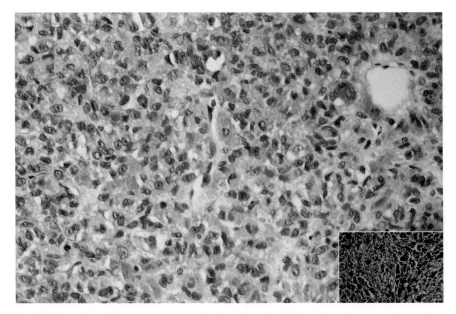

FIG. 10-29. Malignant melanoma composed of large epithelioid cells. Hematoxylin and eosin after bleaching. (*Inset*) Same tumor showing heavily pigmented cells prior to bleaching.

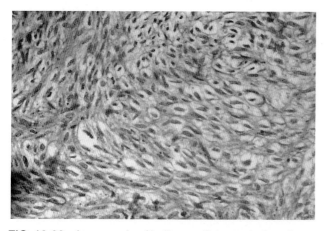

FIG. 10-30. An example of balloon cell degeneration. Some cells contain large amounts of optically empty cytoplasm with a centrally placed nucleus. Hematoxylin and eosin.

composed predominantly of balloon cells, in which case the size of the tumor may overestimate its risk of metastasis.[162] Balloon cell transformation has no known effect on prognosis.

Objective measurements of cellular characteristics have been developed. Several studies have confirmed the usefulness of objective measurement of nucleolar characteristics.[163–165] The **nucleolar area** varies between quiescent cells and cells that are rapidly growing (larger nucleolus) and dividing (absent nucleolus). Therefore, a proliferating tumor has a larger standard deviation of nucleolar size than does normal tissue. The inverse standard deviation of the nucleolar area (ISDNA) is more useful mathematically. There is an inverse relation between the number of epithelioid cells and ISDNA. The advantage of counting epithelioid cells is that no special equipment other than a microscope is required. The disadvantage is that it is not objective, as is the ISDNA.[159,166] The mean of the largest nucleolar area provides similar prognostic value and requires only a micrometer and a microscope.[165]

Comparing studies based on tumor dimensions is difficult because there are no standards for size categories or methods of measurement. Metanalysis of eight studies from 1966 to 1988 showed a 16% mortality from all causes for **small tumors** (less than 10 or 11 mm in basal diameter and less than 2 mm in apical height), 32% for **medium-sized tumors** (3 to 8 mm in apical height but less than 15 or 16 mm in basal diameter), and 53% for **large tumors** (more than 8 mm in apical height or more than 15 or 16 mm in basal diameter).[167] There also appear to be differences in survival within small tumors based on size. In one study, tumors less than 300 mL in volume had a 14% 15-year survival, whereas no fatalities were reported with tumors less than 97 mL in volume.[168]

Anterior location confers a poorer prognosis. In two studies, location anterior to the equator was associated with a 15-year mortality of 59%, compared to 24% for tumors behind the equator.[84,158] This may be due in part

to later detection. A third study of small tumors (less than 1400 mm³) showed a 23% long-term mortality for tumors posterior to the equator, compared to 58% for tumors involving the ciliary body.[85] Ciliary body melanomas are occasionally mistaken for iris melanomas when the anterior segment is involved (Fig. 10-31).

Diffuse growth through the uvea is present in less than 5% of melanomas. Diffuse melanomas cover large areas, expand the choroid, and may be nodular or smooth. Gross tumor is found in the anterior segment in about half the cases.[126] Ring lesions involving the face of the ciliary body should arouse suspicion of a melanoma of the ciliary body and diffuse choroidal melanomas. Tumors with a diffuse growth pattern have a poorer prognosis than confined tumors. Diffuse tumors are often recognized late in their course, frequently have scleral and extrascleral invasion, and contain cells of a more malignant phenotype.

Extrascleral extension occurs in less than 10% of melanomas and may present with microscopic or gross evidence of tumor cells beyond the outer scleral border (Fig. 10-32).[169] Gross extrascleral tumor may appear as fine pigment dusting or as a large tumor nodule. Rarely, the extrascleral portion may be larger than the intraocular portion. Tumor extends beyond the confines of the eye usually through emissarial canals that transmit ciliary nerves and vessels, or vortex veins (Fig. 10-33), and less commonly via the optic nerve. Erosion through the sclera to the extraocular space is rare, although some degree of inner scleral invasion is nearly always observed. Extrascleral extension is more common in larger tumors, those composed of mixed or epithelioid cell types, and diffuse melanomas.[126,170] Extrascleral extension adversely affects survival: 5-year survival has been reported to be 27% to 52% in different series.[169,170] In one study, mortality was doubled with extrascleral extension of tumor, and orbital recurrence was as high as 40%.[171] Surgical transection or nonencapsulation have an additional adverse effect on survival in tumors with extrascleral extension.[169]

Optic nerve invasion occurs in 3% to 8% of all melanomas and is associated with extrascleral extension in about 40% of eyes.[172] Eighty-one percent of peripapillary melanomas have extension into the optic nerve, meningeal coverings, or both.[173] Invasion of the optic nerve by peripapillary melanomas occurs directly through the lamina cribrosa or from the meninges. Optic nerve invasion can occur from shed cells of tumors remote to the optic nerve; it may be facilitated by glaucomatous optic nerve damage.[174] A long section of optic nerve must be excised when peripapillary growth occurs.[173] Optic nerve invasion has an adverse effect on survival (up to 83% mortality) but appears to be coincident with orbital extension and its associated poor prognosis.[172,173]

Electron microscopic evaluation of melanoma tumor blood vessels found that the basement membranes are often thick, multilaminar, composed of excess collagen,

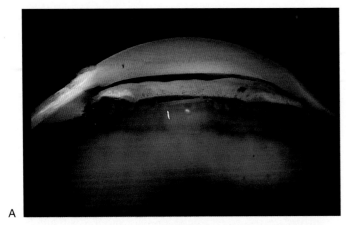

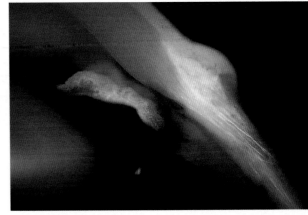

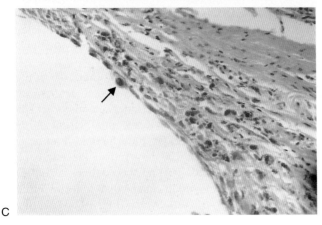

FIG. 10-31. Ring melanoma of the ciliary body. **(A)** There is dense pigmentation of the entire chamber angle. **(B)** Higher magnification shows pigmentation in the chamber angle, iris root, and ciliary body. This enucleation specimen was obtained after malignant melanoma cells were discovered at the surgical margins of an iridocyclectomy specimen. An iris melanoma was suspected; however, the bulk of the tumor was found to be located in the ciliary body at the time of iridocyclectomy. **(C)** Tumor cells (*arrow*), pigment-laden macrophages, and pigment are present in the angle and trabecular meshwork.

and fragmented. These changes can be associated with new blood vessel formation and probably explain the fluorescein angiographic features of melanomas. These changes are similar to those caused by previous radiation exposure but have been seen in untreated melanomas.[175,176]

Recently, investigators have identified nine **vascular patterns** within choroidal melanomas.[175] Only four of these patterns are seen in choroidal nevi. Melanomas containing vascular patterns other than the types found in nevi have a worse prognosis than those with patterns found in nevi. The investigators found that the presence

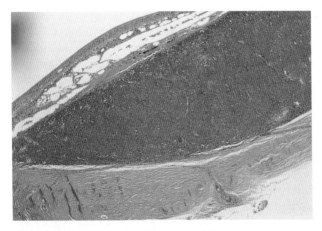

FIG. 10-32. Malignant melanoma with extrascleral extension. Tumor cells exiting the sclera through emisarial canal adjacent to the optic nerve. There is extensive cystoid degeneration of the retina overlying the tumor and a subretinal fibrous membrane replacing the retinal pigment epithelium. Hematoxylin and eosin.

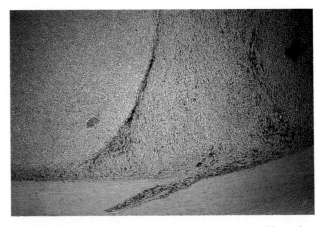

FIG. 10-33. Malignant melanoma with emissarial invasion. Densely pigmented cells are exiting through an emissarial canal surrounding a long posterior ciliary artery. The tumor is composed of distinct clones of cells. Pigmented cells are present on the right and nonpigmented cells are present on the left. Hematoxylin and eosin.

of closed vascular networks was more strongly associated with death from metastatic disease than cell type, tumor size, location, and other factors.

Lymphocytic infiltration is more common in larger tumors and in those of mixed or epithelioid histology. Greater lymphocytic infiltration adversely affects prognosis, although the pattern of infiltration (diffuse versus perivascular) does not seem to be important.[177,178] T lymphocytes are the predominant cell type.

Ploidy analysis (amount of DNA in a tumor cell population) has been found to correlate with tumor progression, recurrence, and metastatic disease in some nonocular tumors. **Euploid** cells (normal amount of DNA) may be diploid (two sets of 23 chromosomes) or tetraploid (four sets of DNA, indicating ongoing cell division). Deviation from these patterns is termed **aneuploidy**. Two methods are available for quantitation of DNA content: **flow cytometry** and **static image analysis**. Aneuploidy has been found in 4% to 37% of choroidal melanomas by flow cytometry, and its presence has been correlated with poorer prognosis.[179,180] **Tetraploidy** has been correlated with increased tumor size and sparse pigmentation. **Image analysis** has shown that the more cells within a melanoma deviate from diploid, the more malignant the tumor. This technology had less prognostic power than nucleolar characterics or tumor size in one study.[181] Flow cytometry and image analysis do not always give identical results for any given tumor.[182]

Measurement of nucleolar organizer units distinguishes uveal nevi from melanocytes. The measurements correlate with other known prognostic factors such as tumor size, cell type, and mitoses. Its ability to add new prognostic information is under study.[164]

Age less than 60 is associated with a lower 5- and 10-year mortality from metastasis.[84] Patients less than age 20 have a similar prognosis overall.[77] Pregnancy and race have not been shown to influence prognosis adversely.[99,115]

Occasionally, diagnostic uncertainty over the melanotic origin of uveal tumors may require the use of **immunohistochemistry**. Antibodies to **S-100** and **HMB-45** proteins are the most commonly used. S-100 proteins are a family of calcium-binding proteins most prevalent in neural glial cells.[72] In paraffin-embedded tissue, positive staining of uveal melanomas was found in about 80% of tumors, whereas none of three metastatic, nonmelanotic, nonneural tumors stained.[183] Several other nonmelanocytic cell types have shown S-100 positively, which limits its usefulness. Monoclonal antibody (MAB-079), specific for subtypes S-100α and S-100β, may be beneficial in differentiating metastatic cutaneous and primary uveal melanomas in the eye or in distant metastatic sites.[72] HMB-45 monoclonal antibodies react against glycoconjugated proteins in premelanosomes. This antibody was positive in 99% of 69 uveal melanomas, compared to 91% for S-100, and is more specific. Nevertheless, it is unreliable in distinguishing benign from malignant uveal melanocytic tumors.[184]

Treatment

Data are inconclusive as to whether **enucleation** or **plaque radiation therapy** is more effective in prolonging life or achieving cure.

The **Collaborative Ocular Melanoma Study** is a three-part, international, multicenter, prospective randomized study. The first part is a randomized trial of patients with medium-sized tumors (3 to 8 mm in height and less than 16 mm in largest basal diameter) treated by enucleation versus iodine-125 plaque irradiation. The second part is a randomized trial of patients with large melanomas (more than 8 mm thick or 16 mm in greatest basal diameter) treated with enucleation alone or preenucleation external beam radiation and enucleation. The final part is a prospective observational study of small melanomas (1 to 3 mm in height and at least 5 mm in largest basal diameter) to determine if a randomized trial of treatment is indicated in the future.[185]

Simple observation of small choroidal tumors is a reasonable approach. Two studies have demonstrated no adverse effect attributed to delay in treatment of small tumors.[168,186] These data suggest that although it is generally safe to watch small tumors, metastasis can occur early in the evolution of these lesions. About 33% of small indeterminate tumors enlarge over time. Greater tumor thickness, the presence of ocular symptoms, orange pigment overlying the tumor, low internal reflectivity on ultrasound, and hot spots on fluorescein angiogram are correlated with growth.[187]

Some physicians have questioned the efficacy of **enucleation** and suggest it may actually increase mortality.[188,189] Metastatic disease discovered at the time of diagnosis of the primary melanoma is rare (less than 6%). There are limited data on the natural history of untreated melanoma, and in some series the mortality rates differ little between enucleated eyes and those observed. Most studies show that peak yearly mortality rates (up to 12%) occur at about 2 years after enucleation. Mortality rates then taper over ensuing years until 7 to 8 years after enucleation, when they parallel estimated rates for untreated melanomas at 1% per year. Tumor-associated antibodies are seen to fall after enucleation; in contrast, antibody levels were found to increase after photocoagulation and plaque radiation therapy. Anesthetic agents and the surgical procedure itself also have been suspected of altering the immune status. A final argument against enucleation is that tumor cells can be shed into the bloodstream during surgery, and their numbers are critical to the incidence of metastasis.[190,191] Pressures up to 500 mm Hg can occur during enucleation and may force tumor cells through and into fragile tumor vessels. "**No-touch**" surgical methods of extraction combine minimal manipulation of the globe with or without cryocoagulation and extraction.[192,193] Animals treated with atraumatic surgery showed fewer metastases and survived longer.[194] Immune impairment further enhanced metastasis in animals.

Proponents of enucleation note that small tumors have a much better prognosis than large tumors and that prognosis is much better for tumors without extrascleral extension. Similar patterns of mortality (ie, a temporal relation between discovery and metastasis) occur in nonocular tumors treated without surgery and in patients with known metastasis.[195] One study in humans showed none of 11 patients with melanoma had a blood sample positive for tumor cells 15 minutes after surgery. One of two choroidal melanomas treated with photocoagulation and three of 18 retinoblastomas treated by enucleation had blood samples positive for tumor cells.[190]

One explanation for the high mortality in the 2 to 3 years after enucleation is that the detection of primary disease and metastasis are simply close in time.[196] Doubling times for choroidal melanomas have been estimated to vary from 3 to 30 months.[197] An intraocular mass creates signs and symptoms while the tumor is relatively small, compared to tumors in other parts of the body. Because metastases are at least one doubling time behind the primary, they are small and undetectable by most screening tests. Very few doubling times would then be needed to allow detection or cause symptoms. If tumor cells do not metastasize until the time of enucleation, much longer periods of time would be required to create a mass of significant size.

Opponents have pointed out that metastatic lesions do not necessarily have similar doubling times and may grow to larger size, even though they evolve later than the intraocular tumor. Furthermore, if patients already had undetected metastases at the time of enucleation, metastasis would have had to occur in some patients when the tumor was still very small.[198]

Radiation is the most common form of treatment for choroidal melanomas in many centers. Two methods of delivery are used: plaque and external beam therapy. Radiation therapy is indicated for small or medium-sized tumors in patients with the desire to preserve vision. One-eyed patients with larger tumors and useful vision also may be considered for this therapy. Juxtapapillary tumors are not good candidates for radiation therapy due to the high incidence of radiation-induced optic neuropathy. Short-term survival rates appear to be similar to enucleation; however, a few patients eventually require enucleation due to treatment failure or complications.

Many radioisotopes have been used in brachytherapy of choroidal melanoma. Iodine-125 is the most commonly used and was chosen for the Collaborative Ocular Melanoma Study because of its equivalent dose penetration to cobalt-60 and greater ease of shielding emitted radiation.[199]

Local resection is possible for some ciliary body and choroidal melanomas. Resection of choroidal tumors can include the whole eye wall with overlying retina or a lamellar scleral and choroid dissection from overlying retina, through a scleral flap. Survival rates appear to be equal to enucleation and radiation therapy. Long-term visual outcomes are good if perioperative complications are avoided.[200]

Laser therapy is used for a few choroidal melanomas. It is especially useful as a vision-sparing procedure for small, flat extrafoveal lesions near the optic nerve, as it avoids the optic neuropathy associated with radiation treatment. Overall, it is associated with more immediate complications and requires more treatment visits than the application of radioactive plaques. Both xenon arc and argon lasers have been used. Argon laser has a lower success rate but is associated with fewer complications.[201]

There appears to be little role for **exenteration** in the treatment of tumors with extrascleral extension discovered either at the time of surgery or on pathologic examination.[172,202] There is no benefit to exenteration for orbital recurrence of malignant melanoma other than for palliation.[169]

As yet, no **chemotherapeutic regimens** have been found to cause a cure for uveal melanoma, although prolonged survival has been demonstrated in some patients. **Immunotherapy** was successful in one case.[203] Oncologists have not commonly used these treatments in the primary management of uveal melanomas because metastatic disease seldom is discovered at the time uveal melanoma is diagnosed. Identifying patients with risk factors for metastatic disease will be more important in the management of uveal melanoma when effective medical treatment, alone or in conjunction with other treatment modalities, is developed.

Optic Nerve

Magnocellular Nevus (Melanocytoma)

A magnocellular nevus is a unique melanocytic nevus most often found on the optic nerve head. Far fewer have been found in the iris, ciliary body, choroid, and sclera.[204–206] Unlike choroidal melanoma, these tumors are more common in blacks and other groups with dark ocular pigmentation, although true occurrence rates are unknown.[207]

Clinically, these lesions are jet black with feathery margins. They typically cover less than half the disc area but may enlarge to cover areas up to two disc diameters in size. Magnocellular nevi can demonstrate disturbing growth but usually remain benign histologically. Rarely, malignant transformation occurs. Vision loss and visual field and afferent pupillary defects secondary to invasion and compression of the optic nerve head (Fig. 10-34)

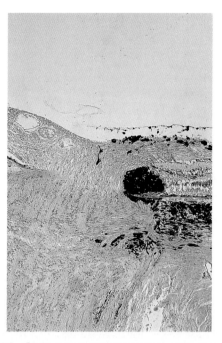

FIG. 10-34. Optic nerve melanocytoma with densely pigmented cells within the choroid, sclera, optic nerve head, and meninges. The posterior vitreous and attached pigmented cells are artifactually detached. Hematoxylin and eosin.

also are reported. Lesions simulating magnocellular nevi include malignant melanoma of the optic nerve head and pigment epithelial adenoma.[208,209]

These benign tumors are composed of two **cell types.** The predominant cell in most tumors is a **large round** or **polyhedral cell** with densely packed, large melanin granules (macromelanosomes). Bleached preparations are needed to view the nuclei, which are small, dark, and oval and have small or absent nucleoli. The second cell type is smaller, **spindle-shaped,** and less pigmented. Their nuclei are elongated and usually have small nucleoli. Melanosomes are smaller and less numerous. These cells are found throughout the tumor in small numbers and are more numerous at the margins of tumors, especially in actively growing lesions. Ultrastructurally, the large cells are packed with large melanin granules and sparse cytoplasmic organelles. The spindle cells have small melanin granules and plentiful organelles. Mitotic figures are rare in both cell types.[210,211]

REFERENCES

1. Wobmann PR, Fine BS. The clump cells of Koganei. A light and electron microscopic study. *Am J Ophthalmol* 1972;73:90.
2. Holmberg A. The ultrastructure of the capillaries in the ciliary body. *Arch Ophthalmol* 1959;62:949.
3. Shields JA. Primary cysts of the iris. *Trans Am Ophthalmol Soc* 1981;79:771.
4. Kozart DM, Scheie HG. Spontaneous cysts of the ciliary epithelium. *Trans Am Acad Ophthalmol Otolaryngol* 1970;74:534.
5. Okun E. Gross and microscopic pathology in autopsy eyes. IV. Pars plana cysts. *Am J Ophthalmol* 1961;51:1221.
6. Rodrigues MC, Spaeth GL, Krachmer JH, Laibson PR. Iridoschisis associated with glaucoma and bullous keratopathy. *Am J Ophthalmol* 1983;95:73.
7. Moses RA. Detachment of the ciliary body—anatomic and physical considerations. *Invest Ophthalmol Vis Sci* 1965;4:935.
8. Gass JDM, Jallow S. Idiopathic serous detachment of the choroid, ciliary body and retina (uveal effusion syndrome). *Ophthalmology* 1982;89:1018.
9. Ward RC, Gragoudas ES, Pon DM, Albert DM. Abnormal scleral findings in the uveal effusion syndrome. *Am J Ophthalmol* 1985;106:139.
10. Vine AK. Uveal effusion in Hunter's syndrome. *Retina* 1986;6:57.
11. Gass JDM. Uveal effusion syndrome: a new hypothesis concerning pathogenesis and technique of surgical treatment. *Retina* 1983;3:159.
12. Bateman JB, Foos RY. Coronal adenomas. *Arch Ophthalmol* 1979;97:2379.
13. Burch PG, Maumenee AE. Iridocyclectomy for benign tumors of the ciliary body. *Am J Ophthalmol* 1967;63:447.
14. Zaidman GW, Johnson BL, Salamon SM, Mondino BJ. Fuchs' adenoma affecting the peripheral iris. *Arch Ophthalmol* 1983;101:771.
15. Brown HH, Glasgow BJ, Foos RY. Ultrastructural and immunohistochemical features of coronal adenomas. *Am J Ophthalmol* 1991;112:34.
16. Glasgow BJ. Intraocular fine needle aspiration biopsy of coronal adenomas. *Diagn Cytopathol* 1991;7:239.
17. Zimmerman LE. The remarkable polymorphism of tumors of the ciliary body: the Norman McAlister Gregg lecture. *Trans Aust Coll Ophthalmol* 1970;2:114.
18. Croxatto JO, Zimmerman LE. Malignant nonpigmented intraocular tumors of neuroectodermal origin in adults: a review of 21 cases. In Spencer WH, ed. *Ophthalmic pathology: an atlas and textbook.* Philadelphia: WB Saunders, 1985:1255.
19. Andersen SR. Medulloepithelioma of the retina. *Int Ophthalmol Clin* 1962;2:483.
20. Rodrigues M, Hidayat A, Karesh J. Pleomorphic adenocarcinoma of ciliary epithelium simulating an epibulbar mass. *Am J Ophthalmol* 1988;106:595.
21. Jakobiec FA, Zimmerman LE, Spencer WH, et al. Metastatic colloid carcinoma versus primary carcinoma of the ciliary epithelium. *Ophthalmology* 1987;94:1469.
22. Grossniklaus HE, Zimmerman LE, Kachmer ML. Pleomorphic adenocarcinoma of the ciliary body: immunohistochemical and electron microscopic features. *Ophthalmology* 1990;97:763.
23. Rennie IG, Faulkner MK, Parsons MA. Adenoma of the pigmented ciliary epithelium. *Br J Ophthalmol* 1994;78:484.
24. Lieb WE, Shields JA, Eagle RC, et al. Cystic adenoma of the pigmented ciliary epithelium: clinical, pathologic, and immunohistopathologic findings. *Ophthalmology* 1990;97:1489.
25. Desroches G, Abrams GW, Gass JDM. Reactive lymphoid hyperplasia of the uvea: a case with ultrasonographic and computed tomographic studies. *Arch Ophthalmol* 1983;101:725.
26. Ryan SJ, Frank RN, Green WR. Bilateral inflammatory pseudotumors of the ciliary body. *Am J Ophthalmol* 1971;72:586.
27. Shields CL, Shields JA, Augsburger JJ. Choroidal osteoma. *Surv Ophthalmol* 1988;33:17.
28. Trimble SN, Schatz H. Choroidal osteoma after intraocular inflammation. *Am J Ophthalmol* 1983;96:759.
29. Katz RS, Gass JDM. Multiple choroidal osteomas developing in association with recurrent orbital inflammatory pseudotumor. *Arch Ophthalmol* 1983;101:1724.
30. Kline LB, Skalka HW, Davidson JD, Wilmes FJ. Bilateral choroidal osteomas associated with fatal systemic illness. *Am J Ophthalmol* 1982;93:192.
31. Cunha SL. Osseous choristoma of the choroid: a familial disease. *Arch Ophthalmol* 1984;102:1052.
32. Noble KG. Bilateral choroidal osteoma in three siblings. *Am J Ophthalmol* 1990;109:656.
33. Eting E, Savir H. An atypical fulminant course of choroidal osteoma in two siblings. *Am J Ophthalmol* 1992;113:52.

34. Trimble SN, Schatz H, Schneider GB. Spontaneous decalcification of a choroidal osteoma. *Ophthalmology* 1988;95:631.

35. DePotter P, Shields JA, Shields CL, Rao VM. Magnetic resonance imaging in choroidal osteoma. *Retina* 1991;11:221.

36. Williams AT, Font RL, Van Dyk HJ, Riekhof FT. Osseous choristoma of the choroid simulating a choroidal melanoma. *Arch Ophthalmol* 1978;96:1874.

37. Gass JDM, Guerry RK, Jack RL, Harris G. Choroidal osteoma. *Arch Ophthalmol* 1978;96:428.

38. Witschel H, Font RL. Hemangioma of the choroid: a clinicopathologic study of 71 cases and a review of the literature. *Surv Ophthalmol* 1976;20:415.

39. Shields JA, Stephens RF, Eagle RC, et al. Progressive enlargement of a circumscribed choroidal hemangioma: a clinicopathologic correlation. *Arch Ophthalmol* 1992;110:1276.

40. Shields JA, Shields CL, Eagle RC, DePotter P. Observations on seven cases of intraocular leiomyoma: the 1993 Byron Demorest Lecture. *Arch Ophthalmol* 1994;112:521.

41. Jakobiec FA, Silbert G. Are most iris melanomas really nevi? A clinicopathologic study of 189 lesions. *Arch Ophthalmol* 1981;99:2117.

42. Ashton N. Primary tumors of the iris. *Br J Ophthalmol* 1964;48:650.

43. Jakobiec FA, Witschel H, Zimmerman LE. Choroidal leiomyoma of vascular origin. *Am J Ophthalmol* 1976;82:205.

44. Meyer SL, Fine BS, Font RL, Zimmerman LE. Leiomyoma of the ciliary body: electron microscopic verification. *Am J Ophthalmol* 1968;66:1061.

45. Jakobiec FA, Font RL, Tso MOM, Zimmerman LE. Mesectodermal leiomyoma of the ciliary body: a tumor of presumed neural crest origin. *Cancer* 1977;39:2102.

46. Foss AJE, Pecorella I, Alexander RA, et al. Are most intraocular "leiomyomas" really melanocytic lesions? *Ophthalmology* 1994;101:919.

47. Shields JA, Sanborn GE, Kurz GH, Augsburger JJ. Benign peripheral nerve tumor of the choroid: a clinicopathologic correlation and review of the literature. *Ophthalmology* 1981;88:1322.

48. Shields JA, Font RL, Eagle RC, et al. Melanotic schwannoma of the choroid: immunohistochemistry and electron microscopic observations. *Ophthalmology* 1994;101:843.

49. Messmer EP, Font RL. Applications of immunohistochemistry to ophthalmic pathology. *Ophthalmology* 1984;91:701.

50. Duke-Elder WS, ed. *System of ophthalmology*. Vol. X. St. Louis: CV Mosby, 1967:387.

51. Allen RA, Straatsma BR. Ocular involvement in leukemia and allied disorders. *Arch Ophthalmol* 1961;66:490.

52. Kincaid MC, Green WR. Ocular and orbital involvement in leukemia. *Surv Ophthalmol* 1983;27:211.

53. Leonardy NJ, Rupani M, Dent G, Klintworth GK. Analysis of 135 autopsy eyes for ocular involvement in leukemia. *Am J Ophthalmol* 1990;109:436.

54. Deitch RD, Wilson FM. Leukemic reticuloendotheliosis with presenting ocular complaints. *Arch Ophthalmol* 1963;69:560.

55. Decker EB, Burnstine RA. Leukemic relapse presenting as acute unilateral hypopyon in acute lymphoblastic leukemia. *Ann Ophthalmol* 1993;25:346.

56. Ridgeway EW, Jaffe N, Walton DS. Leukemic ophthalmopathy in children. *Cancer* 1976;38:1744.

57. Engle HM, Green WR, Michels RG, et al. Diagnostic vitrectomy. *Retina* 1981;1:121.

58. Nelson CC, Hertzberg BS, Klintworth GK. A histopathologic study of 716 unselected eyes in patients with cancer at the time of death. *Am J Ophthalmol* 1983;95:788.

59. Kohno T, Uchida H, Inomata H, et al. Ocular manifestations of adult T-cell leukemia/lymphoma. *Ophthalmology* 1993;100:1794.

60. Kumar SR, Gill PS, Wagner DG, et al. Human T-cell lymphotropic virus type I-associated retinal lymphoma: a clinicopathologic report. *Arch Ophthalmol* 1994;112:954.

61. Kim EW, Zakov N, Albert DM, et al. Intraocular reticulum cell sarcoma: a case report and literature review. *Graefes Arch Clin Exp Ophthalmol* 1979;209:167.

62. Spencer WH, ed. *Ophthalmic pathology: an atlas and textbook*. Philadelphia: WB Saunders, 1985:1656.

63. Albert DM, Rubenstein RA, Scheie HG. Tumor metastasis to the eye. I. Incidence in 213 adult patients with generalized malignancy. *Am J Ophthalmol* 1967;63:723.

64. Jensen OA. Metastatic tumors of the eye and orbit: a histopathological analysis of a Danish series. *Acta Pathol Microbiol Scand* 1970;212(suppl):201.

65. Ferry AP, Font RL. Carcinoma metastatic to the eye and orbit. I. A clinicopathologic study of 227 cases. *Arch Ophthalmol* 1974;92:276.

66. Block RS, Gartner S. The incidence of ocular metastatic carcinoma. *Arch Ophthalmol* 1971;85:673.

67. Stephens RF, Shields JA. Diagnosis and management of cancer metastatic to the uvea: a study of 70 cases. *Ophthalmology* 1979;86:1336.

68. Shields JA, Shields CL. *Intraocular tumors: a text and atlas*. Philadelphia: WB Saunders, 1992.

69. Shields JA, Shields CL, Kiratli H, DePotter P. Metastatic tumors to the iris in 40 patients. *Am J Ophthalmol* 1995;119:422.

70. Shields JA. Metastatic tumors to the uvea. *Int Ophthalmol Clin* 1993;33:155.

71. Shields JA, Shields CL, Ehya H, et al. Fine-needle aspiration biopsy of suspected intraocular tumors: the 1992 Urwick lecture. *Ophthalmology* 1993;100:1677.

72. Kan-Mitchell J, Rao N, Albert DM, et al. S-100 phenotypes of uveal melanomas. *Invest Ophthalmol Vis Sci* 1990;31:1492.

73. Lewis RA, Riccardi VM. Von Recklinghausen neurofibromatosis. Incidence of iris hamartomas. *Ophthalmology* 1981;88:348.

74. Collins FS, Ponder BA, Seizinger BR, Epstein CJ. The von Recklinghausen neurofibromatosis region on chromosome 17—genetic and physical maps come into focus. *Am J Hum Genet* 1989;44:1.

75. Rouleau GA, Wertelecki W, Haines JL, et al. Genetic linkage of bilateral acoustic neurofibromatosis to a DNA marker on chromosome 22. *Nature* 1987;329:246.

76. Rodriguez-Sains RS. Ocular findings in patients with dysplastic nevus syndrome: an update. *Dermatol Clin* 1991;9:723.

77. Barr CC, McLean IW, Zimmerman LE. Uveal melanomas in children and adolescents. *Arch Ophthalmol* 31981;99:2133.

78. Rootman J, Gallagher RP. Color as a risk factor in iris melanoma. *Am J Ophthalmol* 1984;98:558.

79. Grossniklaus HE, Oakman JH, Cohen C, et al. Histopathology, morphometry, and nuclear DNA content of iris melanocytic lesions. *Invest Ophthalmol Vis Sci* 1995;36:745.

80. Yanoff M, Zimmerman LE. Histogenesis of malignant melanoma of the uvea. III. The relationship of congenital ocular melanocytosis and neurofibromatosis to uveal melanomas. *Arch Ophthalmol* 1967;77:331.

81. Yanoff M. Glaucoma mechanisms in ocular malignant melanomas. *Am J Ophthalmol* 1970;70:898.

82. Marcus DM, Mawn LA, Egan KM, Albert DM. Nucleolar organizer regions in iris nevi and melanoma. *Am J Ophthalmol* 1992;114:202.

83. Geisse LJ, Robertson DM. Iris melanomas. *Am J Ophthalmol* 1985;99:638.

84. Shammas HF, Blodi FC. Prognostic factors in choroidal and ciliary body melanomas. *Arch Ophthalmol* 1977,95:63.

85. McLean IW, Foster WD, Zimmerman LE. Prognostic factors in small malignant melanomas of choroid and ciliary body. *Arch Ophthalmol* 1977;95:48.

86. Shields JA, Sanborn GE, Augsburger JJ. The differential diagnosis of melanoma of the iris: a clinical study of 200 patients. *Ophthalmology* 1983;90:716.

87. Gass JDM. Problems in the differential diagnosis of choroidal nevi and malignant melanomas: the XXXIII Edward Jackson Memorial Lecture. *Am J Ophthalmol* 1977;83:299.

88. Hale PN, Allen RA, Straatsma BR. Benign melanomas (nevi) of the choroid and ciliary body. *Arch Ophthalmol* 1965;74:532.

89. Naumann G, Yanoff M, Zimmerman LE. Histogenesis of malignant melanomas of the uvea. I. Histopathologic characteristics of nevi of the choroid and ciliary body. *Arch Ophthalmol* 1966;76:784.

90. Hayreh SS. Choroidal melanomata: fluorescein angiographic and histopathological study. *Br J Ophthalmol* 1970;54:145.

91. Smith LT, Irvine AR. Diagnostic significance of orange pigment

accumulation over choroidal tumors. *Am J Ophthalmol* 1973;76: 212.

92. Augsburger JJ, McCarthy EF, Gonder JR, Shields JA. Macular choroidal nevi. *Int Ophthalmol Clin* 1981;21:99.

93. Gonder JR, Augsburger JJ, McCarthy EF, Shields JA. Visual loss associated with choroidal nevi. *Ophthalmology* 1982;89:961.

94. Flindall RJ, Drance SM. Visual field studies of benign choroidal melanomata. *Arch Ophthalmol* 1969;81:41.

95. McLean IW, Zimmerman LE, Evans RM. Reappraisal of Callender's spindle A type of malignant melanoma of choroid and ciliary body. *Am J Ophthalmol* 1978;86:557.

96. Greer CH. Congenital melanoma of the anterior uvea. *Arch Ophthalmol* 1966;76:77.

97. Egan KM, Seddon JM, Glynn RJ, et al. Epidemiologic aspects of uveal melanoma. *Surv Ophthalmol* 1988;32:239.

98. Hudson HL, Valluri S, Rao NA. Choroidal melanomas in Hispanic patients. *Am J Ophthalmol* 1994;118:57.

99. Margo CE, McLean IW. Malignant melanomas of the choroid and ciliary body in black patients. *Arch Ophthalmol* 1984;102:77.

100. Seddon JM, Gragoudas ES, Glynn RJ, et al. Host factors, UV radiation, and risk factors of uveal melanoma. A case control study. *Arch Ophthalmol* 1990;108:1274.

101. Yanoff M, Zimmerman LE. Histogenesis of malignant melanoma of the uvea. II. Relationship of uveal nevi to malignant melanomas. *Cancer* 1967;20:493.

102. Walker JP, Weiter JJ, Albert DM, et al. Uveal malignant melanoma in three generations of the same family. *Am J Ophthalmol* 1979; 88:723.

103. Simons KB, Hale LM, Morrison HM, et al. Choroidal malignant melanoma in siblings. *Am J Ophthalmol* 1983;96:675.

104. Shields JA, Augsburger JJ, Arbizo V, et al. Malignant melanoma of the choroid in a husband and wife. *Br J Ophthalmol* 1984;68: 623.

105. Cannon-Albright LA, Goldgar DE, Meyer LJ, et al. Assignment of a locus for familial melanoma, MLM, to chromosome 9p13-p22. *Science* 1992;258:1148.

106. Magauran RG, Gray B, Small KW. Chromosome 9 abnormality in choroidal melanoma. *Am J Ophthalmol* 1994;117:109.

107. Kamb A, Gruis NA, Weaver-Feldhaus J, et al. A cell cycle regulator potentially involved in genesis of many tumor types. *Science* 1994;264:436.

108. Albert DM, Chang MA, Lamping K, et al. The dysplastic nevus syndrome: a pedigree with primary malignant melanomas of the choroid and skin. *Ophthalmology* 1985;92:1728.

109. Nik NA, Glew WB, Zimmerman LE. Malignant melanoma of the choroid in the nevus of Ota of a black patient. *Arch Ophthalmol* 1982;100:1641.

110. Pomeranz GA, Bunt AH, Kalina RE. Multifocal choroidal melanoma in ocular melanocytosis. *Arch Ophthalmol* 1981;99:857.

111. Font RL, Ferry AP. The phakomatoses. *Int Ophthalmol Clin* 31972;12:1.

112. Albert DM. The association of viruses with uveal melanomas. *Trans Am Ophthalmol Soc* 1979;77:367.

113. Albert DM, Puliafito CA, Fulton AB, et al. Increased incidence of choroidal malignant melanoma occurring in a single population of chemical workers. *Am J Ophthalmol* 1980;89:323.

114. El Baba F, Blumenkranz M. Malignant melanoma at the site of penetrating ocular trauma. *Arch Ophthalmol* 1986;104:405.

115. Shields CL, Shields JA, Eagle RC, et al. Uveal melanoma and pregnancy: a report of 16 cases. *Ophthalmology* 1991;98:1667.

116. Lischko AM, Seddon JM, Gragoudas ES, et al. Evaluation of prior primary malignancy as a determinant of uveal melanoma. *Ophthalmology* 1989;96:1716.

117. Barr CC, Zimmerman LE, Curtin VT, Font RL. Bilateral diffuse melanocytic uveal tumors associated with systemic malignant neoplasms: a recently recognized syndrome. *Arch Ophthalmol* 1982; 100:249.

118. Servodidio CA, Abramson DH. Presenting signs and symptoms of choroidal melanoma: what do they mean? *Ann Ophthalmol* 1992;24:190.

119. Jensen OA. Malignant melanomas of the uvea in Denmark, 1943–1952. *Acta Ophthalmologica* 1963;75(suppl):17.

120. Erie JC, Robertson DM. Serous detachments of the macula associated with presumed small choroidal melanomas. *Am J Ophthalmol* 1986;102:176.

121. Cunliffe IA, Rennie IG. Choroidal melanoma presenting as vitreous hemorrhage. *Eye* 1987;7:711.

122. Pizzuto D, de Luise V, Zimmerman N. Choroidal malignant melanoma appearing as acute panophthalmitis. *Am J Ophthalmol* 1986; 101:249.

123. Yap EV, Robertson DM, Buettner H. Scleritis as an initial manifestation of choroidal malignant melanoma. *Ophthalmology* 1992;99: 1693.

124. Rose GE, Hoh HB, Harrad RA, Hungerford JL. Intraocular malignant melanomas presenting with orbital inflammation. *Eye* 1993; 7:539.

125. Foos RY. Early diagnosis of ciliary body melanomas. *Arch Ophthalmol* 1969;81:336.

126. Font RL, Spaulding AG, Zimmerman LE. Diffuse malignant melanoma of the uveal tract: a clinicopathologic report of 54 cases. *Trans Am Acad Ophthalmol Otolaryngol* 1968;72:877.

127. Font RL, Zimmerman LE, Armaly MF. The nature of the orange pigment over a choroidal melanoma: histochemical and electron microscopical observations. *Arch Ophthalmol* 1974;91:359.

128. Shields JA, Rodrigues MM, Sarin LK, et al. Lipofuscin pigment over benign and malignant choroidal tumors. *Trans Am Acad Ophthalmol Otolaryngol* 1976;81:871.

129. Char DH, Stone RD, Irvine AR, et al. Diagnostic modalities in choroidal melanoma. *Am J Ophthalmol* 1980;89:223.

130. Nicholson DH, Frazier-Byrne S, Chiu MT, et al. Echographic and histologic tumor height measurements in uveal melanoma. *Am J Ophthalmol* 1985;100:454.

131. Lemay M, Roxburgh STD, Lee WR. The role of ultrasound in the investigation and management of suspected ocular melanoma. *Doc Ophthalmol Proc* 1981;29:85.

132. Pavlin CJ, Japp B, Simpson ER, et al. Ultrasound determination of radioactive plaques to the base of choroidal melanomas. *Ophthalmology* 1989;96:538.

133. Mafee MF, Peyman GA, Peace JH, et al. Magnetic resonance imaging in the evaluation and differentiation of uveal melanoma. *Ophthalmology* 1987;94:341.

134. Peyster RG, Augsburger JJ, Shield JA, et al. Choroidal melanoma: comparison of CT, funduscopy, and US. *Radiology* 1985;156:675.

135. Kolodny NH, Gragoudas ES, D'Amico DJ, Albert DM. Magnetic resonance imaging and spectroscopy of intraocular tumors. *Surv Ophthalmol* 1989;33:502.

136. Bond JB, Haik BG, Mihara F, Gupta KL. Magnetic resonance imaging of choroidal melanoma with and without gadolinium contrast enhancement. *Ophthalmology* 1991;98:459.

137. Shields JA, McDonald PR, Leonard BC, Canny CLB. The diagnosis of uveal melanomas in eyes with opaque media. *Am J Ophthalmol* 1977;83:95.

138. Wollensak J, Heinrich M. In vivo and in vitro measurements of P32-uptake in the ocular tissue in cases of malignant melanoma. *Graefes Arch Clin Exp Ophthalmol* 1981;217:35.

139. Glasgow BJ, Foos RY. *Ocular cytopathology*. Stoneham: Butterworth-Heinnemann, 1993:89.

140. Augsburger JJ, Shields JA, Folberg R, et al. Fine needle aspiration biopsy in the diagnosis of intraocular cancer. *Ophthalmology* 1985; 92:39.

141. Char DH, Miller TR, Crawford JB. Cytopathologic diagnosis of benign lesions simulating choroidal melanomas. *Am J Ophthalmol* 1991;112:70.

142. Glasgow BJ, Straatsma RB, Kreiger AE. Fine-needle aspiration of posterior segment intraocular tumors. *Ophthalmol Clin North Am* 1995;8:67.

143. Karcioglu ZA, Gordon RA, Karcioglu GL. Tumor seeding in ocular fine needle aspiration biopsy. *Ophthalmology* 1985;92:1763.

144. Glasgow BJ, Brown HH, Zaragoza AM, Foos RY. Quantitation of tumor seeding from fine needle aspiration biopsy of ocular melanomas. *Am J Ophthalmol* 1988;105:538.

145. Staman JA, Fitzgerald CR, Dawson WW, et al. The EOG and choroidal malignant melanomas. *Doc Ophthalmol* 1970;49:201.

146. Scheidler J, Leinsinger G, Kirsch C-M, et al. Immunoimaging of choroidal melanoma: assessment of its diagnostic accuracy and limitations in 101 cases. *Br J Ophthalmol* 1992;76:457.

147. Michelson JB, Felberg NT, Shields JA. Evaluation of metastatic

cancer to the eye: carcinoembryonic antigen and gamma glutamyl transpeptidase. *Arch Ophthalmol* 1977;95:692.

148. Pach JM, Robertson DM. Metastasis from untreated uveal melanomas. *Arch Ophthalmol* 1986;104:1624.

149. Wagoner MD, Albert DM. The incidence of metastasis from untreated ciliary body and choroidal melanoma. *Arch Ophthalmol* 1982;100:939.

150. Tobal K, Sherman LS, Foss AJ, Lightman SL. Detection of melanocytes from uveal melanoma in peripheral blood using polymerase chain reaction. *Invest Ophthalmol Vis Sci* 1993;34:2622.

151. Shields JA, Augsburger JJ, Brown GC, Stephens RF. The differential diagnosis of posterior uveal melanoma. *Ophthalmology* 1980;87:518.

152. Ferry AP. Lesions mistaken for malignant melanomas of the posterior uvea: a clinicopathologic analysis of 100 cases with ophthalmoscopically visible lesions. *Arch Ophthalmol* 1964;72:463.

153. Albert DM, Marcus DM. Accuracy of diagnosis of choroidal melanomas in the Collaborative Ocular Melanoma Study: COMS report no. 1. *Arch Ophthalmol* 1990;108:1268.

154. Shields JA, Zimmerman LE. Lesions simulating malignant melanoma of the posterior uvea. *Arch Ophthalmol* 1973;89:466.

155. Davidorf FH, Letson AD, Weiss ET, Levine E. Incidence of misdiagnosis and unsuspected choroidal melanomas. *Arch Ophthalmol* 1983;101:410.

156. Callender GR. Malignant melanotic tumors of the eye: a study of histologic types in 111 cases. *Trans Am Acad Ophthalmol Otolaryngol* 1931;36:131.

157. McLean IW, Foster WD, Zimmerman LE, Gamel JW. Modifications of Callender's classification of uveal melanoma at the Armed Forces Institute of Pathology. *Am J Ophthalmol* 1983;96:502.

158. Seddon JM, Albert DM, Lavin PT, Robinson N. A prognostic factor study of disease-free interval and survival following enucleation for uveal melanoma. *Arch Ophthalmol* 1983;101:1894.

159. Seddon JM, Polivogianis L, Hsieh C, et al. Death from uveal melanoma: number of epithelioid cells and inverse SD of nucleolar area as prognostic factors. *Arch Ophthalmol* 1987;105:801.

160. Shields JA, Augsburger JJ, Dougherty MJ. Orbital recurrence of choroidal melanoma 20 years after enucleation. *Am J Ophthalmol* 1984;97:767.

161. Gamel JW, McLean IW. Quantitative analysis of the Callender classification of uveal melanoma cells. *Arch Ophthalmol* 1977;95:686.

162. Jakobiec FA, Shields JA, Desjardins L, Iwamoto T. Balloon cell melanomas of the ciliary body. *Arch Ophthalmol* 1979;97:1687.

163. Gamel JW, McLean IW. Modern developments in histopathologic assessment of uveal melanomas. *Ophthalmology* 1984;91:679.

164. Marcus DM, Minkovitz JB, Wardwell SD, Albert DM. The value of nucleolar organizer regions in uveal melanoma. *Am J Ophthalmol* 1990;110:527.

165. Huntington AC, Haugan P, McLean IW, Gamel JW. The mean of the 10 largest nucleoli as a measure of malignant potential in ciliochoroidal melanoma. ARVO abstracts. *Invest Ophthalmol Vis Sci* 1988;29:210.

166. Gamel JW, McLean IW. Computerized histopathologic assessment of malignant potential. II. A practical method for predicting survival following enucleation for uveal melanoma. *Cancer* 1983;52:1032.

167. Diener-West M, Hawkins BS, Markowitz JA, Schachat AP. A review of mortality from choroidal melanoma. II. A meta-analysis of 5-year mortality rates following enucleation, 1966 through 1988. *Arch Ophthalmol* 1992;110:245.

168. Thomas JV, Green WR, Maumenee AE. Small choroidal melanomas: a long-term follow-up. *Arch Ophthalmol* 1979;97:861.

169. Pach JM, Robertson DM, Taney BS, et al. Prognostic factors in choroidal and ciliary body melanomas with extrascleral extension. *Am J Ophthalmol* 1986;101:325.

170. Shammas HF, Blodi FC. Orbital extension of choroidal and ciliary body melanomas. *Arch Ophthalmol* 1977;95:2002.

171. Starr HJ, Zimmerman LE. Extrascleral extension and orbital recurrence of malignant melanomas of the choroid and ciliary body. *Int Ophthalmol Clin* 1962;2:369.

172. Affeldt JC, Minckler DS, Azen SP, Yeh L. Prognosis in uveal melanoma with extrascleral extension. *Arch Ophthalmol* 1980;98:1975.

173. Shammas HF, Blodi FC. Peripapillary choroidal melanomas: extension along the optic nerve and its sheaths. *Arch Ophthalmol* 1978;96:440.

174. Spencer WH. Optic nerve extension of intraocular neoplasms. *Am J Ophthalmol* 1975;80:465.

175. Folberg R, Rummelt V, Parys-Van Ginderdeuren R, et al. The prognostic value of tumor blood vessel morphology in primary uveal melanoma. *Ophthalmology* 1993;100:1389.

176. Rummelt V, Folberg R, Rummelt C, et al. Microcirculation architecture of melanocytic nevi and malignant melanomas of the ciliary body and choroid: a comparative histopathologic and ultrastructural study. *Ophthalmology* 1994;101:718.

177. de la Cruz PO, Specht CS, McLean IW. Lymphocytic infiltration in uveal melanoma. *Cancer* 1990;65:112.

178. Whelchel JC, Farah SE, McLean IW, Burnier MN. Immunohistochemistry of infiltrating lymphocytes in uveal melanoma. *Invest Ophthalmol Vis Sci* 1993;34:2603.

179. Meecham WJ, Char DH. DNA content abnormalities and prognosis in uveal melanomas. *Arch Ophthalmol* 1986;104:1626.

180. Fuglestad SJ, Campbell RJ, Tsushima K, et al. Malignant melanoma of the choroid. Nuclear DNA ploidy pattern studied by flow cytometry. ARVO abstracts. *Invest Ophthalmol Vis Sci* 1987;28:59.

181. McLean IW, Gamel JW. Prediction of metastasis of uveal melanoma: comparison of morphometric determination of nuclear size and spectrophotometric determination of DNA. *Invest Ophthalmol Vis Sci* 1988;29:507.

182. Coleman K, Baak JPH, Dorman A, et al. Deoxyribonucleic acid ploidy studies in choroidal melanomas. *Am J Ophthalmol* 1993;115:376.

183. Cochran AJ, Holland GN, Wen D-R, et al. Detection of cytoplasmic S-100 protein in primary and metastatic intraocular melanomas. *Invest Ophthalmol Vis Sci* 1983;24:1153.

184. Steuhl K-P, Rohrbach JM, Knorr M, Thiel H-J. Significance, specificity, and ultrastructural localization of HMB-45 antigen in pigmented ocular tumors. *Ophthalmology* 1993;100:208.

185. Straatsma BR, Fine SL, Earle JD, et al. Enucleation versus plaque irradiation for choroidal melanoma. *Ophthalmology* 1988;95:1000.

186. Augsburger JJ, Vrabec TR. Impact of delayed treatment in growing posterior uveal melanomas. *Arch Ophthalmol* 1993;111:1382.

187. Butler P, Char DH, Zarbin M, Kroll S. Natural history of indeterminate pigmented choroidal tumors. *Ophthalmology* 1994;101:710.

188. Zimmerman LE, McLean IW. An evaluation of enucleation in the management of uveal melanomas. *Am J Ophthalmol* 1979;87:741.

189. Zimmerman LE, McLean IW. Metastatic disease from untreated uveal melanomas. *Am J Ophthalmol* 1979;88:524.

190. Stanford GR, Reese AB. Malignant cells in the blood of eye patients. *Trans Am Acad Ophthalmol Otolaryngol* 1971;75:102.

191. Fisher ER, Fisher B. Experimental studies of factors influencing hepatic metastases: I. The effect of number of tumor cells injected and time of growth. *Cancer* 1959;12:926.

192. Wilson RS, Fraunfelder FT. "No-touch" cryosurgical enucleation: a minimal trauma technique for eyes harboring intraocular malignancy. *Trans Am Acad Ophthalmol* 1978;85:1170.

193. Fraunfelder FT, Boozman FW, Wilson RS, Thomas AH. No-touch technique for intraocular malignant melanomas. *Arch Ophthalmol* 1977;95:161.

194. Niederkorn JY. Enucleation-induced metastasis of intraocular melanoma in mice. *Ophthalmology* 1984;91:692.

195. Seigel D, Myers M, Ferris F, Steinhorn SC. Survival rates after enucleation of eyes with malignant melanoma. *Am J Ophthalmol* 1979;87:761.

196. Manschot WA, van Peperzeel HA. Choroidal melanoma: enucleation or observation? A new approach. *Arch Ophthalmol* 1980;98:71.

197. Gass JDM. Comparison of uveal melanoma growth rates with mitotic index and mortality. *Arch Ophthalmol* 1985;103:924.

198. Zimmerman LE, McLean IW, Foster WD. The Manschot-van Peperzeel concept of the growth and metastasis of uveal melanomas. *Doc Ophthalmol* 1980;50:101.

199. Earle J, Kline RW, Robertson DM. Selection of iodine-125 for

the Collaborative Ocular Melanoma Study. *Arch Ophthalmol* 1987;105:763.

200. Foulds WS, Damato BE. Alternatives to enucleation in the management of choroidal melanoma. *Aust N Z J Ophthalmol* 1986;14:19.

201. Shields JA, Glazer LC, Mieler WF, et al. Comparison of xenon arc and argon laser photocoagulation in the treatment of choroidal melanomas. *Am J Ophthalmol* 1990;109:647.

202. Kersten RC, Tse D, Anderson RL, Blodi FL. Role of orbital exenteration in malignant melanoma with extrascleral extension. *Ophthalmology* 1983;90:63.

203. Mitchell MS, Liggett PE, Green RL, et al. Sustained regression of a primary choroidal melanoma under the influence of a therapeutic melanoma vaccine. *J Clin Oncol* 1994;12:396.

204. Frangieh GT, El Baba F, Traboulsi EI, Green WR. Melanocytoma of the ciliary body: presentation of four cases and review of nineteen reports. *Surv Ophthalmol* 1985;29:328.

205. Lee JS, Smith RE, Minckler DS. Scleral melanocytoma. *Ophthalmology* 1982;89:178.

206. Haas BD, Jakobiec FA, Iwamoto T, et al. Diffuse choroidal melanocytoma in a child: a lesion extending the spectrum of melanocytic hamartomas. *Ophthalmology* 1986;93:1632.

207. Reidy JJ, Apple DJ, Steinmetz RL, et al. Melanocytoma: nomenclature, pathogenesis, natural history and treatment. *Surv Ophthalmol* 1985;29:319.

208. Erzurum SA, Jampol LM, Territo C, O'Grady R. Primary malignant melanoma of the optic nerve simulating a melanocytoma. *Arch Ophthalmol* 1992;110:684.

209. Shields JA, Eagle RC, Shields CL, DePotter P. Pigmented adenoma of the optic nerve head simulating a melanocytoma. *Ophthalmology* 1992;11:1705.

210. Juarez CP, Tso MOM. An ultrastructural study of melanocytomas (magnocellular nevi) of the optic disk and uvea. *Am J Ophthalmol* 1980;90:48.

211. Zimmerman LE. Melanocytes, melanocytic nevi, and melanocytomas. *Invest Ophthalmol Vis Sci* 1965;4:11.

Ophthalmic Pathology with Clinical Correlations,
edited by Joseph W. Sassani, M.D.
Lippincott-Raven Publishers, Philadelphia © 1997.

CHAPTER 11

Pathology of the Retina

Marilyn C. Kincaid

The purpose of this chapter is to review the lesions of the retina. It is impossible in a short space to cover the myriad retinal diseases that have been described and documented over the years; instead, we will emphasize pathologic processes. To understand these properly, it is important to have a thorough understanding of normal retinal structure and its development.

ANATOMY AND EMBRYOLOGY

The retina is the area of the eye responsible for receiving light and for converting the patterns of light and shadow to neural impulses for interpretation by the cerebral cortex. It is a wonderfully complex and highly ordered structure.

Retinal anatomy is commonly thought of, or at least taught, as having ten layers. This has the advantage of providing a list, but simply memorizing ten layers by rote is not conducive to understanding retinal function. It is more logical to consider the retina first in terms of its development, and then in terms of the neural connections.

The retina is an extension or outpouching of the telencephalon, the part of the brain that ultimately becomes the cerebral cortex. Thus, the retina really belongs to the central nervous system. The neuroepithelial cells of the outpouching, the optic vesicle, are arranged as a sphere. The cells then invaginate, much as a balloon can be invaginated by a fist, to become the optic cup. This bilayer of neuroectodermal cells becomes the sensory retina and other epithelial structures lining the uveal tract within the eye (Fig. 11-1).[1] The inner layer develops into the iris pigment epithelium, the ciliary body nonpigmented epithelium, and the sensory retina. The outer layer becomes the iris dilator muscle, the ciliary body pigmented epithelium, and the retinal pigmented epithelium. (By convention, **outer** means toward the sclera and **inner** means

toward the center of the eye.) Reflecting their embryonal development, the cells of the two layers are arranged apex to apex, with the basement membranes at the bases of the cell layers.

The outer layer, the retinal pigment epithelium, remains a monolayer. Its basement membrane forms part of Bruch's membrane, a complex structure that also includes an inner collagenous layer, an elastic layer, an outer collagenous layer, and the basement membrane of the choriocapillaris of the choroid.

Pigmentation throughout the ocular **neuroectoderm** begins early in embryonic development and is completed by about the sixth week of gestation. Both round and lancet-shaped melanin granules are present. In contrast, the melanization of the uveal melanocytes, which are derived from cells of the **neural crest,** begins much later in fetal life and is not really complete until months to years after birth. This stromal melanization thus progresses along the same timetable, and to approximately the same degree, as pigmentation of the skin and hair.[2]

The microvillous processes of the retinal pigment epithelium surround the photoreceptor outer segments, which are shed and regenerated constantly at a rate dependent on incident light. The shed material is engulfed and digested by the retinal pigment epithelium. There are no structural junctions between the retinal pigment epithelial cells and the photoreceptors, in contrast to the tight junctions present between the two epithelial layers of the ciliary body and the iris. Instead, the retinal pigment epithelium constantly pumps fluid from the subretinal space, creating a net negative pressure to maintain photoreceptor apposition.[3]

The sensory retina is distinctive for its highly ordered architecture, as seen by light microscopy. Even at low power, three distinct bands of nuclei are readily evident (Fig. 11-2).

Photoreceptor cells are of two types, rods and cones. These names are derived from the shape of the inner

M. C. Kincaid: Departments of Ophthalmology and Pathology, St. Louis University Eye Institute, St. Louis University School of Medicine, St. Louis, Missouri 63104.

Supported in part by an unrestricted grant from Research to Prevent Blindness, Inc.

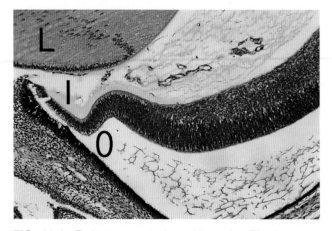

FIG. 11-1. Embryo eye at about 12 weeks. The two neuroectodermal layers, inner (*I*) and outer (*O*), are continuous at the pupillary margin (*M*). The lens (*L*) is in the upper left corner.

segments. Rods and cones are elongated cells whose nuclei make up the outer nuclear layer of the retina. Photoreceptors have specialized light-gathering ends, the outer segments, which consist of stacks of flat lipid-bilayer discs. The inner segments, which connect the discs to the cell body, are filled with mitochondria and other organelles of synthesis and transport.[4]

The photoreceptors synapse with the cells of the inner nuclear layer. The synapses take place in the outer plexiform layer, which lies between the outer and the inner nuclear layers.

The inner nuclear layer is made up of the cell bodies

of horizontal, bipolar, and amacrine cells. These cells are richly interconnected and in turn synapse with the ganglion cells in the inner plexiform layer.

The ganglion cell layer is the innermost layer of cell nuclei. These cells are relatively large, with abundant cytoplasm. In the peripheral retina, this layer is only a single cell layer thick. The anatomic macula is the area where the ganglion cell layer is two or more cells thick, and more centrally this layer can be seven or eight cells thick. The ganglion cells each send a single axon through the nerve fiber layer to the optic nerve. The next synapse takes place in the lateral geniculate body.

The innermost layer of the sensory retina is the internal limiting membrane, a true basement membrane secreted by the Müller cells. These elongated cells extend nearly the full retinal thickness, from the photoreceptor nuclei inward. They are support cells for the retina and may also have neural functions.

Macula

The pathologist and the clinician use the terms fovea and macula differently. The **anatomic macula** is the area where the ganglion cell layer is thicker than one nuclear layer (Fig. 11-3). This area is about 5 mm in diameter, roughly the area encircled by the superior and inferior temporal retinal vessels, corresponding approximately to the clinician's **posterior pole.** The anatomic boundary of the **fovea** is where the retina is thickest; it is about 1.5 mm in diameter, about the size of the optic disc, and includes the entire pit. The area of the anatomist's fovea thus corresponds to what the clinician refers to as the macula. The anatomic **foveola** is the floor of the pit, about 350 μm in diameter. It is thus slightly smaller than the

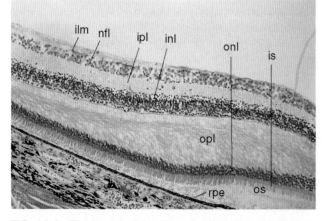

FIG. 11-2. The layers of the normal retina. The choriocapillaris (*cc*) lies just beneath the retinal pigment epithelium (*rpe*). The photoreceptor outer segments (*os*) and inner segments (*is*) have their nuclei in the outer nuclear layer (*onl*). Synapses occur in the outer plexiform layer (*opl*) between the photoreceptors and the cells of the inner nuclear layer (*inl*). In turn, they synapse in the inner plexiform layer (*ipl*) with the cells of the ganglion cell layer. Axons from the ganglion cell layer make up the nerve fiber layer (*nfl*). The internal limiting membrane (*ilm*) is a true basement membrane.

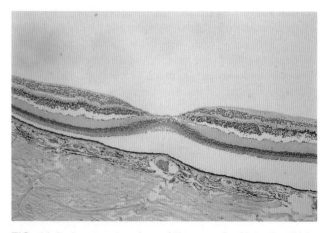

FIG. 11-3. Low-power view of the macula. Note the thickness of the ganglion cell layer close to the fovea. The inner nuclear layer and ganglion cell layer are discontinuous at the foveal pit. The detachment and the split in the sensory retina are artifact.

foveal avascular zone, which is about 500 μm in diameter.[5]

In the foveola, the only photoreceptors are cones, although they resemble long slender rods, thereby allowing greater packing. The only other cells present here are Müller cells because the remaining layers of the sensory retina, including retinal blood vessels, have been pushed aside. The cell processes extending from the cones in the foveola into the outer plexiform layer are therefore obliquely oriented, forming **Henle's fiber layer.** Fluids can more easily collect in this region of the outer plexiform layer because the obliquely oriented fibers are more readily displaced than the more vertically oriented fibers in the peripheral retina.

Retinal Periphery

The ora serrata is the junction between the sensory retina and the nonpigmented ciliary epithelium. Clinically, it appears scalloped, particularly nasally. The nonpigmented ciliary epithelium is attached to the pigmented ciliary epithelium by tight junctions between cells; thus, sensory retinal detachment does not progress anterior to the ora.

Lange's fold (Fig. 11-4) is a fixation artifact not present in the living eye.[6] It is an inward and anterior fold of the peripheral retina at the ora serrata, seen microscopically as well as grossly after fixation. It can be seen as late as age 20 years, but it is most common in infant eyes up to age 2 years. In the very young eye, the far peripheral sensory retina is not adherent to the underlying retinal pigment epithelium; this adhesion normally develops with age.[7]

Blood Supply

The retina receives a dual blood circulation. The inner half of the sensory retina, extending outward to include

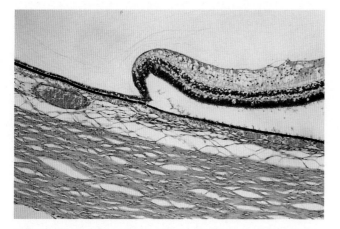

FIG. 11-4. Lange's fold is an inward folding of sensory retina at the ora serrata.

about half of the inner nuclear layer, is supplied directly by the retinal vasculature. The retinal vessels, like those of the brain, are end vessels and do not normally anastomose. Also like those of the brain, the retinal capillaries are impermeable to relatively small molecules such as fluorescein.

Vascularization of the retina begins during the 16th week of gestation at the optic nerve head[8] and normally reaches the ora serrata nasally at the time of birth. It is not quite complete temporally at term, because the distance from the optic nerve head to the ora is greater.

The large arterioles and venules of the retinal circulation travel in the nerve fiber layer and ganglion cell layer. The capillaries extend outward to the inner nuclear layer. Close to the foveal avascular zone, the capillaries form a single layer, but elsewhere the capillaries are present in two or more distinct layers.[9]

The terms artery and vein are used clinically and histologically to designate the **central retinal blood vessels** and their diseases, although the respective blood vessels remain arteries and veins for only a short distance from the optic disc, peripherally becoming arterioles and venules.

The outer half of the sensory retina and the retinal pigment epithelium are nourished through diffusion from the choroidal circulation. The choroid is the most posterior portion of the uveal tract, which also includes the iris and ciliary body. The choroid is composed of fibrocytes, uveal melanocytes, and a rich supply of anastomosing blood vessels. The largest vessels are outermost, and the choriocapillaris is the innermost layer, adjacent to Bruch's membrane. The capillaries of the choriocapillaris are the largest in the body, about 20 μm in diameter. In the posterior pole, the capillaries are arranged in a lobular pattern, with a feeding arteriole in the center of each lobule and several venules peripherally.[10]

The two circulations do not overlap, in part because there are two barriers, referred to as blood–retinal barriers.[11] The intact retinal pigment epithelium blocks the inward migration of substances from the choriocapillaris into the subretinal space. The specific blockage sites are the junctions binding each retinal pigment epithelial cell to adjacent cells. Anatomically, these junctions include a zonula adherens and adjacent zonula occludens, both situated near the apex of the cell and encircling it.[3] This blockade constitutes the outer blood–retinal barrier.[11]

The inner blood–retinal barrier is the retinal vascular endothelium, including the capillary endothelium. The site of the barrier is the specialized tight junctions (zonulae occludentes) between individual endothelial cells. Thus, the permeability of these capillaries is similar to those of the brain, and different from that elsewhere in the body.[11]

CONGENITAL LESIONS

The congenital retinal and pigment epithelial lesions discussed here include abnormalities of development.

Albinism

Albinism includes a group of disorders, variably inherited, in which there is hypopigmentation. The eye and the skin, or the eye alone, can be involved. These disorders have in common poor vision and nystagmus, although the degree of dysfunction varies, even within a single pedigree.[12] On clinical examination, no macular reflex is present and the retinal vessels may enter the normally avascular area.[2]

Histologically, the ganglion cell layer thickens properly in the macular area, but no foveal pit is identified, even with careful serial sectioning.[2] In the most severe forms, no melanin is seen in either the neuroectoderm (pigment epithelial layers) or the uveal stroma. However, the neuroectoderm must be melanized for normal induction of the foveal pit during embryonic development.

The most severe form of oculocutaneous albinism is tyrosinase-negative albinism, inherited as an autosomal recessive trait. These patients have no tyrosinase, an enzyme required for the first step in melanin formation. The skin is very fair, the hair is pale blond, and the irises are gray, with diffuse transillumination defects. Hair bulbs obtained from these patients show no melanosomes.[13]

Other types of albinism are less severe; patients have minimal pigmentation but the appearance can be variable, even in the same kindred.[14] These patients have tyrosinase activity but show other defects in the synthesis or storage of melanin.

Chédiak-Higashi syndrome and Hermansky-Pudlak syndrome are two special types of albinism that show other systemic abnormalities that can be life-threatening. **Chédiak-Higashi syndrome** is inherited as an autosomal recessive trait. In addition to the albinism, the neutrophils cannot lyse ingested bacteria, making these children vulnerable to infection. The cells of the uveal stroma and the pigmented epithelium contain macromelanosomes, some larger than the cell nucleus. The disturbance thus appears to be one of packaging of melanosomes.[15] **Hermansky-Pudlak syndrome** includes albinism and a hemorrhagic disorder.[14] Thus, for both syndromes, the ophthalmologist may be in a position to make the initial diagnosis of a life-threatening disorder and arrange appropriate referral.

Ocular albinism is characterized by a more nearly normal degree of cutaneous pigmentation. The neuroepithelium is involved, but the melanocytes of the neural crest are relatively spared. The classic type of ocular albinism is Nettleship-Falls, inherited as a sex-linked recessive trait. Histologically, both the epidermis and ocular pigment epithelium contain macromelanosomes, huge round melanosomes that may be larger than the cell nucleus. Female carriers can have characteristic pigmentary changes in the fundus as well as macromelanosomes, but they are asymptomatic.[16] Other types are inherited differently and may not have macromelanosomes.

Albinoidism is a reduction in the number of melanosomes of the neural crest–derived tissues. The pigment epithelium, derived from neuroectoderm, is more nearly normal, so that patients have a normal fovea, good vision, and no nystagmus;[13] however, there may be iris transillumination defects.[17]

Pigment Epithelial Hypertrophy

The sensory retina is transparent, so that color seen through it clinically is that of the retinal pigment epithelium and choroid. With hypertrophy, the retinal pigment epithelium is focally darker in color, visible ophthalmoscopically as a dark gray-black flat area. The retinal pigment epithelial cells are increased in number, are larger, and contain more pigment granules than normal. The additional granules are large and spherical. Hyperpigmentation may occur either as a solitary lesion or in a grouped pattern. Sometimes the distribution of the cells resembles the footprints of an animal, hence the term "bear tracks." Lacunae of depigmentation may occur focally or diffusely. These conditions are benign and stationary;[18] however, these lesions can be part of two important syndromes.

Gardner syndrome is a form of hereditary gastrointestinal polyposis with nongastrointestinal manifestations that include benign soft-tissue tumors, osteomas, and bilateral congenital retinal pigment epithelial hypertrophy.[19] The other disorder, **Turcot syndrome,** includes adenomatous polyps of the colon, hypertrophic pigment epithelium, and epithelial tumors of the central nervous system. All these findings may be part of a spectrum.[20] Because the gastrointestinal polyps are adenomatous, they have malignant potential, so ophthalmic examination is potentially lifesaving if it assists in the diagnosis of these syndromes.[21]

Coloboma

During embryonic life, the hyaloid vessels enter the eye inferonasally through the **fetal fissure,** which extends from the optic nerve posteriorly to the iris anteriorly. These vessels nourish the developing lens. Later, the vessels regress and the fissure closes. Normally, closure of the fetal fissure occurs so perfectly that no defect of retina, choroid, or sclera is identifiable clinically or histologically. Rarely, the fissure closes incompletely, resulting in a **coloboma,** which can vary from a tiny, clinically insignificant defect to complete failure of fissure closure, leading to **microphthalmos with cyst.**[22]

The defects resemble bare sclera ophthalmoscopically, but histologically there are a thin glial lining and remnants of the retinal vasculature. The retina also may contain dysplastic rosettes (see the following section on retinal dysplasia), especially at the margins of the coloboma. The pigment epithelium and the choriocapillaris also are absent in the colobomatous defect, and there is an absolute scotoma. Colobomas are bilateral in 60% of patients; they can be an isolated finding or part of a syndrome such as trisomy 13.[22]

Retinal Dysplasia

Retinal dysplasia is an abnormality in the formation of the retina: instead of the normal linear arrangement of the layers of nuclei, the cells form rosettes with varying degrees of differentiation, involving one, two, or all three nuclear layers. Here the term dysplasia implies a malformation, not a premalignant condition. Clinically, the involved areas appear translucent and grayish, rather than transparent. Retinal dysplasia can be a solitary abnormality or associated with various other ocular malformations; it also can be focal or diffuse.

Myelinated Nerve Fibers

The optic nerve fibers normally acquire myelin sheaths just posterior to the lamina cribrosa on their way to the brain, but occasionally some nerve fibers are myelinated in the retina. They appear whitish with feathery margins and follow the orientation of the nerve fiber layer. **Myelinated nerve fibers** are typically congenital lesions, although they can progress slowly.[23] Patients with extensive myelination also may have myopia, amblyopia, and strabismus. The degree of visual field defect varies but usually is surprisingly minimal. The lesion generally extends into the retina from the disc margin, but it can be located anywhere in the retina. Because myelination is never continuous across the lamina cribrosa, there is always some discontinuity in the myelin sheath, even with myelinated fibers that do extend to the disc.[24]

The oligodendroglial cells are believed to be responsible for myelination; they normally populate the optic nerve but not the retina. Rarely, myelinated nerve fibers may be acquired.[25] Demyelination of the myelinated fibers has occurred in multiple sclerosis and other demyelinating diseases.

VASCULAR DISEASE

Of all the blood vessels of the body, the retinal vessels are unique in that they can be observed in their natural state through the ophthalmoscope. The lesions produced by vascular pathology can likewise be observed and pho-tographed. Fluorescein angiography adds a dynamic aspect to the investigation of vascular pathology and physiology.

Many systemic vascular diseases involve the vessels of the retina, so the status of these observable vessels may reflect that of the circulation elsewhere. No retinal vascular lesions are unique to a specific disease; instead, the overall pattern and distribution of the lesions and the patient's history of systemic disease favor one diagnosis over another.

Hemorrhages

Extravasated blood settles according to the local retinal architecture. Therefore, **hemorrhages** can be described as flame-shaped when they are located in the nerve fiber layer and ''dot-blot'' when they are found in deeper layers (Fig. 11-5).

Many blood dyscrasias and retinal diseases can cause retinal hemorrhages, and they may be the predominant lesion. In leukemia, for example, the decreased platelet count and anemia together are believed to be responsible for the hemorrhages.[26] Increased blood viscosity, typical of polycythemia and macroglobulinemia, also causes a fundus picture primarily of hemorrhages.[27] Disseminated intravascular coagulation is another cause of a predominantly hemorrhagic fundus picture.[28] The intraretinal hemorrhages of sickle-cell retinopathy are peripheral and undergo a distinctive resolution.[29]

Aneurysms

Microaneurysms are focal outpouchings of the retinal capillaries. Clinically, they appear as small red dots, usually smaller than dot-blot hemorrhages. They are an initial

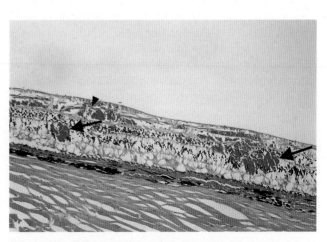

FIG. 11-5. Retinal blood, here appearing black, can be at any level. Superficial hemorrhages in the nerve fiber layer (*arrowhead*) appear flame-shaped; deeper hemorrhages appear as dots or blots (*arrows*).

sign of diabetic retinopathy[30] and are seen in many other diseases as well. They represent damage to the capillary wall with breakdown of the blood–retinal barrier, and thus they tend to leak fluid into the surrounding retina, as demonstrated by fluorescein angiography. Histologically, there is loss of endothelial cells and pericytes, with a focal saccular or fusiform distention of the wall.[31,32]

Larger vessels also can develop aneurysmal dilatation.[33] Arterial macroaneurysms typically occur in patients with hypertension or other vascular disease.[34] The affected vessel is focally dilated and may leak or bleed. The hemorrhage takes on a dumbbell configuration, with blood both beneath the retina and just beneath the internal limiting membrane. This blood may break through the internal limiting membrane, resulting in vitreous hemorrhage. Eyes examined histologically after hemorrhage show clot formation in the aneurysm.[35]

Exudates

Exudates are another consequence of the breakdown of the blood–retinal barrier. They occur when the capillaries leak proteins and lipids into the surrounding retina, seen clinically as yellow, shiny material. Sometimes these occur in a circular, or circinate, pattern surrounding a leakage site such as a microaneurysm. If the leaking microaneurysm is occluded by photocoagulation, the exudates may gradually resorb.[36] Histologically, exudates appear as amorphous collections of eosinophilic material found predominantly in the outer plexiform layer. The anatomy of the outer plexiform retinal layer in the macular region can cause exudates to take on a "macular star" configuration.

Cystoid Macular Edema

Cystoid macular edema is the result of many different diseases and conditions that lead to diffuse abnormal permeability of retinal capillaries. In fully developed cystoid edema, tiny cysts arranged like the petals of a flower are present around the foveola. Fluorescein angiography demonstrates diffuse capillary leakage with pooling into the cystoid spaces. The pathology is incompletely understood, in part because few cases come to enucleation. Clinical causes are diverse and include vascular disease (such as diabetes, central vein occlusion, and phlebitis), intraocular surgery (such as cataract surgery),[37] intraocular tumors, trauma, and accelerated hypertension.[38]

The cystoid spaces usually are found in Henle's fiber layer (Fig. 11-6). In the foveal region, these fibers of the outer plexiform layer are slanted and allow fluid to collect between them; however, the cystoid spaces also can form in the outer nuclear, inner nuclear, inner plexiform, and even the ganglion cell layer. The specific layers involved may depend on the disease.[38]

The cystoid spaces can be intracellular or extracellular.

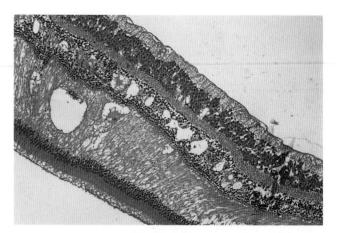

FIG. 11-6. Macular cystoid spaces can occur in the outer plexiform layer and inner nuclear layer.

In one study, the fluid was found within damaged Müller cells, and extracellular fluid was a late change.[39,40] Another study demonstrated extracellular fluid within intact cells.[41] Trypsin digestion of perifoveal vessels shows foci of capillary endothelial proliferation, similar to the microvascular abnormalities seen in diabetic retinal disease. These appear to be the leakage sites.[42]

Ischemia

The retina, like any other tissue, becomes ischemic from lack of blood supply. Either the retinal or the choroidal circulation, or both, can be involved. There is essentially no overlap of the two blood supplies, as demonstrated by the clinical and histologic findings after occlusion.

Choroidal vascular insufficiency affects the outer retinal layers. It is relatively rare posteriorly, but peripherally, outer retinal ischemia is extremely common, recognized clinically as cobblestone or paving-stone degeneration. These lesions appear as well-demarcated round pale areas because of the lack of retinal pigment epithelial cells and their pigment.[43] They increase in frequency with age and are also found more often in axial myopia. Histologically, the retinal pigment epithelium and the outer half of the sensory retina are obliterated, so that the thinned inner nuclear layer is directly adherent to Bruch's membrane (Fig. 11-7). The larger Elschnig spots are histologically identical.[44]

Occlusion of the central retinal artery or its branches results in ischemic infarction of the inner retinal layers. These occlusions are usually embolic. **Emboli** most commonly consist of calcific fragments, platelet aggregates, and cholesterol crystals,[45] although many other materials, including amniotic fluid, bacteria, air, and talc, used by intravenous drug abusers, also can embolize to the eye.[46] Cholesterol emboli often are found in patients with ulcerated atheromatous plaques of the carotid arteries, although

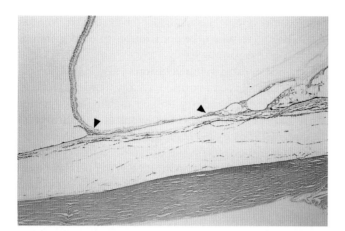

FIG. 11-7. Cobblestone degeneration involves the choriocapillaris, pigment epithelium, and outer retina. The boundaries are abrupt (*arrowheads*). The retinal detachment, to the right, is artifact, but it shows that a true retinal detachment would also probably not extend more anteriorly because of the chorioretinal adhesion.

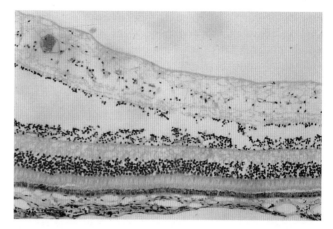

FIG. 11-8. The inner retinal layers are edematous in acute central retinal artery occlusion; this edema partially involves the inner nuclear layer. Outer layers are intact. The splitting is an artifact.

these emboli tend to be nonocclusive because of the flat shape of the cholesterol crystals. Clinically, cholesterol emboli appear as bright, shiny yellow particles within the vessels and are called Hollenhorst plaques.[47] Calcific emboli appear more grayish, and platelet emboli are also grayish-white.[48]

Nonembolic causes of infarction include atherosclerosis and inflammatory processes of the arterial or capillary walls that narrow and occlude the lumen, such as **cranial (temporal) arteritis**[49] or retinitis of various causes.[50]

Branch or central artery occlusion typically occurs suddenly. The inner layers of the normally transparent retina swell, becoming translucent and grayish with loss of underlying detail. This edema begins within a few hours after occlusion and peaks in 24 hours. Visual acuity is profoundly depressed or completely lost. Because there are no inner retinal layers in the foveal pit, the fovea remains transparent. The normally perfused choroid and pigment epithelium remain visible, giving rise to the clinically observed **cherry-red spot.**

Histologically, acute swelling of the inner retinal layers extends from the nerve fiber layer outward to include part of the inner nuclear layer. The outer layers, including the retinal pigment epithelium, remain intact (Fig. 11-8).[51] Ultimately, the inner layers are lost, and the retinal vessels become somewhat hyalinized. Because these occlusions are abrupt and complete, there is no reactive gliosis. Histologically, the inner layers are thinned and homogenized, and the outer layers, including part of the inner nuclear layer, remain intact. In contrast, with atrophy of the optic nerve, including glaucomatous atrophy, only the ganglion cell and nerve fiber layers are lost.

Branch arteriolar occlusion is similar in appearance and clinical course. The involved area is sharply demarcated from adjacent normally perfused areas.

Retinal capillary closure results in very localized ischemia and infarction of inner retinal layers, seen clinically as "cotton-wool spots," in which focal swelling causes loss of transparency, so the retina appears white with feathery margins. **Cotton-wool spots** are common in a number of diseases, including diabetes mellitus, lupus, leukemia, and other blood dyscrasias.[52] Histologically, cotton-wool spots are swollen axons in the nerve fiber layer (Fig. 11-9). These fusiform swellings have been called cytoid bodies because the eosinophilic central density superficially resembles a cell nucleus.[53] Ultrastructurally, these fusiform densities consist of accumulated metabolic cell products where antegrade and retrograde axoplasmic flow has ceased.[54] Other causes of axoplasmic flow interruption not caused by ischemia produce the same clinical and histologic picture.

Cotton-wool spots are transient because the edema is an acute change. After resolution of the edema, capillary

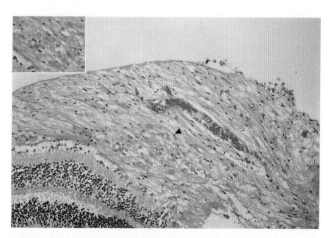

FIG. 11-9. Cytoid bodies are rounded areas (*arrowhead* and *inset*) seen histologically in cotton-wool spots. They represent focal axoplasmic swellings.

nonperfusion is recognized by focal or diffuse nonperfusion on fluorescein angiography. Many diseases in addition to diabetes cause capillary dropout, including retinal vasculitis[55] and sickle-cell retinopathy.[56,57]

Panocular Vascular Insufficiency

Panocular vascular insufficiency, or hypotensive retinopathy, results from inadequate perfusion from any cause. In turn, this decreased perfusion involves both the retinal and the choroidal circulations, and thus is devastating to all intraocular structures. Symptoms include amaurosis fugax and ocular pain.[43]

Atherosclerosis of the carotid artery is the most common cause of diffuse circulatory compromise,[43] but there are others. Takayasu disease is a rare granulomatous occlusive disease of the major arteries, occurring most frequently in young Japanese women. The corresponding Takayasu syndrome refers to any process, such as syphilis, affecting the aortic arch with resulting circulatory compromise.

As would be expected with involvement of both retinal circulations, all retinal layers are affected. Cobblestone degeneration may extend posteriorly, even past the equator, indicating diffuse outer retinal ischemic atrophy from choroidal insufficiency. There is also inner retinal ischemic atrophy from decreased retinal perfusion. Optic nerve head neovascularization has been reported. Anterior segment changes include iris neovascularization, iris necrosis, and cataract.[43]

Retinal Vein Occlusion

Retinal vein occlusion involves the same inner retinal layers as retinal arterial occlusion but appears quite different because of the resulting venous congestion. Variable intraretinal hemorrhage occurs at all levels of the sensory retina. Retinal vein occlusion is usually thrombotic, with the thrombus at the level of the lamina cribrosa in central vein occlusion or at an arterial-venous crossing in branch vein occlusion.

Central retinal vein occlusion can be divided into two types, ischemic and nonischemic.[58] **Nonischemic central vein occlusion** is characterized by a variable number of flame-shaped and dot and blot hemorrhages but few or no cotton-wool spots. There is disc swelling with venous dilatation and tortuosity. As documented by fluorescein angiography, capillary perfusion is nearly normal; thus, the sequelae of ischemia, including iris neovascularization and neovascular glaucoma, are rare in the nonischemic type. The visual prognosis is good. Late sequelae include perivenous sheathing and dilated veins at the optic nerve head.[59] Nonischemic vein occlusion may progress to ischemic occlusion, but this is unusual, especially in younger patients. In younger patients, particularly men, nonisch-

emic central vein occlusion tends to be caused by venous phlebitis, and it runs a benign course. In older persons, arteriosclerosis is most likely.[58]

Ischemic central vein occlusion is also called hemorrhagic vein occlusion because typically there is extensive retinal hemorrhage, called a "blood and thunder" fundus. There may be numerous cotton-wool spots, but even if they are obscured by the hemorrhage, fluorescein angiography helps to document the extensive capillary closure and ischemia. Iris neovascularization is frequently associated and characteristically occurs between 6 weeks and 6 months (so-called "90-day glaucoma").[59]

With either type of vein occlusion, hemorrhage in the macula can result in permanent visual loss. For obscure reasons, primary open angle glaucoma is associated with central vein occlusion in 8% to 20% of patients, either before or after the occlusion.[60]

Histologically, central vein occlusion appears acutely as hemorrhagic necrosis with massive hemorrhage extending outward to involve all layers of the retina. The hemorrhage may also extend under the internal limiting membrane, separating it from the underlying nerve fiber layer. Cytoid bodies and optic nerve head edema may be present.

Histologic examination later in the evolution of the occlusion may show exudates in the outer plexiform layer, along with gliosis. Hemosiderosis of the retina is due to the breakdown of the extravasated blood. Both arterial and venous blood vessel walls can be markedly thickened and altered (Fig. 11-10). The thrombus is organized and may be recanalized.[60]

The histology of branch vein occlusion is similar.[61] Nearly all branch vein occlusions occur when the artery crosses *over* the vein, rather than under the vein, as viewed ophthalmoscopically.[62]

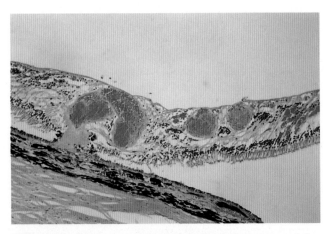

FIG. 11-10. There is considerable retinal alteration and disruption in chronic central vein occlusion, extending outward to involve outer retinal layers. The vascular walls are thickened.

Hypertensive and Arteriosclerotic Retinopathy

Arteriolar sclerosis and hypertension usually occur together, but they are in fact separate phenomena. They are graded separately from I through IV.[63]

Hypertension causes thickening of the arterioles so that the blood column, which is all that is visible ophthalmoscopically, appears narrower than normal in grade I. Grade II includes increased narrowing and focal spasms of the arterioles. Grade III adds hemorrhages at any level of the retina, cotton-wool spots, and hard exudates that may form a macular star clinically. In grade IV, all these changes are seen, along with papilledema.

The choroidal vasculature also can be involved in malignant hypertension. The retinal pigment epithelium can proliferate in a patchy pattern. **Elschnig spots** are areas of choriocapillaris occlusion and are thus similar to cobblestone degeneration except for their larger size and more posterior location.[44] **Siegrist lines**—increased pigmentation along a sclerotic choroidal vessel—are uncommon.[64]

Arteriolar sclerotic changes are also graded from I to IV. Grade I consists of subintimal hyalin deposition and thickening of the vascular wall, seen clinically as an increased light reflex. Grade II adds arteriolar-venular crossing defects. The arterioles and venules normally share a common adventitial sheath where they cross.[62] With thickening and increased rigidity of the arteriolar wall, the venular wall is compressed. Clinically, this appears as a gap in the course of the venule where the arteriole crosses it. Grades III and IV include the above changes and also increased thickening of the arteriole, so that the blood column is narrowed. The increased light reflex gives a coppery appearance to the vessel, called "copper-wire" change in grade III and "silver-wire" change in grade IV. The vessel may nonetheless remain patent to fluorescein angiography.[44,63]

Neovascularization

Over time, areas of the retina observed to be nonperfused may later be a site of **neovascularization.** New vessels may form on the optic nerve head or anywhere else in the retina; the distribution is characteristic for a given disease. For example, neovascularization in sickle-cell anemia is typically anterior to the equator;[57] in diabetic retinopathy, new vessels occur in the posterior pole.[65] Clinically, these vessels overlie the retina and appear fine, delicate, and irregular. They leak fluorescein, and with time increasing fibrous ingrowth tends to accompany them.

Histologically, the vessels are anterior to the internal limiting membrane and usually occupy the space between it and the formed vitreous. The individual vessels are lined with endothelium.[66] Angiogenesis appears to be a complex regulatory process initiated by viable but ischemic tissue.[67]

INFLAMMATION

Inflammation and infection can occur primarily as a retinitis or, alternatively, the retina may be involved secondarily by an inflammatory process occurring primarily elsewhere in the eye, such as a keratitis, uveitis, or scleritis. Inflammation is discussed in Chapter 3.

DEGENERATIONS

Peripheral Microcystoid Degeneration

Peripheral microcystoid degeneration occurs in two forms, typical and reticular (Fig. 11-11). **Typical peripheral microcystoid degeneration** is virtually universal in all eyes except those of young children. It increases in area with age, beginning at the ora serrata and extending circumferentially and posteriorly. Clinically and grossly, typical peripheral microcystoid degeneration appears as a grayish translucent area with myriad tiny interconnecting channels. It is generally more extensive temporally and tends to be symmetric between the two eyes.[68]

Histologically, the cystoid spaces occur at the level of the outer plexiform and inner nuclear layers of the retina. With time, the spaces may spread vertically to involve retinal layers above and below. The cysts contain a hyaluronidase-sensitive acid mucopolysaccharide.

Reticular cystoid degeneration is much less common. It is seen posterior to typical cystoid degeneration. Because these cystoid spaces are closer to the inner retinal

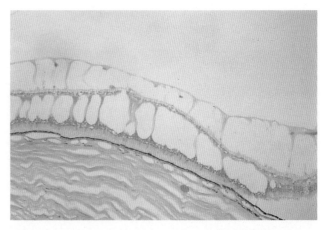

FIG. 11-11. Typical and reticular cystoid degeneration can coexist. Typical peripheral cystoid degeneration is more anterior and closer to the ora serrata and involves the outer plexiform layer. Reticular peripheral cystoid degeneration principally involves the ganglion cell layer and nerve fiber layer.

surface, the vasculature, including the capillaries, appears prominent. The borders of the lesion tend to follow the larger vessels, in contrast to the rounded borders of typical cystoid degeneration. The inner portion of the reticular cystoid spaces is less transparent, giving the clinical appearance of beaten metal.

Reticular cystoid degeneration is found in about 13% of eyes and is bilateral in 46% of those. There is no clear relation with aging. Histologically, the cystoid spaces are at the level of the nerve fiber layer. Thus, the inner aspect of reticular cystoid degeneration is quite thin, including only nerve fiber layer remnants, retinal vessels, and internal limiting membrane.[68]

Retinoschisis

Retinoschisis is a splitting of the layers of the sensory retina. Arbitrarily, cystoid degeneration is called schisis when the spaces measure more than 1.5 mm linearly.[68] Typical degenerative schisis forms from typical cystoid degeneration, involving the same retinal layers. It tends to be clinically benign without increasing in area. Schisis results in an absolute scotoma, in contrast to retinal detachment, which shows a relative scotoma.

Reticular schisis forms from reticular degeneration. With time, the inner layer consists of only the internal limiting membrane and retinal vessels. This inner layer may form a large bullous separation. This type of schisis is significant both because of the propensity to extend posteriorly, and because both inner and outer layers may develop holes (Fig. 11-12).[68] **Juvenile X-linked retinoschisis,** which typically involves the inferotemporal quadrant and the macula, involves the same retinal layers.[69]

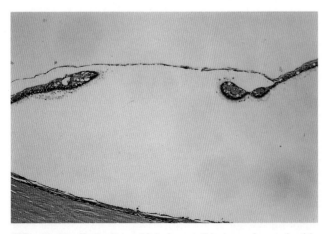

FIG. 11-12. Reticular schisis has a thin inner layer. In this figure, there is a hole in the outer layer of the schisis, with rounded margins.

Degenerations of the Photoreceptor-Pigment Epithelial Unit

Regardless of the underlying disease, neovascularization of the retinal vasculature is a consequence of retinal ischemia.[67] The stimulus for subretinal neovascularization, originating from choroidal vessels, is much less well understood. A variety of diseases and degenerations, most notably age-related macular degeneration, can be associated with subretinal neovascularization.

Age-Related Macular Degeneration

Age-related macular degeneration is one of the leading causes of legal blindness among older adults. Despite its name, age-related macular degeneration and associated visual loss are by no means inevitable; many older people retain excellent vision. However, even in these persons, some age-associated changes typically occur in the photoreceptors, retinal pigment epithelium, and Bruch's membrane. The cause of age-related macular degeneration is obscure and probably multifactorial. In addition to age itself, light toxicity probably plays a role,[70] and cataract may be partially protective.[71] Increased vascular resistance has been suggested.[72] Black persons appear to have less risk, especially for the exudative complications.[73]

Over a person's lifetime, there is considerable stress on the ability of the retinal pigment epithelium to digest the volume of material accumulated from the constantly shed photoreceptor outer segments. As it does in all tissue, lipofuscin, an indigestible end result of cytoplasmic catabolism, accumulates in the retinal pigment epithelium with increasing age.[74] The lipid-rich outer segments are the major source of lipofuscin, an autofluorescent pigment formed from peroxidized lipids. With increasing age, the amount of intracellular lipofuscin increases and the melanosomes reciprocally decrease in number.[74,75] After age 90, virtually no intact melanosomes remain, the remaining melanin being either combined with lipofuscin to form melanolipofuscin, or found within lysosomes.[71]

Bruch's membrane gradually thickens with age, especially posteriorly, although the degree of thickening varies greatly from person to person.[71] Bruch's membrane also becomes somewhat more disorganized, so that the individual layers are more difficult to discern.[76] The retinal pigment epithelium seems to be the source of the changes. Transport of metabolic end products from the retinal pigment epithelium to the choriocapillaris may be slowed by changes in the outer layers of Bruch's membrane, leading to drusen formation.[77] The macula tends to have more severe changes than the periphery; this may relate in part to the effect of focused light.[71]

Histologically, there is increased basophilia of Bruch's membrane, indicating both calcification and a progressive increase in lipid deposition.[77] With increased age, wide-banded collagen is also deposited in Bruch's membrane, not only between the retinal pigment epithelium and its basement membrane but also in the two collagenous zones of Bruch's membrane and between the outer collagenous zone and the basement membrane of the endothelium of the choriocapillaris. Wide-banded collagen deposition may be considered a nonspecific aging change.[78]

With age, foveal cones may become less numerous, but this is not inevitable. Photoreceptor cell nuclei are sometimes seen histologically at the level of the inner segments, evidently migrating outward from the outer nuclear layer.[71]

Drusen

Drusen are the initial clinical findings in age-related macular degeneration. Typical hard, or hyaline, drusen contain complex lipids, undigestible end products of outer segment digestion by the retinal pigment epithelium. By themselves, they do not cause visual loss, and many persons with drusen never show other changes of macular degeneration;[79] however, statistically they are a risk factor for other changes of macular degeneration and visual loss.[80]

The retinal pigment epithelium is intact but thinned overlying the drusen, so they may appear as window defects on fluorescein angiography, showing early hyperfluorescence and staining but no leakage. Some drusen are too small to be seen clinically but are found only by scanning electron microscopy.[81]

Histologically, **hard drusen** are dense, rounded, homogeneous bodies beneath the basement membrane of the retinal pigment epithelium (Fig. 11-13). They have a uniform consistency and contain lipid. Ultrastructurally, they contain finely granular material, vesicles, and sometimes wide-banded collagen.[82] Peripheral drusen, found in the equatorial region, appear similar clinically and histologically.[83,84]

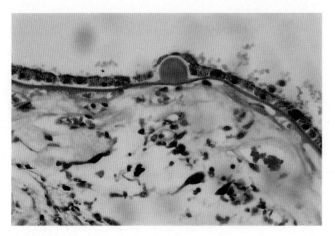

FIG. 11-13. A typical hard druse is rounded and shows thinning of the overlying pigment epithelium.

There are several theories concerning the formation of hard drusen. They may represent focal metabolic abnormalities of the retinal pigment epithelium. A process called apoptosis may explain their formation.[85] Apoptosis is a type of programmed cell death, and it occurs throughout the body as part of both physiologic and pathologic processes. Examples include the regression of glands of lactation in the breast after the baby is weaned, and normal regression of temporary structures during embryogenesis. Photoreceptors degenerate by apoptosis after a variety of injuries.[86]

In contrast to hard drusen, **soft drusen** have less well-defined boundaries clinically; histologically, they are identical to small retinal pigment epithelial detachments.[87] The involved area is larger and more irregular than that of a hard druse, and the material appears somewhat granular and less uniform. Eyes with soft or confluent drusen are more likely to develop visual loss.[76] Ultrastructurally, soft drusen consist of vesicles, membranous debris, and wide-spaced collagen and are associated with diffuse deposits of material beneath the pigment epithelium called basal laminar deposits.[88] The thickening appears to weaken Bruch's membrane, predisposing it to splitting and hence to the sequelae of age-related macular degeneration, including retinal pigment epithelial detachment, neovascularization, and scarring.[89]

With time, the retinal pigment epithelial cells overlying drusen atrophy, and the drusen become fibrotic and sometimes calcify.[79] These calcified drusen probably correspond to what are seen clinically as small, hard, glistening deposits.[87]

Window Defects

Window defects take their name from the abnormality seen on fluorescein angiography. These defects transmit fluorescein during choroidal filling and fade as the choroidal fluorescence fades. They do not change size or shape during the angiogram, nor do they stain late. These characteristics imply an intact retinal pigment epithelium with intercellular junctions in place but with thinning and loss of pigment. There can be loss of overlying photoreceptor cells as well.[90]

Window defects exist in many conditions and can also be an isolated angiographic finding. In age-related macular degeneration, they may correspond to the thinned pigment epithelium over the apex of hard drusen,[91] and they can be a precursor to areolar atrophy.[90]

Areolar Atrophy

Areolar atrophy is the so-called "dry" type of macular degeneration. Clinically, the involved areas are pale and well demarcated and allow an enhanced view of the underlying larger choroidal vessels. These areas transmit fluorescein brightly because the retinal pigment epithelium is lost. Histologically, these areas show loss of the photoreceptors and the retinal pigment epithelium, with adhesion of the outer plexiform layer against Bruch's membrane. Thus, areolar atrophy represents loss of the retinal pigment epithelium-photoreceptor complex. Pre-existing drusen can also disappear in the areas of areolar atrophy.[91]

Most investigators agree that this type of atrophy is distinct from outer ischemic atrophy. The missing layers in outer ischemic atrophy are those normally supplied by the choroidal circulation. In contrast, in areolar atrophy, the inner nuclear layer and the outer plexiform layer remain intact, and the latter is adjacent to Bruch's membrane.[82] Choriocapillaris degeneration occurs to a variable degree in areolar atrophy,[92] and often the choriocapillaris is not lost.[87] The normal hexagonal lobular pattern of the choroidal circulation tends to be replaced by a tubular vascular pattern.[76]

The ''wet'' complications can occur along with areolar atrophy, in the same patient and even in the same eye. In a postmortem study, one third of all patients who had choroidal neovascularization also had areolar atrophy.[91]

Serous Retinal Pigment Epithelial Detachment

If soft drusen enlarge and coalesce, they form what clinically appears to be a **serous detachment of the retinal pigment epithelium** but what is actually a separation between the split layers of Bruch's membrane. This detachment represents a further step in the progressive weakening of Bruch's membrane, and such an eye is at high risk for choroidal neovascularization.[82]

The detached inner aspect of Bruch's membrane is also weakened by the degenerative process. In some cases, it ruptures, appearing clinically and histologically as a rip or tear in the retinal pigment epithelium. Clinically, one also may see a linear rolled edge of retinal pigment epithelium adjacent to a pale area of retina. On fluorescein angiography, the rolled edge of retinal pigment epithelium is hypofluorescent, the denuded area hyperfluorescent.[93] Histologically, the tear involves both the retinal pigment epithelium and the inner aspect of Bruch's membrane, with margins that are scrolled and folded.[94]

Subretinal Neovascularization and Disciform Scarring

Other diseases besides age-related macular degeneration can lead to the subretinal fibrovascular plaque known as a disciform scar; thus, it appears to be a final common pathway. The recognizable difference in age-related macular degeneration seems to be the deposits on the inner aspect of Bruch's membrane.[95] Other diseases that can give rise to **subretinal neovascularization** and scarring

include myopia,[96] angioid streaks,[97] and presumed ocular histoplasmosis. Some **subretinal neovascular** membranes have no identifiable cause and are considered idiopathic.[95]

Splitting of Bruch's membrane is a first step in disciform degeneration, even though degenerative changes may not necessarily be followed by neovascularization. When neovascularization does occur, new vessels extend from the choroid into the area between the two halves of the split Bruch's membrane. The stimulus for this ingrowth is unknown but does not appear to be ischemia. The new vessels may initially be occult and difficult to identify if the overlying retinal pigment epithelium is intact or hypertrophic. Clinical clues include subretinal blood and exudation, which if extensive lead to hemorrhagic or exudative retinal pigment epithelial detachment.[82] Vessels growing inward from the choroid initially have the characteristics of capillaries. With time, the vessels enlarge, taking on arteriolar and venular characteristics, with intervening capillaries.[87]

In an experimental model of photic injury, capillary endothelium itself was shown to digest Bruch's membrane, allowing inward vascular growth. Thus, the vessels can create their own defect in Bruch's membrane.[98]

In time, the exudative or hemorrhagic detachment becomes organized and fibrotic, forming what is clinically recognized as a fibrovascular disciform scar (Fig. 11-14). Sometimes, hemosiderin can be identified in these scars, indicating a prior hemorrhage.[82]

The overlying retinal pigment epithelium also may proliferate, leading to a second component of the scar. This portion forms between the inner portion of Bruch's membrane and the sensory retina. Histologically, the retinal pigment epithelium may remain recognizable as pigmented cells retaining their polarity, or it may undergo

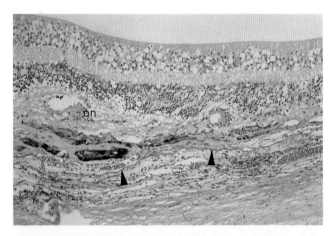

FIG. 11-14. In disciform degeneration there is loss of the photoreceptors. Only some of the outer nuclear layer (*on*) nuclei remain. The pigment epithelium has proliferated, with some retention of pigmentation. Bruch's membrane is split; the outer portion (*arrowheads*) overlies intact choriocapillaris. Blood vessels are seen interior to this portion of Bruch's, within the disciform scar.

fibrous metaplasia to form an avascular fibrous scar. Clinically, these two patterns correspond to dark hypofluorescent areas and pale hyperfluorescent areas, respectively. Usually there is a combination of both, explaining the variegated pattern of disciform scars seen clinically.[82]

If there is a tear or defect in the retinal pigment epithelium and its accompanying inner layer of Bruch's membrane, the two separate areas of scarring become continuous. Such a defect allows vascularization of the previously avascular inner portion of the disciform scar.[82] Also, retinal vessels can anastomose to the choroidal vessels in the scar, although this is uncommon.[99]

The sensory retina overlying the disciform scar generally shows loss of the photoreceptors, especially when the scar is thick.[88] Other degenerative changes include cystoid degeneration and lamellar and full-thickness macular holes.[100]

Recently, surgeons have attempted to excise disciform membranes in an effort to improve vision for patients with age-related macular degeneration and other diseases. Histologically, these membranes appear similar regardless of the prior disease process and contain vascular channels beneath the pigment epithelium, collagen, and inflammatory cells.[95] Immunohistochemical evidence of growth factors also has been demonstrated and possibly implicated in angiogenesis,[101] although the stimulus for these factors remains unknown.

The boundaries of some neovascular membranes may be poorly defined angiographically, and histologic examination of these membranes demonstrates a subsensory retinal component.[95] Moreover, blood vessels are distributed unevenly in these membranes.[102] Recurrent or subsequent neovascularization is not uncommon after surgery and may be related to incomplete excision.[95]

Angioid Streaks

Angioid streaks are idiopathic in about half of all patients, but they are also associated with several diseases of connective tissue. The most common association is with pseudoxanthoma elasticum, an autosomal dominant disorder of elastic tissue.[103] Other reported associations include sickle-cell anemia,[56] other hemolytic anemias,[97] and Paget disease.[103]

Angioid streaks, as the name implies, resemble blood vessels. They appear as irregular, reddish-brown, crack-like lesions radiating outward from the optic disc. They superficially resemble blood vessels because of their shape and color. The overlying pigment epithelium may be disrupted or depigmented, so the streaks transmit fluorescence. Secondary subretinal neovascularization, and ultimately a disciform scar, can lead to visual loss in some patients.

Histologically, the streaks correspond to discontinuities in Bruch's membrane, which is thickened and calcified at the level of the elastic layer (Fig. 11-15).[103] Calcification appears to cause the increased brittleness of Bruch's membrane,[97] which in turn may help predispose to the subretinal neovascularization.

Macular Holes

Macular holes are often an idiopathic finding, and their pathogenesis is controversial. They can be lamellar or full thickness. Clinically, they appear as discrete, small, round areas of retinal discontinuity in the fovea. An epiretinal membrane and small drusen are often present. Patients with full-thickness holes typically have poor vision, but patients with lamellar holes, where there is no full-thickness retinal discontinuity, may have good acuity.[104] Some eyes appear to have an operculum overlying the hole, but histologically this seems to be a detached proliferation of fibrous astrocytes and Müller cells rather than retinal tissue.[105]

Tangential vitreous traction in the macular region is believed to cause detachment and then hole formation. Other theories of pathogenesis include coalescence of cystoid edema and involutional thinning.[106] Macular holes can resolve spontaneously; increasingly, surgical removal of adherent cortical vitreous to repair the holes has been successful.

Histologically, macular holes show rounded margins, as do all true retinal breaks (Fig. 11-16). Sometimes, proliferated retinal pigment epithelium binds the margins, creating a chorioretinal adhesion. Epiretinal membranes may be present.[104] Vitrectomy specimens and whole eyes obtained postmortem after spontaneous healing and surgical repair have been examined histologically. Eyes with spontaneous resolution have shown glial and retinal pigment epithelial proliferation closing the defect.[100] An eye obtained after surgical repair showed much closer approx-

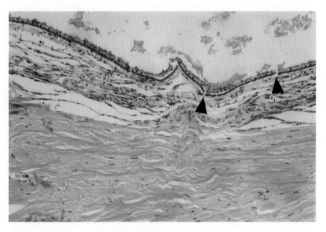

FIG. 11-15. Angioid streaks involve thickening and calcification of Bruch's membrane, with focal fractures (*arrowheads*).

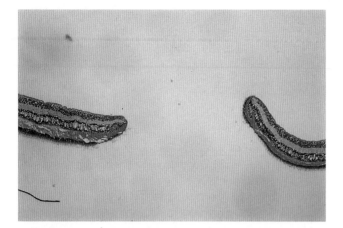

FIG. 11-16. A macular hole with rounded margins. Photoreceptor segments extend close to the hole margins. Courtesy of W. Richard Green, M.D., Wilmer Ophthalmological Institute, Johns Hopkins University.

imation of the margins of the hole, with less extensive glial repair.[106]

HEREDITARY RETINAL DYSTROPHIES

Vitreoretinal Dystrophies

Vitreoretinal dystrophies comprise a group of hereditary diseases with ocular, and sometimes systemic, findings.[107]

Lattice Degeneration

Lattice degeneration is a common peripheral vitreoretinal degeneration, usually located circumferentially at or anterior to the equator.[108] It is characterized by inner retinal thinning, a pocket of overlying fluid vitreous, sclerotic retinal vessels traversing the involved area, and secondary retinal pigment epithelial hyperplasia and migration (Fig. 11-17). The retina can thin to the point of hole formation, and scanning electron microscopy demonstrates a smooth membrane consisting of everted photoreceptor remnants.[109] Radial perivascular lattice shares the same clinical and histologic features but extends along a vessel.[110]

Familial Exudative Vitreoretinopathy

Familial exudative vitreoretinopathy is an autosomal dominant dystrophy that superficially resembles Coats' disease or retinopathy of prematurity. The retina typically has preretinal acellular fibrous membranes peripherally, with retinal traction and macular dragging.[111] Later there is intraretinal exudation, leading to total detachment.[112] The peripheral retina tends to be avascular, and the vascu-

lature elsewhere is abnormal in configuration. It has been suggested that the abnormalities of retinopathy of prematurity resemble those of familial exudative retinopathy.[113]

Stickler Syndrome

The arthro-ophthalmopathy of **Stickler** is an autosomal dominant condition involving the eye and sometimes the orofacial region, the skeletal system, and joints. High myopia, strabismus, presenile cataract, and open angle glaucoma are seen, but the striking finding is vitreous degeneration with syneresis, a so-called "optically empty" vitreous cavity. Fundus changes, which can be progressive, include perivascular pigmentation overlying atrophic retinal pigment epithelium, lattice degeneration, and retinal breaks. Over 50% of patients develop retinal detachment; these can be difficult to repair. Histologically, advanced cases show complete retinal detachment with preretinal membranes that extend through the retinal holes into the retroretinal space.[114] Recent genetic studies have identified several mutations in a gene that codes for a collagen precursor. The result could be an unstable form of the collagen triple helix.[115]

Wagner Disease

Many cases now thought to be Stickler syndrome were originally described as **Wagner disease.** It is now believed that Wagner disease, another autosomal dominant vitreoretinal dystrophy, is rare. It is characterized by low to moderate myopia, degenerative fundus changes simulating retinitis pigmentosa, and gliotic membrane formation, but without retinal detachment.[107]

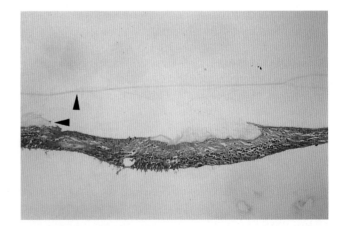

FIG. 11-17. Lattice degeneration involves discrete areas of the retina. A pocket of fluid vitreous overlies the area (*arrowheads*) and is firmly adherent at the margins. Photoreceptors are lost and the remainder of the retina is thinned. Courtesy of W. Richard Green, M.D., Wilmer Ophthalmological Institute, Johns Hopkins University.

Photoreceptor Dystrophies

The dystrophies of the outer retina have been intensively studied, and in recent years many of the causative genes have been identified.

Retinitis Pigmentosa

The clinical picture of **retinitis pigmentosa** appears to represent a final common pathway for a vast number of inherited ocular, central nervous system, and systemic diseases involving carbohydrate, lipid, or protein metabolism.[116] It also can be an isolated condition, inherited as an autosomal recessive, autosomal dominant, or X-linked recessive trait.[117] The bone spicule appearance can be an isolated degenerative change in the peripheral fundus.[118]

In primary retinitis pigmentosa, the clinical manifestations are least severe in the autosomal dominant form and most severe in the X-linked form. In all patients, an early symptom is decreased night vision. Gradually, the visual fields become more constricted. The electroretinogram is abnormal in both the light-adapted and dark-adapted states.[119] The fundus shows a characteristic spicule arrangement of pigment, waxy pallor of the optic disc, and marked attenuation of the arterioles.[117] Female carriers of the X-linked form can have normal fundi, or patchy involvement of the fundus with some visual reduction.[120] Fluorescein angiography shows the pigment epithelial changes as mottling, with focal window defects.[121]

Histologically, the earliest changes occur in the equatorial zone, extending from there both peripherally and centrally. Nuclei of the photoreceptors migrate outward, with subsequent degeneration of photoreceptors. Pigment epithelial cells migrate into the retina, mostly around vessels but also in small clusters. The endothelial cells of the surrounded retinal vessels tend to thin and develop fenestrations. This finding explains the leakage observed on fluorescein angiography. The vascular walls are thickened and gliotic.[122] The remaining retina adheres to Bruch's membrane. There can be cystoid macular edema or hole formation, and there often are epiretinal membranes. Other macular abnormalities include disciform changes. There is gliosis overlying the optic disc,[123] and there can be retinal gliosis in advanced cases.[124] The photoreceptor loss is greatest in the areas of poorest vision clinically.[119] The inner retina remains relatively more intact, but there is some loss of ganglion cells.[125] Carriers of X-linked retinitis pigmentosa can show many of the same histologic features.[120] The overlying vitreous contains cells that have been shown to include pigment epithelial cells, uveal melanocytes, macrophages, and retinal astrocytes, along with free pigment.[126]

Rhodopsin, the light-receiving protein of the rod outer segments, is altered in many patients. Several specific mutations have been identified. Patients with the same genetic mutation may be affected to variable degrees.[127] Alterations in the gene for peripherin are responsible for other retinitis pigmentosa pedigrees. **Peripherin,** found at the edges of the stacked disc membranes of the outer segment, may be essential for assembly and stability of the membranes. Further identification of these genetic mutations may allow corrective therapy.[128]

Stargardt Disease and Fundus Flavimaculatus

Formerly, **Stargardt disease** and **fundus flavimaculatus** were believed to be separate entities, but more recently they have been considered to be part of the same disease. Usually, it is inherited as an autosomal recessive trait, but it can be autosomal dominant.[129] Genetic studies have shown only one genetic defect for families with the autosomal recessive form, but several different genes have been found for the autosomal dominant form.[130]

Clinically, the retina shows poorly defined yellow-white linear or fishtail opacities at the level of the retinal pigment epithelium. Fluorescein angiography shows hypofluorescence of new lesions, but later, as the lesions are resorbed, they may be hyperfluorescent. If there is macular involvement, there is gradual, progressive visual loss secondary to atrophic degeneration, with a bull's-eye appearance to the macula.[131]

Histologic studies have shown accumulation of a form of lipofuscin in the retinal pigment epithelium, resulting in markedly enlarged cells, especially posteriorly.[131] Similar findings are found in the autosomal dominant form.[129] This accumulation begins within the first few months of life.[132] However, in a case without maculopathy, no lipofuscin was found in the retinal pigment epithelium, although the cells did contain lipid membranes.[133]

Vitelliform Dystrophy

Vitelliform dystrophy, or **Best disease,** is inherited as an autosomal dominant trait. In its classic form, a striking yellow deposit is seen at the macula or elsewhere in the posterior pole. The deposit is smooth and round and has been likened to the yolk of an egg. At this stage, visual acuity is surprisingly good, and it does not decrease until the yolk "scrambles," becoming irregular in appearance. The hallmark of the disorder is a depressed electrooculogram with a normal electroretinogram, and these findings can be used to diagnose patients who do not yet show a fundus abnormality.[134]

There is controversy about whether the primary defect lies in the photoreceptors or in the retinal pigment epithelium. Lipofuscin accumulates within the apices of the retinal pigment epithelial cells. In the macular region, an acellular fibrillar material has been found beneath the retinal pigment epithelium.[135,136] These findings, therefore, may represent disordered shedding of photoreceptor outer segments[136] or diffusely impaired metabolism of the retinal pigment epithelial cells.[135,137] There can be secondary subretinal neovascularization. Recently, genetic linkage analysis of several pedigrees has indicated that a gene for a protein expressed in the photoreceptor outer segment is likely to be the cause.[130]

An adult form of vitelliform dystrophy, a retinal pigment epithelial dystrophy, causes a mild loss of visual acuity in middle age, a normal or only slightly abnormal electro-oculogram, and pale macular lesions. Histologically, the retinal pigment epithelium may show atrophy and hypertrophy with fibrosis,[138] or retinal pigment epithelial nodular proliferation.[139] The cases may represent different stages of the same disease.

Pattern Dystrophies

Several congenital abnormalities of the retinal pigment epithelium have been described. Depending on the arrangement of the pigment, they have been given picturesque names such as butterfly-shaped dystrophy and macroreticular dystrophy. They are typically inherited as an autosomal dominant trait, and patients maintain good visual acuity, color vision, and dark adaptation. The dystrophies are probably variants of a single disease process, because families with different presentations within the same pedigree have been reported.[140,141] Several mutations in the peripherin gene have been identified in these patients.[130]

Choroidal Dystrophies

In **choroidal dystrophies,** there is primary selective atrophy of the choriocapillaris. Loss of the choriocapillaris in turn causes loss of retinal pigment epithelium and outer retina. There are several diseases in this group, characterized by the location of the involved area. In all, however, the junction between involved and uninvolved regions is sharp and abrupt. The involved areas are pale, with prominent choroidal vasculature, suggesting the appearance of sclerotic vessels.[142]

Gyrate atrophy is the only one of these diseases with an identified enzyme defect. The involved enzyme is ornithine aminotransferase, an enzyme found in the mitochondrial matrix. The ocular findings are characteristic and consist of confluent, sharply demarcated areas of depigmentation in the midperiphery. Histologically, the retina shows abrupt photoreceptor and pigment epithelial loss in the atrophic area, with focal pigment epithelial hyperplasia.[143]

SYSTEMIC DISEASES INVOLVING THE RETINA

Crystalline Retinopathy

Bietti's dystrophy is a congenital condition involving the cornea and the retina, although onset of symptoms is typically in the third decade. The inheritance pattern is most likely autosomal recessive. It has been reported in patients all over the world.[144] The retinal changes cause loss of vision, which is variable but can be profound. The retinal pigment epithelium is atrophic, and there is variable choriocapillaris atrophy. Small shiny crystals at all levels in the retina at the posterior pole are the most striking feature. Visual fields are initially normal[145] but later become constricted. Color vision can be abnormal with a suggestion of tritan deficiency.[144] Because the retinal disease may be localized or diffuse, Bietti's may represent a group of conditions. The cornea also contains sparkling, refractile crystals seen most densely at the corneal periphery, becoming more rarefied centrally. Similar crystals and deposits are present in circulating lymphocytes, suggesting a metabolic abnormality;[144] however, serum levels of lysosomal enzymes are normal. Thus, this condition is probably not a lysosomal storage disorder.[145]

Calcium oxalate crystals can accumulate in the retina from the inborn metabolic error primary hyperoxaluria,[146] secondary to methoxyflurane abuse or other poisoning,[147] or from renal failure and malnutrition.[148] They appear as whitish, variably refractile particles in deep retina, associated with small, round areas of pigment hyperplasia. With time, there is additional pigment proliferation in a geographic pattern with decreased visual acuity. Histologically, birefringent calcium oxalate crystals are seen within sensory retina, particularly within vessel walls.[148]

Storage Diseases

Mucopolysaccharidoses are a group of metabolic disorders of the metabolism of the glycosaminoglycans keratan sulfate, dermatan sulfate, and heparan sulfate, allowing accumulation of one or more of these substances in several ocular and nonocular tissues. The diseases differ in their systemic manifestations and can often be identified clinically. Acid mucopolysaccharide is found in inclusions in the retinal pigment epithelium and in the retinal ganglion cells. These inclusions can be so numerous that the cells are markedly distended, and the pigment epithelium is hypopigmented.[149] Other changes can include loss of photoreceptors[150] and inclusions in vascular endothelium and pericytes.[149] Hyperplasia and migration of retinal pigment epithelial cells into the retina occur to a variable extent in the different types.

The sphingolipidoses and some of the mucolipidoses are characterized ophthalmoscopically by a **cherry-red spot.** As with central retinal artery occlusion, there is swelling and distention of the inner retina, but in these diseases the material is not edema fluid, but rather a metabolic product stored in the ganglion cells. Sometimes, after significant atrophy of the ganglion cell layer, the cherry-red spot may no longer be evident, even though abnormal inclusions can still be identified ultrastructurally.[151,152]

The **sphingolipidoses** are inborn errors of metabolism in which one of the sphingolipids accumulates in neural tissues. The enzyme defects are known and can be assayed. Many of these diseases are characterized by retinal thickening and cherry-red spot, or by formation of a macular halo.[153,154] Mucolipidoses are diseases that combine clinical features of the mucopolysaccharidoses and the sphingolipidoses, but without mucopolysacchariduria. The enzyme defect is known for some of these diseases.[151]

TRAUMA

Toxic Retinal Degenerations

Some drugs, most notably **chloroquine** but also others such as **clofazimine,** cause a **bull's-eye retinopathy** that appears to be dose-dependent. Along with the fundus appearance, other signs of toxicity include an abnormal electroretinogram and changes in color vision.[155] Chloroquine has been shown histologically to cause inclusions in the ganglion cells and inner nuclear cells, although these changes are not visible clinically. Late retinal pigment epithelial changes also occur.[156]

Severe visual loss with a fundus pattern similar to gyrate atrophy has been reported with thioridazine toxicity.[157]

Tamoxifen, an antiestrogen drug, has produced a retinopathy characterized by white refractile opacities in superficial retinal layers. Histologically, small spherical lesions containing glycosaminoglycans have been found in nerve fiber and inner plexiform layers. Ultrastructurally, these lesions consist of branching filaments, possibly representing axonal degenerative products.[158]

Canthaxanthin, a carotenoid used as a dye to simulate a suntan, can be deposited in the retina, although it does not seem to cause visual loss.[159]

Postirradiation Retinopathy

The eye may be injured by radiant energy directed at tumors within or near the globe. With modern methods of shielding, damage can be reduced, but it may be impossible to protect the eye entirely. Radiation energy damages the capillary endothelium, leading to loss of the intraretinal blood–retinal barrier and resulting in hemorrhages and exudates that can be massive.[160] Secondary complications include retinal ischemia with neovascularization and vitreous hemorrhage.[161,162]

Light Energy Retinopathy

Sungazing or eclipse watching with inadequate protection leads to retinal damage. Light in the visible and ultraviolet range can be focused by the lens onto the retina, and damage occurs at the level of the photoreceptors, with retinal pigment epithelial alteration. Sometimes, however, the macula can recover, and the patient may regain good vision.[163]

The operating microscope has been shown to cause retinal light toxicity, although there is controversy about the long-term clinical significance. Because the microscope illumination is not quite coaxial, the lesions noted clinically are just superior to the fovea. Thus, central vision may be preserved, but a paracentral scotoma is present, with pigment epithelial changes.[164] Similar lesions have been created by endoillumination during vitrectomy.[165]

The damage appears to be primarily photochemical,[166] but because lowering the temperature is somewhat protective, there is probably also a thermal component.[167] Shorter wavelengths, in the ultraviolet and blue range, seem especially damaging, putting aphakic patients at particular risk,[164] but the near-infrared light emitted by operating microscopes also is toxic.[166]

An important type of light injury is that deliberately applied to the retina. Lasers emitting light in the visible spectrum are used to treat retinal vascular disease and subretinal neovascularization. The radiant energy passes through the transparent retina and is absorbed by melanin pigment, hemoglobin, or both, depending on the wavelength chosen. The result is a focal scar of the outer retina or, if intense enough, full-thickness retina.[168]

The choriocapillaris is effectively closed by photocoagulation, as demonstrated by studies of vascular casts.[169] After panretinal photocoagulation, the oxygen tension on the inner retinal surface is greater over areas of scarring, presumably due in part to greater oxygen diffusion from the larger vessels of the choroid. This effect would alleviate retinal ischemia and help explain how photocoagulation causes retinal neovascular regression.[170]

In the juxtafoveal area, krypton red is associated with less inner retinal damage than argon green;[171,172] however, the wavelength used appears to be unimportant in extrafoveal areas of the retina.[172]

Traumatic Retinopathy

The traumatic insult stimulates hyperplasia of the retinal pigment epithelium, which in turn migrates into the sensory retina, simulating the bone-spicule appearance of retinitis pigmentosa; however, it can occur as a localized phenomenon anywhere in the retina. Once the acute stimulus has resolved, there is no progression of the pigmentation.[173]

Choroidal ruptures—tears of the choroid, Bruch's membrane, and retinal pigment epithelium—can result from direct trauma or contusion. Clinically, they appear as well-circumscribed crescentic pale areas at the posterior pole and are arranged concentrically around the optic disc. Sometimes there is pigment epithelial proliferation.[174]

Fresh choroidal ruptures are accompanied by hemorrhages, and fibroblastic proliferation can start as soon as 4 days after trauma. The proliferation can be massive and can extend into the vitreous. The retina shows outer atrophy to full-thickness discontinuity with scarring, depending on the traumatic insult.[174]

Commotio retinae, sometimes called **Berlin edema,** is a contrecoup injury to the retina produced by blunt trauma. The force is transmitted from the point of impact to the retina at the opposite pole of the globe. Clinically, the lesion appears whitish and indistinct. After several days, pigmentary changes occur. Histologically, these changes occur in deep retina and are the result of disruption of photoreceptor cell outer segments.[175]

Purtscher retinopathy is a condition associated with head trauma, chest compression, long bone fractures, or rapid deceleration. After such injuries, the retina shows edema, hemorrhages, and cotton-wool patches. Nontraumatic causes have been recently described, including acute pancreatitis, childbirth,[176] and chronic renal failure.[177] The cause of the fundus appearance seems to be microemboli composed of aggregates of granulocytes, induced by activation of the complement system.[176]

RETINAL DETACHMENT

The correct term for retinal detachment is **retinal separation** because the detachment occurs between the two embryonic neuroectodermal layers. Retinal "detachment" simply recapitulates the normal embryonic separation between the inner neuroectodermal layer, the sensory retina, and the retinal pigment epithelium, the outer neuroectodermal layer (see Fig. 11-1). A true retinal detachment would occur below the basement membrane of the retinal pigment epithelium, separating it from the rest of Bruch's membrane. Because the attachment between the two neuroectodermal layers is physiologic and biochemical, rather than anatomic,[7] detachments also are common artifacts in histologic preparations of the eye.

Retinal detachment is caused by fluid seepage from the underlying tissues into the subsensory retinal space, traction from the vitreous, or both. For fluid to leak into the subsensory retinal space, one or more defects in the retinal pigment epithelium must exist so that the integrity of the blood–retinal barrier is lost. This phenomenon occurs frequently with primary and metastatic tumors of the choroid, inflammatory diseases of the choroid or sclera, and idiopathic central serous choroidopathy. This leakage results in a bullous detachment of the sensory retina that shifts according to the position of the patient.[178]

Central serous choroidopathy, also called **central serous retinopathy, pigment epitheliopathy,** or **chorioretinopathy,** is an idiopathic disorder usually occurring in young men. On fluorescein angiography, early frames demonstrate a "smokestack" as the fluorescein enters the subretinal space through the leakage site. The borders of the detachment are indistinct, in contrast to detachment of the pigment epithelium, which has sharp margins. The condition can recur, and the cause is not understood.[179] Sometimes there is secondary subretinal fibrosis.[180]

Several conditions, including scleritis, inflammation or tumors of the choroid,[178] and subretinal neovascularization, especially in older patients (Fig. 11-18),[91] can cause secondary leakage through defects in the retinal pigment epithelium.

The other major cause of retinal detachment is **vitreous traction,** which can lead to detachment with or without formation of a hole in the sensory retina. When vitreous traction causes a tear leading to detachment, it is called **rhegmatogenous,** from the Greek word for tear or rent. Rhegmatogenous detachments can result from abnormalities of the vitreous, retina, or both. A hole or defect in the retina by itself does not usually cause detachment; there must also be traction at the margin of the defect. Thus, for example, holes in the center of lattice degeneration do not lead to retinal detachment, because the overlying vitreous is fluid.[181]

The vitreous normally is adherent around the optic nerve head, around the fovea, and along the major retinal vessels. The densest vitreous adhesion is at its base, overlying the ora serrata and adjacent pars plana. With aging, the vitreous liquefies and the remaining formed vitreous falls anteriorly, peeling away from its more posterior attachments. If there is a focal area of increased adherence, the detaching vitreous may pull out a portion of partial- or full-thickness retina. One sign of vitreous traction is retinal pit formation, partial-thickness retinal defects that appear as tiny holes alongside retinal vessels. Histologically, they represent focal inner retinal tissue loss.[182] A full-thickness defect in the sensory retina is a hole or tear. The vitreous may remain attached to the flap of the tear, sometimes producing continued traction.

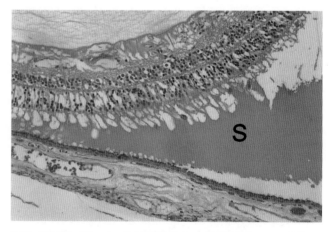

FIG. 11-18. Serous fluid (*S*) beneath the sensory retina. The pigment epithelium appears intact in this area.

Several conditions predispose to retinal detachment. **High myopia** is believed to cause increased stretch on the retina because of the enlarged eye. Retinal detachment is also more common after cataract extraction. Heredity also plays a role. Lattice degeneration causes retinal thinning, but additionally there is a firm vitreous adhesion on either side of the lattice so that traction at this adhesion makes a detachment more likely.[181]

Retinal dialysis is the term for tearing of the retina from its attachment at the ora serrata. It is usually associated with penetrating or blunt trauma. Retinal dialysis involves a disturbance of the overlying vitreous base, and histologic preparations show vitreous attached to the margin of the dialysis.[183]

Several pathologic changes occur after long-standing retinal detachment. The photoreceptors typically atrophy because they have been separated from their nutrient supply from the choriocapillaris. The proliferating retinal pigment epithelium generates an unusual type of drusen called **dendritic drusen** (Fig. 11-19). Large intraretinal cysts can develop in longstanding retinal detachments.[183] Preretinal[184] and retroretinal membranes[185] are formed by glial and pigment epithelial tissue. Some of the cells in these membranes, including fibrous astrocytes, fibrocytes, and retinal pigment epithelial cells, develop myofibroblastic differentiation. Actin filaments line up along the cytoplasmic membrane, giving the cells contractile properties. As the membranes shrink, they cause fixed folds in the thickened, detached retina[184] called proliferative vitreoretinopathy. Growth factors stimulating collagen synthesis have been identified in the vitreous of patients with proliferative vitreoretinopathy.[186] Elevated intraocular pressure may sometimes be due to retinal debris, including photoreceptor fragments, obstructing the trabecular meshwork.[187,188]

Eyes with long-standing retinal detachment may ultimately become phthisical; that is, they may shrink and become internally disorganized. Bone formation is often

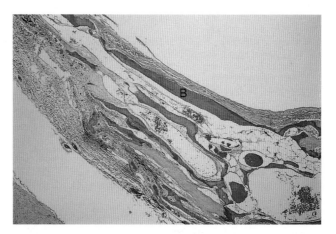

FIG. 11-20. In a phthisical eye, there is considerable fibrous metaplasia with bone formation (*B*). The choroid and retina are not recognizable. The tissue is artifactually detached from sclera, seen to the lower left.

observed (Fig. 11-20). The cell of origin for the bone is uncertain but may be the pigment epithelial cell.

Scleral buckling surgery is the usual means for correcting a retinal detachment. The purpose of the surgery is to relieve vitreous traction with the buckle by indenting the sclera, and to create retinal adhesion in the region of the tear by means of a chorioretinal scar. Histologically, pigment epithelial hyperplasia and migration are seen in the area of the scar, with variable amounts of retinal gliosis. Vitrectomy is increasingly becoming part of retinal detachment surgery, particularly to cut and remove fibrous traction bands. Complications of surgery include cystoid macular edema, ciliochoroidal effusion, and choroidal neovascularization.[189] The visual results can be disappointing, even when anatomic success is achieved, particularly when the macula is detached. Outer retinal atrophy and macular edema are both causes of decreased vision, but sometimes eyes with poor vision have no obvious cause.[190] The process of apoptosis has been identified as at least part of the reason for photoreceptor regression in eyes with retinal detachment; this helps explain why the duration of retinal detachment determines the degree of visual recovery.[86]

REFERENCES

1. Moore KL. *The developing human: clinically oriented embryology.* Philadelphia: WB Saunders, 1982.
2. Mietz H, Green WR, Wolff SM, et al. Foveal hypoplasia in complete oculocutaneous albinism: a histopathologic study. *Retina* 1992;12:254.
3. Duvall J. Structure, function, and pathologic responses of pigment epithelium: a review. *Sem Ophthalmol* 1987;2:130.
4. Bok D. Retinal photoreceptor-pigment epithelium interactions. *Invest Ophthalmol Vis Sci* 1985;26:1659.
5. Orth DH, Fine BS, Fagman W, et al. Clarification of foveomacular nomenclature and grid for quantitation of macular disorders. *Trans Am Acad Ophthalmol Otolaryngol* 1977;83:OP506.
6. Kalina RE. A histopathologic postmortem and clinical study of

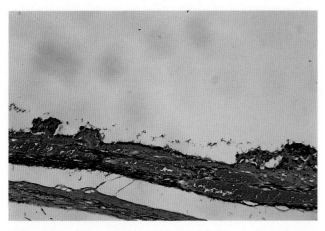

FIG. 11-19. With chronic retinal detachment, the pigment epithelium can proliferate and form drusen with unusual branching shapes, called dendritic drusen.

peripheral retinal folds in infant eyes. *Am J Ophthalmol* 1971;71:446.

7. Gartner S, Henkind P. Lange's folds: a meaningful ocular artifact. *Ophthalmology* 1981;88:1307.

8. Garner A. Retinal angiogenesis: mechanism in health and disease. *Sem Ophthalmol* 1987;2:71.

9. Iwasaki M, Inomata H. Relation between superficial capillaries and foveal structures in the human retina. *Invest Ophthalmol Vis Sci* 1986;27:1698.

10. Yoneya S, Tso MOM. Angioarchitecture of the human choroid. *Arch Ophthalmol* 1987;105:681.

11. Cunha-Vaz J. The blood-ocular barriers. *Surv Ophthalmol* 1979;23:279.

12. Castronuovo S, Simon JW, Kandel GL, et al. Variable expression of albinism within a single kindred. *Am J Ophthalmol* 1991;111:419.

13. King RA, Lewis RA, Townsend D, et al. Brown oculocutaneous albinism: clinical, ophthalmological, and biochemical characterization. *Ophthalmology* 1985;92:1496.

14. Summers CG, King RA. Ophthalmic features of minimal pigment oculocutaneous albinism. *Ophthalmology* 1994;101:906.

15. Valenzuela R, Morningstar WA. The ocular pigmentary disturbance of human Chédiak-Higashi syndrome: a comparative light- and electron-microscopic study and review of the literature. *Am J Clin Pathol* 1981;75:591.

16. Wong L, O'Donnell FE Jr, Green WR. Giant pigment granules in the retinal pigment epithelium of a fetus with X-linked ocular albinism. *Ophthal Paediatr Genet* 1983;2:47.

17. Hittner H, King R, Riccardi V, et al. Oculocutaneous albinoidism as a manifestation of reduced neural crest derivatives in the Prader-Willi syndrome. *Am J Ophthalmol* 1982;94:328.

18. Lloyd WC III, Eagle RC Jr, Shields JA, et al. Congenital hypertrophy of the retinal pigment epithelium: electron microscopic and morphometric observations. *Ophthalmology* 1990;97:1052.

19. Traboulsi EI, Maumenee IH, Krush AJ, et al. Pigmented ocular fundus lesions in the inherited gastrointestinal polyposis syndromes and in hereditary nonpolyposis colorectal cancer. *Ophthalmology* 1988;95:964.

20. Munden PM, Sobol WM, Weingeist TA. Ocular findings in Turcot syndrome (glioma-polyposis). *Ophthalmology* 1991;98:111.

21. Traboulsi EI, Maumenee IH, Krush AJ, et al. Congenital hypertrophy of the retinal pigment epithelium predicts colorectal polyposis in Gardner's syndrome. *Arch Ophthalmol* 1990;108:525.

22. Pagon RA. Ocular coloboma. *Surv Ophthalmol* 1981;25:223.

23. Ali BH, Logani S, Kozlov KL, et al. Progression of retinal nerve fiber myelination in childhood. *Am J Ophthalmol* 1994;118:515.

24. Straatsma BR, Foos RY, Heckenlively JR, et al. Myelinated retinal nerve fibers. *Am J Ophthalmol* 1981;91:25.

25. Baarsma GS. Acquired medullated nerve fibres. *Br J Ophthalmol* 1980;64:651.

26. Rosenthal AR. Ocular manifestations of leukemia: a review. *Ophthalmology* 1983;90:899.

27. Khouri GG, Murphy RP, Kuhajda FP, et al. Clinicopathologic features in two cases of multiple myeloma. *Retina* 1986;6:169.

28. Ortiz JM, Yanoff M, Cameron JD, et al. Disseminated intravascular coagulation in infancy and in the neonate: ocular findings. *Arch Ophthalmol* 1982;100:1413.

29. Gagliano DA, Goldberg MF. The evolution of salmon-patch hemorrhages in sickle cell retinopathy. *Arch Ophthalmol* 1989;107:1814.

30. Murphy RP, Nanda M, Plotnick L, et al. The relationship of puberty to diabetic retinopathy. *Arch Ophthalmol* 1990;108:215.

31. de Venecia G, Davis M, Engerman R. Clinicopathologic correlations in diabetic retinopathy. I. Histology and fluorescein angiography of microaneurysms. *Arch Ophthalmol* 1976;94:1766.

32. Bresnick GH, Davis MD, Myers FL, et al. Clinicopathologic correlations in diabetic retinopathy. II. Clinical and histologic appearances of retinal capillary microaneurysms. *Arch Ophthalmol* 1977;95:1215.

33. Rabb MF, Burton TC, Schatz H, et al. Fluorescein angiography of the fundus: a schematic approach to interpretation. *Surv Ophthalmol* 1978;22:387.

34. Fichte C, Streeten BW, Friedman AH. A histopathologic study of retinal arterial aneurysms. *Am J Ophthalmol* 1978;85:509.

35. Perry HD, Zimmerman LE, Benson WE. Hemorrhage from isolated aneurysm of a retinal artery: report of two cases simulating malignant melanoma. *Arch Ophthalmol* 1977;95:281.

36. Reeser F, Fleischman J, Williams GA, et al. Efficacy of argon laser photocoagulation in the treatment of circinate diabetic retinopathy. *Am J Ophthalmol* 1981;92:762.

37. Kincaid MC, Green WR, Iliff WJ. Granulomatous reaction to Choyce-style intraocular lens. *Ophthalmic Surg* 1982;13:292.

38. Tso MOM. Pathology of cystoid macular edema. *Ophthalmology* 1982;89:902.

39. Fine BS, Brucker AJ. Macular edema and cystoid macular edema. *Am J Ophthalmol* 1981;92:466.

40. Yanoff M, Fine BS, Brucker AJ, et al. Pathology of human cystoid macular edema. *Surv Ophthalmol* 1984;28(Suppl):505.

41. Gass JDM, Anderson DR, Davis EB. A clinical, fluorescein angiographic, and electron microscopic correlation of cystoid macular edema. *Am J Ophthalmol* 1985;100:82.

42. Michael JC, de Venecia G. Retinal trypsin digest study of cystoid macular edema associated with peripheral choroidal melanoma. *Am J Ophthalmol* 1995;119:152.

43. Kahn M, Green WR, Knox DL, et al. Ocular features of carotid occlusive disease. *Retina* 1986;6:239.

44. Tso MOM, Jampol LM. Pathophysiology of hypertensive retinopathy. *Ophthalmology* 1982;89:1132.

45. Patrinely JR, Green WR, Randolph ME. Retinal phlebitis with chorioretinal emboli. *Am J Ophthalmol* 1982;94:49.

46. Kresca LJ, Goldberg MF, Jampol LM. Talc emboli and retinal neovascularization in a drug abuser. *Am J Ophthalmol* 1979;87:334.

47. Brownstein S, Font RL, Alper MG. Atheromatous plaques of the retinal blood vessels: histologic confirmation of ophthalmoscopically visible lesions. *Arch Ophthalmol* 1973;90:49.

48. Jarrett WH II, North AW. Dynamic platelet embolization of the retinal arteriole. *Arch Ophthalmol* 1995;113:531.

49. Diamond JP. Treatable blindness in temporal arteritis. *Br J Ophthalmol* 1991;75:432.

50. Cohen SM, Davis JL, Gass JDM. Branch retinal arterial occlusions in multifocal retinitis with optic nerve edema. *Arch Ophthalmol* 1995;113:1271.

51. Zimmerman LE. Embolism of central retinal artery. *Arch Ophthalmol* 1965;73:822.

52. Enzenauer RJ, Stock JG, Enzenauer RW, et al. Retinal vasculopathy associated with systemic light chain deposition disease. *Retina* 1990;10:115.

53. Wolter JR. Axonal enlargements in the nerve-fiber layer of the human retina. *Am J Ophthalmol* 1968;65:1.

54. Ashton N, Harry J. The pathology of cotton wool spots and cytoid bodies in hypertensive retinopathy and other diseases. *Trans Ophthalmol Soc UK* 1963;83:91.

55. Chang TS, Aylward GW, Davis JL, et al. Idiopathic retinal vasculitis, aneurysms, and neuro-retinitis. *Ophthalmology* 1995;102:1089.

56. Nagpal KC, Goldberg MF, Rabb MF. Ocular manifestations of sickle hemoglobinopathies. *Surv Ophthalmol* 1977;21:391.

57. McLeod DS, Goldberg MF, Lutty GA. Dual-perspective analysis of vascular formations in sickle cell retinopathy. *Arch Ophthalmol* 1993;111:1234.

58. Hayreh SS, Zimmerman MB, Podhajsky P. Incidence of various types of retinal vein occlusion and their recurrence and demographic characteristics. *Am J Ophthalmol* 1994;117:429.

59. Hayreh SS. Classification of central retinal vein occlusion. *Ophthalmology* 1983;90:458.

60. Green WR, Chan CC, Hutchins GM, et al. Central retinal vein occlusion: a prospective histopathologic study of 29 eyes in 28 cases. *Retina* 1981;1:27.

61. Frangieh GT, Green WR, Barraquer-Somers E, et al. Histopathologic study of nine branch retinal vein occlusions. *Arch Ophthalmol* 1982;100:1132.

62. Weinberg D, Dodwell DG, Fern SA. Anatomy of arteriovenous crossings in branch retinal vein occlusion. *Am J Ophthalmol* 1990;109:298.

63. Scheie HG. Evaluation of ophthalmoscopic changes of hypertension and arteriolar sclerosis. *Arch Ophthalmol* 1953;49:117.

64. Kishi S, Tso MOM, Hayreh SS. Fundus lesions in malignant hy-

pertension. I. A pathologic study of experimental hypertensive choroidopathy. *Arch Ophthalmol* 1985;103:1189.

65. Diabetic Retinopathy Study Research Group. Photocoagulation treatment of proliferative diabetic retinopathy. Clinical application of Diabetic Retinopathy Study (DRS) findings, DRS report number 8. *Ophthalmology* 1981;88:583.

66. Kincaid MC, Green WR, Fine SL, et al. An ocular clinicopathologic correlative study of six patients from the Diabetic Retinopathy Study. *Retina* 1983;3:218.

67. D'Amore PA. Mechanisms of retinal and choroidal neovascularization. *Invest Ophthalmol Vis Sci* 1994;35:3974.

68. Foos RY. Senile retinoschisis: relationship to cystoid degeneration. *Trans Am Acad Ophthalmol Otolaryngol* 1970;74:33.

69. Laatikainen L, Tarkkanen A, Saksela T. Hereditary X-linked retinoschisis and bilateral congenital retinal detachment. *Retina* 1987; 7:24.

70. Tso MOM. Pathogenetic factors of aging macular degeneration. *Ophthalmology* 1985;92:628.

71. Feeney-Burns L, Burns RP, Gao C-L. Age-related macular changes in humans over 90 years old. *Am J Ophthalmol* 1990;109:265.

72. Friedman E, Krupsky S, Lane AM, et al. Ocular blood flow velocity in age-related macular degeneration. *Ophthalmology* 1995;102: 640.

73. Schachat AP, Hyman L, Leske MC, et al. Features of age-related macular degeneration in a black population. *Arch Ophthalmol* 1995;113:728.

74. Weiter JJ, Delori FC, Wing GL, et al. Retinal pigment epithelial lipofuscin and melanin and choroidal melanin in human eyes. *Invest Ophthalmol Vis Sci* 1986;27:145.

75. Feeney-Burns L. The pigments of the retinal pigment epithelium. *Curr Top Eye Res* 1980;2:119.

76. Eagle RC Jr. Mechanisms of maculopathy. *Ophthalmology* 1984; 91:613.

77. Feeney-Burns L, Ellersieck MR. Age-related changes in the ultrastructure of Bruch's membrane. *Am J Ophthalmol* 1985;100:686.

78. van der Schaft TL, de Bruijn WC, Mooy CM, et al. Is basal laminar deposit unique for age-related macular degeneration? *Arch Ophthalmol* 1991;109:420.

79. Sarks SH. Drusen and their relationship to senile macular degeneration. *Austral J Ophthalmol* 1980;8:117.

80. Holz FG, Wolfensberger TJ, Piguet B, et al. Bilateral macular drusen in age-related macular degeneration. *Ophthalmology* 1994; 101:1522.

81. Ulshafer RJ, Allen CB, Nicolaissen B Jr, et al. Scanning electron microscopy of human drusen. *Invest Ophthalmol Vis Sci* 1987;28: 683.

82. Green WR, McDonnell PJ, Yeo JH. Pathologic features of senile macular degeneration. *Ophthalmology* 1985;92:615.

83. Lewis H, Straatsma BR, Foos RY, et al. Reticular degeneration of the pigment epithelium. *Ophthalmology* 1985;92:1485.

84. van der Schaft TL, Mooy CM, de Bruijn WC, et al. Histologic features of the early stages of age-related macular degeneration: a statistical analysis. *Ophthalmology* 1992;99:278.

85. Burns R, Feeney-Burns L. Clinico-morphologic correlations of drusen of Bruch's membrane. *Trans Am Ophthalmol Soc* 1980; 78:206.

86. Chang C-J, Lai WW, Edward DP, et al. Apoptotic photoreceptor cell death after traumatic retinal detachment in humans. *Arch Ophthalmol* 1995;113:880.

87. Green WR. Clinicopathologic studies of senile macular degeneration. In: Nicholson DH, ed. *Ocular pathology update.* New York: Masson, 1980.

88. Green WR, Enger C. Age-related macular degeneration histopathologic studies: the 1992 Lorenz E. Zimmerman lecture. *Ophthalmology* 1993;100:1519.

89. Kenyon KR, Maumenee AE, Ryan SJ, et al. Diffuse drusen and associated complications. *Am J Ophthalmol* 1985;100:119.

90. Keno DD, Green WR. Retinal pigment epithelial window defect. *Arch Ophthalmol* 1978;96:854.

91. Green WR, Key SN III. Senile macular degeneration: a histopathologic study. *Trans Am Ophthalmol Soc* 1977;75:180.

92. Henkind P, Gartner S. The relationship between retinal pigment epithelium and the choriocapillaris. *Trans Ophthalmol Soc UK* 1983;103:444.

93. Yeo JH, Marcus S, Murphy RP. Retinal pigment epithelial tears: patterns and prognosis. *Ophthalmology* 1988;95:8.

94. Toth CA, Pasquale AC III, Graichen DF. Clinicopathologic correlation of spontaneous retinal pigment epithelial tears with choroidal neovascular membranes in age-related macular degeneration. *Ophthalmology* 1995;102:272.

95. Grossniklaus HE, Hutchinson AK, Capone A Jr, et al. Clinicopathologic features of surgically excised choroidal neovascular membranes. *Ophthalmology* 1994;101:1099.

96. Hampton GR, Kohen D, Bird AC. Visual prognosis of disciform degeneration in myopia. *Ophthalmology* 1983;90:923.

97. Jampol LM, Acheson R, Eagle RC Jr, et al. Calcification of Bruch's membrane in angioid streaks with homozygous sickle cell disease. *Arch Ophthalmol* 1987;105:93.

98. Heriot WJ, Henkind P, Bellhorn RW. Choroidal neovascularization can digest Bruch's membrane: a prior break is not essential. *Ophthalmology* 1984;91:1603.

99. Green WR, Gass JDM. Senile disciform degeneration of the macula: retinal arterialization of the fibrous plaque demonstrated clinically and histopathologically. *Arch Ophthalmol* 1971;86:487.

100. Guyer DR, Green WR, de Bustros S, et al. Histopathologic features of idiopathic macular holes and cysts. *Ophthalmology* 1990;97: 1045.

101. Reddy VM, Zamora RL, Kaplan HJ. Distribution of growth factors in subretinal neovascular membranes in age-related macular degeneration and presumed ocular histoplasmosis syndrome. *Am J Ophthalmol* 1995;120:291.

102. Bynoe LA, Chang TS, Funata M, et al. Histopathologic examination of vascular patterns in subfoveal neovascular membranes. *Ophthalmology* 1994;101:1112.

103. Dreyer R, Green WR. The pathology of angioid streaks: a study of twenty-one cases. *Trans PA Acad Ophthalmol Otolaryngol* 1978;31:158.

104. Frangieh GT, Green WR, Engel HM. A histopathologic study of macular cysts and holes. *Retina* 1981;1:311.

105. Madreperla SA, McCuen BW II, Hickingbotham D, et al. Clinicopathologic correlation of surgically removed macular hole opercula. *Am J Ophthalmol* 1995;120:197.

106. Funata M, Wendel RT, de la Cruz Z, et al. Clinicopathologic study of bilateral macular holes treated with pars plana vitrectomy and gas tamponade. *Retina* 1992;12:289.

107. Maumenee IH. Vitreoretinal degeneration as a sign of generalized connective tissue diseases. *Am J Ophthalmol* 1979;88:432.

108. Straatsma BR, Zeegen PE, Foos RY, et al. Lattice degeneration of the retina. Edward Jackson memorial lecture. *Am J Ophthalmol* 1974;77:619.

109. Robinson MR, Streeten BW. The surface morphology of retinal breaks and lattice retinal degeneration: a scanning electron microscopic study. *Ophthalmology* 1986;93:237.

110. Parelhoff ES, Wood WJ, Green WR, et al. Radial perivascular lattice degeneration of the retina. *Ann Ophthalmol* 1980;12:25.

111. Brockhurst RJ, Albert DM, Zakov ZN. Pathologic findings in familial exudative vitreoretinopathy. *Arch Ophthalmol* 1981;99: 2143.

112. Boldrey EE, Egbert P, Gass JDM, et al. The histopathology of familial exudative vitreoretinopathy: a report of two cases. *Arch Ophthalmol* 1985;103:238.

113. van Nouhuys CE. Signs, complications, and platelet aggregation in familial exudative vitreoretinopathy. *Am J Ophthalmol* 1991; 111:34.

114. Blair NP, Albert DM, Liberfarb RM, et al. Hereditary progressive arthro-ophthalmopathy of Stickler. *Am J Ophthalmol* 1979;88:876.

115. Ahmad NN, Dimascio J, Knowlton RG, et al. Stickler syndrome: a mutation in the nonhelical 3' end of type II procollagen gene. *Arch Ophthalmol* 1995;113:1454.

116. Wilson DJ, Green WR. Systemic diseases with retinitis pigmentosa-like changes. *MD Med J* 1986;35:1011.

117. Pagon RA. Retinitis pigmentosa. *Surv Ophthalmol* 1988;33:137.

118. Bastek JV, Siegel EB, Straatsma BR, et al. Chorioretinal juncture: pigmentary patterns of the peripheral fundus. *Ophthalmology* 1982;89:1455.

119. Bunt-Milam AH, Kalina RE, Pagon RA. Clinical–ultrastructural study of a retinal dystrophy. *Invest Ophthalmol Vis Sci* 1983;24: 458.

120. Szamier RB, Berson EL. Retinal histopathology of a carrier of X-chromosome–linked retinitis pigmentosa. *Ophthalmology* 1985; 92:271.

121. Meyer KT, Heckenlively JR, Spitznas M, et al. Dominant retinitis pigmentosa: a clinicopathologic correlation. *Ophthalmology* 1982; 89:1414.

122. Li Z-Y, Possin DE, Milam AH. Histopathology of bone spicule pigmentation in retinitis pigmentosa. *Ophthalmology* 1995;102: 805.

123. Gartner S, Henkind P. Pathology of retinitis pigmentosa. *Ophthalmology* 1982;89:1425.

124. Lahav M, Craft J, Albert DM. Advanced pigmentary retinal degeneration: an ultrastructural study. *Retina* 1982;2:65.

125. Stone JL, Barlow WE, Humayun MS, et al. Morphometric analysis of macular photoreceptors and ganglion cells in retinas with retinitis pigmentosa. *Arch Ophthalmol* 1992;110:1634.

126. Albert DM, Pruett RC, Craft JL. Transmission electron microscopic observations of vitreous abnormalities in retinitis pigmentosa. *Am J Ophthalmol* 1986;101:665.

127. Berson EL, Rosner B, Sandberg MA, et al. Ocular findings in patients with autosomal dominant retinitis pigmentosa and a rhodopsin gene defect (pro-23-his). *Arch Ophthalmol* 1991;109:92.

128. Bird AC. Retinal photoreceptor dystrophies. Edward Jackson memorial lecture. *Am J Ophthalmol* 1995;119:543.

129. Lopez PF, Maumenee IH, de la Cruz Z, et al. Autosomal-dominant fundus flavimaculatus. Clinicopathologic correlation. *Ophthalmology* 1990;97:798.

130. Zhang K, Nguyen T-HE, Crandall A, et al. Genetic and molecular studies of macular dystrophies: recent developments. *Surv Ophthalmol* 1995;40:51.

131. Eagle RC Jr, Lucier AC, Bernardino VB Jr, et al. Retinal pigment epithelial abnormalities in fundus flavimaculatus: a light and electron microscopic study. *Ophthalmology* 1980;87:1189.

132. Steinmetz RL, Garner A, Maguire JI, et al. Histopathology of incipient fundus flavimaculatus. *Ophthalmology* 1991;98:953.

133. McDonnell PJ, Kivlin JD, Maumenee IH, et al. Fundus flavimaculatus without maculopathy: a clinicopathologic study. *Ophthalmology* 1986;93:116.

134. Mohler CW, Fine SL. Long-term evaluation of patients with Best's vitelliform dystrophy. *Ophthalmology* 1981;88:688.

135. O'Gorman S, Flaherty WA, Fishman GA, et al. Histopathologic findings in Best's vitelliform macular dystrophy. *Arch Ophthalmol* 1988;106:1261.

136. Frangieh GT, Green WR, Fine SL. A histopathologic study of Best's macular dystrophy. *Arch Ophthalmol* 1982;100:1115.

137. Weingeist TA, Kobrin JL, Watzke RC. Histopathology of Best's macular dystrophy. *Arch Ophthalmol* 1982;100:1108.

138. Patrinely JR, Lewis RA, Font RL. Foveomacular vitelliform dystrophy, adult type: a clinicopathologic study including electron microscopic observations. *Ophthalmology* 1985;92:1712.

139. Jaffe GJ, Schatz H. Histopathologic features of adult-onset foveomacular pigment epithelial dystrophy. *Arch Ophthalmol* 1988;106: 958.

140. Hsieh RC, Fine BS, Lyons JS. Patterned dystrophies of the retinal pigment epithelium. *Arch Ophthalmol* 1977;95:429.

141. de Jong PTVM, Delleman JW. Pigment epithelial pattern dystrophy: four different manifestations in a family. *Arch Ophthalmol* 1982;100:1416.

142. Noble KG. Pathology of the hereditary macular dystrophies. *Sem Ophthalmol* 1987;2:110.

143. Wilson DJ, Weleber RC, Green WR. Ocular clinicopathologic study of gyrate atrophy. *Am J Ophthalmol* 1991;111:24.

144. Wilson DJ, Weleber RG, Klein ML, et al. Bietti's crystalline dystrophy: A clinicopathologic correlative study. *Arch Ophthalmol* 1989;107:213.

145. Harrison RJ, Acheson RR, Dean-Hart JC. Bietti's tapetoretinal degeneration with marginal corneal dystrophy (crystalline retinopathy): case report. *Br J Ophthalmol* 1987;71:220.

146. Small KW, Letson R, Scheinman J. Ocular findings in primary hyperoxaluria. *Arch Ophthalmol* 1990;108:89.

147. Novak MA, Roth AS, Levine MR. Calcium oxalate retinopathy associated with methoxyflurane abuse. *Retina* 1988;8:230.

148. Wells CG, Johnson RJ, Qingli L, et al. Retinal oxalosis: a clinicopathologic report. *Arch Ophthalmol* 1989;107:1638.

149. McDonnell JM, Green WR, Maumenee IH. Ocular histopathology of systemic mucopolysaccharidosis, type II-A (Hunter syndrome, severe). *Ophthalmology* 1985;92:1772.

150. Lavery MA, Green WR, Jabs EW, et al. Ocular histopathology and ultrastructure of Sanfilippo's syndrome, type III-B. *Arch Ophthalmol* 1983;101:1263-1274, 1983.

151. Cibis GW, Harris DJ, Chapman AL, et al. Mucolipidosis I. *Arch Ophthalmol* 1983;101:933.

152. Usui T, Sawaguchi S, Abe H, et al. Late-infantile type galactosialidosis: histopathology of the retina and optic nerve. *Arch Ophthalmol* 1991;109:542.

153. Matthews JD, Weiter JJ, Kolodny EH. Macular halos associated with Niemann-Pick type B disease. *Ophthalmology* 1986;93:933.

154. Zarbin MA, Green WR, Moser HW, et al. Farber's disease: light and electron microscopy of the eye. *Arch Ophthalmol* 1985;103: 73.

155. Craythorn JM, Swartz M, Creel DJ. Clofazimine-induced bull's eye retinopathy. *Retina* 1986;6:50.

156. Ramsey MS, Fine BS. Chloroquine toxicity in the human eye: histopathologic observations by electron microscopy. *Am J Ophthalmol* 1972;73:229.

157. Miller FS III, Bunt-Milam AH, Kalina RE. Clinical–ultrastructural study of thioridazine retinopathy. *Ophthalmology* 1982;89:1478.

158. Kaiser-Kupfer MI, Kupfer C, Rodrigues MM. Tamoxifen retinopathy: a clinicopathologic report. *Ophthalmology* 1981;88:89.

159. Chang TS, Aylward GW, Clarkson JG, et al. Asymmetric canthaxanthin retinopathy. *Am J Ophthalmol* 1995;119:801.

160. Brown GC, Shields JA, Sanborn G, et al. Radiation retinopathy. *Ophthalmology* 1982;89:1494.

161. Midena E, Segato T, Piermarocchi S, et al. Retinopathy following radiation therapy of paranasal sinus and nasopharyngeal carcinoma. *Retina* 1987;7:142.

162. Boozalis GT, Schachat AP, Green WR. Subretinal neovascularization from the retina in radiation retinopathy. *Retina* 1987;7:156.

163. Tso MOM, Wallow IHL, Powell JO, et al. Recovery of the rod and cone cells after photic injury. *Trans Am Acad Ophthalmol Otolaryngol* 1972;76:1247.

164. McDonald HR, Irvine AR. Light-induced maculopathy from the operating microscope in extracapsular cataract extraction and intraocular lens implantation. *Ophthalmology* 1983;90:945.

165. Kuhn F, Morris R, Massey M. Photic retinal injury from endoillumination during vitrectomy. *Am J Ophthalmol* 1991;111:42.

166. Michels M, Sternberg P Jr. Operating microscope-induced retinal phototoxicity: pathophysiology, clinical manifestations and prevention. *Surv Ophthalmol* 1990;34:237.

167. Rinkoff J, Machemer R, Hida T, et al. Temperature-dependent light damage to the retina. *Am J Ophthalmol* 1986;102:452.

168. Swartz M. Histology of macular photocoagulation. *Ophthalmology* 1986;93:959.

169. Wilson DJ, Green WR. Argon laser panretinal photocoagulation for diabetic retinopathy: scanning electron microscopy of human choroidal vascular casts. *Arch Ophthalmol* 1987;105:239.

170. Landers MB III, Stefansson E, Wolbarsht ML. Panretinal photocoagulation and retinal oxygenation. *Retina* 1982;2:167.

171. Thomas EL, Apple DJ, Swartz M, et al. Histopathology and ultrastructure of krypton and argon laser lesions in a human retinachoroid. *Retina* 1984;4:22.

172. Smiddy WE, Fine SL, Green WR, et al. Clinicopathologic correlation of krypton red, argon blue-green, and argon green laser photocoagulation in the human fundus. *Retina* 1984;4:15.

173. Bastek JV, Foos RY, Heckenlively J. Traumatic pigmentary retinopathy. *Am J Ophthalmol* 1981;92:621.

174. Aguilar JP, Green WR. Choroidal rupture: a histopathologic study of 47 cases. *Retina* 1984;4:269.

175. Sipperley JO, Quigley HA, Gass JDM. Traumatic retinopathy in primates: the explanation of commotio retinae. *Arch Ophthalmol* 1978;96:2267.

176. Blodi BA, Johnson MW, Gass JDM, et al. Purtscher's-like retinopathy after childbirth. *Ophthalmology* 1990;97:1654.

177. Stoumbos VD, Klein ML, Goodman S. Purtscher's-like retinopathy in chronic renal failure. *Ophthalmology* 1992;99:1833.

178. Kincaid MC, Green WR, Kelley JS. Acute ocular leukemia. *Am J Ophthalmol* 1979;87:698.

179. Yannuzzi LA, Shakin JL, Fisher YL, et al. Peripheral retinal de-

tachments and retinal pigment epithelial atrophic tracts secondary to central serous pigment epitheliopathy. *Ophthalmology* 1984;91: 1554.

180. Schatz H, McDonald HR, Johnson RN, et al. Subretinal fibrosis in central serous chorioretinopathy. *Ophthalmology* 1995;102:1077.

181. Foos RY, Simons KB. Vitreous in lattice degeneration of retina. *Ophthalmology* 1984;91:452.

182. Meyer E, Kurz GH. Retinal pits: a study of pathologic findings in two cases. *Arch Ophthalmol* 1963;70:640.

183. Smiddy WE, Green WR. Retinal dialysis: pathology and pathogenesis. *Retina* 1982;2:94.

184. Kampik A, Kenyon KR, Michels RG, et al. Epiretinal and vitreous membranes: comparative study of 56 cases. *Arch Ophthalmol* 1981;99:1445.

185. Schwartz D, de la Cruz Z, Green WR, et al. Proliferative vitreoreti-nopathy: ultrastructural study of 20 retroretinal membranes removed by vitreous surgery. *Retina* 1988;8:275.

186. González-Avila G, Lozano D, Manjarrez M-E, et al. Influence on collagen metabolism of vitreous from eyes with proliferative retinopathy. *Ophthalmology* 1995;102:1400.

187. Matsuo T. Photoreceptor outer segments in aqueous humor: key to understanding a new syndrome. *Surv Ophthalmol* 1994;39:211.

188. Netland PA, Mukai S, Covington HL. Elevated intraocular pressure secondary to rhegmatogenous retinal detachment. *Surv Ophthalmol* 1994;39:234.

189. Wilson DJ, Green WR. Histopathologic study of the effect of retinal detachment surgery on 49 eyes obtained post mortem. *Am J Ophthalmol* 1987;103:167.

190. Barr CC. The histopathology of successful retinal reattachment. *Retina* 1990;10:189.

Ophthalmic Pathology with Clinical Correlations,
edited by Joseph W. Sassani, M.D.
Lippincott-Raven Publishers, Philadelphia © 1997.

CHAPTER 12

Optic Nerve

Martha J. Farber

DEVELOPMENT

Beginning at 3 weeks' gestation, the optic nerve develops within **neuroectodermal tissue** that connects the optic vesicle to the forebrain, the optic stalk.[1] Axons from the retinal ganglion cells grow into the optic stalk beginning around the seventh week of gestation. The optic stalk neuroectoderm is transformed into astrocytes and oligodendrocytes. The astrocytes nourish the axons. Around this same time, mesodermal tissue surrounds the retrolaminar optic nerve, forming the **optic nerve sheath,** which consists of the pia, arachnoid, and dura. The pia extends into the nerve, separating the axons into nerve fiber bundles. The arachnoidal and dural sheaths surround the entire nerve.

Around the fifth month of gestation, the glial cells begin to condense in the area of the **lamina cribrosa,** and the scleral fibers grow into the nerve, forming the **lamina scleralis.** From the 16th to the 31st week of gestation, there is a massive remodeling of the optic nerve axons, resulting in a decrease from a high of 3.7 million axons to 1.2 million when completed. By the seventh month of gestation, the oligodendrocytes in the **retrolaminar** nerve begin myelinating the axons, a process that is not completed until months after birth. By birth, the optic nerve has achieved 75% of its growth, and by age 1 year the optic nerve has reached 95% of its full growth.[2]

ANATOMY

The optic nerve is composed of about 1 million axons that originate from the ganglion cell layer of the retina. Most of these axons synapse in the **lateral geniculate body** and are visual axons. Others synapse in the **superior colliculi** and **pretectal nuclei** and are concerned with pupillary light reflex and general response to light

stimuli. Axons from adjacent areas of retina bundle together as they enter the optic nerve head. Axons from the peripheral retina are in the outer nerve fiber layer, and the more central fibers are adjacent to the internal limiting membrane. Axons from the peripheral ganglion cells are located in the peripheral optic nerve head. The axons do not cross the horizontal meridian. Thus, damage to nerve fiber bundles within the optic nerve is associated with visual field loss that is inferior or superior to the meridian that bisects the optic nerve and macula horizontally. Axons temporal to the macula take a curved path around the macula. The line formed when these axons meet in the horizontal meridian is called the **horizontal raphe.**

The optic nerve is divided into anatomic regions.[3] The **intraocular nerve** (anterior optic nerve head) extends to the lamina cribrosa. The **intraorbital** (retrolaminar) **nerve** extends from the lamina cribrosa to the optic canal. The intracanalicular portion of the nerve courses through the optic canal and becomes the intracranial nerve as it emerges from the optic canal and enters the cranium.

The **intraocular** optic nerve measures about 1.5 mm in diameter and is slightly oval. The axons arriving from the nerve fiber layer complete a 90° turn into the optic nerve head. The axons in the anterior optic nerve head are supported solely by astrocytes and are easily separated by edema. Blood supply in the anterior optic nerve head is from branches of the posterior ciliary vessels and the adjacent choroidal vessels.

The axons pass through the lamina scleralis and then become myelinated, increasing the diameter to 3 to 4 mm. Posterior to the lamina scleralis, the pia separates the nerve fiber bundles, adding more support to the axons. The pia and arachnoid end at the posterior lamina cribrosa. The dura is continuous with the outer sclera. The subdural and subarachnoid spaces are continuous with these spaces surrounding the brain. Spinal fluid is present in the subarachnoid space of the optic nerve. About 10 mm behind the globe, the central retinal artery and vein

M. J. Farber: Department of Ophthalmology, Veterans Administration Medical Center—Albany, New York 12208.

pierce the dura and meninges to enter the optic nerve parenchyma. Branches from the central retinal artery, as well as branches directly from the ophthalmic artery, form the blood supply for the intraorbital optic nerve. Small capillaries course through the pial septae, supplying the nerve fiber bundles with nutrition.

Within the orbit, the optic nerve sheath is cushioned by fat and connective tissue. The intraorbital nerve is 25 mm long. This redundant length allows for some slack in the nerve within the orbit. Although the dural covering of the optic nerve is firmly attached at the optic canal, this laxity in the intraorbital portion of the optic nerve allows for extensive proptosis of the globe before the intraorbital optic nerve is compromised. Nevertheless, because of the firm attachment of the dura at the optic canal, the intracanalicular optic nerve is prone to damage from blunt trauma.

HISTOLOGY

The retinal layers, retinal pigment epithelium, and choroid end abruptly at the optic disc. The axons dip down at right angles into the nerve and are separated into bundles by astrocytes lining up in columns. Some of the astrocytes send processes to the vitreal surface of the optic disc, where a thin basement membrane is formed.

The sclera sends collagen and elastic fibers across the optic nerve canal to support the nerve fiber bundles and the posterior aspect of the globe; this structure is called the **lamina scleralis.** The central retinal artery and vein share a supporting connective tissue sheath that interdigitates with the laminar collagen fibers, creating a secure fixation of the vessels as they travel through the lamina cribrosa. Occlusion of the major blood vessels of the optic nerve most often occurs in this region due to the lack of flexibility.

Within the orbital portion of the optic nerve, the pial septae form the collagenous framework for the nerve fibers and supply the axons and glial cells with blood. Three types of glial cells are present: **astrocytes** and **oligodendrocytes** are derived from neuroectoderm, and **microglia,** derived from the reticuloendothelial system, function as scavenger or macrophage-like cells.

CONGENITAL ABNORMALITIES

Developmental anomalies of the optic nerve head are due to infectious, environmental, or chromosomal effects. They are associated with a wide range of visual deficits and central nervous system abnormalities.[4] Understanding the development of the optic nerve has increased our ability to predict which lesions will have associated defects. Magnetic resonance imaging has made it possible to confirm these defects and predict neurologic or endocrinologic problems.

Optic disc hypoplasia is the most common optic disc anomaly.[5] The degree of hypoplasia can vary from total aplasia to segmental irregularities. Clinically, a "double ring sign" is sometimes detectable; this is a ring of pigmented tissue surrounding the nerve, with a pale halo around the pigment.[6] Histopathology reveals that the halo corresponds to the sclera/lamina cribrosa junction; the inner pigment ring is the extension of the retinal pigment epithelium and retina over the outer lamina cribrosa (Fig. 12-1). The number of retinal ganglion cells and their axons is reduced in optic nerve hypoplasia. The rest of the retina appears normal.

Examination of fetuses with anencephaly at different stages of development has suggested that hypoplasia of the optic nerve is secondary to degeneration of the retinal ganglion cell axons due to faulty central nervous system connections or the influence of toxic substances, not as the result of primary retinal ganglion cell failure. **Superior segmental optic nerve hypoplasia** is pathognomonic of children with insulin-dependent diabetic mothers. Agenesis of the septum pellucidum and pituitary dysplasia (midline defects found in de Morsier syndrome) are associated with optic nerve hypoplasia 25% of the time. Growth hormone deficiency is the most common endocrinologic abnormality associated with optic nerve hypoplasia.

Excavated optic disc anomalies can arise from embryologic problems and give rise to three distinct clinical appearances. When the enlarged optic nerve is centered in a funnel-shaped excavation of the posterior retina, the defect is called the **"morning glory" disc anomaly.** Chorioretinal pigmentation characteristically surrounds the excavation, and a glial tuft of tissue is present within the center of the nerve head (Fig. 12-2).[7] The central retinal vessels have an anomalous branching pattern. The morning glory syndrome is most often seen unilaterally, in white females, and can be associated with **basal en-**

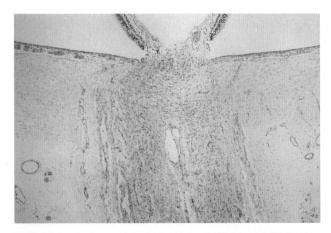

FIG. 12-1. Optic nerve hypoplasia. Note the extension of the choroid and retinal pigment epithelium over the outer lamina scleralis. This gives rise to the double ring sign seen clinically.

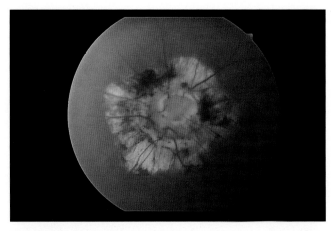

FIG. 12-2. Morning glory disc. Excavated disc is surrounded by chorioretinal pigmentation and a central tuft of glial tissue.

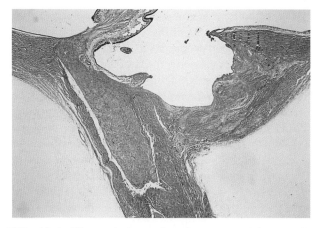

FIG. 12-4. Histopathology of optic nerve coloboma with segmental absence of nerve and adjacent tissue.

cephalocele. Midfacial anomalies, including **hypertelorism,** often are seen.

Histopathologically, there is controversy over what this anomaly represents. The presence of contractile elements in the nerve sheath and surrounding sclera suggests a mesodermal problem. Others have suggested that an anomalously large optic stalk develops at the optic vesicle stage.

Colobomas of the optic disc result from a defect in closure of the embryonic fissure that occurs in the inferonasal quadrant of the globe (Fig. 12-3). The optic disc is excavated inferiorly, and there is loss of the inferior nerve tissue. The coloboma can extend into the inferonasal choroid and retina and can be associated with ciliary body and iris colobomas. Histologic examination reveals segmentally absent nerve and adjacent tissue with thinned sclera, often containing smooth muscle strands (Fig. 12-4).

These two excavated disc anomalies should be differentiated from **posterior staphylomas** resulting from thin peripapillary scleral support and **megalopapilla** (bilateral large optic discs with otherwise normal architecture).

An **optic pit** is another result of developmental anomaly. This round or oval white depression in the optic disc often is found in the temporal disc, but it can be anywhere on the disc. The pathogenesis is uncertain and does not seem to be related to colobomas. There is a defect in the nerve tissue extending into the lamina cribrosa, which often connects to the subarachnoid space. This defect is filled with dysplastic retina.

OPTIC DISC SWELLING

There are several causes of **optic disc swelling** (Fig. 12-5).[8] Unilateral swelling is associated with local interruptions of axonal transport caused by orbital compression or local ischemia, inflammation, or hypotony. Bilateral optic disc swelling is associated with systemic disease (ie, hypertension) or increased intracranial pressure.

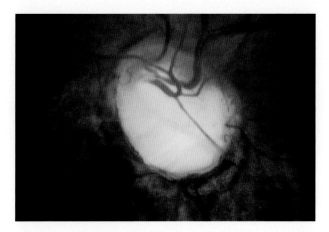

FIG. 12-3. Coloboma of the optic nerve. Inferior excavation of the optic nerve is secondary to failure of complete embryonic fissure closure.

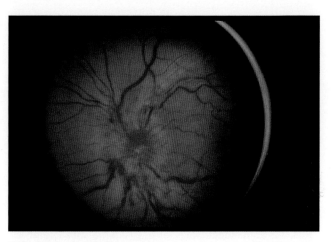

FIG. 12-5. Papilledema due to hypertension with obscuration of central retinal vessels.

Histopathologic examination of the optic nerve in experimentally induced optic disc swelling reveals blockage of axonal transport at the level of the lamina cribrosa, with distention of the nerve fibers of the optic nerve head. These nerve fibers protrude into the vitreous and expand laterally to displace the retina. This displacement of photoreceptors causes the enlarged blind spot seen on visual field testing.[9] With prolonged acute swelling, fluid may accumulate in the peripapillary subretinal space, and wrinkling of the retina in concentric rings around the disc may be apparent (Fig. 12-6). With chronic optic disc edema, atrophy of nerve fibers and their ganglion cells occurs, leading to permanent visual loss. Increased gliosis fills in the nerve head, leading to the appearance of a pale flat nerve.

Optic nerve head drusen, especially if they are not present on the surface but rather are buried in the nerve head, can mimic papilledema. They can be sporadic, inherited as an autosomal dominant trait, or associated with retinitis pigmentosa.[10] Their appearance changes over the years, and as the deposits become located more superficially in the optic nerve head, visual field loss, peripapillary hemorrhages, and subretinal neovascular membranes may develop. The optic nerve head diameter usually is small, with absent cupping (Fig. 12-7).

Histopathologically, drusen are found anterior to the lamina cribrosa. They are calcified laminar aggregates (Fig. 12-8). It is believed that crowding of the axons within a small disc leads to accumulation of extracellular mitochondria, which form a nidus for drusen formation.

ISCHEMIA

Vascular disease affecting the central retinal vessels, posterior ciliary vessels, and the ophthalmic artery can cause **optic nerve infarction.** On histopathologic examination, the nerve fibers are necrotic and surrounded by

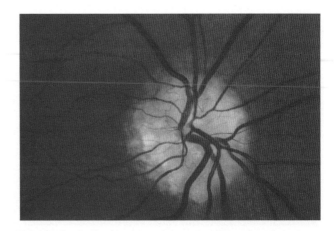

FIG. 12-7. Optic nerve head drusen. Notice the absent cup.

inflammation. Phagocytes remove the necrotic tissue. Gliosis and atrophy result. Cavernous degeneration may involve the necrotic retina anterior to the lamina cribrosa. Thrombosis, cranial arteritis (giant cell arteritis), arteriosclerosis, and infection (*Mucor, Aspergillus*) are possible causes of posterior ciliary artery and small vessel compromise in the optic nerve, leading to infarction.[11]

Occlusion of the central retinal vein occurs most often at the lamina cribrosa. Glaucoma, atherosclerosis, papilledema, diabetes, drusen, and optic nerve tumors all can initiate the occlusion. If vascular compromise is gradual, existing small-caliber blood vessels in the region may dilate, establishing collateral blood flow in time to prevent profound axonal damage. These vessels are called **optociliary shunt vessels** (Fig. 12-9).[12]

Cranial arteritis (giant cell arteritis) is an important cause of optic nerve ischemia.[13] This disease is characterized by granulomatous inflammation in the elastic lamina of larger optic nerve vessels and the posterior ciliary vessels (Fig. 12-10). The vascular lumen, markedly narrowed by the inflammation, then may become occluded by

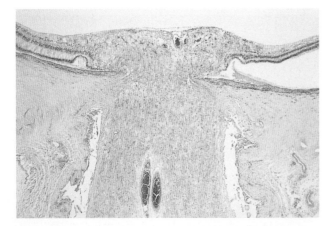

FIG. 12-6. Histopathology of papilledema with lateral displacement of photoreceptors due to nerve fiber swelling and peripapillary subretinal fluid.

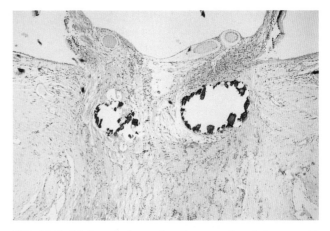

FIG. 12-8. Histopathology of optic nerve head drusen with calcifications noted in the nerve anterior to the lamina cribrosa.

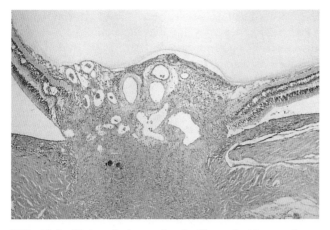

FIG. 12-9. Histopathology of optociliary shunt vessels on the optic nerve head, in this case due to optic nerve glioma.

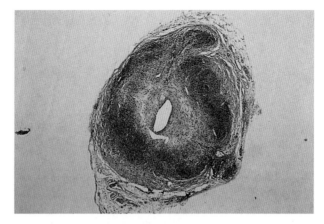

FIG. 12-11. Temporal arteritis markedly narrows the vessel lumen, leading to ischemia.

thrombus or proliferation of vascular endothelial cells (Fig. 12-11).[14] Such vascular occlusion results in pale swelling of the optic nerve head because the area of optic nerve most often involved is at or just posterior to the lamina. Biopsy of a tender temporal artery, which often has a thready pulse, can confirm the diagnosis. The fellow eye can be affected soon after the first eye manifests visual changes; therefore, immediate systemic steroid therapy is warranted. The biopsy remains positive for up to 2 weeks after initiating steroid treatment.

TRAUMA

Optic nerve pathology due to **trauma** can happen anywhere along the nerve.[15] Anteriorly, the optic nerve can be partially or totally avulsed from the globe by violent rotations of the globe. Direct injury to the optic nerve anteriorly does not rule out visual recovery. With blunt head trauma, optic nerve damage is seen in up to 5% of cases. Less frequently, the optic nerve is damaged from direct penetrating trauma. As mentioned before, the slack in the orbital optic nerve permits quite a bit of exophthalmos before the optic nerve is damaged. As the optic nerve passes through the optic canal, it is tightly bound to the dura, which in turn is fused to the periosteum of the bony optic canal. Thus, this intracanalicular portion of the nerve is more susceptible to indirect impact forces that affect the bone, as is the intracranial portion of the optic nerve underlying the falciform dural fold. These injuries can be differentiated from posterior intraorbital optic nerve injuries, which result in intrasheath hemorrhage, by magnetic resonance imaging. Fractures of the optic canal occur, but more commonly the optic nerve is damaged by shearing forces, resulting in optic nerve sheath hemorrhage and axonal damage (Fig. 12-12).[16]

Secondary mechanisms also can lead to optic nerve damage. Ongoing vascular compromise and swelling may result in further loss of axons that may not have suffered permanent damage at the time of the initial injury. Delayed visual loss, which occurs in less than 10% of cases

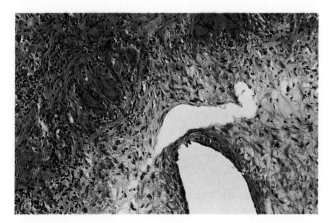

FIG. 12-10. Histopathology of temporal arteritis with granulomatous inflammation in the area of the elastic lamina.

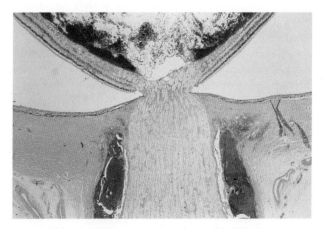

FIG. 12-12. Histopathology of subdural hemorrhage due to child abuse. The hemorrhage is believed to be secondary to shearing forces on the bridging vessels.

of optic nerve trauma, has the greatest potential for recovery with aggressive therapy.

INFLAMMATION

Inflammation of the optic nerve can result from both infectious and noninfectious causes. Optic neuritis produces visual loss because inflammation of the optic nerve causes axonal damage. One cause of this condition is **multiple sclerosis,** a demyelinating disease of the central nervous system.[17] The cause of multiple sclerosis remains unknown. Histopathologic studies of the optic nerve in multiple sclerosis reveal discrete zones of demyelination and loss of oligodendrocytes, the cells that make myelin.[18] These zones surround blood vessels, and there is perivascular lymphocytic cuffing and prominent glial proliferation. Up to 85% of optic neuritis patients eventually develop multiple sclerosis, and about 50% of multiple sclerosis patients have evidence of previous optic neuritis. If the inflammation is in the anterior optic nerve head (papillitis, neuroretinitis), there will be optic nerve head swelling. Often, however, posterior optic neuritis produces no clinical signs except decreased central vision with cecocentral scotomas and an afferent pupillary defect. Patients often report pain when moving the eye. Magnetic resonance imaging is the most sensitive test to diagnose multiple signal abnormalities consistent with multiple sclerosis or to reveal findings consistent with other causes of optic nerve disease. The clinician must exclude other causes of optic neuropathy, such as compressive lesions, before diagnosing retrobulbar optic neuritis.

Noninfectious inflammatory optic nerve swelling can also be caused by **sarcoidosis.**[19] Magnetic resonance imaging reveals a diffuse swelling of the nerve. Histopathology reveals diffuse infiltration of the nerve with noncaseating granulomas. Diagnosis is confirmed by biopsy of other involved tissue (conjunctiva, lacrimal gland, lung, or intraocular tissue). Multiple biopsy sites and microscopic examination of multiple sections is important before excluding this entity.

Collagen vascular diseases, including **Wegener's granulomatosis,** also may involve the optic nerve through direct extension, but more frequently they cause neuronal damage through vascular compromise secondary to a vasculitis.[20] A case of **juvenile xanthogranuloma** has been reported that involved the optic nerve and retina, leading to rubeosis iridis and subsequent enucleation for blind painful eye.[21] Optic nerve atrophy due to diffuse sclerosis of nerve fiber bundles and demyelination is a feature of some inherited metabolic disorders, including **Leigh's disease,** the **leukodystrophies,**[22] and acute **disseminated encephalomyelitis.**

Infectious causes of optic neuritis include bacterial (syphilis, tuberculosis), viral (cytomegalovirus, herpes zoster),[23] fungal (*Cryptococcus*),[24] and parasitic (toxoplasmosis). They may involve the optic nerve through direct extension from adjacent structures (retina, orbit, brain) or arrive via hematogenous spread.

TUMORS

Most **tumors of the optic nerve** are secondary tumors.[25] Of 205 optic nerve tumors at the Massachusetts Eye and Ear Infirmary, 18% were primary. Of the remaining 169 lesions, 79% were direct extensions from intraocular tumors. The optic nerve becomes involved by such lesions through direct invasion from primary tumors of the globe (retinoblastoma, melanoma), orbit, or brain or from hematogenous spread. Intraocular hematogenous spread of tumors, with secondary extension into the optic nerve, is involved in about 40% of cases. Metastases from breast and lung carcinomas are most common. In 13% to 18% of cases, leukemia causes papilledema and pallor, with or without increased intracranial pressure.[26] Optic nerve involvement in leukemia is much more common now that chemotherapy is prolonging the course of this disease. Lymphoma[27] and multiple myeloma[28] also may invade the optic nerve in longstanding cases, but these are rare events.

When **retinoblastoma** invades the optic nerve beyond the lamina cribrosa, the prognosis for survival worsens. Retinoblastomas manifesting glaucoma, seeding, necrosis, and an undifferentiated histologic pattern are associated with an increased incidence of optic nerve invasion. Uveal melanomas with a juxtapapillary location, epithelioid cell types, necrosis, and invasion of retina lead to increased invasion of the optic nerve.[29]

Primary tumors of the optic nerve can be benign or malignant. Gliomas of the optic nerve account for 65% of primary optic nerve tumors.[30] They most often are benign and usually occur in the first decade of life. If confined to the intraorbital optic nerve, mortality is about 5%, but if the chiasm is involved, mortality is 50%. **Malignant optic glioma** is a distinct tumor occurring in middle-aged patients and is often fatal.[31] Gliomas or pilocytic astrocytomas arise from slow-growing astrocytes and oligodendrocytes. Mitotic figures are rare. Growth often is self-limited. Of neurofibromatosis patients, 15% to 20% have gliomas that may be multifocal or bilateral without chiasmal involvement. Clinical manifestations include exophthalmos, optociliary shunt vessels, and optic atrophy. Grossly, the tumor is fusiform. The dura is intact.[32] Two types of growth patterns have been described. One involves lesions that break through into the perineural space and proliferate under an intact dura. They are more often associated with neurofibromatosis. The second growth pattern involves proliferation within the optic nerve parenchyma, with expansion of the

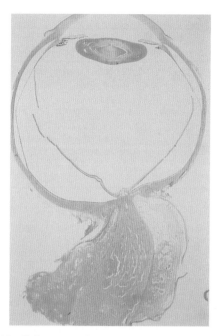

FIG. 12-13. Full-mount photo of optic nerve glioma involving the nerve parenchyma and sheath.

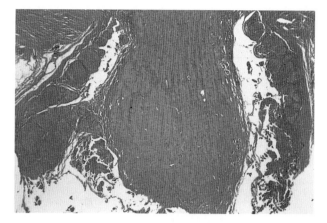

FIG. 12-15. Whorls of meningioma cells within the perineural space.

pial trabeculae (Fig. 12-13).[33] Histologically, the tumor cells are spindle cells with dilated eosinophilic cytoplasmic processes called **Rosenthal fibers** (Fig. 12-14). Growth occurs due to proliferating glia, vascular congestion, meningeal hyperplasia, and reactive gliosis. Arachnoidal hyperplasia often can be confused with meningioma if incisional biopsy is performed for diagnosis.[34] Clinical attention to the existence of extradural extension favors meningioma in these cases.

Primary meningioma of the optic nerve arises from the perineural space and consists of whorls of meningeal cells in which calcified **psammoma bodies** develop (Fig. 12-15).[35] Mitoses are rare. Tumor growth can be stimulated by pregnancy. Meningiomas, the second most common primary optic nerve tumor, are also benign. They

are detected much earlier (first and second decade of life) than intracranial or orbital meningiomas and are more commonly associated with neurofibromatosis. The tumor frequently extends through the dura into the orbital space, thus causing little optic nerve compression and resulting in little visual disturbance until the tumor is large. Meningiomas grow slowly and are more common in women. Left untreated, the tumor continues to grow slowly and can cause optic nerve edema, optociliary shunt vessels, and ultimately disc pallor. Metastases do not occur; however, multiple sites may arise simultaneously or may represent spread along pial trabeculae. Magnetic resonance imaging offers excellent differentiation of the optic nerve tumors.

Melanocytoma, a primary pigmented tumor of the optic nerve, occurs more frequently in heavily pigmented people.[36] It often is located in the anterior optic nerve head and laminar optic nerve. Clinically, it is a deeply pigmented tumor with feathery margins that grows very slowly (Fig. 12-16). The melanocytes that make up the tumor have benign, small, round nuclei with abundant

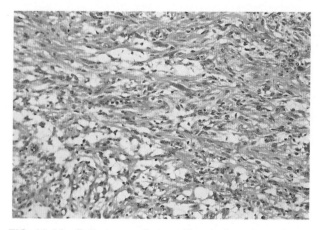

FIG. 12-14. Optic nerve glioma with spindle cells and cytoplasmic eosinophilic processes (Rosenthal fibers).

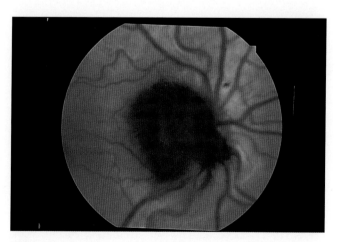

FIG. 12-16. Optic nerve melanocytoma with feathery margins.

TABLE 1. *Optic nerve head lesions*

Optic nerve head lesion	Associated systemic abnormalities	Inheritance	Fluorescein angiogram
Capillary hemangioma	von Hippel-Lindau disease, CNS hemangiomas, pheochromocytoma, renal cell CA	Sporadic, autosomal dominant	Lesion fills during arteriolar phase, leaks late
Cavernous hemangioma	CNS cavernous hemangioma, cutaneous vascular lesions	Autosomal dominant	Lesion is early hypofluorescent with filling with or after the venous phase; no leakage
Astrocytic hamartoma	Tuberous sclerosis, mental deficiency, seizures, adenoma sebaceum, intravenous calcifications	Autosomal dominant	Autofluorescence with prominent vessels that leak late

pigment in the cytoplasm. Metastases have not been reported, but slow growth is possible and can cause visual loss through neuronal or vascular compromise, especially when the laminar optic nerve is involved.[37] Capillary hemangiomas, cavernous hemangiomas, and astrocytic hamartomas all may occur on the anterior optic nerve head.[38] They may be present as isolated tumors, or they may be associated with systemic abnormalities, which are inherited in an autosomal dominant pattern (Table 12-1).

DEGENERATIONS

Optic atrophy can occur from damage to the retinal ganglion cell bodies (**ascending atrophy**) or from injury occurring anywhere along the optic nerve up to the synapse in the lateral geniculate body, which results in **descending atrophy** of the retinal ganglion cell layer. Once the optic nerve fibers are damaged, they are replaced with glial cells and increased connective tissue within the pial septae. The optic nerve decreases in caliber, resulting in widening of the subdural space (Fig. 12-17). Loss of the corresponding ganglion cells occurs, but no transsynaptic degeneration of the inner nuclear or outer nuclear layers of the retina is found.[39]

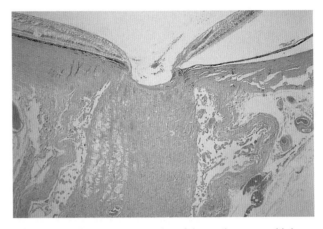

FIG. 12-18. Cavernous atrophy of the optic nerve with large spaces in the retrolaminar nerve due to acute ischemia.

In a special form of optic nerve degeneration called **cavernous atrophy** or **Schnabel's cavernous optic atrophy,** large spaces develop in the retrolaminar optic nerve as a result of hydropic degeneration of nerve fiber bundles, thought to be due to acute ischemia (Fig. 12-18). Alcian blue staining reveals that these spaces are filled with mucopolysaccharides sensitive to hyaluronidase (Fig. 12-19). This material may represent vitreous that

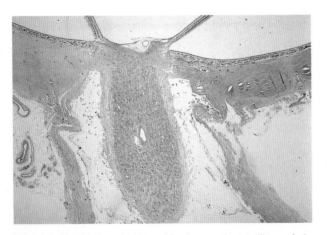

FIG. 12-17. Optic atrophy with decreasing caliber of the nerve parenchyma resulting in widening of the subdural space (×20).

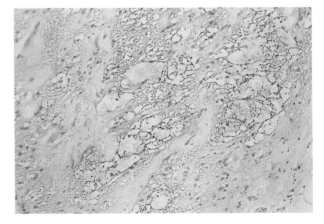

FIG. 12-19. Positive alcian blue staining of cavernous spaces in the optic nerve (×200).

migrates in to fill the spaces. This process is most often associated with high pressures in glaucoma leading to ischemia, but it can be seen with atherosclerosis and other conditions that can cause optic nerve ischemia without high intraocular pressure.[40]

REFERENCES

1. Hogan, Weddell. Optic nerve. In: *Histology of the human eye.* Philadelphia: WB Saunders, 1971:523.
2. Rimmer S, Keating C, Chou T, et al. Growth of the human optic disk and nerve during gestation, childhood and early adulthood. *Am J Ophthalmol* 1993;116:748.
3. Reeh MJ, Wobig JL, Wirtschafter JD. Ophthalmic anatomy: a manual with some clinical applications. San Francisco: American Academy of Ophthalmology, 1981:167.
4. Brodsky MC. Congenital optic disk anomalies. *Surv Ophthalmol* 1994;39:89.
5. Mosier MA, Lieberman MF, Green WR, Knox DL. Hypoplasia of the optic nerve. *Arch Ophthalmol* 1978;96:1437.
6. Lambert SR, Hoyt CS, Narahara MH. Optic nerve hypoplasia. *Surv Ophthalmol* 1987;32:1.
7. Manschot WA. Morning glory syndrome: a histopathological study. *Br J Ophthalmol* 1990;74:568.
8. Spencer. Optic nerve. In: *Ophthalmic pathology: an atlas and textbook,* 3d ed. Philadelphia: WB Saunders, 1986:2337.
9. Hayreh SS. Fluids in the anterior part of the optic nerve in health and disease. *Surv Ophthalmol* 1978;23:1.
10. Friedman AH, Beckerman B, Gold DH, Walsh JB, Gartner S. Drusen of the optic disc. *Surv Ophthalmol* 1977;21:375.
11. Yanoff M, Fine BS. Optic nerve. In: *Ocular pathology: a text and atlas,* 3d ed. Philadelphia: JB Lippincott, 1989:479.
12. Imes RK, Schatz H, Hoyt WF, Montiero MLR, Narahara M. Evolution of optociliary veins in optic nerve sheath meningioma. *Arch Ophthalmol* 1985;103:59.
13. Cullen JF, Coliero JA. Ophthalmic complications of giant cell arteritis. *Surv Ophthalmol* 1976;20:247.
14. Albert DM, Searl SS, Craft JL. Histologic and ultrastructural characteristics of temporal arteritis: the value of the temporal artery biopsy. *Ophthalmology* 1982;89:1111.
15. Steinsapir KD, Goldberg RA. Traumatic optic neuropathy. *Surv Ophthalmol* 1994;38:487.
16. Walsh FB, Hedges TR Jr. Optic nerve sheath hemorrhage. *Am J Ophthalmol* 1951;34:509.
17. Sergott RC, Brown MJ. Current concepts of the pathogenesis of optic neuritis associated with multiple sclerosis. *Surv Ophthalmol* 1988;33:108.
18. Prineas J. Pathology of the early lesion in multiple sclerosis. *Hum Pathol* 1975;6:531.
19. Beck AD, Newman NJ, Grossniklaus HE, Galetta SL, Kramer TR. Optic nerve enlargement and chronic visual loss. *Surv Ophthalmol* 1994;38:555.
20. Belden CJ, Hamed LM, Mancusco AA. Bilateral isolated retrobulbar optic neuropathy in limited Wegener's granulomatosis. *J Clin Neuro-ophthalmol* 1993;13:119.
21. Wertz FD, Zimmerman LE, McKeown CA, et al. Juvenile xanthogranuloma of the optic nerve, disc, retina, and choroid. *Ophthalmology* 1982;89:1331.
22. Cohen SMZ, Green WR, De La Cruz ZC, et al. Ocular histopathologic studies of neonatal and childhood adrenoleukodystrophy. *Am J Ophthalmol* 1983;95:82.
23. Winward KE, Hamed LM, Glaser JS. The spectrum of optic nerve disease in human immunodeficiency virus infection. *Am J Ophthalmol* 1989;107:373.
24. Ofner S, Baker RS. Visual loss in cryptococcal meningitis. *J Clin Neuro-ophthalmol* 1987;7:45.
25. Christmas NJ, Mead MD, Richardson EP, Albert DM. Secondary optic nerve tumors. *Surv Ophthalmol* 1991;36:196.
26. Kincaid M, Green WR. Ocular and orbital involvement in leukemia. *Surv Ophthalmol* 1983;27:211.
27. Guyer DR, Green WR, Schacat AP, et al. Bilateral ischemic optic neuropathy and retinal vascular occlusions associated with lymphoma and sepsis: clinicopathologic correlation. *Ophthalmology* 1990;97:882.
28. Gudas PP Jr. Optic nerve myeloma. *Am J Ophthalmol* 1971;71:1085.
29. Shammas HF, Blodi FC. Peripapillary choroidal melanomas: extension along the optic nerve and its sheaths. *Arch Ophthalmol* 1978;96:440.
30. Dutton JJ. Gliomas of the anterior visual pathway. *Surv Ophthalmol* 1994;38:427.
31. Wulc AE, Bergin DJ, Barnes MD, et al. Orbital optic nerve glioma in adult life. *Arch Ophthalmol* 1987;107:1013.
32. Yanoff M, Davis R, Zimmerman LE. Juvenile pilocytic astrocytoma (glioma) of optic nerve: clinicopathologic study of 63 cases. In: Jakobrec FA, ed. *Ocular and adnexal tumors.* Birmingham, AL: Aesculapius Publishing, 1978:685.
33. Stern J, Jakobiec FA, Housepian EM. The architecture of optic nerve gliomas with and without neurofibromatosis. *Arch Ophthalmol* 1980;98:505.
34. Marquardt MD, Zimmerman LE. Histopathology of meningiomas and gliomas of the optic nerve. *Hum Pathol* 1982;13:226.
35. Dutton JJ. Optic nerve sheath meningiomas. *Surv Ophthalmol* 1992;37:167.
36. Brown G. Tumors of the optic nerve head. *Int Ophthalmol Clin* 1993;33:147.
37. Schuey TF, Blacharski PA. Pigmented tumor and acute visual loss. *Surv Ophthalmol* 1988;33:121.
38. Brown GC, Shields JA. Tumors of the optic nerve head. *Surv Ophthalmol* 1985;29:239.
39. Radius RL. Anatomy of the optic nerve head and glaucomatous optic neuropathy. *Surv Ophthalmol* 1987;32:35.
40. Brownstein S, Font RL, Zimmerman LE, Murphy SB. Nonglaucomatous cavernous degeneration of the optic nerve. *Arch Ophthalmol* 1980;98:354.

Ophthalmic Pathology with Clinical Correlations,
edited by Joseph W. Sassani, M.D.
Lippincott-Raven Publishers, Philadelphia © 1997.

CHAPTER 13

Pathology of the Orbit

Steven A. McCormick and Lois M. McNally

Although orbital disease is relatively uncommon in general ophthalmic practice, familiarity with orbital pathology makes recognition, diagnosis, and management of these problems clinically rewarding. The incidence and prevalence of various lesions varies with the age, race, and sex of the patient. Consequently, accurate diagnosis may be challenging and usually involves various imaging modalities and often specialized pathologic techniques.

Orbital disease processes may be primary, secondary, or metastatic. **Primary processes,** such as inflammatory and lymphoid tumors, hemangiomas, and lacrimal gland fossa lesions, often produce characteristic clinical and radiologic presentations. **Secondary processes** originating in the orbital bones, paranasal sinuses, adjacent meninges, or the cranial cavity are usually discerned radiographically. Metastatic lesions from distant malignancies, which are often problematic, require thorough clinical histories and systemic evaluations for appropriate management. Imaging studies, primarily with computed tomography (CT) or magnetic resonance imaging (MRI),[1] are essential to narrow the differential diagnosis and to plan an appropriate biopsy technique if indicated.

The surgeon must narrow the differential diagnosis to optimize the pathologist's handling of the tissue after it has been obtained. Preoperative consultation with the pathologist is critical to facilitate the use of any specialized techniques needed.

ANATOMIC CONSIDERATIONS

Segments of the frontal, ethmoid, lacrimal, maxillary, sphenoid, and temporal bones and the structures of the

S. A. McCormick: Departments of Pathology, Ophthalmology, and Otolaryngology/Head and Neck Surgery, New York Medical College, Director of Pathology and Laboratory Medicine, The New York Eye and Ear Infirmary, New York, NY 10003.
L. M. McNally: Department of Ophthalmology, State University of New York Health Science Center at Brooklyn, Director of Medical Student Education, Department of Ophthalmology, The New York Eye and Ear Infirmary, New York, NY 10003.

eyelids demarcate the soft-tissue compartment known as the orbit. This enclosed space contains the globe, its supporting soft tissues, and the lacrimal apparatus, all within a mere approximate volume of 30 ml.[2] The orbital walls are lined by the **periorbita,** which continues anteriorly as the **orbital septum** and anatomically forms the anterior soft-tissue border of the orbit. The diversity of tissue types found in the orbit (the orbital segment of the optic nerve, the extraocular muscles, peripheral and cranial nerves, blood vessels, adipose and fibrous connective tissues, and the lacrimal gland) leads to the wide variety of pathologic conditions that may be encountered in the orbit.[2] Epithelial tumors, benign and malignant mesenchymal tumors, neural tumors, vascular lesions, and lymphoid and inflammatory diseases all may present in the orbit. Additionally, many complex connective tissue septa that compartmentalize the orbital soft tissues often dictate the pattern of clinical presentation.[2]

CLINICAL PRESENTATIONS

A common presentation for orbital mass lesions is **exophthalmos.** Inflammatory and infectious processes, hemorrhage, and benign and malignant tumors of the orbit, including the lacrimal gland, may produce exophthalmos. Displacement of the globe offers valuable clues that aid in the differential diagnosis. Retrobulbar and intraconal lesions typically produce axial exophthalmos,[2] whereas superior masses produce downward displacement of the globe. Superolateral orbital processes, such as zygomaticofrontal dermoid cysts or lacrimal gland fossa lesions, usually produce downward and medial exophthalmos.[2] Secondary orbital involvement by carcinomas or abscesses of fronto-ethmoid sinus origin may produce downward and lateral displacement of the globe.[2] Superior displacement of the globe with or without exophthalmos is typical in advanced maxillary sinus processes,[2] which are usually neoplastic in nature. Bilateral exophthalmos, either symmetric or asymmetric, usually indicates an inflammatory process, such as thyroid-related orbitopathy (TRO) or idiopathic orbital inflammation (IOI). Lymphoid hyperplasia, malignant lymphoma, and metastatic lesions may present as bilateral orbital masses.[2]

The degree of exophthalmos and its duration are wide ranging. Massive exophthalmos of rapid onset is unusual in neoplastic disease. Therefore, hemorrhage and inflammatory processes are more likely considerations when the patient's complaint is of short-term duration (days to a few weeks). The notable exception to this rule is rapidly progressive exophthalmos in children, which may indicate aggressive malignancies such as **rhabdomyosarcoma**[3] or, less frequently, involvement by **neuroblastoma**[4] or **granulocytic sarcoma,**[5] either primary or metastatic.

Benign neoplasms of the lacrimal gland may produce massive exophthalmos, but the progression is very slow (many months to years). The change in the patient's appearance is often so gradual that even family members fail to recognize an alarming degree of clinically evident exophthalmos. Similarly, orbital hemangiomas, varices, arteriovenous malformations, and benign neoplasms (eg, fibrous histiocytoma, schwannoma, neurofibroma) usually display an insidious progression of exophthalmos. These tumors are typically large and advanced on initial presentation.

Lymphoid tumors, both benign and malignant, typically present with an onset of intermediate duration.[6] Progressive exophthalmos over a few to several months is typical of these lesions, with the exception of high-grade malignant lymphomas. Likewise, IOI usually presents with a few month's history of exophthalmos, except in acute cases when the onset is abrupt and the presentation may mimic infectious orbital cellulitis.

Exophthalmos may be fluctuating. Lymphangiomas, particularly in the young, may present with increased exophthalmos associated with upper respiratory infections.[7] This is probably secondary to a reactive increase in the lymphoid infiltrate associated with these tumors. A ruptured dermoid cyst may lead to abruptly progressive exophthalmos that may wane as the inflammation subsides. In children, this exuberant inflammatory response may lead to a clinical presentation suggestive of malignancy. Carotid–cavernous sinus fistulae, arteriovenous malformations, and, rarely, varices may exhibit a transient increase in exophthalmos with the Valsalva maneuver.[8]

Pain is a significant complaint in the evaluation of orbital disease. Inflammatory disease of acute onset usually is accompanied by moderate to severe pain, whether the inflammation is of infectious, immune-mediated, or idiopathic etiology (Fig. 13-1). Hemorrhage, with its typically abrupt increase in orbital soft-tissue volume, may be painful. Bone erosion and perineural invasion by malignant tumors, most notably adenoid cystic carcinoma of the lacrimal gland, may incite pain of varying degrees.[9] Benign neoplasms, lymphoid tumors, chronic IOI,

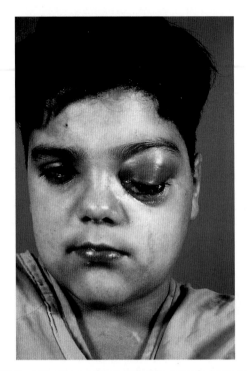

FIG. 13-1. Infectious orbital cellulitis acutely increases the orbital volume, leading to pain and exophthalmos that are important clinical parameters in evaluating orbital pathology. Erythema, massive edema, and conjunctival exudate in this patient provide useful clues in the differential diagnosis.

and TRO typically are painless, despite often-marked exophthalmos.

CLINICAL EVALUATION

Physical examination of the orbit should begin with an assessment of the periorbital structures. Common eyelid and periorbital findings include erythema, edema, skin discoloration, ecchymosis, ptosis, lid retraction, and the presence of a visible or palpable orbital mass. Hertel exophthalmometry allows quantification of the degree of exophthalmos and allows tracking of the progression or recession of a lesion over time. The direction of the globe's displacement (axial, upward, downward, medial, or temporal) should be noted and semiquantified by approximation of the axis and degree of deviation from primary position.[2]

Eyelid retraction and ''lid lag'' are hallmarks of TRO, while entropion associated with exophthalmos is a feature of many cases of chronic IOI. These findings result from secondary effects on the extraocular muscles or the soft tissues of the proximal eyelids. Plexiform neurofibroma of the anterior orbit and eyelid may cause an S-shaped deformity of the eyelid margin.[10] This results from the enlargement and elongation of eyelid nerves as the tumor's proliferation progresses within the neural sheaths.

Gross asymmetry of the facial skeleton should suggest

processes involving the orbital bones, such as fibrous dysplasia[11] or intraosseous meningioma. Again, although the asymmetry may be grossly apparent to the new examiner, the patient may be unaware of the finding because of its insidious progression in these diseases. Osseous metastases in such malignancies as prostate[12] and breast carcinoma[13] or multiple myeloma[14] may present with a more rapid progression of asymmetry of the orbital bones.

A "frozen globe" is noted in some patients with **idiopathic orbital inflammation** (IOI), advanced TRO,[15] and even chronic fungal infections. This finding results from activation or proliferation of fibroblasts, with attendant production of collagen and other extracellular matrix products.[16] Any other sclerosing process, including metastatic scirrhous carcinomas (most notably breast carcinomas), Erdheim-Chester disease, and others, may result in this presentation.

Secondary conjunctival signs often help narrow the clinical differential diagnosis. Elevated, pink subconjunctival infiltrates, sometimes with a cobblestone surface, the so-called "salmon patch," are harbingers of lymphoid neoplasia (Fig. 13-2). When associated with an orbital mass, the diagnosis of malignant lymphoma should be the primary consideration.[17] Biopsy of the conjunctival infiltrate alone is inadequate in this setting. The orbit may harbor atypical or frankly malignant lymphoid infiltrates even if the conjunctival process is histologically benign. On the contrary, an *isolated* salmon patch is more frequently benign lymphoid hyperplasia, although primary conjunctival lymphoma certainly may occur. Primary conjunctival lymphomas are usually low-grade small cell lymphocytic lymphomas and often exhibit plasmacytoid differentiation. Secondary tortuosity and enlargement of conjunctival blood vessels, resulting from altered venous drainage of the orbit, suggest vascular tumors and vascular anomalies within the orbit.[18]

Intraocular signs may accompany orbital tumors, and

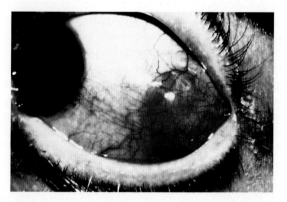

FIG. 13-2. Lymphoid lesions of the conjunctiva may be harbingers of orbital lymphoproliferation. These elevated, salmon-pink infiltrates with intact overlying conjunctiva are usually benign, although malignant lymphoma presents identically. Even if benign, these tumors may coincide with malignant disease in the orbit.

these are readily assessed by dilated fundus examination. Unsuspected intraocular tumors capable of extension into the orbit, notably malignant melanoma,[19] may be encountered. Furthermore, certain chorioretinal lesions are associated with specific orbital tumors, particularly in the phakomatoses. For example, retinal astrocytoma may be associated with optic nerve glioma,[20] eyelid or orbital neurofibroma,[21] or sphenoid wing hypoplasia in type I neurofibromatosis.[22]

Nonspecific findings related to mass effect, such as chorioretinal striae and optic disc abnormalities, may indicate the position and size of a mass lesion, but these do not usually point to specific etiologies. Chorioretinal folds generally indicate compression of the globe by an orbital mass.[23] Similarly, the optic nerve head may reveal edema, pallor, or atrophy, all of which may indicate compressive optic neuropathy. Loss of visual acuity, alteration of color perception, and relative afferent pupillary defects may be present with tumors that exert pressure on the optic nerve. Visual field and color vision testing should be performed to detect more subtle sensory abnormalities resulting from unsuspected optic neuropathy.

Anterior or posterior uveitis, or both, may accompany orbital inflammatory disease, including IOI and TRO. It is often said that uveitis may accompany sarcoidosis of the orbit or lacrimal gland, but in our experience the globe and the orbital structures are rarely simultaneously involved.

Elevation of intraocular pressure with direction of gaze as detected by applanation tonometry may occur with compressive force on the globe by an orbital mass or with a restrictive extraocular myopathy. Assessment of ocular motility and orthoptic measurement of attendant strabismus should be performed to aid diagnosis and document progression. Strabismus may be classified as restrictive, as in TRO; paretic, with lesions interrupting innervation of extraocular muscles; or simply secondary to mass effect.[9]

Palpation of the symptomatic orbit often helps in both localizing anterior processes and noting the character of the swelling. Alteration of the normal resistance of orbital tissues to retrodisplacement of the globe may help define the location of an orbital mass or discern general orbital congestion secondary to an infiltrative process. However, resistance to retropulsion of the eye may be normal in the presence of even large orbital tumors of long standing. Tense and partially cystic masses palpated in the supranasal region invoke mucocele, encephalocele, and neurofibroma in the differential diagnosis. Well-circumscribed, firm masses in the anterior supratemporal region suggest epithelial tumors of the lacrimal gland or dermoid cysts. More diffuse processes in this area suggest lymphoid or inflammatory tumors. Although the anterior orbit may be involved, angiomatous lesions and IOI are usually difficult to localize precisely with palpation. Mass lesions of the superior orbit may displace the lacrimal gland into a more accessible location, and therefore palpation of its smooth, arcuate, and rolled border may suggest pathology deeper in the supratemporal orbit.

Palpation may reveal a pulsatile mass in the orbit. Dural and orbital arteriovenous malformations and carotid–cavernous sinus fistulae are often accompanied by bruits detectable by auscultation over the closed eyelids. Pulsation without bruits may be discerned in neurofibromatosis. This finding can be secondary to either the rich vascularity of an orbital neurofibroma or the sphenoid wing hypoplasia sometimes associated with neurofibromatosis. Similarly, any other lesion that allows a relative pressure transference from the cranium, such as meningoencephaloceles or surgical removal of the orbital floor or roof, may lead to pulsatile exophthalmos.

Imaging Studies

CT and MRI have largely replaced conventional roentgenograms and tomograms in the evaluation of orbital lesions. CT is considered the optimal modality for defining the osseous components of the orbit; the effects of malignant lesions on bone and adjacent soft tissues are well demonstrated (Fig. 13-3). Although MRI is considered a superior technique for evaluating soft tissues, in the orbit most pathologic processes are adequately demonstrated by CT.[1] Consequently, CT remains the primary modality for imaging the orbit, although in certain situations, such as suspected optic nerve lesions, diffuse or ill-defined soft-tissue lesions, and cystic lesions, MRI is a useful adjunct.[1] MRI is contraindicated if there is any suspicion of intraocular or intraorbital metallic foreign bodies, because these may be dislodged and damage adjacent structures during MRI imaging.

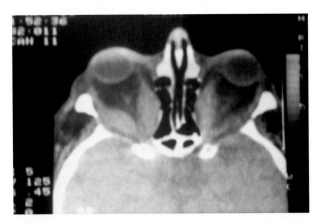

FIG. 13-3. Proptosis is often the presenting sign in patients with tumors of the orbit. Imaging studies, such as this computed axial tomogram, demonstrate the locus of the pathology, thereby aiding in the differential diagnosis. In this case, enlargement of several extraocular muscles suggests thyroid-related orbitopathy rather than a neoplastic lesion or other diffuse inflammatory process.

Ultrasonography and Other Methods

Ultrasound is a valuable tool for imaging the globe, extraocular muscles, and adjacent soft tissues. Because ultrasound often is readily accessible, in experienced hands useful information may be obtained at the patient's initial presentation. The lesion's contours, density, cystic nature, and separation from adjacent structures can be readily determined. Certain lesions may be amenable to ultrasound-guided fine-needle aspiration biopsy in the office setting, occasionally obviating the need for open biopsy. However, this technique is usually unsuitable for the definitive diagnosis of inflammatory disease and for lymphoid tumors.[24]

Plain roentgenograms of the skull are useful only in certain settings, such as primary bone diseases (eg, fibrous dysplasia). Similarly, with the advent of CT and magnetic resonance angiography (MRA), arteriography and venography are rarely used. However, these studies can be useful to evaluate lesions of the cavernous sinus, arteriovenous malformations, varices, and vascular anastomoses within the intracranial compartment. Nevertheless, advanced MRA techniques may render these modalities completely obsolete.

Pathology and Laboratory Studies

Laboratory studies, done before biopsy, can yield important clues to delimit the differential diagnosis. The clinical examination and history, as always, should guide the ordering process. If the differential leans toward inflammatory or lymphoproliferative disease, thyroid function tests, white blood cell count with differential, and serum calcium, alkaline phosphatase, and other chemical studies may be useful. Serologic markers for specific malignancies may be helpful if metastatic disease is suspected. Carcinoembryonic antigen, prostate specific antigen, CA-145 (an ovarian cancer marker), and others are available to help guide the systemic evaluation.

Because diagnostic incisional biopsy of the orbit usually yields only a relatively small amount of tissue, preoperative consultation with the pathologist is of paramount importance. The general pathologist may be unaccustomed to ophthalmic and orbital disease and therefore should be made aware in advance of the clinical diagnoses being entertained. Often, electron microscopy, immunohistochemistry, flow cytometry, and molecular analysis may be necessary for a definitive diagnosis.[25] Most of these techniques require special preparation at the time of biopsy. Frozen section analysis often is required, especially if a lymphoproliferative process is suspected. Accurate diagnosis may be compromised if the specimen is inadequate for the pathologist's analysis. It is good practice to obtain the pathologist's opinion at the time of the procedure as to whether the biopsy is adequate for pathologic evaluation.

CLASSIFICATION OF ORBITAL PATHOLOGY

It is helpful to begin developing a differential diagnosis of orbital pathologic processes according to age at presentation. The incidence of disease processes varies among infants, children, and adults. Furthermore, initial consideration of any orbital process should attempt to place it in one of the classic categories of pathologic processes: congenital, infectious, inflammatory, immune-mediated, neoplastic, or degenerative.

ORBITAL PATHOLOGY IN CHILDREN

Congenital Malformations

Congenital malformations of the orbit and ocular tissue usually are manifest at or shortly after birth. **Craniofacial dysostoses** cause gross asymmetry, easily established by radiographic and clinical parameters. Tissue rarely is obtained in this setting, but it would be composed of architecturally normal elements. Overgrowth of a tissue element that is normally present in a given anatomic location, with varying degrees of disorganization, is known as a **hamartoma** (from the Greek *hamartion,* a bodily defect). Examples include infantile hemangiomas and neurofibromatosis (discussed below). The presence of normal or disorganized tissue elements *not* usually present in a given anatomic location is known as a choristoma (from the Greek *choristos,* separated). Cystic epidermoid lesions, neural choristomas (ectopic brain with or without a cystic component), and ectopic lacrimal gland are examples. All may affect orbital growth and may produce secondary exophthalmos.

Microphthalmos with cyst, caused by incomplete closure of the embryonic choroidal fissure, may cause exophthalmos and orbital malformation (Fig. 13-4). The cystic outpouching of the sclera is lined by disorganized retinal and glial tissue, often with a choroid-like vascular layer. The cyst usually lies inferior to the microphthalmic eye and produces superior exophthalmos. It is important to differentiate microphthalmos with cyst from encephalocele, meningocele, and meningomyelocele before surgical intervention, as these entities usually maintain a connection with the cranial cavity. Other congenital abnormalities of ocular development, such as anophthalmia, synophthalmia, microphthalmia, and congenital cystic eye, each may produce secondary malformations of the orbit.[26]

Congenital Epithelial Cystic Lesions

Most congenital cystic lesions are typical **dermoid cysts.** These are choristomas formed as the embryo devel-

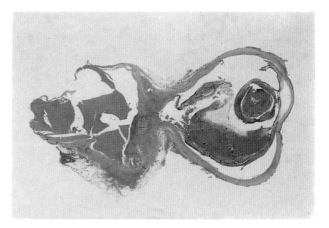

FIG. 13-4. A microphthalmic eye with disorganized contents displays a cystic outpouching of sclera partially lined by a choroid-like layer and filled with disorganized retinoglial tissue. In other cases with severe microphthalmos, the cyst may be much larger than the eye. This pathology results from the incomplete closure of the embryonic fissure during ocular development.

ops by sequestration or "pinching off" of epidermal anlage at the time of closure of the osseous cranial suture lines. Clinically, these lesions are found most commonly in the superolateral orbit along the zygomaticofrontal suture. Although usually discovered in childhood, adult presentation of a dermoid cyst is possible, especially if it is located more deeply in the orbit posterior to the orbital septum. Histologic examination reveals normal skin elements, including epidermis, skin adnexa (eg, hair, sebaceous glands), and dermal tissue (Fig. 13-5).

Simple epithelial inclusion cysts usually are lined by keratinized stratified squamous epithelium and are filled with keratinous debris. Other rarer examples of simple epithelial cysts are lined by respiratory, apocrine, or lacrimal ductal epithelium.

The surgeon must use great care when excising cystic inclusions of the orbit to avoid spilling their contents in the orbit, because a foreign body granulomatous inflammatory reaction can result. The cysts may rupture after minor trauma, inciting a severe inflammatory reaction with rapidly increasing exophthalmos; in this setting, biopsy to rule out malignancy often is performed.[27]

Infectious Cellulitis and Inflammatory Disease in Childhood

In children, **cellulitis** is usually of bacterial etiology. The clinician must distinguish between preseptal and postseptal presentations to institute appropriate therapy. Preseptal cases usually are related temporally to upper respiratory or ear infections; in children under 5 years of age, *Haemophilus influenzae* is the most common etiologic agent. A history of trauma or skin infection may be elicited. The inflammation, edema, and erythema may be

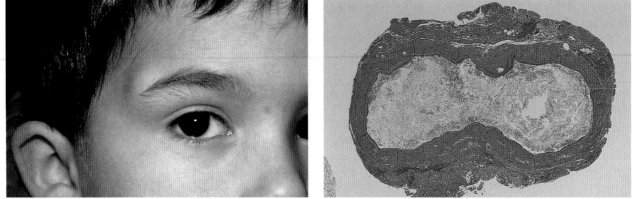

FIG. 13-5. Congenital dermoid cysts usually present overlying the zygomaticofrontal suture (**A**). They display derivatives of the primary epidermal germ layer in the wall of the cyst, including pilosebaceous units. The cyst contains the keratinous debris of desquamation and variable amounts of hair (**B**). Progressive enlargement and minor trauma may lead to rupture, often resulting in an intense inflammatory response mimicking infectious cellulitis.

quite severe, making a thorough examination difficult. If fever and septicemia are present, postseptal involvement is likely, and aggressive evaluation and treatment are necessary. Samples for microbiologic analysis and Gram stain may be taken from the conjunctival exudate or from tissues obtained from debridement.

Fever and signs of sepsis are often noted in more advanced cases of postseptal or orbital cellulitis. Compromised orbital function, including restricted ductions, ptosis, exophthalmos, chemosis, and pain, may be evident. A relative afferent pupillary defect and decreased color vision, indicating compromised optic nerve function, may be found in severe cases. CT scanning may help localize the source of infection.[28] Processes extending from adjacent periorbital structures, most commonly the paranasal sinuses but occasionally dental infections or dacryocystitis, are easily evaluated by CT. These causes are more common in adults.

Exogenous agents, foreign bodies, trauma, or postoperative complications all may result in pre- or postseptal cellulitis. Bacteremia may result in endogenous seeding of the orbital tissues from a distant source. Severe endophthalmitis or panophthalmitis may present as orbital cellulitis due to the extensive inflammation.[29]

Noninfectious causes of orbital inflammation are less common in children than in adults, but TRO and IOI may present in childhood. These entities are discussed in the section dealing with adults.

Benign Neoplasms of the Pediatric Orbit

Neoplastic disease is relatively uncommon in children and in large series represents only a fraction of the orbital pathology presenting in this age group. However, certain specific neoplastic entities are most common in this population.

Vascular Tumors

Capillary hemangioma is the most common benign neoplasm found in the orbit of children (Fig. 13-6). This tumor may be present congenitally, but it typically presents in early infancy, occasionally in association with facial skin hemangiomas. The orbital component may enlarge rapidly, causing great alarm in the parents and the ophthalmologist. Because this presentation may mimic a malignancy, biopsy may be performed.

The natural history of this tumor is spontaneous involution, although exophthalmos during its course may be profound. The eyelid may be involved, resulting in ptosis, occlusion of the pupillary axis, or astigmatism with the threat of subsequent amblyopia. If such clinical findings warrant, excision or treatment with corticosteroid injection is indicated. No controlled studies have been performed, but steroid injection is advocated by many to produce more rapid regression of vasoproliferative activity.

Histologic examination of these lesions reveals cellular proliferation of benign endothelium, pericytes, and stromal elements. In early lesions, the luminal spaces may be obscured by the plump, proliferative endothelial cells that are often vaguely arranged in lobular configurations. At this time, the benign vascular nature of the lesion may not be readily apparent; the tumor may even mimic a solid, malignant mesenchymal tumor. Thin paraffin sections (3 microns) or resin-embedded "thick sections" (1 micron thick) may allow resolution of the capillary lumina. As these vessels mature, cellularity decreases and

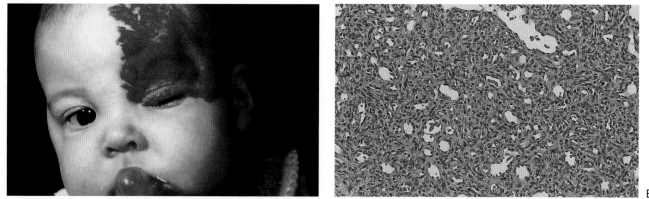

A   B

FIG. 13-6. In children, capillary hemangiomas of the orbit may present with skin involvement (**A**), exhibiting a red "papier-mâché" appearance. Histologically, the lesions are hypercellular initially with small, sometimes imperceptible vascular lumina (**B**). As the lesions mature, the arborizing capillary network is more apparent, with larger-caliber feeder vessels visible at low power.

the underlying network of large, central feeder vessels branching centripetally to form a capillary network is recognized. Immunohistochemistry can detect factor VIII expression in the endothelial cells, confirming their vascular origin.[30]

Lymphangiomas occur in the orbit, eyelid, and conjunctiva of children, adolescents, and young adults; presentation in later life is relatively uncommon. The pathogenesis of these lesions remains enigmatic because lymphatic vessels have not been definitively identified in the human orbit (Fig. 13-7). Consequently, some consider this tumor a choristoma, but others suggest that this lesion does not occur in the orbit and is truly a variant of more typical hemangiomas. Nevertheless, electron microscopy

and careful routine microscopy allow differentiation of lymphangioma from other vascular lesions of the orbit. The tumor is formed by sinuous channels incompletely lined by endothelium, lacking pericyte support. Irregular septate projections into the channels may be present; these have been likened to the pseudovalves of the normal lymphatic vasculature. Lymphoid aggregates, often with well-formed germinal centers, are typically present. The stroma contains a delicate capillary network that is often intimately apposed to the lymphatic channels. These fine vessels may rupture, leading to hemorrhage into the lymphatic vascular spaces and resulting in "chocolate" or "blood cysts" that surgically and histologically suggest cavernous hemangiomas. It is possible, however, to eliminate this diagnosis if endothelial linings are incomplete, if the capillary network in the stroma is well developed, and if aggregates of lymphoid tissue are present. These are features of lymphangioma and are not usually seen in hemangiomas. During upper respiratory infections, the lymphoid tissue component may increase and lead to clinical enlargement, a helpful diagnostic clue. Lymphangiomas are usually not well encapsulated, and involvement of several contiguous orbital structures as well as the paranasal sinuses may make complete excision surgically difficult or impossible.[31,32]

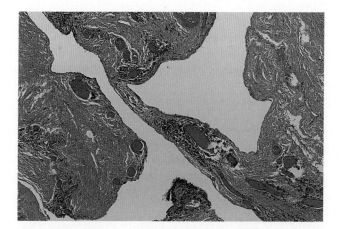

FIG. 13-7. Although lymphatic vasculature has not been convincingly demonstrated in the human orbit, lymphangiomas are well described histopathologically in this location. This tumor displays irregular vascular spaces incompletely lined by widely spaced endothelial cells. The intervening stroma contains a rich capillary network and scattered lymphoid infiltrates, often with germinal center formation. These capillaries may rupture into the lymphatic spaces and partially fill them with blood. This common finding leads to confusion with cavernous hemangiomas.

Neural Tumors

Optic nerve gliomas typically present in the first decade of life with exophthalmos, strabismus, decreased vision, and at times an afferent pupillary defect. Clinically, disc edema, optic atrophy, or retinal striae from posterior pressure may all be seen. Neurofibromatosis is present in 25% to 50% of the patients. Optic nerve gliomas involve the intraorbital segment of the optic nerve in about half the cases; in the other half, they involve the intracranial segment. Neuroimaging reveals a fusiform enlargement of the optic nerve, with or without expansion of the optic canal (Fig. 13-8).[33,34] Pathologically, the tumors are pilocytic (hair-like) astrocytomas, with little or no mitotic activity. The thin cell processes assume a loose, whorled arrangement. Associated reactive arachnoid cells can lead to an erroneous diagnosis of meningioma.[35] Treatment is controversial and must be tailored to the patient's clinical course; observation, excision,[36] and radiation therapy have all been advocated.[37]

Neurofibromas may occur in children, usually in association with neurofibromatosis (discussed below in the section on neurogenic tumors of the adult orbit).

Malignant Neoplasms of the Pediatric Orbit

Rhabdomyosarcoma is the most common primary orbital malignancy in children. It typically presents at 7 to 8 years of age with rapidly expanding unilateral exophthalmos. The rapid growth and attendant signs of mild inflammation may lead to confusion with infectious cellulitis.[38] Imaging studies and biopsy should be performed emergently to rule out or confirm this diagnosis. If this diagnosis is made, a metastatic workup should likewise be performed so that appropriate staging and treatment with orbital irradiation, multiagent chemotherapy, or both may begin.[39] Dramatic advances in survival have been made during the past two decades, largely due to the clinical studies of the Intergroup Rhabdomyosarcoma Study. Consequently, patients should be enrolled in its protocols for appropriate, contemporary therapy. Biopsy specimens reveal a malignant neoplasm with skeletal

muscle differentiation (Fig. 13-9), although this tumor apparently originates from pluripotential mesenchymal cells of the orbit rather than extant skeletal muscle in the orbit. Regardless of histologic subtype, demonstration of skeletal muscle differentiation may be determined in routine sections by detecting cytoplasmic cross-striations or evidence of skeletal muscle differentiation by electron microscopy.[40] Currently, immunohistochemical expression of skeletal muscle myosin or actin is a direct and very effective method of confirming the histologic diagnosis.[41]

There are four histologic subtypes of rhabdomyosarcoma. Embryonal rhabdomyosarcoma, the most common histologic type in children, usually arises in the supranasal orbit. Histologically, the tumor is composed of undifferentiated ovoid to short spindle-shaped cells arranged in clusters and short fascicles. These cells mimic the undifferentiated mesenchyme seen in the developing embryo. Immunochemistry or electron microscopy is usually necessary to confirm the diagnosis.[42–44]

Alveolar rhabdomyosarcoma is less common but has a more aggressive, more malignant behavior. Histologically, it is composed of small to medium-sized round cells, draped from a delicate fibrovascular network. Artifactitious retraction of these cells, which have scant cytoplasm, results in a histologic pattern resembling the alveolar spaces of the lung (hence the name). This type is considered one of the "small round blue cell tumors of infancy," along with primitive neuroectodermal tumors (eg, retinoblastoma, neuroblastoma), Ewing's sarcoma, and others.[45] Special techniques are often necessary to confirm skeletal muscle differentiation.[43,46]

Pleomorphic (or differentiated) **rhabdomyosarcoma** has the highest degree of differentiation, with large cells exhibiting a large, eccentric cytoplasmic body that occasionally contains cross-striations. These have been termed **strap cells.** This type is relatively rare in the orbit but has the best prognosis. It is the type usually reported in the few examples of rhabdomyosarcoma presenting in adults.[43]

Botryoid rhabdomyosarcoma is another subtype not encountered as an orbital primary. It has been described in the conjunctiva and paranasal sinuses with secondary orbital invasion. The exophytic "cluster of grapes" external appearance leads to its name; it is more common in the genitourinary tract.[43]

Metastatic and Secondary Tumors in the Pediatric Orbit

Metastatic malignancy can become manifest in the orbit in children. Often the primary is already known, but exophthalmos secondary to metastasis may be the presenting sign.

Neuroblastoma, a malignant neuroectodermal tumor, usually arises in the adrenal gland (50%) but may be

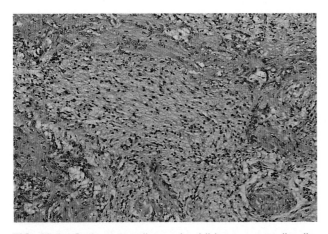

FIG. 13-8. Optic nerve gliomas in children are usually pilocytic astrocytomas, presenting long, slender hair-like cells with elongated nuclei expanding and altering the underlying framework of the optic nerve. Typically, the nerve sheath remains intact, but visual function is compromised by the encroachment of the proliferating glial cells. Fusiform enlargement of the optic nerve is the usual finding in imaging studies. (Courtesy of Norman Charles, M.D.).

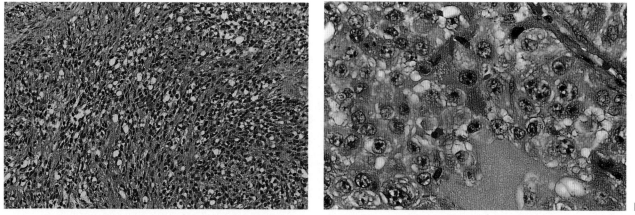

FIG. 13-9. Rhabdomyosarcoma presents as a rapidly growing neoplasm in the orbit in childhood. Histologically, immature cells form short fascicles and sheets resembling embryonal mesenchyme (**A**). Some cells may show evidence of skeletal muscle differentiation with the formation of an eosinophilic cytoplasmic process. These cells, which may possess cross-striations, are called strap cells (**B**).

found in the retroperitoneal space (25%), mediastinum (10%), or neck (5%). It may present as metastatic disease involving the ocular adnexa, sometimes as an atraumatic, spontaneous lid ecchymosis.[47] This metastatic presentation may produce swelling and necrosis in the zygoma, simulating orbital inflammation or cellulitis.[47] Histologically, the tumor consists of sheets of small blue cells with abundant mitoses.[45,48] **Homer-Wright rosettes** may be seen in the primary lesion but are less common in the metastatic deposits. Basophilic stippling of the walls of blood vessels associated with tumor necrosis, well known in retinoblastoma, is a common feature in neuroblastoma. Both of these lesions are capable of at least partial spontaneous regression in occasional cases. The treatment of neuroblastoma consists of local orbital radiation and systemic chemotherapy.[49] If there are no osseous metastases, survival approaches 80% to 85%.

Ewing's sarcoma, a primary bone cancer of uncertain histogenesis, usually arises in the bone of the axial or appendicular skeleton and has a predilection for lung and bone metastasis.[50] Like neuroblastoma, orbital metastasis presents with rapid exophthalmos, hemorrhage, and inflammation from tumor necrosis. Treatment consists of radiation and chemotherapy.

Wilms' tumor, or nephroblastoma, is the most common abdominal tumor in children. It is composed of primitive renal epithelial tubules, stromal elements, and heterologous elements, such as cartilage, bone, adipose tissue, and smooth muscle. The prognosis has been related to the degree of anaplasia of the stromal element. Metastatic lesions to the orbit have been reported.[51] Combination therapy, consisting of surgery, radiation, and chemotherapy, has significantly improved the prognosis, which now approaches a 90% survival rate.

Leukemic infiltrates may occur in the orbit in children. The most common is **acute lymphoblastic leukemia** (ALL). The lymphoblastic cells may infiltrate any orbital

structure and produce exophthalmos. Orbital presentation of ALL has been reported. Aggressive chemotherapy has improved survival rates in recent years.

Granulocytic sarcoma may present with ecchymoses of the lids and orbital signs. Because this lesion has a green coloration on gross inspection, the term chloroma was previously used to describe this malignancy. Histologically, this lesion can be confused with rhabdomyosarcoma, neuroblastoma, or leukemia. The Leder stain for cytoplasmic esterase granules, immunohistochemistry, and electron microscopy often are necessary to establish the myeloid derivation of the neoplasm. As with leukemias, the treatment consists of chemotherapy.[52]

Burkitt's lymphoma is a special variety of small, noncleaved cell lymphocytic lymphoma that may involve the bones of the orbit, causing their destruction. In the endemic African variety, in which the Epstein-Barr virus has been pathogenetically implicated, the tumor frequently presents as an expansile lesion of the jaw bones, often with orbital involvement. Sporadic Burkitt's lymphoma is more common outside of Africa and is apparently not linked to Epstein-Barr virus. In either case, histopathology demonstrates a diffuse infiltrate of atypical, intermediate-sized lymphocytes with little cytoplasm and dark-staining, noncleaved nuclei. High mitotic activity and brisk apoptosis incite a reactive population of benign histocytes imbibing cellular debris. These pale-staining cells are sprinkled throughout the infiltrate, imparting the classic "starry sky" appearance described in this neoplasm. Aggressive chemotherapy is the treatment of choice.[53]

Retinoblastoma may secondarily involve the orbit. Spread may be by extrascleral extension, invasion of emissary canals, or involvement of the optic nerve. This form of spread usually occurs only in neglected cases, after the eye is largely filled by the neoplasm. In this setting, the child may present with signs and symptoms of orbital cellulitis. Orbital recurrence after enucleation may occur.[54]

ORBITAL PATHOLOGY IN ADULTS

Infectious Cellulitis

The presentation of orbital cellulitis in adults is similar to that in children, with fever, sepsis, limitation of ductions, and compromise of optic nerve function. In adults, however, the usual pathogen after trauma is *Staphylococcus aureus,* presumably from contamination by normal commensal organisms of the skin. In cases related to subacute or chronic dacryocystitis, the etiologic organism is usually *Actinomyces* or *Candida* spp. The initial treatment is empiric and is modified based on the results of culture and sensitivity testing.[29]

In diabetics and other immunocompromised hosts, phycomycotic orbital cellulitis can be devastating and even fatal if not diagnosed early and treated aggressively (Fig. 13-10). These fungal infections usually extend from adjacent paranasal sinuses and may present with a cavernous sinus or superior orbital fissure syndrome. Mucormycosis or infections by *Rhizopus* spp. are most common in this clinical setting. These organisms have a predilection to invade vessel walls, precipitating thrombosis and resultant necrosis of the tissue supplied by the affected vessel. Debridement yields necrotic tissue containing large nonseptate branching hyphae, best demonstrated with periodic acid–Schiff or Gomori methenamine-silver stain. Systemic treatment with amphotericin often is necessary; this usually is supplemented with local debridement. In

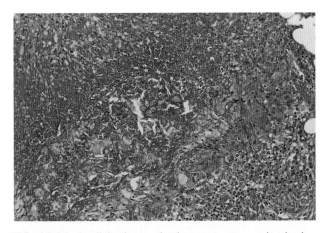

FIG. 13-10. In diabetics or the immunocompromised, phycomycoses may present as an aggressive, necrotizing orbital cellulitis, usually extending from the paranasal sinuses. Special stains [periodic acid–Schiff, (PAS); or Gomori's methenamine silver (GMS)] may be helpful in highlighting the organisms in tissue sections, but, as shown here, these large organisms are readily visible in H&E-stained sections. Necrosis and granulomatous inflammation are present in the orbital tissues.

advanced cases, exenteration may be necessary to ensure patient survival.[55] Extension of the infection into the central nervous system results in a grave prognosis.[56]

Inflammatory Diseases in the Adult Orbit

Thyroid-related retinopathy (TRO) is the most common cause of exophthalmos in adults; it rarely presents in children. In the 25-to-50-year-old age range, women outnumber men 8:1. Thyroid function studies, as measured by thyroxin levels (T3, T4, and free thyroxine index), are performed as part of the diagnostic evaluation; however, thyroid function may be normal, elevated, or decreased. The orbital signs include eyelid retraction, upper eyelid lag during down gaze, and diplopia due to asymmetric muscle restriction and exophthalmos. Optic nerve compression due to massively enlarged extraocular muscles can occur in advanced cases and requires treatment. Decompressive surgery, radiation, or both may be necessary to prevent permanent visual loss.[57] Because TRO affects primarily the extraocular muscles, CT or MRI is an effective modality in the diagnostic evaluation. The inferior rectus is the most frequently involved extraocular muscle, followed by the medial rectus, but any number or combination of the muscles may be involved. Involvement usually is asymmetric. In imaging studies, it usually is possible to demonstrate sparing of the muscle tendons, a characteristic that helps differentiate TRO from other causes of myositis.[58,59]

Diagnostic biopsy usually is unnecessary, and therefore the pathologist rarely has the opportunity to examine tissue from patients with TRO. Histologically, the muscles are infiltrated by varying numbers of lymphocytes, plasma cells, and mast cells. Often the infiltrate is scant and disproportional to the gross enlargement of the muscles (Fig. 13-11). The chronic inflammation is accompanied by edema and extracellular deposition of glycosaminoglycans, which can be demonstrated in tissue sections using the alcian blue stain (pH 2.5). The inflammatory process eventually leads to fibrosis and a permanent restrictive myopathy. The final position of the eyelids and globe and the degree of restriction are highly unpredictable and do not correlate with the results of thyroid function tests. The disease should be quiescent for many months before attempting strabismus surgery to address diplopia. Reconstructive or cosmetic surgery to correct eyelid deformities may be contemplated. The surgical priority is to restore adequate orbital volume in an effort to protect optic nerve function and to prevent exposure keratopathy.

Idiopathic orbital inflammation (IOI) historically was known as inflammatory pseudotumor, but this term is out of favor currently. The clinical presentation is highly variable. In its acute form, IOI presents abruptly with pain lasting days to a few weeks. Patients experience pain, restriction of ductions, and exophthalmos; thus, infectious

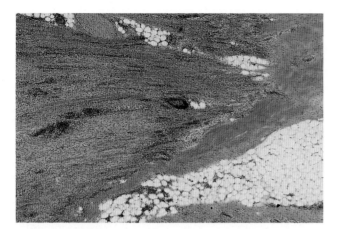

FIG. 13-11. Despite the often massive enlargement of the extraocular muscles in thyroid-related orbitopathy, the muscles may show few pathologic changes. In this case, there is a moderately intense but patchy chronic inflammatory infiltrate composed of lymphocytes and plasma cells. Deposition of glycosaminoglycans separates individual muscle fibers, and eventually collagen is laid down within the muscle, leading to a restrictive myopathy.

orbital cellulitis may be suspected. The onset may be more indolent in the subacute form, progressing over weeks to months without significant external inflammatory signs. A chronic form exists that may progress slowly over several months with essentially no attendant external inflammatory signs. Gradually increasing exophthalmos and limitation of extraocular muscle functions are the principal signs.

One or more typically several orbital structures may be involved by IOI. The primary presentation may be dacryoadenitis, myositis, or more diffuse soft-tissue disease. Even when the inflammatory process is primarily localized to one orbital structure, the infiltrate tends to extend in an irregular fashion beyond the borders of this structure. When the extraocular muscles are involved, there is no tendency to spare the tendons and adjacent adipose tissue, in contrast to TRO. Imaging studies reveal an infiltrate partially respecting anatomic tissue planes, leading to a partially compartmentalized appearance; however, the borders of the infiltrate are typically shaggy and ill defined.

The presumptive diagnosis of IOI, especially in the acute and subacute forms, may be based on clinical presentation and imaging studies. Therapy with corticosteroids may be initiated. Although the response may be dramatic, IOI tends to be a chronic disease; relapses and a protracted clinical course are common. In the chronic form of IOI, biopsy may be necessary to rule out other sclerosing disease processes. This form tends to respond less dramatically to steroid therapy. When steroid therapy fails, low-dose radiation therapy may be necessary to quell the inflammatory process.[60]

IOI is typically a unilateral disease, although bilateral involvement does occur. The radiographic appearance often leads to a differential diagnosis between IOI and lymphoproliferative disease; bilateral involvement suggests the latter.

When biopsy of the orbit is performed, the orbital tissue is found to be infiltrated by a mixture of inflammatory cells in varying proportions, roughly corresponding to the time course of the disease at the time of biopsy (Fig. 13-12). Prior steroid therapy may alter the nature and degree of the inflammatory infiltrate. Histologically, a polymorphous collection of lymphocytes, plasma cells, neutrophils, eosinophils, and macrophages is present. In the acute form, which is rarely biopsied, neutrophils and eosinophils predominate; macrophages and lymphocytes become more prominent in the subacute form. In chronic cases, lymphoid cells predominate, but the presence of a few eosinophils, neutrophils, and macrophages helps to differentiate this lesion from lymphoproliferative disease. Particularly in the lacrimal gland, small lymphoid follicles (germinal centers) may be present, leading to confusion with lymphoid hyperplasia, an entity distinct from IOI.

In practice, biopsies are typically obtained when a patient fails to respond to steroid therapy, often after IOI has progressed to its chronic phase. In these biopsies, collagen deposition may be marked. In sclerosing forms, the lymphoid infiltrate may have regressed to a sparse, angiocentric pattern; the primary tissue manifestation at this point is a collagenized stroma. Occasional cases may present a granulomatous pattern with noncaseating granulomas that mimic sarcoidosis. The lack of systemic findings and a normal level of serum angiotensin-converting enzyme allow the diagnosis of granulomatous IOI.

Sarcoidosis is an idiopathic granulomatous inflammatory disease that may involve diverse organ systems, including the eye and ocular adnexa. The ophthalmologist most frequently encounters sarcoidosis as a uveitis or as an indolent dacryoadenitis; indeed, an orbital mass may be the presenting sign of the systemic disease. Although either the eye or the orbit may be involved, rarely are both affected by the inflammatory process simultaneously. Sarcoidosis is suggested when biopsy reveals a noncaseating granulomatous inflammation of the orbital tissues or lacrimal gland (Fig. 13-13). Typically, congeries of epithelioid macrophages (''histiocytes'') and multinucleated giant cells are present against a background of lymphocytic inflammatory cells. Langhans' giant cells (with multiple nuclei arranged at the periphery of the cell) typically are encountered. Other specific causes of granulomatous inflammation must be ruled out using special stains for organisms that may cause this inflammatory pattern (periodic acid–Schiff or Gomori methenamine-silver for fungi and Ziehl-Neelsen for acid-fast bacilli).[61] In the orbit, caseation necrosis in the granulomas may be seen, suggesting tuberculosis. To rule out infectious agents definitively, microbiologic cultures should be prepared from tissues obtained at biopsy. When cultures and

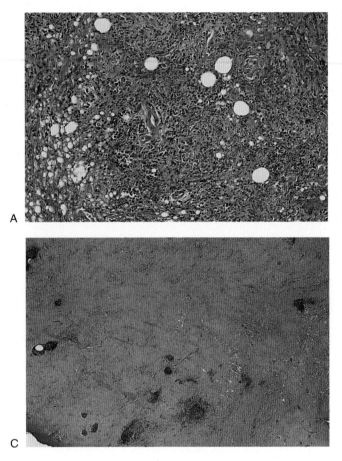

A

B

C

FIG. 13-12. Idiopathic orbital inflammation presents with a wide range of histopathologic patterns. With acute presentations, neutrophils, eosinophils, and macrophages are present in the orbital soft tissues (**A**). As the disease becomes more chronic, lymphocytes and plasma cells become the predominant cell types in the infiltrate (**B**). Sclerosing forms may have relatively few inflammatory foci and are characterized instead by dense fibrosis (**C**).

special stains are negative, a systemic evaluation should be performed, including chest x-ray, serum angiotensin-converting enzyme (usually elevated in sarcoidosis), a PPD (to determine exposure to the tubercle bacillus), and an anergy panel. A gallium scan may reveal systemic

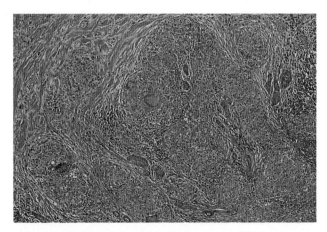

FIG. 13-13. Sarcoidosis frequently involves the lacrimal gland. Typical noncaseating granulomas and a chronic inflammatory infiltrate are present in this case. Several Langhans'-type multinucleated giant cells are present. Another systemic site of involvement should be documented, and infectious causes of granulomatous inflammation, such as tuberculosis and fungal diseases, must be ruled out to document a clinical diagnosis of sarcoidosis. (H&E, ×10)

inflammatory foci suggestive of sarcoidosis. Sarcoidosis is a diagnosis of exclusion: only when systemic disease is documented and infectious agents are ruled out should the diagnosis of sarcoidosis be made.

Several other systemic inflammatory processes, including Wegener's granulomatosis, giant cell (temporal) arteritis, polyarteritis nodosa, and other vasculitides, rarely involve the orbit (Figs. 13-14 and 13-15). Orbital inflammatory signs may be present in these systemic diseases. The lymphoepithelial lesions of the salivary glands associated with Sjögren's syndrome may involve the lacrimal gland and produce glandular enlargement. This involvement may lead to the development of keratoconjunctivitis sicca.

Orbital Lymphoproliferative Disease

Lymphoproliferative diseases of the orbit have been an area of intense investigation during the past two decades, as investigations of lymphoid neoplasia have exploited advances in immunology and molecular genetics in the elucidation of the pathogenesis of malignant lymphoma. The orbit normally does not house lymph nodes; likewise, lymphatic vasculature has not been convincingly demonstrated in the human orbit. Nevertheless,

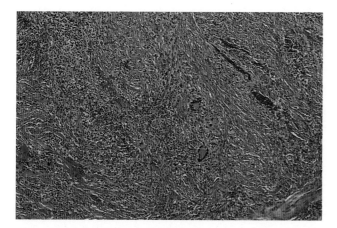

FIG. 13-14. Wegener's granulomatosis presenting in the orbit is often a diagnostic challenge. The histopathologic findings of necrotizing vasculitis, scattered multinucleated giant cells, and a mixed acute and chronic inflammatory infiltrate might be dismissed as nonspecific findings, but correlation of the overall histologic pattern and the clinical signs allows a presumptive diagnosis, as in this case. The serum anti-neutrophil cytoplasmic antibody (ANCA) level is usually elevated in this disease, but it may be negative when there is limited systemic involvement.

lymphoid lesions of the orbit do occur and are often problematic for the pathologist.

Lymphoproliferative disease in the orbit is classified as benign lymphoid hyperplasia (BLH), atypical lymphoid hyperplasia (ALH), and malignant lymphoma (ML) (Fig. 13-16). Clinically, patients present with an indolent, gradually increasing exophthalmos, usually of several weeks' to a few months' duration. Imaging studies (CT or MRI) show a localized, space-occupying lesion that classically molds to adjacent orbital structures and orbital septa. Bone erosion and destruction of soft-tissue structures is rare. Lymphoid lesions may be encountered anywhere in the orbit, but anterior or superior presentation is most common. The lacrimal gland is a frequent site of involvement. In some cases, conjunctival involvement may be present. The typical "salmon patch," a slightly raised, salmon-pink lesion with intact overlying conjunctival epithelium, usually involves the bulbar conjunctiva. If this is the presenting sign, imaging studies of the orbit are indicated because simultaneous contiguous or noncontiguous involvement may be discovered. Because malignant lesions of the orbit may coincide with benign conjunctival lymphoid infiltrates, biopsy of the orbital infiltrate should be performed along with biopsy of the conjunctival lesion.

Histopathologic evaluation of lymphoid tumors requires an adequate specimen. Numerous special techniques are often required to arrive at a correct diagnosis. Of paramount importance is intraoperative handling of the tissue, because lymphoid cells are particularly prone to crush artifact. Therefore, the surgeon must minimize tissue manipulation. The fresh tissue should then be trans-

ported immediately to the pathology laboratory for frozen section analysis.

In our laboratory, touch preparations are made by lightly contacting the tissue (preferably a fresh-cut surface) with a dry glass slide and immediately fixing the slide with alcohol/formalin solution. These slides provide excellent cytomorphology to assess fine microscopic details such as nuclear chromatin patterns. About half of the specimen is then frozen (avoiding organic freezing agents such as isopropanol), and cryosections are prepared. H&E-stained "touch preps" and frozen sections are then examined to confirm the lymphoid nature of the lesion. Often, definitive diagnosis may be rendered at this time, but at a minimum the pathologist should communicate to the surgeon whether or not the specimen is adequate for diagnostic evaluation before the patient is removed from the operating room. We retain the frozen tissue for possible molecular genetic analysis; gene rearrangement studies are easily performed on DNA extracted from nonfixed, previously frozen tissue. The remaining half of the specimen is then fixed in formalin or B5 fixative for routine processing. Because the tissue sample size is often marginally adequate, multiple unstained sections suitable for immunohistochemistry are prepared at the time of initial routine slide preparation. In our laboratory, 10 such slides are prepared to reduce tissue wastage.

Once it is established that a lesion is lymphoproliferative in nature, the primary goal of the pathologist is to classify the lesion as BLH, ALH, or ML. In routine H&E-stained sections, this distinction is often possible, but many cases require immunohistochemistry to determine if a monoclonal population is present. Gene rearrangement studies may be helpful in ALH and even necessary to

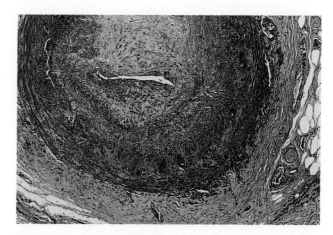

FIG. 13-15. Giant cell arteritis is characterized by a granulomatous inflammatory reaction centered on the elastic lamina of medium-sized arteries, typically involving the superficial and orbital branches of the external carotid artery. Destruction of the elastic lamina results. The inflammatory lesions involve the artery at scattered foci ("skip lesions"); therefore, a 1-cm length of the artery should be sectioned at many levels to detect the underlying pathology.

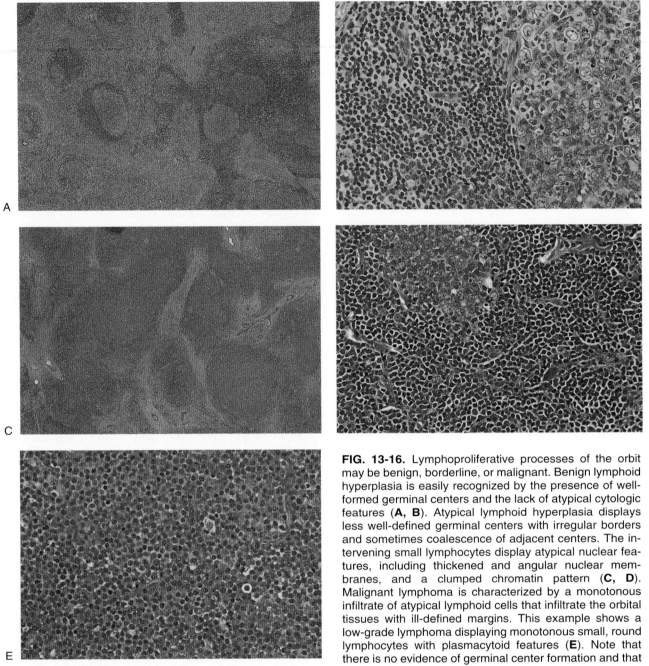

FIG. 13-16. Lymphoproliferative processes of the orbit may be benign, borderline, or malignant. Benign lymphoid hyperplasia is easily recognized by the presence of well-formed germinal centers and the lack of atypical cytologic features (**A, B**). Atypical lymphoid hyperplasia displays less well-defined germinal centers with irregular borders and sometimes coalescence of adjacent centers. The intervening small lymphocytes display atypical nuclear features, including thickened and angular nuclear membranes, and a clumped chromatin pattern (**C, D**). Malignant lymphoma is characterized by a monotonous infiltrate of atypical lymphoid cells that infiltrate the orbital tissues with ill-defined margins. This example shows a low-grade lymphoma displaying monotonous small, round lymphocytes with plasmacytoid features (**E**). Note that there is no evidence of germinal center formation and that the cells are relatively uniform. Special studies, such as immunocytochemistry or molecular genetics, may be used to demonstrate monoclonality.

rule out the presence of a monoclonal and presumably malignant population of cells. The histologic parameters for classifying these lesions are detailed here.

The pathologist should first determine whether well-formed germinal centers are present. In BLH, germinal centers should be prominent and well defined. They are composed of medium-sized and large B cells (immunoblasts) with high mitotic activity. Macrophages (''gitter cells'') are sprinkled throughout as they consume the cellular debris of high cell turnover. Surrounding these active follicles is a mantle zone of small to intermediate-sized lymphocytes that represent the

next stage of B-cell development. Small T cells are present in this region. In BLH, the germinal centers are generally sharply demarcated from this mantle zone. Between the follicles is a mixed infiltrate of small mature B and T cells, as well as a few plasma cells. Using immunohistochemistry, both kappa and lambda light chain expression should be detected in the B cells of the infiltrate. This confirms the polyclonal nature of BLH.

In ALH, follicles are seen, but they are generally not as numerous or as well formed as those in BLH. Often, follicles are large and merge irregularly. At the edges of the follicles, the mantle zone often is expanded and irregular, in contrast to the sharp margins encountered in BLH. The interfollicular zones are often large, displaying a diffuse pattern with monomorphous small to intermediate-sized lymphocytes. Some of these cells may exhibit atypical features, such as irregular nuclear outlines and thickening of the nuclear membranes. In ALH, polyclonality may be demonstrated, but genetic studies may reveal a clonal population of lymphocytes, suggestive of malignancy. These borderline lesions are the most problematic for pathologists and are somewhat controversial in that not all authors agree on the significance of genetic rearrangements in lymphoid lesions.

Frank ML in the orbit is almost always a diffuse B-cell neoplasm displaying a monotonous infiltrate of atypical cells that demonstrate either kappa or lambda light chains by immunohistochemistry.[62] Subclassification usually is possible histologically to determine whether the lesion portends a low-, intermediate-, or high-grade clinical behavior using the Working Formulation (modified Rappaport classification) sponsored by the National Cancer Institute. This system uses tissue patterns and cell types to classify malignant lymphomas. In the orbit, in our experience, mixed cell lymphomas and follicular lymphomas are extremely uncommon. Most are diffuse intermediate cell lymphomas (eg, mucosal-associated lymphoid tissue lymphomas, mantle cell lymphomas), and low-grade, diffuse small cell lymphocytic or lymphoplasmacytic lymphomas are frequently encountered.[63,64] In patients with AIDS, high-grade lesions usually are found; rapidly progressing immunoblastic lymphoma and Burkitt's lymphoma are typically seen in this setting.[65]

At our institution, all patients with a biopsy-proven diagnosis of lymphoproliferative disease are referred for oncologic evaluation to determine whether systemic disease is present. The workup usually includes CT scans of the chest and abdomen and bone marrow biopsy, although the latter may be deferred in BLH. If the biopsy reveals a lymphoma with plasmacytic differentiation, a serum protein electrophoresis may be indicated to detect the presence of a monoclonal gammopathy. Such evaluation is recommended even in the absence of a diagnosis of ML because about 40% of patients with BLH or ALH of the orbit may progress to frank systemic ML. Consequently, long-term follow-up is important for all BLH, ALH, and ML patients.

If after systemic evaluation the disease is found to be localized to the orbit, local radiation with shielding of the globe may be delivered. Our protocol calls for 2000 rads in ALH and 3000 rads in ML. BLH may respond to steroid therapy, but low-dose radiation therapy may be used in certain patients. When systemic involvement is documented, patients are treated by chemotherapy, and the protocol is based on the stage and clinical grade determined by the oncologic evaluation. Local radiation therapy may be used in cases with massive exophthalmos for palliation.

Mesenchymal Neoplasms of the Adult Orbit

The orbit contains numerous mesenchymal structures, including fibroconnective tissue, skeletal and smooth muscle, blood vessels, and nerves, all of which may give rise to benign and malignant tumors. Malignant mesenchymal neoplasms are rare in the adult orbit; benign mesenchymal neoplasms are more common.

Benign soft-tissue tumors are typically slow-growing. They expand the orbital volume by compression and displacement of adjacent structures. Most are encapsulated and well defined in imaging studies. The patient often does not notice the progressive exophthalmos, and evaluation of old photographs may be helpful in assessing the changes that have occurred. The time course may extend over many months, even to several years. CT scans may demonstrate reactive sclerosis of the adjacent orbital bones, but bone erosion is rare.

Vascular Tumors

Cavernous hemangioma is the most common acquired vascular lesion in adults. It occurs more frequently in middle-aged women. These lesions may enlarge during pregnancy. Unlike capillary hemangiomas, these lesions do not spontaneously involute; excision is usually necessary, particularly when orbital function is compromised.[66] The typical example is an intraconal, globoid tumor that displays high-amplitude internal echoes with ultrasonography. Sharp margins are demonstrated in CT scans. Because the vascular spaces within cavernous hemangiomas have little communication with the systemic vasculature, the tumor displays low signal intensity in the T1-weighted MRI, similar to the vitreous. It is hyperintense in T2-weighted images.

During surgery, the tumor presents as a compressible, dark red to purple mass. After fixation, the cut surface reveals a honeycomb appearance due to the macroscopically visible vascular spaces. Histologically, the lesion is usually surrounded by a fibrous capsule. Ovoid vascular spaces are lined by a continuous endothelium and are supported by a delicate stroma. Some examples may contain smooth muscle in the stroma. When this is a prominent component, some authors suggest that the term **venous angioma** be applied. The vascular lumina contain largely intact erythrocytes and may display a plasma level reflecting low flow or "settling" during fixation; thrombosis is uncommon.[67] Cavernous hemangioma can be differentiated from a hemorrhagic lymphangioma by the continuous endothelium, lack of a significant capillary vasculature in the stroma, lack of lymphoid tissue, and the presence of a capsule in the hemangioma (Fig. 13-17).

Hemangiopericytoma is an uncommon neoplasm derived from vascular pericytes, the cells that enrobe and

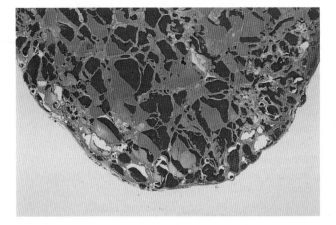

FIG. 13-17. Cavernous hemangioma is the most common mesenchymal tumor in adults. The large, distended, blood-filled vascular spaces are lined by a continuous endothelial layer, and there is usually little intervening stroma.

provide support for vascular structures. These generally well-circumscribed tumors, encountered in the orbit infrequently, are recognized histologically as a highly cellular neoplasm with a rich supporting capillary network. The feeder vessels display an anastomosing vasculature of varying calibers, often revealing a so-called "staghorn" configuration (Fig. 13-18). At surgery, bleeding may be profuse. Benign and malignant forms are recognized, but the greatest difficulty lies with borderline lesions. It may be difficult to predict clinical behavior in these lesions. Hemangiopericytomas should be completely excised because recurrence and malignant degeneration are well-documented phenomena.[68,69]

Other malignant vascular tumors may occur in the orbit, albeit rarely. **Angiosarcoma** is a rare neoplasm in general, and only 3% of 366 cases in one series presented in the orbit.[95] The histologic appearance varies greatly between well-differentiated and poorly differentiated forms. Immunohistochemical demonstration of factor VIII antigen in the neoplastic cells helps confirm the diagnosis. This tumor occurs across all age groups and has a generally poor prognosis. With the advent of AIDS, **Kaposi's sarcoma** has become more prevalent in the orbit and conjunctiva. Viral-mediated oncogenesis is likely, but the causative agent currently is debated. Although skin and mucosal lesions display a wide variety of histologic appearances, the typical orbital lesion is recognized by poorly formed vascular channels exhibiting varying degrees of cellular pleomorphism. Erythrocyte extravasation and hemosiderin deposition typically are present (Fig. 13-19).

Several nonneoplastic tumors of the orbital vasculature may produce signs and symptoms of a mass lesion. All are nonencapsulated. **Arteriovenous malformations** consist of an elastic artery feeding directly into a muscular vein without an intervening capillary bed. Histologically, the vessels are dilated, particularly on the venous side because of exposure to arterial pressure. The walls of the vessels are irregularly thickened and form worm-like configurations (Fig. 13-20). **Arteriovenous fistulae** display similar histopathology but are usually related to trauma. Hemosiderin deposition and partial thrombosis are more commonly seen than in arteriovenous malformations. An orbital varix is an abnormally dilated vein that may gradually enlarge to produce a mass lesion. Partial thrombosis is common, and calcification within the thrombus may be seen in radiographs. Because adjacent structures may be partially enmeshed by each of these vascular malformations, excision may be difficult. Ligation or embolization may be used in some cases.

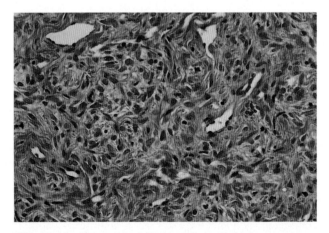

FIG. 13-18. Hemangiopericytoma is a relatively uncommon neoplasm that, nevertheless, should be considered in the differential diagnosis of well-circumscribed mesenchymal lesions of the orbit. Histopathologically, "staghorn" vascular spaces are separated by a cellular infiltrate of round to ovoid cells that represent neoplastic proliferation of pericytes.

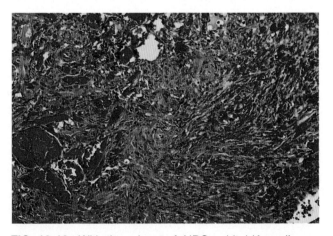

FIG. 13-19. With the advent of AIDS, orbital Kaposi's sarcoma has become more prevalent. This tumor is recognized by poorly developed, slit-like vascular channels lined by endothelial cells with atypical cytologic features. Erythrocyte extravasation and hemosiderin deposition are commonly present, as seen here.

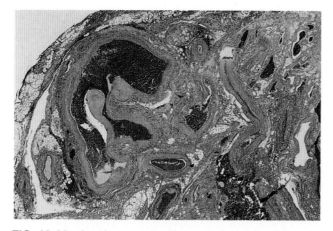

FIG. 13-20. Arteriovenous malformations are characterized by a vermiform collection of variably dilated blood vessels that display features of both elastic arteries and muscular veins. This section demonstrates the discontinuity of the arterial elastic lamina (black staining) in vascular channels with venous and arterial characteristics.

Neurogenic Tumors in the Adult Orbit

Numerous cranial and peripheral nerves course through the orbital soft tissue. Consequently, neurogenic tumors are relatively common in the orbit; most are benign. They present in diverse clinical settings, and historical data, anatomic location, and radiographic findings often lead to a clinical diagnosis before biopsy or excision. True neoplasms are represented by schwannomas (neurilemmomas), optic nerve gliomas (pilocytic astrocytomas), and meningiomas (both of the optic nerve and the orbital apex). Neurofibromas may present as solitary lesions or as one manifestation of neurofibromatosis (von Recklinghausen's disease).

A **schwannoma** is a benign neoplasm arising from Schwann cells, the myelin-producing cells that enrobe the neurites of peripheral nerves. Treatment for these well-defined, encapsulated tumors is surgical excision. Histologic recognition of schwannomas rests with the identification of two tissue patterns, Antoni A and Antoni B, which may be present in varying amounts. Antoni A areas consist of highly cellular interlacing fascicles of long spindle-shaped cells, with nuclei often arranged side by side in a palisading pattern. Highly organized Verocay bodies, seen as two groups of palisading nuclei aligned in parallel, may be present. Antoni B areas consist of similar but less well-organized spindle-shaped cells in an often abundant "myxoid" ground substance rich in mucopolysaccharides and varying amounts of collagen. This tissue pattern may result from degeneration within the neoplasm. The nuclei in both areas are characteristically thin and wavy and have tapered ends (Fig. 13-21).

S-100 protein is readily demonstrated in the neoplastic cells by immunohistochemistry, indicating their derivation from the neural crest.[70] Special stains for neurons, such as with antineurofilament antibodies, are negative within the tumor. As the proliferation of Schwann cells progresses, the native neurons are displaced to the periphery rather than being entrapped within the tumor. In our experience, larger lesions often display central cystic degeneration in imaging studies. This characteristic may lead to confusion with cavernous hemangiomas; the larger coalescent spaces in schwannomas are a helpful diagnostic clue.[71]

Neurofibroma may occur in the adult orbit as a solitary tumor but is most often associated with type I neurofibromatosis. This tumor consists of long, slender, spindle-shaped cells similar to those in schwannomas, but it is less well organized. It contains a variable mixture of cells demonstrating schwannian, neural, perineural, and fibroblastic differentiation (Fig. 13-22). Consequently, S-100 positivity is less intense than in schwannomas, and neuronal cells can be demonstrated using antibodies to neurofilament protein.[32,70] This is a helpful finding in differentiating solitary neurofibroma from schwannoma.

Clinically, neurofibromas associated with neurofibromatosis are usually nonencapsulated tumors that expand and elongate the nerve of origin. This tumoral proliferation leads to a convoluted, plexiform mass that on palpation suggests a "bag of worms." Often, the upper eyelid and anterior orbit are involved, and the eyelid presents with an S-shaped deformity. Congenital glaucoma may be associated with this finding.[72] Plexiform neurofibromas may involve the deeper orbital structures.[73]

Solitary neurofibromas may be encapsulated, spherical tumors similar to schwannomas, or they may be diffusely

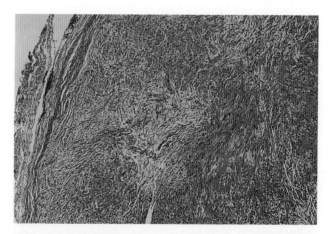

FIG. 13-21. Schwannomas are relatively common orbital tumors representing neoplastic proliferation of the Schwann cells associated with peripheral nerves. They can be recognized by the presence of two histopathologic patterns. Antoni A areas display compact, cellular proliferation of long, spindle-shaped cells with slender, wavy nuclei. Nuclear palisading is a feature in this tissue type in many tumors. Antoni B areas are less cellular and display myxomatous degeneration of the stroma. Cystic degeneration, perceptible in imaging studies, may be present.

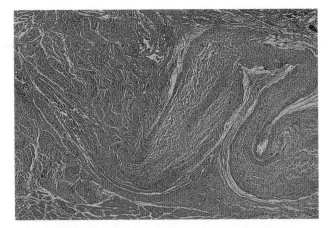

FIG. 13-22. Neurofibromas can be histopathologically similar to schwannomas but in fact are composed of several cellular elements, including Schwann cells, neurites, and perineural fibroblasts. Solitary tumors not associated with neurofibromatosis may be encountered, but the plexiform type shown here is usually associated with this phakomatosis. Here, the neurofibromatous proliferation is partially contained by the nerve sheath, which is elongated and buckled. In some cases with a prominent fibroblastic component, they may be confused with scar tissue. Neurons coursing through the substance of the neoplasm can be demonstrated using immunohistochemical methods.

infiltrative tumors that may be difficult to resect completely.

Meningioma is a benign neoplasm derived from the arachnoid villi. The tumor may arise in the optic nerve sheath or intracranially with secondary involvement of the orbit. Intraosseous meningiomas may arise from rests of meningeal cells trapped in the orbital bones. Meningiomas account for less than 5% of all orbital tumors; they are more common in females in the fourth to sixth de-

cades. As with other space-occupying lesions, ophthalmic findings depend on the site and size of the tumor. Disc pallor, optociliary shunt vessels, and visual loss are the classic presentation for optic nerve meningiomas. Imaging studies reveal fusiform thickening of the optic nerve, with or without enlargement of the optic canal. Calcification or enhancement may be seen at the periphery of the lesion. When the orbital or cranial bones are affected, reactive bony thickening is seen in imaging studies.

The cells of these lesions are usually round to cuboidal meningoepithelial cells, with round nuclei and sharply defined eosinophilic cytoplasm. Concentrically laminated, spheroidal concretions known as psammoma bodies are commonly found within the tumor, but their presence is not essential for diagnosis (Fig. 13-23).[72]

Optic nerve glioma is relatively rare in adults; it usually occurs in children under age 5.[74] It should be considered in the differential of fusiform swellings of the optic nerve (see the section on neural tumors in children).

Fibrohistiocytic and Mesenchymal Tumors

Fibrous histiocytoma is a relatively common benign tumor that usually presents in the supranasal orbit of middle-aged patients.[75] Although the exact histogenesis is obscure, histologically it consists of spindle cells arranged in a storiform, "cartwheel" configuration. These cells may demonstrate fibroblastic, myofibroblastic, or undifferentiated mesenchymal characteristics (Fig. 13-24). Vimentin and, to varying degrees, smooth muscle-

FIG. 13-24. Benign spindle-cell tumors of the orbit may pose diagnostic problems for the pathologist. Fibrous histiocytomas present several clues that allow their immediate recognition. Set within a storiform proliferation of cytologically bland spindle-shaped cells, scattered histiocytoid cells are noted. Some of these may be multinucleated, and lipidized cytoplasm is not uncommon. Despite high cellularity, there is little or no mitotic activity. When cellular pleomorphism and mitotic activity are present, the pathologist must consider a diagnosis of malignant fibrous histiocytoma.

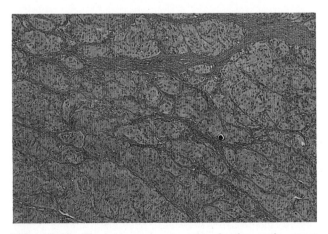

FIG. 13-23. Meningiomas may arise in the optic nerve sheath, in the meninges of the cranial vault, or within the bones of the orbit. Histologically, collections of small round cells with ample cytoplasm, the meningoepithelial cells, are present. Psammoma bodies (*arrow*) may be present in meningiomas and are helpful diagnostic clues.

specific actin (demonstrating myofibroblastic differentiation) may be demonstrated by immunohistochemistry. A diagnostic hallmark is the presence of varying numbers of mononuclear and multinucleated histiocytes that express macrophage cell markers such as lysozyme and CD68. Some of the multinucleated cells may assume the phenotype of Touton giant cells with lipid vacuoles in the cytoplasm external to an organized ring of nuclei.[76]

Most fibrohistiocytic tumors are benign, displaying bland-appearing cells and little or no mitotic activity. When areas of hypercellularity and infiltrative margins are encountered, however, the tumors may have a more aggressive course. When mitotic activity is high and cellular pleomorphism is noted, **malignant fibrous histiocytoma** is diagnosed. This tumor is relatively rare in the orbit, but it may occur after orbital radiation therapy for retinoblastoma. Consequently, it should be considered along with osteogenic sarcoma in the differential diagnosis of tumors occurring after radiation therapy. It should be excised with wide margins to prevent recurrence.

Fibroma, fibromyxoma, myxoma, and **leiomyoma** are extremely rare in the orbit but must be considered in the histologic differential of any spindle-cell neoplasms such as those discussed above. Generally, these tumors display more cytoplasmic differentiation (eg, eosinophilic muscle fibrils in leiomyoma) or more abundant extracellular matrix (eg, collagen in fibroma or mucopolysaccharides in myxoma). Immunohistochemistry and electron microscopy may be needed in some cases to rule out these tumors. Malignant tumors of these types (**leiomyosarcoma** and **fibrosarcoma**) are exceedingly rare in the orbit.

Rare examples of **lipoma** and **liposarcoma** in the orbit have been reported. True examples of lipoma contain fibroblastic or angiomatous components, and liposarcomas exhibit lipoblasts, often with a myxoid background. Most clinical examples of ''lipomas'' of the anterior orbit represent normal orbital adipose tissue that has herniated through rents in the orbital septum. These may be submitted as lipomas after resection during cosmetic surgery.

Nodular fasciitis is a reactive proliferation of myofibroblastic origin that may be confused with several malignant mesenchymal neoplasms. It is more common in the eyelid and conjunctiva, but it may involve the orbit. It presents as a rapidly growing, usually violaceous mass that in biopsy specimens shows pleomorphic, atypical-appearing myofibroblasts in a variable myxoid stroma. Despite its infiltrative margins, the lesion is self-limited and benign. The usually rich chronic inflammatory infiltrate within the proliferation is a helpful diagnostic clue in recognizing this reactive lesion (Fig. 13-25).

Metastatic and Secondary Tumors in the Adult Orbit

Although virtually any primary malignancy may involve the orbit through hematogenous dissemination, the

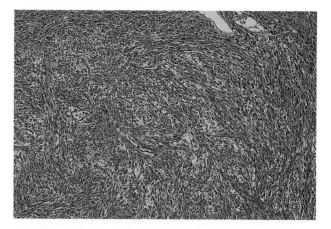

FIG. 13-25. Nodular fasciitis is a reactive, inflammatory tumor that may be confused with malignant neoplasms. It displays cytologically atypical myofibroblasts within an inflamed, often myxoid stroma.

more common primaries are those that are the most frequently encountered for each sex: in men, **prostate** and **lung carcinoma** and in women, **breast carcinoma** (Fig. 13-26).[77-79] When metastatic lesions involve the orbit, they usually occur outside the muscle cone and result in paraxial exophthalmos. In scirrhous carcinomas, notably those of breast origin, enophthalmos may result from retraction of orbital contents secondary to desmoplastic scarring within the tumor.[80] Bone destruction with irregular tumor margins may be a prominent CT feature of metastatic lesions, particularly metastatic prostatic carcinoma. Some metastases are accompanied by an inflammatory or sclerotic component; consequently, imaging studies may reveal an infiltrate resembling idiopathic orbital inflammation. Similarly, cystic lesions may be encountered because of necrosis or hemorrhage with the metastasis. Metastasis to the extraocular muscles has been reported from renal cell carcinoma and cutaneous melanoma. These metastatic tumors may mimic TRO or myositis.

It is always important to elicit any history of previous malignancy in patients with orbital masses. Despite long disease-free intervals, certain carcinomas notoriously present with late, solitary metastasis. **Renal cell carcinoma,** which may produce metastases years or even decades after resection of the primary, and **breast carcinoma** are notable examples.

Secondary tumors arise in structures adjacent to the orbit, including the paranasal sinuses and the cranium; these may present clinically with primarily orbital signs. Imaging studies usually reveal that the orbital process is an extension from a contiguous structure. Extraorbital meningiomas with secondary orbital involvement are readily distinguished; the hyperostosis associated with meningioma is an especially prominent feature in CT scans. Generally, orbital extension most often is seen in

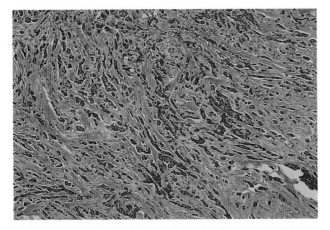

FIG. 13-26. Metastatic tumors in the orbit may reveal histologic features that suggest their origin. Here, "Indian filing" of the metastatic carcinoma was consistent with a breast primary. The patient had had excision of a breast mass 10 years earlier.

meningiomas arising from the sphenoid ridge and the basofrontal region.

Similarly, tumors that originate from the paranasal sinuses are well visualized with CT. Typically, malignant or aggressive lesions extend from the maxillary sinus; infectious and hemorrhagic lesions originate in the ethmoid and frontal sinuses. Examples include **squamous cell carcinoma** and **inverting papillomas.**

Uveal malignant melanoma may rarely present primarily with exophthalmos. Examples of small choroidal tumors with massive orbital extension have been documented, and melanoma may recur in the orbit after treatment of the primary lesion. Primary orbital melanoma occurs rarely in patients with oculodermal melanocytosis.

Basal cell carcinoma, squamous cell carcinoma, and **sebaceous cell carcinoma** of the eyelid may extend into and invade the orbit,[81] but their cutaneous manifestation is typically readily apparent. Although not neoplastic, mucoceles and pyoceles may produce exophthalmos secondary to progressive, cystic enlargement into the orbit from the paranasal sinuses.[82]

BENIGN AND MALIGNANT EPITHELIAL NEOPLASMS OF THE LACRIMAL GLAND

Although inflammatory and lymphoproliferative lesions of the lacrimal gland are more common, epithelial neoplasms are encountered. The lacrimal gland is developmentally related to the salivary glands; consequently, the neoplasms seen here mirror those that occur much more commonly in the parotid, submandibular, sublingual, and accessory salivary glands.

Benign Epithelial Neoplasms

Pleomorphic adenoma ("benign mixed tumor" in older nomenclature) is the most common benign epithelial tumor of the lacrimal gland.[83] It is composed of epithelial proliferations of ductal cells that may form tubules or acinar or solid sheets and occasionally undergo squamous differentiation. At the periphery of these structures, myoepithelial differentiation is evidenced by more spindle-shaped cells lying individually or in narrow bands within variable amounts of lightly basophilic, myxoid stroma (Fig. 13-27). Formerly, these cells were thought to represent a second, stromal cell type within the tumor—hence the designation "mixed" tumor. However, it is now clear that this component is evidence of the normal myoepithelial potentiality of ductal cells. Tumors vary in the proportion of these tissue types.

Pleomorphic adenoma usually presents in middle age within the orbital lobe of the gland, with inferomedial displacement of the globe. Occasional examples have been seen in the palpebral lobe with presentation as an eyelid or conjunctival mass. Imaging studies reveal a well-circumscribed ovoid or spherical lesion within the gland. This globoid enlargement is in contrast to the plump elongation and molding to the eyeball seen when lymphoproliferative processes involve the gland. Larger tumors may produce adjacent bone remodeling, but bone erosion is absent.[84] Gross inspection reveals a rubbery to firm mass with delicate encapsulation and a smooth or lobulated surface; the adjacent normal glandular tissue is compressed.

Imaging studies usually suggest the diagnosis. Surgical removal of the tumor should proceed without breaching the tumor's capsule because pleomorphic adenomas often recur if not removed intact. The recurrence rate in this situation approaches 100%, and malignant degeneration in recurrences is well documented.[85–88] Incisional biopsy should be avoided, and the use of fine-needle aspiration biopsy for preoperative diagnosis is controversial.

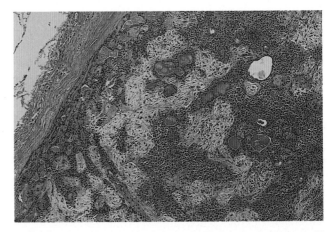

FIG. 13-27. Pleomorphic adenoma ("benign mixed tumor") is derived from the ductal elements of the lacrimal gland. It is composed of mixed elements displaying epithelial (ductal, acinar, and tubular) differentiation and myoepithelial differentiation. In the latter areas, a myxomatous stroma is prominent.

In contrast to the salivary glands, **monomorphic adenoma, Warthin's tumor** (cystadenoma lymphomatosum), and **oncocytoma,** other examples of benign epithelial neoplasms, are very rare in the lacrimal gland.

Malignant Epithelial Neoplasms

Adenoid cystic carcinoma is the most common primary malignant lesion of the lacrimal gland. It may be encountered at essentially any age, although it is rare in children. Similar to its benign counterpart, pleomorphic adenoma, imaging studies of adenoid cystic carcinoma reveal globoid enlargement of the gland, but usually with less well-defined borders, irregular extensions, and mottled bony erosion of the lacrimal gland fossa compared to pleomorphic adenoma. Classically, this tumor presents with pain, possibly because of its propensity to invade and extend along peripheral nerves (perineural invasion) and its effects on adjacent bones. Cystic degeneration and necrosis may be recognized. When there is a high index of suspicion, fine-needle aspiration biopsy may be helpful in establishing the diagnosis preoperatively. This allows optimized surgical treatment planning.

Adenoid cystic carcinoma is characterized by a lace-like, cribriform glandular arrangement of cells displaying ductular differentiation. Typically, cytologic pleomorphism is slight, giving a false sense of benignancy. Back-to-back glands with no intervening stroma form the so-called "Swiss cheese" pattern that is easily recognized (Fig. 13-28).[89,90] A basaloid or solid histologic pattern may be present in varying proportions; the presence of this presumably more primitive tissue pattern has been associated with a poorer prognosis in some series. Areas with substantial amounts of extracellular matrix material and hemorrhagic necrosis are common.

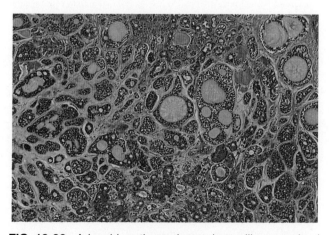

FIG. 13-28. Adenoid cystic carcinoma is readily recognized by its "Swiss cheese" histologic pattern. This pattern results from back-to-back proliferation of glandular elements with no intervening stroma, the so-called cribriform pattern. Necrosis and hemorrhage are common features.

Treatment is by complete excision; however, some authors have recommended more radical approaches, such as orbital exenteration with or without partial orbitectomy (removal of parts of the orbital bones of the lacrimal gland fossa). However, no solid evidence exists that more radical treatment improves the long-term prognosis. Adenoid cystic carcinoma portends a fairly uniform poor prognosis, although survival may exceed several years. Metastatic disease and locally aggressive recurrence may occur late. Chemotherapy or radiation therapy regimens have been unsuccessful in controlling the ultimate outcome.[91-93]

Mucoepidermoid carcinoma, a less common malignancy, may arise in the lacrimal gland or in the mucous glands of the lacrimal sac. It is a mixed neoplasm displaying areas with squamous differentiation and others with glandular differentiation. The histochemical stain mucicarmine helps detect the mucin-producing cells in this tumor that are essential for diagnosis.[94]

SUMMARY

Although the range of pathology that may present in the orbit is vast, systematic evaluation of the patient, imaging studies, and history allow the formation of a reasonable differential diagnosis in most cases. Familiarity with the pathologic classification of orbital disease processes, awareness of incidence rates based on age, and a sound knowledge of anatomy and patterns of disease presentation combine to allow the clinician to narrow these differential diagnostic considerations. Working with the pathologist before and after biopsy or excision leads to optimized diagnostic evaluation and, ultimately, optimized patient care.

REFERENCES

1. Albert DM, Jakobiec FA, eds. *Principles and practice of ophthalmology, clinical practice,* vol. 5. Philadelphia: WB Saunders, 1994.
2. Rootman J. *Diseases of the orbit.* Philadelphia: JB Lippincott, 1988.
3. Bale PM, Parson RE, Stevens MM. Diagnosis and behavior of juvenile rhabdomyosarcoma. *Hum Pathol* 1983;14:596.
4. Musarella MA, Chen HSL, DeBoer G, et al. Ocular involvement in neuroblastoma: prognostic implications. *Ophthalmology* 1984;91:936.
5. Zimmerman LE, Font RL. Ophthalmic manifestations of granulocytic sarcoma (myeloid sarcoma or chloroma). *Am J Ophthalmol* 1975;80:975.
6. Knowles DM, Jakobiec FA. Ocular adnexal lymphoid neoplasms: clinical, histopathologic, electron microscopic, and immunologic characteristics. *Hum Pathol* 1982;13:148.
7. Iliff WJ, Green WR. Orbital lymphangioma. *Ophthalmology* 1979;86:914.
8. Flanagan JC. Vascular problems of the orbit. *Ophthalmology* 1979;86:896.
9. Zimmerman LE, Sanders TE, Ackerman LV. Epithelial tumors of the lacrimal gland: prognostic and therapeutic significance of histologic types. *Int Ophthalmol Clin* 1962;2:337.
10. Kobrin JL, Blodi FC, Weingeist TA. Ocular and orbital manifestation of neurofibromatosis. *Surv Ophthalmol* 1979;24:45.

11. Moore RT. Fibrous dysplasia of the orbit. *Surv Ophthalmol* 1969; 13:321.

12. Wolter JR, Hendrix RC. Osteoblastic prostate carcinoma metastatic to the orbit. *Am J Ophthalmol* 1981;91:648.

13. Bullock JD, Yanes B. Ophthalmic manifestations of metastatic breast cancer. *Ophthalmology* 1980;87:961.

14. Mewis-Levin L, Garcia CA, Olson JD. Plasma cell myeloma of the orbit. *Ann Ophthalmol* 1981;13:477.

15. Jellinek EH. The orbital pseudotumor syndrome and its differentiation from endocrine exophthalmos. *Brain* 1969;92:35.

16. Rootman J, Nugent R. The classification and management of acute orbital pseudotumors. *Ophthalmology* 1982;89:1040.

17. Knowles DM, Jakobiec FA. Ocular adnexal lymphoid neoplasms. *Hum Pathol* 1982;13:148.

18. Hedges TR. Carotid cavernous fistula: a re-evaluation of orbital signs. *Ophthalmic Surg* 1975;4:75.

19. Shields CL, Shields JA, Yarian DL, et al. Intracranial extension of choroidal melanoma via the optic nerve. *Br J Ophthalmol* 1987;71: 172.

20. Marshall D. Glioma of the optic nerve as manifestation of von Recklinghausen's disease. *Am J Ophthalmol* 1954;37:15.

21. Shields JA, Shields CL, Lieb WE, et al. Multiple orbital neurofibromas unassociated with von Recklinghausen's disease. *Arch Ophthalmol* 1990;108:80.

22. Shields JA, Shields CL. The phakomatoses. In: Nelson LB, Calhoun JC, Harley RD, eds. *Pediatric ophthalmology*, 3d ed. Philadelphia: WB Saunders, 1991:427.

23. Friberg TR, Grove AS. Choroidal folds and refractive errors associated with orbital tumors: an analysis. *Arch Ophthalmol* 1983;101: 598.

24. Ossoinig KC. Standardized echography: basic principles, clinical application and results. *Int Ophthalmol Clin* 1979;19:127.

25. Messmer EP, Font RL. Applications of immunohistochemistry to ophthalmic pathology. *Ophthalmology* 1984;91:701.

26. Makley TA Jr, Battles M. Microphthalmos with cyst. *Surv Ophthalmol* 1969;13:200.

27. Shields JA, Bakewell B, Augsburger JJ, et al. Space-occupying orbital masses in children. *Ophthalmology* 1986;93:379.

28. Weiss A, Friendly D, Eglin K, et al. Bacterial periorbital and orbital cellulitis in childhood. *Ophthalmology* 1983;90:195.

29. Macy JI, Mandelbaum SH, Minckler DS. Orbital cellulitis. *Ophthalmology* 1980;87:1309.

30. Haik BG, Jakobiec FA, Ellsworth RM, et al. Capillary hemangioma of the lids and orbit: an analysis of the clinical features and therapeutic results in 101 cases. *Ophthalmology* 1979;86:760.

31. Iliff WJ, Green WR. Orbital lymphangiomas. *Ophthalmology* 1979; 86:914.

32. Jones IS, Desjardins L. Management of orbital neurofibromatosis and lymphangiomas. In: Jakobiec FA, ed. *Ocular and adnexal tumors*. Birmingham, Ala.: Aesculapius Publishing Co., 1978:735.

33. Holman RE, Grimson BS, Drayer BP, et al. Magnetic resonance imaging of optic gliomas. *Am J Ophthalmol* 1985;100:596.

34. Jakobiec FA, Depot MJ, Kennerdell JS, et al. Combined clinical and computed tomographic diagnosis of orbital glioma and meningioma. *Ophthalmology* 1984;91:137.

35. Marquardt MD, Zimmerman LE. Histopathology of meningiomas and gliomas of the optic nerve. *Hum Pathol* 1986;13:226.

36. Tenny RT, Laws ER Jr, Younge BR, et al. The neurosurgical management of optic glioma: results in 104 patients. *J Neurosurg* 1982; 57:452.

37. Brand WN, Hoover SV. Optic glioma in children: review of 16 cases given megavoltage radiation therapy. *Child's Brain* 1979;5: 459.

38. Bale PM, Parsons RE, Stevens MM. Diagnostic and behavior of juvenile rhabdomyosarcoma. *Hum Pathol* 1983;14:596.

39. Abramson DH, Ellsworth RM, Tretter P, et al. The treatment of orbital rhabdomyosarcoma with irradiation and chemotherapy. *Ophthalmology* 1979;86:1330.

40. Kahn HJ, Yeger H, Kassim O, et al. Immunohistochemical and electron microscopic assessment of childhood rhabdomyosarcoma. *Cancer* 1983;51:1897.

41. Azumi N, Ben-Ezra J, Battifora H. Immunophenotypic diagnosis of leiomyosarcomas and rhabdomyosarcomas with monoclonal antibodies to muscle-specific actin and desmin in formalin-fixed tissue. *Mod Pathol* 1988;1:469.

42. Cameron D, Wick MR. Embryonal rhabdomyosarcoma of the conjunctiva. *Arch Ophthalmol* 1986;104:1203.

43. Newton WA, Soule EH, Hamoudi AB, et al. Histopathology of childhood sarcomas, intergroup rhabdomyosarcoma studies I and II: clinicopathologic correlation. *J Clin Oncol* 1988;6:67.

44. Ashton N, Morgan G. Embryonal sarcoma and embryonal rhabdomyosarcoma of the orbit. *J Clin Pathol* 1965;18:699.

45. Triche TJ, Askin FB. Neuroblastoma and the differential diagnosis of small-, round-, and blue-cell tumors. *Hum Pathol* 1983;14:569.

46. Tsokos M, Howard R, Coasta J. Immunohistochemical study of alveolar and embryonal rhabdomyosarcoma. *Lab Invest* 1983;48: 148.

47. Albert DM, Rubenstein RA, Scheie HG. Tumor metastasis to the eye. II. Clinical study in infants and children. *Am J Ophthalmol* 1967;63:727.

48. Triche TJ. Round cell tumors in childhood; the application of newer techniques to the differential diagnosis. *Perspect Pediatr Pathol* 1982;7:270.

49. Green AA, Hayes FA, Hushu HO. Sequential cyclophosphamide and doxorubicin for induction of complete remission in children with disseminate neuroblastoma. *Cancer* 1981;48(10):2310.

50. Enzinger FM, Weiss SW. *Soft tissue tumors,* 3d ed. St. Louis: CV Mosby, 1995.

51. Fratkin JD, Purcell JJ, Krachmer JH, et al. Wilms' tumor metastatic to the orbit. *JAMA* 1977;238:1841.

52. Zimmerman LE, Font RL. Ophthalmologic manifestations of granulocytic sarcoma (myeloid sarcoma or chloroma). *Am J Ophthalmol* 1975;80:975.

53. Jakobiec FA, Jones IS. Lymphomatous plasmacytic, histiocytic and hematopoietic tumors. In: Jones IS, Jakobiec FA, eds. *Diseases of the orbit.* Hagerstown, Md.: Harper & Row, 1979:309.

54. Rootman J, Ellsworth RM, Hofbauer J, et al. Orbital extension of retinoblastoma: a clinicopathological study. *Can J Ophthalmol* 1978;13:72.

55. Yohai RA, Bullock JD, Aziz AA, Markert RJ. Survival factors in rhino-orbital-cerebral mucormycosis. *Surv Ophthalmol* 1994; 39(1):3.

56. Macy JI, Mandelbaum SH, Minckler DA. Orbital cellulitis. *Ophthalmology* 1980;87:1309.

57. Hurbli T, Char DS, Harris J, et al. Radiation therapy for thyroid eye disease. *Am J Ophthalmol* 1985;99:633.

58. Volpe R. Autoimmunity in Graves' and Hashimoto's disease. In: Gorman CA, Waller RR, Dyer JA, eds. *The eye and orbit in thyroid disease.* New York: Raven Press, 1984:59.

59. Wall JR. Autoimmunity in Graves' ophthalmopathy. In: Gorman CA, Waller RR, Dyer JA, eds. *The eye and orbit in thyroid disease.* New York: Raven Press, 1984:103.

60. Orcutt JC, Garner A, Henk JM, Wright JE. Treatment of idiopathic inflammatory orbital pseudotumours by radiotherapy. *Br J Ophthalmol* 1983;67:570.

61. Khalil MK, Lindley S, Matouk E. Tuberculosis of the orbit. *Ophthalmology* 1985;92:1624.

62. Jakobiec FA, Neri A, Knowles DM. Genotypic monoclonality in immunophenotypically polyclonal orbital lymphoid tumors. *Ophthalmology* 1987;94:980.

63. Knowles DM, Jakobiec FA, McNally L, et al. Lymphoid hyperplasia and malignant lymphoma occurring in the ocular adnexa (orbit, conjunctiva, and eyelids). *Hum Pathol* 1990;21:959.

64. McNally L, Jakobiec FA, Knowles DM. Clinical, morphologic, immunophenotypic, and molecular genetic analysis of bilateral ocular adnexal lymphoid neoplasms in 17 patients. *Am J Ophthalmol* 1987;103:555.

65. Antle CM, White VA, Horsman DE, et al. Large cell orbital lymphoma in a patient with acquired immune deficiency syndrome. *Ophthalmology* 1990;97:1494.

66. Harris GJ, Jakobiec FA. Cavernous hemangioma of the orbit: an analysis of 66 cases. *J Neurosurg* 1979;51:219.

67. Ruchman MC, Flanagan J. Cavernous hemangiomas of the orbit. *Ophthalmology* 1983;90:1328.

68. Boniuk M, Messmer EP, Font RL. Hemangiopericytoma of the meninges of the optic nerve: a clinico-pathologic report including electron microscopic observations. *Ophthalmology* 1985;92:1780.

69. Henderson JW, Farrow GM. Primary orbital hemangiopericytoma: an aggressive and potentially malignant neoplasm. *Arch Ophthalmol* 1978;96:666.

70. Weiss WS, Langloss JM, Enzinger FM. Value of S-100 protein in the diagnosis of soft tissue tumors, with particular reference to benign and malignant Schwann cell tumors. *Lab Invest* 1983; 49:299.

71. Schmitt E, Spoerri O. Schwannomas of the orbit. *Acta Neurochirur* 1980;53:79.

72. Marquardt MD, Zimmerman LE. Histopathology of meningiomas and gliomas of the optic nerve. *Hum Pathol* 1982;13:226.

73. Gurland JE, Tenner M, Hornblass A, Wolintz AH. Orbital neurofibromatosis. *Arch Ophthalmol* 1976;94:1723.

74. Woog JJ, Albert DM, Solt LC, et al. Neurofibromatosis of the eyeball and orbit. *Int Ophthalmol Clin* 1982;22:157.

75. Marback RL, Kincaid MC, Green WC, Iliff WJ. Fibrous histiocytoma of the lacrimal sac. *Am J Ophthalmol* 982;93:511.

76. Font RL, Hidayat AA. Fibrous histiocytoma of the orbit. *Hum Pathol* 1982;13:199.

77. Ferry AP, Font RL. Carcinoma metastatic to the eye and orbit: I. A clinicopathologic study of 227 cases. *Arch Ophthalmol* 1974; 92:276.

78. Font RL, Ferry AP. Carcinoma metastatic to the eye and orbit: III. A clinicopathologic study of 28 cases metastatic to the orbit. *Cancer* 1976;38:1326.

79. Buys R, Abramson DH, Kitchin FD, et al. Simultaneous ocular and orbital involvement from metastatic bronchogenic carcinoma. *Ann Ophthalmol* 1982;14:1165.

80. Bullock JD, Yanes B. Ophthalmic manifestations of metastatic breast cancer. *Ophthalmology* 1980;87:961.

81. Weimar VM, Ceilley RI. Basal-cell carcinoma of a medial canthus with invasion of supraorbital and supratrochlear nerves: report of a case treated by Mohs' technique. *J Dermatol Surg Oncol* 1979;5: 279.

82. Iliff CE. Mucoceles in the orbit. *Arch Ophthalmol* 1973;89:392.

83. Wright JE, Stewart WB, Krohel GB. Clinical presentation and management of lacrimal gland tumors. *Br J Ophthalmol* 1979;63:600.

84. Jakobiec FA, Yeo JH, Trokel SL, Abbott GF, et al. Combined clinical and computed tomographic diagnosis of lacrimal gland lesions. *Am J Ophthalmol* 1982;94:785.

85. Stewart WB, Krohel GB, Wright JE. Lacrimal gland and fossa lesion: an approach to diagnosis and management. *Ophthalmology* 1979;86:886.

86. Zimmerman LE, Sanders TE, Ackerman LV. Epithelial tumors of the lacrimal gland: prognostic and therapeutic significance of histologic types. *Int Ophthalmol Clin* 1962;2:337.

87. Perzin K, Jakobiec FA, LiVolsi V, Desjardins L. Lacrimal gland malignant mixed tumors (carcinomas arising in benign mixed tumors): a clinicopathologic study. *Cancer* 1980;45:2593.

88. Waller RR, Riley FC, Henderson JW. Malignant mixed tumor of the lacrimal gland: occult source of metastatic carcinoma. *Arch Ophthalmol* 1973;90:297.

89. Wright JE, Stewart WB, Krohel GB. Clinical presentation and management of lacrimal gland tumors. *Br J Ophthalmol* 1979;63:600.

90. Font RL, Gamel JW. Adenoid carcinoma of the lacrimal gland: a clinicopathologic study of 79 cases. In: Nicholson DH, ed. *Ocular pathology update.* New York: Masson, 1980:277.

91. Forrest AW. Epithelial lacrimal gland tumors: pathology as a guide to prognosis. *Trans Am Acad Ophthalmol Otolaryngol* 1954;58:848.

92. Gamel JW, Font RL. Adenoid cystic carcinoma of the lacrimal gland: the clinical significance of a basaloid pattern. *Hum Pathol* 1982;13:219.

93. Perzin K, Gullane P, Clairmont A. Adenoid cystic carcinoma arising in salivary glands: a correlation of histologic features and clinical course. *Cancer* 1978;42:265.

94. Malhotra GS, Paul SD, Batra DV. Mucoepidermoid carcinoma of the lacrimal gland. *Ophthalmologica* 1967;153:184.

95. Enzinger FM, Weiss SW. Malignant vascular tumors. In: *Soft tissue tumors,* 3rd ed. St. Louis: Mosby, 1995;642.

Subject Index